CLINICAL GUIDELINES IN ADULT HEALTH
Second Edition

Constance R. Uphold
PhD, RNCS, ARNP

Mary Virginia Graham
PhD, RNCS, ARNP

Veterans Affairs Medical Center and
Family Nurse Practitioner Program
College of Nursing
University of Florida
Gainesville, Florida

1999
Barmarrae Books
Gainesville, Florida

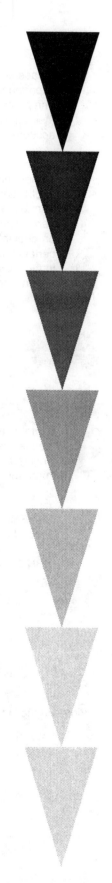

MESSAGE FROM THE AUTHORS AND PUBLISHER

Please keep in mind that medicine is an ever-changing science. As new research and clinical experience broaden our knowledge, changes in treatment including drug therapies are required. The authors and the publisher of this work have checked with sources believed to be reliable in their efforts to provide information that is complete and in accord with the standards of practice accepted at the time of publication.

However, in view of the possibility of human error or changes in medical sciences, neither the authors nor the publisher nor any other party who has been involved in the preparation or publication of this work are responsible for any errors or omissions or for the results obtained from use of such information. Readers are encouraged to confirm the information contained herein with other sources. For example, and in particular, readers are advised to consult the product information sheet included in the package of each drug they plan to administer to make certain that the information contained in this book is accurate and changes have not been made in the recommended dose or in the contraindications for administration. For medications that are administered infrequently, following this procedure is of critical importance.

First Edition 1994
Second Edition 1999

ISBN 0-9646151-5-0

Printed in the United States of America.

PREFACE

Since the publication of the first edition of <u>Clinical Guidelines in Adult Health</u>, the field or primary care has become a major force in the health care system. An interdisciplinary array of health care clinicians including nurse practitioners, physician assistants, and physicians are playing a central role in the provision of comprehensive, personalized, cost-effective health care.

Like the previous edition, this edition was designed to help these clinicians quickly access up-to-date information regarding health maintenance and commonly occurring primary care problems. The book contains the latest approaches to diagnosis, evaluation, and management in primary care. Diagnostic criteria and guidelines from national health advisory boards and authoritative sources are incorporated throughout.

The second edition of <u>Clinical Guidelines in Adult Health</u> has been extensively updated and expanded with additional tables and illustrations to help the reader quickly locate information. New health maintenance guidelines which focus on developmental assessment as well as approaches to behavioral problems are included. Twenty new topics including erectile dysfunction, abnormal liver enzymes, head injury, and shoulder pain have been added.

Each chapter has been reviewed by a practicing clinician with specialized knowledge and experience. We hope <u>Clinical Guidelines in Adult Health</u> is a helpful reference and provides clinicians with valuable information to assist them in understanding and managing health problems of families across the lifespan.

Constance R. Uphold
Mary Virginia Graham

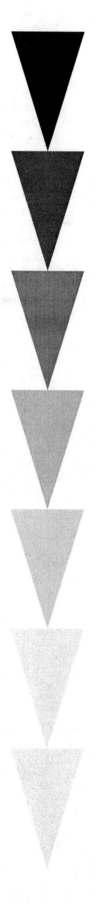

REVIEWERS

M. Katherine Crabtree, DNSc, RNCS, ANP
Associate Professor
Primary Health Care Nurse Practitioner Specialty
Oregon Health Sciences University School of
    Nursing
Portland, Oregon

Jean E. DeMartinis, PhD, RNCS, ARNP
Assistant Professor
Director, Cardiac Health, Wellness &
    Rehabilitation Nursing Curriculum
Creighton University School of Nursing
Omaha, Nebraska

J. Jordan Goodman, PhD, RNCS, ARNP
Coordinator, Clinical Programs
Division of Endocrinology and Metabolism
University of Florida
Gainesville, Florida

Lori A. Graham, MN, RNCS, FNP
Graduate Student
University of Florida
Gainesville, Florida

Susan Greishaw, MSN, ARNP
Gainesville Family Physicians
Gainesville, Florida

Betsy Hernandez, MSN, RNCS, ARNP
Coordinator of Clinical Programs
Community Health and Family Medicine
University of Florida
Gainesville, Florida

Carol Massey Lavin, ARNP
Coordinator of Clinical Services
University of Florida Clinic at Fanning Springs
Gainesville, Florida

Donna J. Lilly, MSN, ARNP
Comprehensive Epilepsy Program
University of Florida
Gainesville, Florida

Nancy Hurley Pontes, MSN, RNCS, FNP
Doctoral Student
Columbia University School of Nursing
New York, New York

Mary C. Schwartz Ryngaert, MSN, RNCS, ARNP
Pediatric Nurse Practitioner
The Kid's Health Team
Gainesville, Florida

Cynthia S. Selleck, DSN, RNCS, ARNP
Associate Professor
Department of Family Medicine
University of South Florida
Tampa, Florida

Tish Smyer, DNSc, RN
Associate Professor
South Dakota State University College of
    Nursing
Brookings, South Dakota

Paula J. Watt-Gilstrap, MS, RNCS, FNP
Program Manager for Nursing Programs
    and Services
Joseph F. Sullivan Center for Nursing
    and Wellness
Clemson University
Clemson, South Carolina

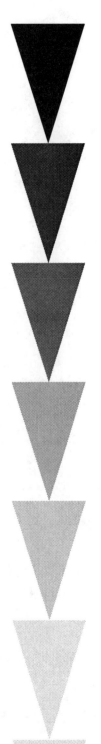

AUTHOR'S NOTE: We would like to thank **Gail Luparello** for her meticulous, creative work and dedication in the preparation of this text

We wish to dedicate this book to our families: Bill,
Lindsay, Nicholas, Charles, Myrtle, and Jay, Lori,
Robin, and Cecile

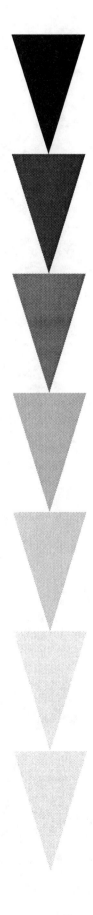

TABLE OF CONTENTS

CHAPTER 1

Health Maintenance

PERIODIC HEALTH EVALUATION FOR ADULTS

I. Definition: Age-specific preventive services performed by primary care clinicians on ASYMPTOMATIC adults in the context of routine care

II. Overview of preventive health services and age-specific charts

   A. The age-specific charts for adults are organized into three age groups: 11-24 years, 25-64 years, and 65 years and older
      1. Conditions likely to benefit from early identification but are not recommended for routine screening are listed in a separate table below (see CONDITIONS FOR WHICH CLINICIANS SHOULD REMAIN ALERT)
      2. Recommendations for the care of pregnant women are not included here

   B. Preventive services for the general population are contained in the top half of each chart
      1. Interventions listed are based on leading causes of death as well as leading causes of morbidity in each age group
      2. Potential effectiveness of each of the interventions in terms of improving clinical outcomes is a major factor in determination of which interventions to include

   C. Preventive services for members of high-risk groups are contained in the lower half of each chart
      1. Interventions listed are grouped together by general patient characteristics that broadly define high-risk populations
      2. Patients must meet the individual high-risk definition indicated by the annotated high-risk (HR) code after each intervention (**Note:** Patient may share characteristics of the general high-risk groupings without actually meeting the individual high-risk definitions for **every** intervention within that group)

   D. A periodicity schedule for health promotion visits has not been established for the following reasons
      1. For many interventions, evidence of an optimal periodicity is lacking
      2. Periodicity for certain interventions varies with patient characteristics such as age, gender, and risk factors

   E. Preventive services are divided in three categories: Screening tests, counseling interventions, and immunizations and chemoprophylaxis
      1. **Screening tests** are those preventive services utilizing special tests or standardized examination procedures to identify patients requiring special intervention
      2. **Counseling interventions** involve the provision of information and advice to patients regarding personal behaviors (e.g., seat belt use) that could reduce the risk of subsequent illness or injury
      3. **Immunizations** include both vaccines and immunoglobulins (passive immunizations) given to persons with no evidence of infectious disease
      4. **Chemoprophylaxis** refers to the use of drugs or biologics given to ASYMPTOMATIC persons to reduce the risk of developing a disease (e.g., folic acid supplements for women of childbearing age)

   F. Screening recommendations across age groups are summarized in a table at the end of this section on pages 10 and 11 (see SUMMARY OF SCREENING RECOMMENDATIONS)

III. History

    A. Use the Age Specific Charts developed by the US Preventive Services Task Force and contained in the <u>Guide to Clinical Preventive Services</u> (1996) and reprinted on pages 5 through 10 by permission to guide history taking

    B. Obtain complete health history at the initial visit and update it periodically

    C. Use the five counseling areas in each of the charts to guide history taking (**Note: Sample questions are provided for each area; however, these are by no means the only questions that should be asked!**)
        1. Injury prevention: Sample Questions: "Do you always use a seat belt?" "Do you have a smoke detector in your house?" "Do you check it frequently?" "Do you change the batteries at least once a year?" "Do you have a firearm in the household?" "Where is it kept?"
        2. Substance use: Sample Questions: "Do you use tobacco?" "Do you ever drink alcohol?"
        3. Sexual behavior: Sample Questions: "Are you sexually active?" "Do you always use condoms?" "Have you ever had a sexually transmitted disease?"
        4. Diet and exercise: Sample Questions: "What is your diet like?" "Tell me what you had for breakfast today." "Do you exercise regularly?" "What do you do and how often?"
        5. Dental health: Sample Questions: "Do you brush your teeth after every meal?" "Do you see a dentist regularly?"
        6. Note: The counseling areas are arranged in a priority listing in the age charts; note that different priority is given to each of the areas depending on the age group

    D. Patient with complaints or with significant past medical history, family history, or social history require problem identification and individualized screening measures

    E. For the asymptomatic patient (the patient for whom the periodic health examination is designed), most of the visit should be spent in history taking and counseling

IV. Physical Examination

    A. Use the Age Specific Charts developed by the US Preventive Services Task Force, <u>Guide to Clinical Preventive Services</u> (1996), and reprinted on pages 5 through 10 by permission to guide physical exam

    B. Physical exam recommendations are incorporated in the **Screening** section which also contains recommendations relating to laboratory testing and history questions that are used to screen (e.g., problem drinking)

    C. In evaluation of asymptomatic adults, inessentials are eliminated from the physical examination; *counsel more, examine less*

V. Laboratory Screening Procedures

    A. Use the Age Specific Charts developed by the US Preventive Services Task Force, <u>Guide to Clinical Preventive Services</u> (1996), and reprinted on pages 5 through 10 by permission to guide laboratory screening

    B. Commonly performed laboratory tests are often a waste of time and money when done routinely instead of selectively

VI.   Counseling

    A.   Use the Age Specific Charts developed by the US Preventive Services Task Forces, <u>Guide to Clinical Preventive Services</u> (1996), and reprinted on pages 5 through 10 by permission to guide counseling

    B.   Consider leading causes of morbidity and mortality for the age group as well as characteristics of the particular patient receiving services to guide counseling interventions aimed at changing behavior

VII.   Immunizations and Chemoprophylaxis

    A.   Use the Age Specific Charts developed by the US Preventive Services Task Forces, <u>Guide to Clinical Preventive Services</u> (1996), and reprinted on pages 5 through 10 by permission to guide immunization and chemoprophylaxis services

    B.   More detailed information on immunizations is contained in the tables at the end of this section on pages 10 through 12 (see SUMMARY FOR ADULT IMMUNIZATIONS)

INTERVENTIONS CONSIDERED AND RECOMMENDED FOR THE PERIODIC HEALTH EXAMINATION AGES 11-24 YEARS

LEADING CAUSES OF DEATH

MOTOR VEHICLE/ OTHER UNINTENTIONAL INJURIES	SUICIDE
	MALIGNANT NEOPLASMS
HOMICIDE	HEART DISEASES

Interventions for the General Population

SCREENING
Height & weight
Blood pressure[1]
Papanicolaou (Pap) test[2] (females)
Chlamydia screen[3] (females <20 yr)
Rubella serology or vaccination hx[4] (females >12 yr)
Assess for problem drinking

COUNSELING
Injury Prevention
Lap/shoulder belts
Bicycle/motorcycle/ATV helmets*
Smoke detector*
Safe storage/removal of firearms*

Substance Use
Avoid tobacco use
Avoid underage drinking & illicit drug use*
Avoid alcohol/drug use while driving, swimming, boating, etc.*

CHEMOPROPHYLAXIS
Multivitamin with folic acid (females)

Sexual Behavior
STD prevention: abstinence*; avoid high-risk behavior*; condoms/femal barrier with spermicide*
Unintended pregnancy: contraception

Diet and Exercise
Limit fat & cholesterol; maintain caloric balance; emphasize grains, fruits, vegetables
Adequate calcium intake (females)
Regular physical activity*

Dental Health
Regular visits to dental care provider*
Floss, brush with fluoride toothpaste daily*

IMMUNIZATIONS
Tetanus-diphtheria (Td) boosters (11-16 yr)
Hepatitis B[5]
MMR (11-12 yr)[6]
Varicella (11-12 yr)[7]
Rubella[4]

Interventions for High-Risk Populations

POPULATION	POTENTIAL INTERVENTIONS (see detailed high-risk definitions)
High-risk sexual behavior	RPR/VDRL (HR1); screen for gonorrhea (female)(HR2), HIV (HR3), chlamydia (female)(HR4); hepatitis A vaccine (HR5)
Injection or street drug use	RPR/VDRL (HR1); HIV screen (HR3); hepatitis A vaccine (HR5); PPD (HR6); advice to reduce infection risk (HR7)
TB contacts: immigrants; low income	PPD (HR6)
Native Americans/Alaska Natives	Hepatitis A vaccine (HR5); PPD (HR6); pneumococcal vaccine (HR8)
Travelers to developing countries	Hepatitis A vaccine (HR5)
Certain chronic medical conditions	PPD (HR6); pneumococcal vaccine (HR8); influenza vaccine (HR9)
Settings where adolescents and young adults congregate	Second MMR (HR10)
Susceptible to varicella, measles, mumps	Varicella vaccine (HR11); MMR (HR12)
Blood transfusion between 1975-1985	HIV screen (HR3)
Institutionalized persons; health care/lab workers	Hepatitis A vaccine (HR5); PPD (HR6); influenza vaccine (HR9)
Family h/o skin cancer; nevi; fair skin, eyes, hair	Avoid excess/midday sun, use protective clothing* (HR13)
Prior pregnancy with neural tube defect	Folic acid 4.0 mg (HR14)
Inadequate water fluoridation	Daily fluoride supplement (HR15)

(continued)

[1]Periodic BP for persons aged ≥21 yr. [2]If sexually active at present or in the past: q ≤3 yr. If sexual history is unreliable, begin Pap tests at age 18 yr. [3]If sexually active. [4]Serologic testing, documented vaccination history, and routine vaccination against rubella (preferably with MMR) are equally acceptable alternatives. [5]If not previously immunized; current visit, 1 and 6 mo later. [6]If no previous second dose of MMR. [7]If susceptible to chickenpox.

*The ability of clinician counseling to influence this behavior is unproven.

Source: US Preventive Services Task Force. (1996). Guide to clinical preventive services. (2nd ed.). Baltimore: Williams & Williams
(Reprinted by permission)

Detailed High-Risk Definitions

HR1 = Persons who exchange sex for money or drugs, and their sex partners; persons with other STDs (including HIV); and sexual contacts of persons with active syphilis. Clinicians should also consider local epidemiology

HR2 = Females who have: two or more sex partners in the last year; a sex partner with multiple sexual contacts; exchanged sex for money or drugs; or a history of repeated episodes of gonorrhea. Clinicians should also consider local epidemiology

HR3 = Males who had sex with males after 1975; past or present injection drug use; persons who exchange sex for money or drugs, and their sex partners; injection drug-using, bisexual, or HIV-positive sex partner currently or in the past; blood transfusion during 1978-1985; persons seeking treatment for STDs. Clinicians should also consider local epidemiology

HR4 = Sexually active females with multiple risk factors including: history of prior STD; new or multiple sex partners; age under 25; nonuse or inconsistent use of barrier contraceptives; cervical ectopy. Clinicians should consider local epidemiology of the disease in identifying other high-risk groups

HR5 = Persons living in, traveling to, or working in areas where the disease is endemic and where periodic outbreaks occur (e.g., countries with high or intermediate endemicity; certain Alaska Native, Pacific Island, Native American, and religious communities); men who have sex with men; injection or street drug users. Vaccine may be considered for institutionalized persons and workers in these institutions, military personnel, and day-care, hospital, and laboratory workers. Clinicians should also consider local epidemiology

HR6 = HIV positive, close contacts of persons with known or suspected TB, health care workers, persons with medical risk factors associated with TB, immigrants from countries with high TB prevalence, medically underserved low-income populations (including homeless), alcoholics, injection drug users, and residents of long-term facilities

HR7 = Persons who continue to inject drugs

HR8 = Immunocompetent persons with certain medical conditions, including chronic cardiac or pulmonary disease, diabetes mellitus, and anatomic asplenia. Immunocompetent persons who live in high-risk environments or social settings (e.g., certain Native American and Alaska Native populations)

HR9 = Annual vaccination of: residents of chronic care facilities; persons with chronic cardiopulmonary disorders, metabolic diseases (including diabetes mellitus), hemoglobinopathies, immunosuppression, or renal dysfunction; and health care providers for high-risk patients

HR10 = Adolescents and young adults in settings where such individuals congregate (e.g., high schools and colleges), if they have not previously received a second dose

HR11 = Healthy persons aged ≥13 yr without a history of chickenpox or previous immunization. Consider serologic testing for presumed susceptible persons aged ≥13 yr

HR12 = Persons born after 1956 who lack evidence of immunity to measles or mumps (e.g., documented receipt of live vaccine on or after the first birthday, laboratory evidence of immunity, or a history of physician-diagnosed measles or mumps)

HR13 = Persons with a family or personal history of skin cancer, a large number of moles, atypical moles, poor tanning ability, or light skin, hair, and eye color

HR14 = Women with prior pregnancy affected by neural tube defect who are planning pregnancy

HR15 = Persons aged <17 yr living in areas with inadequate water fluoridation (<0.6 ppm)

INTERVENTIONS CONSIDERED AND RECOMMENDED FOR THE PERIODIC HEALTH EXAMINATION AGES 25-64 YEARS

LEADING CAUSES OF DEATH

MALIGNANT NEOPLASMS
HEART DISEASES
MOTOR VEHICLE AND OTHER
  UNINTENTIONAL INJURIES

HIV INFECTION
SUICIDE AND HOMICIDE

Interventions for the General Population

SCREENING
Blood pressure
Height and weight
Total blood cholesterol (men age 35-64, women age 45-64)
Papanicolaou (Pap) test (women)[1]
Fecal occult blood test[2] and/or sigmoidoscopy ($\geq$50 yr)
Mammogram ± clinical breast exam[3] (women 50-69 yr)
Assess for problem drinking
Rubella serology or vaccination hx[4] (women of childbearing age)

COUNSELING
Substance Use
Tobacco cessation
Avoid alcohol/drug use while driving, swimming, boating, etc.*

Diet and Exercise
Limit fat & cholesterol; maintain caloric balance; emphasize grains, fruits, vegetables
Adequate calcium intake (women)
Regular physical activity*

Injury Prevention
Lap/shoulder belts
Motorcycle/bicycle/ATV helmets*
Smoke detector*
Safe storage/removal of firearms*

Sexual Behavior
STD prevention: avoid high-risk behavior*; condoms/female barrier with spermicide*
Unintended pregnancy: contraception

Dental Health
Regular visits to dental care provider*
Floss, brush with fluoride toothpaste daily*

IMMUNIZATIONS
Tetanus-diphtheria (Td) boosters
Rubella[4] (women childbearing age)

CHEMOPROPHYLAXIS
Multivitamin with folic acid (women planning or capable of pregnancy)
Discuss hormone prophylaxis (peri- and postmenopausal women)

Interventions for High-Risk Populations

POPULATION	POTENTIAL INTERVENTIONS (see detailed high-risk definitions)
High-risk sexual behavior	RPR/VDRL (HR1); screen for gonorrhea (female)(HR2), HIV (HR3), chlamydia (female)(HR4); hepatitis B vaccine (HR5); hepatitis A vaccine (HR6)
Injection or street drug use	RPR/VDRL (HR1); HIV screen (HR3); hepatitis B vaccine (HR5); hepatitis A vaccine (HR6); PPD (HR7); advice to reduce infection risk (HR8)
Low income; TB contacts: immigrants; alcoholics	PPD (HR7)
Native Americans/Alaska Natives	Hepatitis A vaccine (HR6); PPD (HR7); pneumococcal vaccine (HR9)
Travelers to developing countries	Hepatitis B vaccine (HR5); hepatitis A vaccine (HR6)
Certain chronic medical conditions	PPD (HR7); pneumococcal vaccine (HR9); influenza vaccine (HR10)
Blood product recipients	HIV screen (HR3); hepatitis B vaccine (HR5)
Susceptible to measles, mumps, or varicella	MMR (HR11); varicella vaccine (HR12)
Institutionalized persons	Hepatitis A vaccine (HR6); PPD (HR7); pneumococcal vaccine (HR9); influenza vaccine (HR10)
Health care/lab workers	Hepatitis B vaccine (HR6); hepatitis A vaccine (HR6); PPD (HR7); influenza vaccine (HR10)
Family h/o skin cancer; nevi; fair skin, eyes, hair	Avoid excess/midday sun, use protective clothing* (HR13)
Previous pregnancy with neural tube defect	Folic acid 4.0 mg (HR14)

(continued)

[1]Women who are or have been sexually active and who have a cervix: q $\leq$ 3 yr. [2]Annually. [3]Mammogram q1-2 yr, or mammogram q-2 yr with annual clinical breast examination. [4]Serologic testing, documented vaccination history, and routine vaccination against rubella (preferably with MMR) are equally acceptable.

*The ability of clinician counseling to influence this behavior is unproven.

Source: US Preventive Services Task Force. (1996). <u>Guide to clinical preventive services</u>. (2nd ed.). Baltimore: Williams & Williams
(Reprinted by permission)

INTERVENTIONS CONSIDERED AND RECOMMENDED FOR THE PERIODIC HEALTH EXAMINATION AGES 25-64 YEARS	LEADING CAUSES OF DEATH

LEADING CAUSES OF DEATH

MALIGNANT NEOPLASMS   HIV INFECTION
HEART DISEASES   SUICIDE AND HOMICIDE
MOTOR VEHICLE AND OTHER
    UNINTENTIONAL INJURIES   (CONTINUED)

Detailed High-Risk Definitions

HR1 = Persons who exchange sex for money or drugs, and their sex partners; persons with other STDs (including HIV); and sexual contacts of persons with active syphilis. Clinicians should also consider local epidemiology

HR2 = Women who exchange sex for money or drugs, or who have had repeated episodes of gonorrhea. Clinicians should also consider local epidemiology

HR3 = Men who had sex with men after 1975; past or present injection drug use; persons who exchange sex for money or drugs, and their sex partners; injection drug-using, bisexual, or HIV-positive sex partner currently or in the past; blood transfusion during 1978-1985; persons seeking treatment for STDs. Clinicians should also consider local epidemiology

HR4 = Sexually active women with multiple risk factors including: history of STD; new or multiple sex partners; nonuse or inconsistent use of barrier contraceptives; cervical ectopy. Clinicians should consider local epidemiology

HR5 = Blood product recipients (including hemodialysis patients), persons with frequent occupational exposure to blood or blood products, men who have sex with men, injection drug users and their sex partners, persons with multiple recent sex partners, persons with other STDs (including HIV), travelers to countries with endemic hepatitis B

HR6 = Persons living in, traveling to, or working in areas where the disease is endemic and where periodic outbreaks occur (e.g., countries with high or intermediate endemicity; certain Alaska Native, Pacific Island, Native American, and religious communities); men who have sex with men; injection or street drug users. Consider for institutionalized persons and workers in these institutions, military personnel, and day-care, hospital, and laboratory workers. Clinicians should also consider local epidemiology

HR7 = HIV positive, close contacts of persons with known or suspected TB, health care workers, persons with medical risk factors associated with TB, immigrants from countries with high TB prevalence, medically underserved low-income populations (including homeless), alcoholics, injection drug users, and residents of long-term care facilities

HR8 = Persons who continue to inject drugs

HR9 = Immunocompetent institutionalized persons aged ≥50 yr and immunocompetent persons with certain medical conditions, including chronic cardiac or pulmonary disease, diabetes mellitus, and anatomic asplenia. Immunocompetent persons who live in high-risk environments or social settings (e.g., certain Native American and Alaska Native populations)

HR10 = Annual vaccination of: residents of chronic care facilities; persons with chronic cardiopulmonary disorders, metabolic diseases (including diabetes mellitus), hemoglobinopathies, immunosuppression, or renal dysfunction; and health care providers for high-risk patients

HR11 = Persons born after 1956 who lack evidence of immunity to measles or mumps (e.g., documented receipt of live vaccine on or after the first birthday, laboratory evidence of immunity, or a history of physician-diagnosed measles or mumps)

HR12 = Healthy adults without a history of chickenpox or previous immunization. Consider serologic testing for presumed susceptible adults

HR13 = Persons with a family or personal history of skin cancer, a large number of moles, atypical moles, poor tanning ability, or light skin, hair, and eye color

HR14 = Women with previous pregnancy affected by neural tube defect who are planning pregnancy

Interventions for the General Population

SCREENING
Blood pressure
Height and weight
Fecal occult blood test[1] and/or sigmoidoscopy
Mammogram ± clinical breast exam[2] (women ≤69 yr)
Papanicolaou (Pap) test (women)[3]
Vison screening
Assess for hearing impairment
Assess for problem drinking

COUNSELING
Substance Use
Tobacco cessation
Avoid alcohol/drug use while driving, swimming,
    boating, etc.*

Diet and Exercise
Limit fat & cholesterol; maintain caloric balance;
    emphasize grains, fruits, vegetables
Adequate calcium intake (women)
Regular physical activity*

Injury Prevention
Lap/shoulder belts
Motorcycle and bicycle helmets*
Fall prevention*
Safe storage/removal of firearms*
Smoke detector*
Set hot water heater to <120-130°F*
CPR training for household members

Dental Health
Regular visits to dental care provider*
Floss, brush with fluoride toothpaste daily*

Sexual Behavior
STD prevention: avoid high-risk behavior*; use condoms*

IMMUNIZATIONS
Pneumococcal vaccine
Influenza[1]
Tetanus-diphtheria (Td) boosters

CHEMOPROPHYLAXIS
Discuss hormone prophylaxis (peri- and postmenopausal women)

Interventions for High-Risk Populations

POPULATION	POTENTIAL INTERVENTIONS (see detailed high-risk definitions)
Institutionalized persons	PPD (HR1); hepatitis A vaccine (HR2); amantadine/rimantadine (HR4)
Chronic medical conditions; TB contacts; low income; immigrants; alcoholics	PPD (HR1)
Persons ≥75 yr; or ≥70 yr with risk factors for falls	Fall prevention intervention (HR5)
Cardiovascular disease risk factors	Consider cholesterol screening (HR6)
Family h/o skin cancer; nevi; fair skin, eyes, hair	Avoid excess/midday sun, use protective clothing* (HR7)
Native Americans/Alaska Natives	PPD (HR1); hepatitis A vaccine (HR2)
Travelers to developing countries	Hepatitis A vaccine (HR2); hepatitis B vaccine (HR8)
Blood product recipients	HIV screen (HR3); hepatitis B vaccine (HR8)
High-risk sexual behavior	Hepatitis A vaccine (HR2); HIV screen (HR3); hepatitis B vaccine (HR8); RPR/VDRL (HR9); advice to reduce infection risk (HR10)
Injection or street drug use	PPD (HR1); hepatitis A vaccine (HR2); HIV screen (HR3); hepatitis B vaccine (HR8); RPR/VDRL (HR9); advice to reduce infection risk (HR10)
Health care/lab workers	PPD (HR1); hepatitis A vaccine (HR2); amantadine/rimantadine (HR4); hepatitis B vaccine (HR8)
Persons susceptible to varicella	Varicella vaccine (HR11)

(continued)

(continued)

[1]Annually. [2]Mammogram q1-2 yr, or mammogram q`-2 yr with annual clinical breast examination. [3]All women who are or have been sexually active and who have a cervix. Consider discontinuation of testing after age 65 yr if previous regular screening with consistently normal results.

*The ability of clinician counseling to influence this behavior is unproven.

Source: US Preventive Services Task Force. (1996). Guide to clinical preventive services. (2nd ed.). Baltimore: Williams & Williams
(Reprinted by permission)

Detailed High-Risk Definitions

HR1 = HIV positive, close contacts of persons with known or suspected TB, health care workers, persons with medical risk factors associated with TB, immigrants from countries with high TB prevalence, medically underserved low-income populations (including homeless), alcoholics, injection drug users, and residents of long-term care facilities

HR2 = Persons living in, traveling to, or working in areas where the disease is endemic and where periodic outbreaks occur (e.g., countries with high or intermediate endemicity; certain Alaska Native, Pacific Island, Native American, and religious communities); men who have sex with men; injection or street drug users. Consider for institutionalized persons and workers in these institutions, and day-care, hospital, and laboratory workers. Clinicians should also consider local epidemiology

HR3 = Men who had sex with men after 1975; past or present injection drug use; persons who exchange sex for money or drugs, and their sex partners; injection drug-using, bisexual, or HIV-positive sex partner currently or in the past; blood transfusion during 1978-1985; persons seeking treatment for STDs. Clinicians should also consider local epidemiology

HR4 = Consider for persons who have not received influenza vaccine or are vaccinated late; when the vaccine may be ineffective due to major antigenic changes in the virus; for unvaccinated persons who provide home care for high-risk persons; to supplement protection provided by vaccine in persons who are expected to have a poor antibody response; and for high-risk persons in whom the vaccine is contraindicated

HR5 = Persons aged 75 years and older; or aged 70-74 with one or more additional risk factors including: use of certain psychoactive and cardiac medications (e.g., benzodiazepines, antihypertensives); use of ≥4 prescription medications; impaired cognition, strength, balance, or gait. Intensive individualized home-based multifactorial fall prevention intervention is recommended in settings where adequate resources are available to deliver such services

HR6 = Although evidence is insufficient to recommend routine screening in elderly persons, clinicians should consider cholesterol screening on a case-by-case basis for persons ages 65-75 with additional risk factors (e.g., smoking, diabetes, or hypertension)

HR7 = Persons with a family or personal history of skin cancer, a large number of moles, atypical moles, poor tanning ability, or light skin, hair, and eye color

HR8 = Blood product recipients (including hemodialysis patients), persons with frequent occupational exposure to blood or blood products, men who have sex with men, injection drug users and their sex partners, persons with multiple recent sex partners, persons with other STDs (including HIV), travelers to countries with endemic hepatitis B

HR9 = Persons who exchange sex for money or drugs and their sex partners; persons with other STDs (including HIV); and sexual contacts of persons with active syphilis. Clinicians should also consider local epidemiology

HR10 = Persons who continue to inject drugs

HR11 = Healthy adults without a history of chickenpox or previous immunization. Consider serologic testing for presumed susceptible adults

SUMMARY OF SCREENING RECOMMENDATIONS

Type	Current Expert Opinion
Blood Pressure	Adults believed to be normotensive should receive blood pressure measurement at least every 2 years
Height and Weight	Periodic measurement of height and weight; frequency for measurement is a matter of clinical discretion. Calculate BMI (body weight in kg divided by the square of height in meters). Healthy range is 18.5-24.9 for adults of both genders, all ages
Pap Test	Regular pap tests are recommended for all women who are or have been sexually active and who have a cervix. Pap tests should begin at age when woman becomes active and should be performed at least every 3 years (More often in high risk groups). Discontinue regular testing on women after age 65 if they have had regular previous screening in which the smears have been consistently normal. Women who have had a hysterectomy in which the cervix was removed do not need pap testing, unless the reason for the removal of cervix was because of cervical cancer

(continued)

SUMMARY OF SCREENING RECOMMENDATIONS (CONTINUED)

Type	Current Expert Opinion
Chlamydia Screen	Routine screening for asymptomatic infection with *Chlamydia trachomatous* during pelvic exam is recommended for all sexually active female adolescents and for other women at high risk for infection
Rubella Serology or Vaccination hx (females >12)	Screening for rubella susceptibility by history of vaccination or by serology is recommended for all women of childbearing age at their first clinical encounter
Total Blood Cholesterol	Periodic screening (every 5 years) for high blood cholesterol, using specimens obtained from fasting or nonfasting individuals for all men 35-65 and women 45-65
Fecal Occult Blood Test	Screening for colorectal cancer is recommended for all persons aged 50 and older with **annual** fecal occult blood testing, or sigmoidoscopy (periodicity unspecified) or both
Mammogram	Routine screening for breast cancer every 1-2 years with mammography alone or with clinical breast exam (CBE) for women aged 50-69
Alcohol Abuse	Screening for problem drinking recommended for all adult and adolescent patients using a careful history or a standardized screening questionnaire such as the CAGE
Vision Screening	Routine vision screening is recommended among the elderly, using Snellen acuity testing, with the optimal frequency left to clinical discretion
Hearing Impairment	Screening older adults for hearing impairment by periodically questioning them about their hearing is recommended with the optimal frequency left to clinical discretion

SUMMARY OF RECOMMENDATIONS FOR ADULT IMMUNIZATION

Vaccine name	For whom it is recommended	What is the usual schedule	Schedule for those who have fallen behind
Influenza *"flu shot"*	✦ People who are 65 years of age or older. ✦ People under 65 with medical problems such as heart disease, lung disease, diabetes, renal dysfunction, hemoglobinopathies, immunosuppression, and/or those living in chronic care facilities. Adults working or living with these people should be vaccinated as well. ✦ Healthy pregnant women who will be in their 2nd or 3rd trimesters during the influenza season. ✦ Pregnant women who have underlying medical conditions should be vaccinated before the flu season, regardless of the stage of pregnancy. ✦ Anyone who wishes to reduce the likelihood of becoming ill with influenza.	✦ October through November is the optimal time to receive a flu shot to maximize protection, but the vaccine may be given at any time during the influenza season.	May be given anytime during the influenza season, including the winter months, as long as cases are still occurring in the community.
Pneumococcal *pneumococcal shot"*	✦ All adults 65 years of age and older. ✦ People under 65 who have chronic illness or other high risk factors including chronic cardiac and pulmonary diseases, anatomic or functional asplenia, chronic liver disease, alcoholism, diabetes mellitus, CSF leaks. Others at high risk include immunocompromised persons including those with HIV infection, leukemia, lymphoma, Hodgkin's disease, multiple myeloma, generalized malignancy, chronic renal failure, or nephrotic syndrome, those receiving immunosuppressive chemotherapy (including corticosteroids), and those who received an organ or bone marrow transplant.	✦ Routinely given as a one-time dose. ✦ Revaccination is recommended 5 years later for people at highest risk of fatal pneumococcal infection, or if the 1st dose was given prior to age 65.	
Hepatitis B (Hep-B) (HBV)	✦ Many high-risk adults need vaccination including: household contacts and sexual partners of hepatitis B carriers; users of injectable drugs; heterosexuals with more than one sexual partner in 6 months; men who have sex with men; patients in hemodialysis units; recipients of certain blood products; health care workers and public safety workers who are exposed to blood; clients and staff of institutions for the developmentally disabled; inmates of long-term correctional facilities, and certain international travelers. **Note:** Prior serologic testing may be recommended depending on the specific level of risk and/or likelihood of previous exposure. *Editor's note: It is especially prudent to screen individuals who have emigrated from endemic areas. When HBsAg "carriers" are identified, offer them appropriate disease management. In addition, their household members and intimate contacts should be screened and, if found susceptible, vaccinated.*	✦ Commonly used timing options for vaccination: 0, 1, 6 months 0, 2, 4 months 0, 1, 4 months	✦ There must be one month between doses #1 and #2, and two months between doses #2 and #3. Overall there must be at least four months between doses #1 and #3. ✦ If the series is delayed between doses, do not start the series over. Simply continue from where you left off.

(continued)

Vaccine name	For whom it is recommended	What is the usual schedule	Schedule for those who have fallen behind
Hepatitis A (Hep-A)	✦ Adults who travel outside of the U.S. (except for Northern and Western Europe, New Zealand, Australia, Canada, and Japan). ✦ People with chronic liver disease; drug users; men who have sex with men; people with clotting disorders; people who work with hepatitis A virus in experimental lab settings (this does not refer to routine medical laboratories); and food handlers where health authorities or private employers determine vaccination to be cost-effective. **Note:** prevaccination testing is likely to be cost effective for persons >40 years of age as well as for younger persons in certain groups with a high prevalence of HAV infection.	✦ #1 ✦ #2: If using Havrix, give second dose 6-12 months after the first dose. If using Vaqta, give second dose 6 months after the first dose.	✦ #2 dose should be given no sooner than 6 months after #1.
Td (Tetanus, diphtheria)	After the primary series has been completed, a booster dose is recommended every 10 years. Make sure your patients have received a primary series of 3 doses.	Booster dose every 10 years after completion of the primary series of 3 doses.	The primary series is: ✦ #1 ✦ #2 given 1 month later ✦ #3 given 6-12 months after #2
MMR Measles, Mumps, Rubella	✦ Adults born in 1957 or later need one dose of the MMR if there is no proof of immunity or documentation of a dose given on or after 1st birthday. ✦ Adults in high-risk groups, such as health care workers, students entering post secondary schools, and international travelers may need a second dose. **Note:** Adults born before 1957 are usually considered immune but proof of immunity may be considered for health care workers.	✦ #1 ✦ #2, if recommended, is given no sooner than 1 month after #1.	#2 may be given as early as 1 month after dose #1.
Varicella *"Chickenpox shot"* (Var)	✦ All susceptible adults should be vaccinated. **Note:** Adults with reliable histories of chickenpox (such as self or parental report of disease) can be assumed to be immune. For those who have no reliable history, serologic testing may be cost effective to determine immunity since most adults are immune.	All adults need two doses. Give dose #2 4-8 weeks after dose #1.	✦ Give #2 no sooner than 4 weeks after #1.
Polio vaccine IPV	Not routinely recommended for adults 18 years of age and older. **Note:** Adults living in the U.S. who never received or completed a primary series of polio vaccine, need not be vaccinated, unless they intend to travel to areas where exposure to wild-type virus is likely. Health care workers should have completed a primary series.	Refer to ACIP recommendations regarding unique situations, schedules, and dosing information. If polio vaccine is indicated for adults, IPV is generally preferred.	

For specific ACIP immunization recommendations refer to the full statements which are published in the *MMWR*. To obtain a complete set of ACIP statements, contact your state health department or call 800/232-2522. The references most frequently used in creating this table include recent ACIP statements, *General Recommendations on Immunization, MMWR*, 1/28/94, and *Update on Adult Immunization, MMWR*, 11/15/91.

This table was developed to combine the recommendations of adult immunization onto one page. It was devised especially to assist health care workers in determining appropriate use and scheduling of vaccines. It can be posted in immunization clinics or clinicians' offices. The table will be revised approximately once a year because of the changing nature of national immunization recommendations.

Source: Immunization Action Coalition (website: http:\\www.immunize.org)

NUTRITION IN ADULTHOOD

I. Provide dietary counseling to adults based on these guidelines

   A. Keep total fat intake ≤30% of total daily calories and limit intake of saturated fats to <10% of total fat calories

   B. Keep protein intake at moderate levels (about 12% of total daily calories) and avoid foods high in sugar

   C. Eat a variety of foods; learn how to prepare low-fat meals that are quick and easy to prepare

   D. Limit sodium intake to no more than 2400 mg/day (a little more than 1 tsp salt)

   E. Maintain an adequate calcium intake; obtain vitamins and minerals from foods, not from supplements

F.   Maintain a desirable weight

G.   Drink alcohol only in moderation, or avoid altogether

H.   Reduce or eliminate caffeine from diet

I.   Drink eight 8-oz. glasses of water each day

J.   1 g fat = 9 calories; 1 g carbohydrate = 4 calories; 1 g protein = 4 calories

II.   Base counseling on consideration of changing nutritional needs of adults through the life cycle

     A.   In adulthood, growth stops, so energy needs decrease

     B.   Loss of muscle mass is the most important change that occurs with aging and is more pronounced in men than in women (until after menopause)
          1.   As muscle tissue is lost, the person eats less as fewer calories are needed
          2.   Persons who maintain a physically active lifestyle do not lose as much muscle as their inactive counterparts

     C.   For the elderly, lack of sun exposure and natural decline in body's ability to make its own Vitamin D can lead to deficiency in this vitamin

     D.   After age 80, the ability to secrete enough stomach acid to fully absorb folic acid, calcium, iron, and Vitamin$_{12}$ is compromised

     E.   The role of antioxidants in the aging process remains unclear but the elderly may benefit from antioxidant supplements if their diet is not rich in Vitamins C and E, beta carotene and the mineral selenium

     F.   Drinking enough water is important for everyone regardless of age, but becoming dehydrated presents special problems for the elderly

     G.   During pregnancy, more calories are needed (weight gain of 25-30 pounds is recommended)

     H.   In lactating women, about 500 extra Cal/day are needed to support milk production

III.   Use the environment in your office to promote good nutrition

     A.   Subscribe to health-oriented magazines and newsletters such as the following:

The University of California at Berkeley Wellness Letter, PO Box 420148, Palm Coast, FL 32142

Tufts University Diet & Nutrition Letter, PO Box 57857, Boulder, CO 80322-7587

     B.   Use resources in the following table to obtain free or low-cost materials on health, diet, and nutrition.

RESOURCES ON HEALTH, DIET, AND NUTRITION

American Academy of Family Physicians
PH: 800/944-0000
▸*A catalog of education, services, and products*

American Heart Association
National Center
7272 Greenville Ave
Dallas TX 75231-4596
▸*"Nutritious Nibbles: A Guide to Healthy Snacking"*

US Department of Health and Human Services, Public Health Service (PHS)
Office of Disease Prevention and Health Promotion
Washington DC 20201
▸*Listing of PHS publications*

American Cancer Society
1599 Clifton RD.. NE
Atlanta GA 30329-4251
PH: 800/ACS-2345
▸*"Nutrition, Common Sense, and Cancer"*
▸*"Taking Control: 10 Steps to a Healthier Life and Reduced Cancer Risk"*

(continued)

American Dietetic Association
National Center for Nutrition and Dietetics
216 W Jackson Blvd Suite 800
Chicago IL 60606-6995
PH: 312/899-0040
▸"Eat Right America: The Good Nutrition Reading List"

Department of Agriculture Human Nutrition Information Service
6505 Belcrest Rd. Room 344
Hyattsville MD 20782
PH: 301/436-7725
▸"Eating Right: The Dietary Guidelines Way," a listing of educational materials that can be ordered at modest prices.

Huffington Library
American Academy of Family Physicians Foundation
8880 Ward Pkwy, Box 8418
Kansas City MO 64114-0418
PH: 800/274-2237, ext 4400
▸A free health education database that lists favorably reviewed patient education materials.

Office of Cancer Communications
Bldg 31, Room 10A24
National Cancer Institute
Bethesda MD 20892
PH: 800/4-CANCER
▸"Diet, Nutrition, and Cancer Prevention: The Good News"
▸"Eat More Fruits and Vegetables: 5 A Day for Better Health"
▸The NCI's publication lists.

Food & Nutrition Information Center
National Agricultural Library/USDA
10301 Baltimore Avenue Room 304
Beltsville, MD 20705-2351
301/504-5719 or www.fnic@nalusda.gov
▸A wonderful resource for nutritional information

National Heart, Lung, and Blood Institute (NHLBI)
Education Programs Information Center
Box 30105
Bethesda MD 20824-0105
PH: 301/951-3260
▸"NHLBI's Kit Yellow Pages," a catalog of materials from federal government sources and nonprofit organizations.

National Dairy Council
O'Hare International Center
10255 W Higgins Road Suite 900
Rosemont IL 60018-5616
PH: 708/803-2000
▸"Healthy Dividends: A Plan for Balancing Your Fat Budget"
▸A catalog of printed nutrition education materials, wall posters, slides, videos, and films.

Nutrition Screening Initiative
2626 Pennsylvania Ave NW Suite 301
Washington DC 20037
PH: 202/625-1662
▸"Determine Your Nutritional Health," a screening checklist for older people developed by the Initiative, a project sponsored by the American Dietetic Assn.., the American Academy of Family Physicians, and the National Council on the Aging, Inc.
▸"Nutrition Screening Manual for Professionals Caring for Older Americans," a reference guide linked with the checklist.

C.   Use attractive posters on walls to promote healthy eating habits; available from the following sources:

Poster	Source
Food Guide Pyramid ▸ Full color, 23 ½ x 28 inches ▸ Cost: free	U.S. Department of Agriculture, Human Nutrition Information Service, 6505 Belcrest Rd., Room 363, Hyattsville MD 20782
Food Guide Pyramid ▸Full color, 22 x 34 inches ▸Cost: $1.50	National Live Stock and Meat Board, 444 N Michigan Ave, Chicago IL 60611
5 a Day for Better Health ▸Full color ▸Cost: free	Produce for Better Health Foundation, 1500 Casho Mill Rd., Box 6035, Newark DE 19714-6035
Guide to Good Eating ▸Full color, 26 ½ x 36 ½ inches ▸Cost: low	National Dairy Council, O'Hare International Center, 10255 W Higgins Rd., Suite 900, Rosemont IL 60018-5616

IV.   Instruct patients in how to use the Food Guide Pyramid to put dietary guidelines into action (see Figure 1.1 on page 15)

A.   Most of the daily (see WHAT'S IN A SERVING on page 16) servings of food should be chosen from the food groups that are the largest in the picture and closest to the base of the pyramid

B.   Most of the foods eaten each day should come from the grain products group (6-11 servings), the vegetable group (3-5 servings), and the fruit group (2-4 servings)

C.   Only moderate amounts of foods should come from the milk group (2-3 servings) and meat and beans group (2-3 servings)

D.   Foods high in fat and sugar should be used sparingly

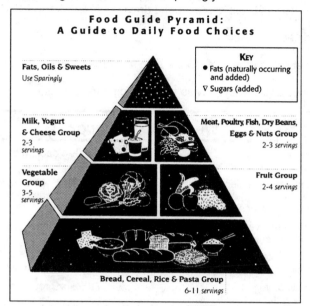

Figure 1.1. Food Guide Pyramid.

Source: US Department of Agriculture. Department of Health and Human Services. (1995). Nutrition and you health: Dietary guidelines for Americans. Washington, DC: Author, p. 4.

V.   Use the DASH diet to counsel patients

A.   The DASH (Dietary Approaches to Stop Hypertension) diet evolved from a study to reduce hypertension
1.   The diet did lower blood pressure in persons with slightly elevated BPs
2.   May also help reduce risk of cancer and osteoporosis
3.   The DASH diet is in the table below and is online at http://dash.bwh.harvard.edu

DASH DIET	
Food/Servings	**Food Examples**
Grains & grain products--7 to 8 daily	Whole wheat breads, English muffins, pita bread, bagels, cereals, oatmeal, grits
Fruits & vegetables--4 to 5 fruit servings daily; 4 to 5 vegetable servings daily	Apricots, bananas, grapes, oranges, grapefruit, melons, strawberries, tomatoes, peas, carrots, potatoes, broccoli, squash, leafy greens
Dairy foods (low-fat or nonfat)--2 to 3 daily	Skim or 1% milk, nonfat or low-fat yogurt, nonfat or part-skim cheese
Meats, poultry & fish--2 or fewer daily	Lean meats only; trim visible fat, remove skin from poultry; broil, roast or boil
Nuts, seeds & legumes--4 to 5 a week	Almonds, peanuts, mixed nuts, sunflower seeds, kidney beans, lentils

Adapted from Joint National Committee on Detection, Evaluation, and Treatment of High Blood Pressure. (1997). The sixth report of the joint national committee on detection, evaluation, and treatment of high blood pressure (JNV VI). Archives of Internal Medicine, 157, 24-14-2446.

VI.   Counseling tips for your patients who dine out frequently are as follows

A.   Take the edge off hunger by starting the meal with healthy appetizers such as raw fruits/vegetables or a broth based soup

B.   Select steamed, broiled or baked main dishes and avoid fried or sauteed foods

C.   Remove skin from chicken, cut the fat off red meats

D.   Avoid foods with thick, rich sauces; instead, choose foods with sauces that are thin and stock-based (Avoid hollandaise, bearnaise and gravies)

E.   Request steamed vegetables

F.   Always request salad dressings on the side and order only low-fat selections

G.   To save calories and money, advise patients to share a portion with their companions

WHAT'S IN A SERVING?		
Bread group	1 slice bread 1 oz ready-to-eat cereal	½ c cooked cereal, rice, or pasta
Fruit group	1 medium-sized piece of fruit or 1 melon wedge ½ c chopped, cooked, or canned fruit	3/4 c 100% fruit juice 1/4 c dried fruit
Vegetable group	1 c raw leafy vegetables 3/4 c vegetable juice	½ c other vegetables (cooked or raw)
Meat group	2-3 oz cooked lean meat, fish, or poultry 1-1 ½ c of cooked dry beans	1 egg 2 tbsp peanut butter
Milk group	1 c milk or yogurt 1 ½ oz natural cheese	2 oz processed cheese

VII.   Document your discussions/recommendations in patient record and follow up on subsequent visits

A.   Providing positive reinforcement is important

B.   Refer patients with special problems to nutritionist

DENTAL HEALTH MAINTENANCE

I.   Tooth Preservation is a Lifelong Process

A.   Maintaining good oral hygiene is important throughout life because poor oral hygiene can lead to gingival recession, increased tooth mobility, and eventual tooth loss

B.   Older persons are especially vulnerable to tooth loss and oral disease, because of changes that normally occur as a result of aging
1.   Periodontal structures degenerate with aging, exposing roots of the tooth
2.   Root surface caries due in part to a decline in mineralization of the root surface are much more prevalent in the elderly than in the younger adult
3.   A decrease in saliva production, called dry mouth or xerostomia, is also believed to increase tooth decay (**Note:** Most cases of diminished saliva in the elderly are caused by medications such as sedatives, antihistamines, decongestants, and some antihypertensives)

II.   Tooth Care Steps: Brushing and Flossing

A.   Brushing at margin of teeth and gums with a soft-textured, multi-tufted nylon bristle toothbrush is recommended after every meal or at least twice a day
1.   Recommend placing brush on gumline at a 45 degree angle, and then brushing gums and teeth with an elliptical motion
2.   Stress that thoroughness, rather than vigor, is the key
3.   For patients who have difficulty holding the toothbrush, suggest use of a sponge on adhesive tape to enlarge toothbrush handle diameter
4.   Use of fluorinated toothpaste in any age group speeds up remineralization, the process by which tooth enamel absorbs calcium and phosphorous

5. **Note:** While some recent studies suggest that fluoride accumulated in bone over a lifetime may increase risk of hip fracture and osteoporosis in persons over 65, the data are conflicting, and intake of appropriate levels of fluoride do not appear to have this effect

B. Flossing teeth after every meal can reduce plaque formation and may be even more important than brushing
   1. Explain that waxed or unwaxed products are equally effective
   2. For a better grip on dental floss, suggest use of a commercial dental floss holder

C. For patients who cannot brush or floss after a meal, teach them to swish vigorously with a mouthful of water
   1. Swishing with water washes away food particles and reduces mouth bacteria by 30%
   2. In addition, swishing helps neutralize enamel-attacking acids

D. Persons with dentures should be counseled to do the following:
   1. Remove and rinse dentures after every meal and thoroughly clean with brush at least once a day
   2. Thoroughly clean oral cavity (with dentures removed) daily, using soft toothbrush to brush all intraoral surfaces especially those that underlie the dentures
   3. When cleaning dentures, do so over a water-filled sink to reduce risk of breakage if dropped in sink

III. Dental Visits

A. Regular visits to a dentist for evaluation and oral health counseling should be scheduled at least once a year; patients with dentures need visits every 2 years for evaluation of proper fit and gum and bond conditions

B. Because older persons are more likely to see a primary care provider than a dentist, a thorough oral exam must be performed as a routine part of health maintenance visits
   1. All removable prosthesis should be removed
   2. A tongue depressor or a piece of gauze may be used to keep tongue out of the way during exam

IV. Nutrition

A. Oral health is significantly influenced by diet

B. High sugar foods are to be discouraged in the diet
   1. Advise patients to avoid foods that have a high sugar content, particularly ones that are sticky
   2. Suitable between meal snacks are fresh fruits and vegetables which have a low caries potential index

PREPARTICIPATION SPORTS EXAMINATION

I.   Definition: A sports-specific evaluation emphasizing recent injuries and/or any health condition affecting sports participation

II.   Overview of Evaluation

    A.   Objectives of evaluation
        1.   Help maintain the health and safety of athletes during both training and competition
        2.   Identify those athletes who need further conditioning, require further evaluation prior to clearance, or who require exclusion from a specific sport
        3.   Meet legal and insurance requirements

    B.   Timing of evaluation
        1.   Ideally, timing of the preparticipation examination should occur at least 6 weeks prior to preseason practice
        2.   Adequate time is needed to provide for conditioning, rehabilitation, or further evaluation, if needed

III.   History

    A.   The history is the cornerstone of the evaluation and a thorough history will identify approximately 75% of problems affecting athletic participation

    B.   If possible, the athlete should complete the history form prior to the examination, and the health care provider should review the history with the athlete at the time of the exam

    C.   Use a history form such as the one that follows which emphasizes the areas of greatest concern for sports participation

PREPARTICIPATION PHYSICAL EVALUATION

HISTORY | **DATE OF EXAM** _____

Name _____ Sex _____ Age _____ Date of birth _____
College _____ _____ Sport(s) _____
Address_____ Phone _____
Personal health care provider _____
In case of emergency, contact
Name _____ Relationship _____ Phone (H) _____ (W) _____

Explain "Yes" answers below.
Circle questions you don't know the answers to.

Yes No

1. Have you had a medical illness or injury since your last check up or sports physical? ☐ ☐
   Do you have an ongoing or chronic illness? ☐ ☐

2. Have you ever been hospitalized overnight? ☐ ☐

3. Are you currently taking any prescription or nonprescription (over-the-counter) medications or pills or using an inhaler? ☐ ☐
   Have you ever taken any supplements or vitamins to help you gain or lose weight or improve your performance? ☐ ☐

4. Do you have any allergies (for example, to pollen, medicine, food, or stinging insects)? ☐ ☐
   Have you ever had a rash or hives develop during or after exercise? ☐ ☐

5. Have you ever passed out during or after exercise? ☐ ☐
   Have you ever been dizzy during or after exercise? ☐ ☐
   Have you ever had chest pain during or after exercise? ☐
   Do you get tired more quickly than your friends do during exercise? ☐ ☐
   Have you ever had racing of your heart or skipped heartbeats? ☐ ☐
   Have you had high blood pressure or high cholesterol? ☐ ☐
   Have you ever been told you have a heart murmur? ☐
   Has any family member or relative died of heart problems or of sudden death before age 50? ☐
   Have you had a severe viral infection (for example, myocarditis or mononucleosis) within the last month? ☐ ☐
   Has a physician ever denied or restricted your participation in sports for any heart problems?

6. Do you have any current skin problems (for example, itching, rashes, acne, warts, fungus, or blisters)? ☐ ☐

7. Have you ever had a head injury or concussion? ☐ ☐
   Have you ever been knocked out, become unconscious, or lost your memory? ☐ ☐
   Have you ever had a seizure? ☐ ☐
   Do you have frequent or severe headaches? ☐ ☐
   Have you ever had numbness or tingling in your arms, hands, legs, or feet? ☐ ☐
   Have you ever had a stinger, burner, or pinched nerve? ☐ ☐

8. Have you ever become ill from exercising in the heat? ☐ ☐

9. Do you cough, wheeze, or have trouble breathing during or after activity? ☐ ☐
   Do you have asthma? ☐ ☐
   Do you have seasonal allergies that required medical treatment? ☐ ☐

Yes No

10. Do you use any special protective or corrective equipment or devices that aren't usually used for your sport or position (for example, knee brace, special neck roll, foot orthotics, retainer on your teeth, hearing aid? ☐ ☐

11. Have you had any problems with your eyes or vision? ☐ ☐

12. Have you ever had a sprain, strain, or swelling after injury? ☐ ☐
    Have you broken or fractured any bones or dislocated any joints? ☐ ☐
    Have you had any other problems with pain or swelling in muscles, tendons, bones, or joints? ☐ ☐
    If yes, check appropriate box and explain below.

    ☐ Head ☐ Elbow ☐ Hip
    ☐ Neck ☐ Forearm ☐ Thigh
    ☐ Back ☐ Wrist ☐ Knee
    ☐ Chest ☐ Hand ☐ Shin/calf
    ☐ Shoulder ☐ Finger ☐ Ankle
    ☐ Upper arm ☐ Foot

13. Do you want to weigh more or less than you do now? ☐ ☐
    Do you lose weight regularly to meet weight requirements for your sport? ☐ ☐

14. Do you feel stressed out? ☐ ☐

15. Record dates of your most recent immunizations (shots) for:
    Tetanus _____ Measles _____
    Hepatitis B _____ Chickenpox _____

FEMALES ONLY

16. When was your first menstrual period? _____
    When was your most recent menstrual period? _____
    How much time do you usually have from the start of one period to the start of another? _____
    How many periods have you had in the last year? _____
    What was the longest time between periods in the last year? _____

Explain "Yes" answers here: _____
_____
_____
_____
_____
_____
_____
_____
_____
_____
_____
_____

Source: American Academy of Family Physicians. (1997). <u>Preparticipation physical evaluation</u>. New York: McGraw-Hill, p. 47. (Reprinted by permission)

I hereby state that, to the best of my knowledge, my answers to the above questions are complete and correct.

Signature of athlete _____ Date _____

IV.   Physical Examination

   A.   The physical exam is a screening tool emphasizing the areas of greatest concern in sports participation and areas identified in the history

   B.   Use a physical examination form such as the one that follows which emphasizes the areas of greatest concern for sports participation

   C.   Orthopedic screening deserves special attention. Use the general musculoskeletal screening examination that follows

PREPARTICIPATION PHYSICAL EVALUATION

PHYSICAL EXAMINATION

Name _____ Date of birth _____

Height _____ Weight _____ % Body fat (optional) _____ Pulse _____ BP ____ / ____ (____ / ____ , ____ / ____)

Vision R 20/ _____ L 20/ _____   Corrected: Y   N   Pupils: Equal _____ Unequal _____

	NORMAL	ABNORMAL FINDINGS	INITIALS*
MEDICAL			
Appearance			
Eyes/Ears/Nose/Throat			
Lymph Nodes			
Heart			
Pulses			
Lungs			
Abdomen			
Genitalia (males only)			
Skin			
MUSCULOSKELETAL			
Neck			
Back			
Shoulder/arm			
Elbow/forearm			
Wrist/hand			
Hip/thigh			
Knee			
Leg/ankle			
Foot			

*Station-based examination only

❏   **Cleared**
❏   **Cleared after completing evaluation/rehabilitation for:** _____
_____
_____

❏   **Not cleared for:** _____   **Reason:** _____
Recommendations: _____
_____
_____

Name of health care provider (print/type) _____ **Date** _____
Address _____ **Phone** _____
Signature of health care provider _____

Source: American Academy of Family Physicians. (1997). Preparticipation physical evaluation. New York: McGraw-Hill, p. 48. (Reprinted by permission)

GENERAL MSK SCREENING EXAMINATION

Instructions	Observations
Stand facing examiner	Acromioclavicular joints, general habitus, symmetry of trunk, upper extremities
Look at ceiling, floor, over both shoulders; touch ears to shoulders	Cervical spine motion
Shrug shoulders (examiner resists)	Trapezius strength
Abduct shoulders 90° (examiner resists at 90°)	Deltoid strength
Full external rotation of arms	Shoulder range of motion
Flex and extend elbows	Elbow range of motion
Arms at sides, elbows 90° flexed; pronate and supinate wrists	Elbow and wrist range of motion
Spread fingers; make fist	Range of motion, hands and fingers
Tighten (contract) quadriceps; relax quadriceps	Symmetry and knee effusion; ankle effusion
"Duck walk" 4 steps (away from examiner with buttocks on heels)	Mobility of hip, knee and ankle; strength & balance
Back to examiner, bending forward at waist	Shoulder symmetry, scoliosis
Knees straight, touch toes	Scoliosis, hip motion, hamstring tightness
Raise up on toes, raise heels	Calf symmetry, leg strength

Adapted from American Academy of Family Physicians. (1997). Preparticipation physical evaluation. New York: McGraw-Hill.

V. Diagnostic Tests

    A.   Routine laboratory screening tests in asymptomatic athletes are not required

    B.   Findings from the health history or physical examination may indicate a need to arrange specific diagnostic test

VI. Plan/Management

    A.   Individuals with the following conditions may **not** participate in sports
        1.   **Carditis**. This condition may result in sudden death with exertion
        2.   **Fever**. Fever can increase cardiopulmonary effort, reduce exercise capacity, increase heat intolerance, and predispose to orthostatic hypotension during exercise
        3.   **Diarrhea**. Unless mild, diarrhea may increase the risk of dehydration and heat illness

    B.   Individuals with the following conditions **always require further evaluation** before clearance can be obtained; some sports may not be possible for some persons

CONDITIONS THAT REQUIRE FURTHER EVALUATION TO ASSESS THE SAFETY OF A GIVEN SPORT FOR A PARTICULAR ATHLETE

Cardiovascular Disorders	Hypertension Congenital heart disease Dysrhythmia	Mitral valve prolapse Heart murmur
Neurologic Disorders	Cerebral palsy Convulsive disorder, poorly controlled	History of serious head or spine trauma, severe of repeated concussions, or craniotomy
Respiratory Disorders	Pulmonary compromise, including CF	Acute upper respiratory infection
Hematologic Disorders	Bleeding disorders	Sickle cell disease

(continued)

CONDITIONS THAT REQUIRE FURTHER EVALUATION TO ASSESS THE SAFETY OF A GIVEN SPORT FOR A PARTICULAR ATHLETE (CONTINUED)		
Eyes	Loss of an eye	History of serious eye injury
Genitourinary	Absence of one kidney	
Musculoskeletal	Any MSK disorder	Atlantoaxial instability
Skin	Boils Herpes simplex Impetigo	Scabies Molluscum contagiosum
Gastrointestinal	Enlarged spleen	Enlarged liver
Behavioral	Obesity Anorexia nervosa	Bulimia nervosa

C.   Individuals with the following conditions should not be excluded from participation in sports solely on the basis of the condition

CONDITIONS NOT NECESSARILY PRECLUDING PARTICIPATION IN SPORTS	
Endocrine	Diabetes mellitus (with proper attention to diet, hydration, and insulin therapy)
Immunocompromised	HIV infection (all sports may be played so long as the person is able)
Genitourinary	Absence of one ovary Absent or undescended testicle
Respiratory	Asthma (with proper medication and education, only athletes with severe asthma will need to modify participation)
Hematologic	Sickle cell trait
Neurological	Convulsive disorder, well controlled (risk of convulsion during participation is minimal)

D.   A preparticipation clearance form such as the one that follows can be used to make recommendations regarding participation

PREPARTICIPATION PHYSICAL EVALUATION

CLEARANCE FORM

❏ **Cleared**

❏ **Cleared after completing evaluation/rehabilitation for:** _____

_____

_____

_____

❏ **Not cleared for:** _____ **Reason:** _____

Recommendations: _____

_____

_____

Name of health care provider (print/type) _____ **Date** _____

Address _____ **Phone** _____

Signature of health care provider _____

Source: American Academy of Family Physicians. (1997). <u>Preparticipation physical evaluation</u>. New York: McGraw-Hill, p. 49. (Reprinted by permission)

E. Be aware of the medicolegal considerations when performing preparticipation physical evaluations
    1. Many athletes are unwilling to accept restrictions in sport participation
        a. A second medical opinion may be sought or an attorney may be retained
        b. Under the Rehabilitation Act of 1973, and the Americans with Disabilities Act of 1990, athletes may have the legal right to participate against medical advice
    2. Health care providers who recommend restricted participation or exclusion from a sport should consult with experts in the medical condition in question to assist in determining the risk to the athlete of participating in the desired sport
        a. This approach limits the likelihood that the athlete will be inappropriately excluded from the sport
        b. This approach also reassures the athlete if restriction or exclusion is indeed the correct course
        c. Finally, such an approach provides liability protection for the health care provider who is making the recommendation

REFERENCES

American Academy of Family Physicians. (1997). Preparticipation physical evaluation. Minneapolis, MN: McGraw Hill.

Brangman, S.A. (1992). The mouth. In R.J. Ham & P.D. Sloan (Eds.), Primary care geriatrics: A case-based approach. St. Louis: Mosby.

Gardner, P., & Schaffner, W. (1993). Immunization of adults. New England Journal of Medicine, 328(17), 1252-1257.

Gordon, S.R. (1990). Oral and dental problems. In R.W. Schrier (Ed.), Geriatric medicine. Philadelphia: Saunders.

Immunization Action Coalition. (1997, Oct). Summary of recommendations for adult immunizations. St. Paul, MN: Author.

Johns Hopkins Medical Letter. (1993). Dental Care: Keeping your mouth healthy. Health After 50, 5(5), 4-6.

Joint National Committee on Detection, Evaluation, and Treatment of High Blood Pressure. (1997). The sixth report of the joint national committee on detection, evaluation, and treatment of high blood pressure (JNC VI). Archives of Internal Medicine, 157, 24-13-2446.

Lipschitz, D.A., Ham, R.J., & White, J.V. (1992). An approach to nutrition screening for older Americans. American Family Physician, 45(2), 601-608.

Snelling, A.M. (1997, Apr). A concise guide to nutrition counseling. Patient Care, 47-53.

US Department of Agriculture, Department of Health and Human Services. (1995). Nutrition and your health: Dietary guidelines for Americans. Washington, DC: Author.

US Preventive Services Task Force. (1996). Guide to clinical preventive services (2nd ed.). Baltimore: Williams & Wilkins.

General

FEVER

I. Definition of fever: Traditionally defined as body temperature greater than 38.0°C (100.4°F) rectally, 37.8°C (100°F) orally, or 37.2°C (99°F) axillary; more recently defined as early morning body temperature (measured orally) ≥37.2° (≥99.0°) or a temperature of ≥37.8° (≥100°) (see table that follows for conversion of temperature)

CONVERSION OF TEMPERATURE		
37°C	=	98.6°F
38°C	=	100.4°F
39°C	=	102.2°F
40°C	=	104.0°F

A. Fever without localizing sign (source): unexplained fever of brief duration or lasting <5-7 days; source of acute febrile illness is not apparent after a careful history and physical examination

B. Fevers of unknown origin (FUO): fever persisting for 3 weeks, > 101°F and eluding one week of intensive diagnostic testing

II. Pathogenesis of Fever

A. Fever occurs when bacteria, viruses, toxins, or other agents are phagocytosed by leukocytes

B. Then, interluekin-1 and other chemical mediators (previously referred to as endogenous pyrogens) are produced and activate the production of prostaglandins

C. Prostaglandins act on the thermoregulatory mechanism in the hypothalamus and upwardly readjust the body's thermostat

D. Raising the hypothalamic set-point initiates the process of heat production and conservation by increasing metabolism, triggering peripheral vasoconstriction, and less frequently by triggering shivering which increases heat production from the muscles

E. Infection is the most common cause of fever in both adults and children; most infections are viral in etiology

F. Other causes include the following:
   1. Hypersensitivity to drugs
   2. Recent immunizations with certain vaccines
   3. Vascular occlusive and/or inflammatory events such as deep vein thrombophlebitis, pulmonary emboli, or myocardial infarction
   4. Acute hemolytic episodes associated with acute autoimmune hemolytic anemia or sickle cell anemia
   5. Neoplasms
   6. Collagen-vascular diseases
   7. Central nervous system abnormalities

G. Occasionally, a patient may have a factitious fever or a high reading on the thermometer which was artificially produced by the patient for secondary gains

H. True fever must be differentiated from hyperthermia
   1. Hyperthermia occurs when there is increased body temperature but no alteration in the hypothalamic set point

2. Hyperthermia may be due to increased metabolic heat (e.g., thyrotoxicosis), excessive environmental temperature (e.g., heat stroke), defective heat loss because of environmental conditions (e.g. high humidity, overdressing, sitting in unventilated, sunny car, exercise), or dermatologic disorder (e.g., ectodermal dysplasia)

III. Clinical Presentation

A. Fever, by itself, is not a illness; rather, a sign that the body is fighting an infection or reacting to a stimulus; normal temperatures are characterized by the following:
   1. Temperature is usually highest around 6 pm and lowest around 6 am
   2. Normal temperature deviations occur with physical activity, stress, ovulation, and environmental heat

B. Typical symptoms include malaise, fatigue, myalgias, and tachycardia (pulse rate is often elevated by about 10-15 beats per 1°C of fever)

C. Central nervous system symptoms may occur ranging from mild changes in alertness to delirium, particularly in elderly and chronically-ill patients

D. Although each 1°F raises the basal metabolic rate by 7%, most patients can tolerate fevers well with a few exceptions such as patients with underlying cardiac disease or chronically, debilitating diseases, immunocompromised patients, and the elderly who are at a greater risk for developing dehydration

E. Bacteremia, meningitis, and seizures are serious conditions related to fevers

IV. Diagnosis/Evaluation

A. History
   1. Inquire about onset, duration, and pattern of fever; ascertain that the patient knows how to correctly measure temperature; inquire about type of thermometer used
   2. Inquire about associated symptoms such as anorexia, chills, headache, nasal congestion, earache, sore throat, cough, abdominal pain, vomiting, diarrhea, painful urination
   3. Explore hydration status by asking about amount of fluid intake and frequency and amount of fluid output
   4. Ask about comfort level of patient
   5. Explore possibilities of heat illness (heat stroke) or from other types of environmental exposure
   6. Ask whether patient started any new medications or had a recent immunization
   7. Ask whether other household members are ill or have fevers
   8. Inquire about recent travel, pet scratches, or exposure to ticks
   9. Inquire about last dosage of an antipyretic and other self-treatment measures
   10. Past medical history should include a list of current medications, discussion of previous illnesses and diseases, particularly any cardiac or chronically debilitating disorders
   11. A complete review of systems may be needed to uncover source of fever and to determine severity of debility due to elevated body temperature

B. Physical Examination
   1. Measure temperature
      a. Always confirm initial temperature measurement; retake temperature before ordering diagnostic tests or prescribing treatment to reduce fever
      b. Rectal temperatures are gold standard as they are accurate, reproducible, and not affected by environmental factors; rectal temperatures are approximately 1° higher than oral temperatures and 2 to 2.5° higher than axillary temperatures
      c. Oral temperatures are reliable but may vary with rapid breathing and recent ingestion of hot or cold fluids
      d. The infrared ear thermometer estimates the temperature of the tympanic membrane (TM); improper placement and aiming, incomplete probe penetration into external ear canal, and obstruction/tortuosity of the external ear canal can lead to underestimating TM temperature

2. Measure respiratory rate, pulse, and blood pressure
3. Observe general appearance, looking for subtle signs such as changes in alertness
4. Observe skin for color, rashes, petechiae or purpura
5. Assess for signs of dehydration such as skin turgor and capillary refill
6. Assess neck for nuchal rigidity
7. Check for lymphadenopathy
8. Assess for swollen joints
9. May need to do a complete physical examination to find localized infection such as otitis media, pharyngitis, sinusitis, meningitis, cervical adenitis, pneumonia, or urinary tract infection

C. Differential Diagnosis: See pathogenesis for ETIOLOGIES OF FEVER
1. The height (unless extremely high) of the temperature, the duration of the fever, and whether the fever responds to antipyretics are usually not helpful in differentiating the cause
2. Fevers almost always result in increases in pulse rates; absence of a pulse rate increase suggests factitious fever, mycoplasmal infection or typhoid fever
3. It is important to differentiate true fever from hyperthermia
4. Fever pattern provides clues to diagnosis:
    a. Continuous or sustained fever with slight remissions (not exceeding 2.0°F): lobar and gram-negative pneumonia, the rickettsioses, typhoid fever, CNS disorders
    b. Intermittent fever with wide fluctuations (usually normal or low in morning and peaking between 4:00 and 8:00 pm): localized pyogenic infections, bacterial endocarditis, malaria
    c. Intermittent fever with two daily peaks: salmonelloses, miliary tuberculosis, gonococcal and meningococcal endocarditis
    d. Sporadic episodes of fever or periods of normal temperature and recurrence of fever: cholangitis
    e. Weekly or longer periods of fever and equally long afebrile periods with repetition of cycle: Hodgkin's disease, brucellosis, occasionally tuberculosis
    f. Highest temperature elevation in early morning hours: occasionally in miliary tuberculosis, salmonelloses, hepatic abscess, bacterial endocarditis
    g. Sharply increased elevation of temperature with exacerbation of other clinical abnormalities occurs several hours after antibiotic treatment of syphilis, leptospirosis and tick-borne relapsing fever

D. Diagnostic Tests: Recommended diagnostic tests depend on patient's age, clinical presentation, and previous medical history
1. In the majority of cases, the history and physical examination will uncover likely causes of the fever and suggest selective diagnostic tests
2. For patients who have a localized infection but also have 1 of the following: look toxic, have an extremely elevated temperature, are immunodeficient, or have an underlying chronic disease, consider ordering the following
    a. Urine analysis for specific gravity and the presence of ketones to determine hydration status
    b. CBC with differential and erythrocyte sedimentation rate (ESR) to determine likelihood of a bacterial etiology and/or blood cultures to rule out bacteremia and need for more aggressive treatments such as hospitalization and parenteral antimicrobial therapy
3. Fevers of unknown origin (FUO) require an extensive diagnostic evaluation.

V. Plan/Management

A. Immediately transport the following patients to the hospital:
1. Patients who are disoriented or delirious
2. Patients with meningismus, petechiae or purpura

B. Consider consultation and hospitalization for following patients:
1. Patients with extremely elevated temperatures
2. Patients who are immunodeficient or have a history of cardiac or another serious disease

3. Very old patients
4. Patients who are taking corticosteroid or immunosuppressive therapy
5. Patients who have prosthetic devices
6. IV drug abusers
7. Patients who are dehydrated
8. Any patient who appears toxic (rigors, hypotension, oliguria, CNS abnormalities, petechial rash, marked leukocytosis or leukopenia, cardiorespiratory distress, new significant cardiac murmurs)
9. Any patient whose fever lasts longer than 7-10 days

C. Treat cause of fever; antibiotics should be prescribed when there is an identified bacterial infection

D. Antipyretics: Controversy exists concerning when to treat a fever with antipyretics.
1. Reasons for not treating a low-grade or moderate fever in an otherwise well patient include the following: Antipyretics do not alter the course or duration of disease; may mask the signs and symptoms of a serious disease and confuse the clinical picture; and can be potentially harmful in some patients (e.g., side effects, toxicity)
2. However, most clinicians agree that antipyretics should be given in the following situations:
   a. When fevers are 103°F and higher
   b. In patients for whom side effects of fever may be harmful (e.g. patients with compensated cardiac disease and chronic debilitating disorders, patients who become dehydrated rapidly, patients who are alcoholics)
   c. Patients who are uncomfortable and unable to rest
3. In hyperthermic states such as thyrotoxicosis, heat stroke and overdressing, the set point has not been changed and antipyretic medications are not effective because they act to lower set point
4. The drug of choice is acetaminophen (Tylenol); Adults: 325-650 mg every 4-6
   a. Do not use in liver disease or transplant patients
   b. Strictly follow correct doses to prevent liver damage; maximum effect at 2 hours
5. Aspirin (325-650 mg every 4-6 hours) is a second choice for fever management in adults but should never be given to children and adolescents who have a fever because of the dangers of Reye syndrome
   a. Adverse effects: gastric irritation and risk of bleeding
   b. Risk of asthma exacerbation and anaphylactic reaction, particularly in patients with history of asthma and nasal polyps
6. Ibuprofen (Motrin) is another therapeutic option
   a. Dosage is 400 mg every 6 hours
   b. Overdose is rare and less toxic than salicylates and tylenol
   c. Avoid in patients with aspirin allergies, ulcers, renal insufficiency, and bleeding disorders

E. Sponging may be performed but usually is unnecessary and may even be harmful because it can cause discomfort and chilling
1. If temperature is extremely high or if aggressive fever management is necessary such as a child with history of febrile seizures, sponge patient after giving antipyretic
2. Sponging is an important part of the management plan in the following cases: patients with severe liver disease who cannot take acetaminophen, neurologic problems in which temperature regulation mechanisms are abnormal, heat stroke, or in environments with excessive temperatures
3. When sponging, water should be lukewarm and should not cause the patient to shiver (colder temperatures are used for heat illness such as heat stroke)

F. Patient Education
1. Teach the correct method to measure temperature; keep thermometer in place for at least 2 minutes
2. Reinforce when to call a health care provider about an elevated temperature

      a.   Immediately call when there is delirium (disorientation or confusion), seizures, stiff neck, petechial or purpural rash, signs of dehydration (can teach how to assess capillary refill) and high fever of >103°F (39.4°C)

      b.   Call health care provider if patient has associated symptoms such as swollen joints, severe cough, is not eating/drinking well, is lethargic and is very restless during sleep

3.   Instruct to drink extra fluids; for patients who are dehydrated, teach to drink fluids every 15-60 minutes

4.   Daily activities should be modified to provide for additional rest, light meals, and avoidance of strenuous activities depending on patient's condition

5.   Remind patients to avoid overdressing when they have a fever

6.   Tell patients to never use alcohol for sponging

7.   Inform patients that elevated temperatures are a normal body defense mechanism, not a disease; height of the temperature except when extremely high does not correlate well with serious diseases; assure everyone that there are almost always no adverse effects from fevers

G.   Follow Up

    1.   Variable and depends on age, diagnosis, and clinical presentation of patient as well as the amount of friend and family support available

    2.   For elderly and chronically-ill patients consider scheduling return visit for following morning or have telephone contact within 24 hours to assess condition

    3.   Instruct patients to return for further evaluation if fever persists for more than 2 or 3 days

LYMPHADENOPATHY

I.   Definition: Lymph node enlargement

II.   Pathogenesis

    A.   Following mechanisms result in lymphadenopathy

        1.   Proliferation in response to an antigen

        2.   Invasion of cells from cells outside the node such as malignant cells

        3.   Transformation of primary nodular tissue into neoplastic cells

    B.   Causes of generalized lymphadenopathy

        1.   Infections (most common cause)

           a.   Viral: Human immunodeficiency virus, mononucleosis, cytomegalovirus, hepatitis B, measles, rubella, rubeola

           b.   Bacterial: Group A. Streptococci, cat-scratch disease, secondary syphilis

           c.   Mycobacterial: atypical mycobacterial infection, miliary tuberculosis

           d.   Fungal: histoplasmosis

           e.   Protozoal: toxoplasmosis

        2.   Collagen vascular disorders: systemic lupus erythematosus, rheumatoid arthritis

        3.   Endocrine disorders: hyperthyroidism, hypopituitarism, hypoadrenocorticism

        4.   Neoplasms: leukemia, lymphoma, immunoblastic lymphadenopathy, metastases

        5.   Hypersensitivity states: serum sickness, drug reactions (phenytoin and less commonly: hydralazine, para-aminosalicylic acid, propylthiouracil, and allopurinol)

        6.   Miscellaneous: sarcoidosis, lipid storage disease, Kawasaki disease

    C.   Causes of localized lymphadenopathy: local infection, growth, or recent immunization in area drained by involved lymph node (also see table IV.B.1)

        1.   Anterior auricular: viral conjunctivitis, rubella, scalp infection

        2.   Submandibular or cervical (unilateral): buccal cavity infection, pharyngitis, nasopharyngeal tumor, thyroid malignancy

        3.   Cervical (bilateral): mononucleosis, sarcoidosis, toxoplasmosis, pharyngitis

4. Supraclavicular (right): pulmonary, mediastinal, and esophageal malignancies
5. Supraclavicular (left): malignancies (intra-abdominal, renal, testicular, ovarian)
6. Axillary: breast malignancy or infection, upper extremity infection
7. Epitrochlear: syphilis (bilateral), hand infection (unilateral)
8. Inguinal: syphilis, genital herpes, lymphogranuloma venereum, chancroid, lower extremity or local infection
9. Hilar adenopathy: sarcoidosis, fungal infection, lymphoma, bronchogenic carcinoma, tuberculosis
10. Any region: benign reactive hyperplasia, lymphomas, cat scratch disease, leukemia, sarcoidosis, malignancies

III. Clinical presentation: The following key factors are helpful in arriving at a diagnosis:

A. Generalized versus localized lymphadenopathy
1. Generalized adenopathy is due to systemic disease
2. Localized adenopathy is caused by either local infection, tumor, or systemic disease

B. Location of node (see PATHOGENESIS); supraclavicular node, often called "sentinel" node suggests Hodgkin's disease

C. Character of node
1. Size: a large node (>1 cm.) usually represents a specific pathology
2. Metastatic cancer: hard, painless, matted, fixed, often >3 cm.
3. Reactive: discrete, mobile, rubbery, and mildly tender
4. Lymphadenitis: tender, warm, red, fluctuant
5. Infection: firm, red, warm
6. Lymphoma, leukemia: firm or rubbery nodes

D. Age of patient
1. In patients <30 years, most cases are benign and caused by infection
2. Benign reactive hyperplasia or transient node enlargement from unknown causes occurs frequently in children and young adults
3. Palpable nodes in the anterior cervical triangle are common and usually normal, especially in children and young adults
4. Posterior cervical node enlargement in the older child, adolescent, and young adult may be mononucleosis
5. Risk of cancer increases with age

E. Onset and duration
1. Nodes of acute onset and duration are typically due to viral or pyogenic infection
2. Chronicity suggests neoplastic disease, sarcoidosis, tuberculosis, and fungal infections although lymphadenitis may take several months to resolve

F. Rate of change: usually nodes that are rapidly growing are more pathologic than slow-growing nodes

G. Associated symptoms
1. Low-grade fevers with night sweats and weight loss characterize lymphoma, HIV infection or tuberculosis
2. Fatigue and weight loss suggest systemic infection, cancer, or connective tissue disease
3. Hilar lymph node enlargement may cause compression of thoracic structures and result in cough, dyspnea, and wheezing

H. Associated signs
1. Splenomegaly: mononucleosis, lymphoma, or leukemia
2. Thyromegaly: hyperthyroidism
3. Tender, warm, or enlarged joints: collagen vascular disease and leukemia
4. Rash: viral exanthems, Kawasaki disease, collagen and vascular diseases

I. Epidemiologic leads
  1. Recent exposure to cats is predisposing factor in cat-scratch disease
  2. History of multiple sexual partners and IV drug use may be associated with sexually transmitted disease or HIV infection
  3. Alcohol or tobacco abuse in elderly patient with cervical lymphadenopathy may represent head and neck carcinoma
  4. Occupational diseases such as silicosis or asbestosis may result in hilar and mediastinal lymphadenopathy

IV. Diagnosis/Evaluation

  A. History
    1. Ask about onset, duration, and rate of growth of all palpable nodes
    2. Question about tenderness of node
    3. Ask about recent infections and trauma
    4. Inquire about systemic symptoms such as weight loss, night sweats, fatigue, and diarrhea
    5. Question about exposure to animals, travel to foreign countries, occupation, and explore other risk factors such as substance abuse and sexual exposure
    6. Ask about medications
    7. Explore past medical history and family history

  B. Physical examination
    1. Assess all palpable nodes, noting size, localization, consistency, tenderness, warmth, and fixation (see table that follows)

PALPABLE LYMPH NODES AND LYMPHATIC DRAINAGE	
Node	**Drainage Area**
Occipital	Posterior scalp, neck
Mastoid	Mastoid area
Submental	Apex of tongue and lower lip
Submaxillary	Buccal cavity, tongue, cheek, lips
Cervical	Head, neck, and oropharynx
Axillary	Greater part of arm, shoulder, superficial anterior and lateral thoracic and upper abdominal wall
Supraclavicular	Right: Inferior neck and mediastinum Left: Inferior neck, mediastinum, and upper abdomen
Epitrochlear	Hand, forearm, and elbow
Inguinal	Leg and genitalia
Femoral	Leg
Popliteal	Posterior leg and knee

      a. Normal, palpable nodes are discrete, freely mobile, and nontender
      b. Normal size of nodes is < 1cm. with two exceptions:
        (1) Inguinal nodes are normal up to 1.5 cm.
        (2) Epitrochlear nodes are abnormal if >0.5 cm.
    2. For localized lymphadenopathy, carefully assess all body parts within the lymphatic drainage area (see preceding table)
    3. For generalized lymphadenopathy a careful, comprehensive physical examination is needed

  C. Differential Diagnosis; potential causes range from simple and benign to complicated and serious; for a large proportion of enlarged nodes, no specific cause is found (see pathogenesis for range of etiologies)

D. Diagnostic Tests (If benign cause of lymphadenopathy is suspected, close observation is indicated); when the diagnosis is uncertain, stepwise testing with the following tests is needed:
1. CBC
   a. Atypical lymphocytes: mononucleosis or other viral syndromes
   b. Increased granulocytes: bacterial infection
   c. Increased eosinophils: hypersensitivity states
   d. Decreased red blood cells and platelets: malignancy
2. Chest x-ray which will detect pulmonary disease and hilar adenopathy is needed for seriously ill patients and those with supraclavicular lymphadenopathy or respiratory complaints
3. Serologic tests
   a. Monospot or Epstein-Barr virus: mononucleosis
   b. VDRL: syphilis
   c. HIV antibody: HIV infection
   d. Antinuclear antibody and rheumatoid factor: collagen diseases
   e. Other serologic tests: cytomegalovirus and toxoplasmosis infections
4. Tuberculin skin test for myobacterial disease
5. Cultures
   a. Throat for cervical adenopathy
   b. Urethral and cervical for inguinal adenopathy
   c. Aspirated lymph tissue for suspected fungal or mycobacterial infection
   d. Blood culture for suspected bacteremia
6. Lymph node biopsy provides a definitive diagnosis; indicated when simple testing fails to provide a diagnosis or for cases when cancer, tuberculosis or sarcoidosis is suspected
   a. The following characteristics suggest the need for an early biopsy:
      (1) Node > 2 cm
      (2) Abnormal chest x-ray
      (3) Enlarged supraclavicular node
      (4) Associated signs and symptoms of weight loss and hepatosplenomegaly
      (5) Absence of respiratory tract symptoms
   b. Nodes that remain constant in size for 4-8 weeks and those that fail to resolve in 8-12 weeks need a biopsy
7. Ultrasound and computed tomography are sometimes helpful in differentiating lymphadenopathy from nonlymphatic enlargement
8. Bone marrow examination is needed for patients with severe anemia, neutropenia, thrombocytopenia or peripheral smear for malignant blast cells

V. Plan/Management

A. Treatment depends on diagnosis; see sections on CERVICAL ADENITIS, PHARYNGITIS, etc.

B. Consider consultation for patients suspected of having serious disease or one of the following:
1. Undiagnosed adenopathy lasting longer than 2 months
2. Firm, matted, rapidly enlarging, nontender nodes
3. Associated signs and symptoms such as night sweats, weight loss, bone pain, hepatosplenomegaly, and fever of unknown etiology
4. Associated complete cell count abnormality, positive PPD, or abnormal chest x-ray

C. Follow Up
1. Diagnosis will determine when patient should return for follow-up
2. For cases in which the cause of lymphadenopathy is uncertain, watchful waiting with follow up every 3-5 days for 2 weeks is appropriate

PAIN

I. Definition: Unpleasant sensory and emotional experience related to actual or potential tissue damage

II. Pathogenesis

    A. Peripheral stimulation occurs when free nerve endings or nociceptors found in various parts of body (i.e., skin, blood vessels, viscera, muscles) are stimulated and then action potentials are transmitted along afferent nerve fibers to the spinal cord

    B. Gate control theory of pain
        1. The perception of pain is an interplay between the nociceptive pain fibers and the nonociceptive or non-transmitting neurons that synapse in the spinal cord
        2. Clinically, this is important because certain treatments such as acupuncture, topical irritants, and transcutaneous electrical nerve stimulation (TENS) can stimulate the large nonociceptive neurons and produce an analgesic effect

    C. Pain-initiated processes as well as other information are carried through the ascending spinal cord pathways (particularly the spinothalamic tract) to the brain

    D. In the brain, pain is perceived as a partial summation of two processes:
        1. Positive feedback is the nociceptive stimulus which activates pain transmission
        2. Negative feedback is the brain's modulatory network composed of the endogenous opiate system (opiate receptors, endorphins) which inhibits pain

    E. Other neurotransmitter substances such as acetylcholine, dopamine, norepinephrine, and serotonin play a role in pain transmission as well

    F. The brain also controls pain sensation through an organized descending or efferent pain transmission system

III. Clinical Presentation

    A. Acute pain
        1. Arises from injury, trauma, spasm or disease of body parts
        2. Usually is short-lived and decreases as damaged area heals
        3. Associated with hyperactivity of the sympathetic nervous system resulting in the following: tachycardia, tachypnea, elevated blood pressure, diaphoresis and dilated pupils

    B. Chronic pain
        1. Pain which lasts longer than 6 months and is rarely accompanied with hyperactivity of sympathetic nervous system
        2. Can be characterized by its location
            a. Visceral locations (initiated in abdomen or thorax)
            b. Somatic pain (initiated in muscles and connective tissue)
            c. Neurologic causes (i.e., diabetic neuropathy)
        3. Chronic pain typology:
            a. Pain that persists beyond the normal healing time for an acute injury
            b. Chronic disease pain
            c. Pain without identifiable organic cause
            d. Cancer pain
        4. Symptoms of depression often accompany chronic pain

    C. Although research findings are contradictory, some studies found an age-related reduction in pain sensitivity; elderly patients with recent changes in cognition, function, and behavior should have a thorough pain assessment

IV. Diagnosis/Evaluation

    A. History
        1. Mnemonic may be used to obtain patient's subjective description of pain
            a. P: palliative or precipitating factors such as stress, exertion
            b. Q: quality of pain such as sharpness, crushing, throbbing, burning
            c. R: region or radiation of pain
            d. S: subjective descriptions of severity of pain such as awakens at night or takes breath away
            e. T: temporal nature such as daytime, during meals; constant vs. intermittent
        2. May use a visual analog scale to quantify pain or ask patient to relate where pain falls on a line from zero (no pain) to 10 (worst pain ever experienced)
        3. Inquire about drug use and its efficacy
        4. Ask about previous personal or family history of chronic pain
        5. Particularly in the elderly, ask about recent changes in cognition, behavior such as agitation and withdrawal; inquire about sleep alterations, bowel changes, depression, problems with gait and balance
        6. Assess patient's level of functioning in all spheres of living such as family relationships, social relationships, employment, and hobbies to help determine secondary gains
        7. Complete review of systems to determine relationship of pain to other parts of body

    B. Physical Examination
        1. Assess vital signs
        2. Observe general appearance for signs of distress
        3. Observe patient's affect
        4. Inspect, palpate, percuss and auscultate, as appropriate, all areas and surrounding structures which patient perceives as painful

    C. Diagnostic tests are variable depending of patient's condition

    D. Differential Diagnosis
        1. Malingering for ongoing litigation or secondary gains
        2. Anxiety or depression

V. Plan/Management

    A. General principles of pain management
        1. Cultivating a sense of control by the patient over the pain is important in both acute and chronic situations; remember in elderly there is increased sensitivity to adverse effects of all pain medications
        2. Particularly in chronic situations, it is important to get the patient engaged in an active, productive life
        3. Essential to involve the patient's family and friends in the management plan

    B. Pharmacologic principles of treating pain
        1. Identify source of pain and treat as appropriate
        2. Use the least potent analgesic with the fewest side effects
        3. Give analgesics for adequate trial time and properly titrate the dose which means considering individual patient characteristics and needs
        4. Use analgesics on a regular dosing schedule and not on a "prn" basis which promotes anxiety and contributes to future drug dependence
        5. Prevent persistent pain and relieve breakthrough pain; Order rescue medication equivalent to half the standing dose to start on a prn basis
        6. Recognize and treat side effects; avoid excessive sedation
            a. Use neurostimulants to reduce sedative effects such as caffeine, dextroamphetamine, methylphenidate
            b. Regular laxative therapy with docusate sodium and sennosides (Senokot) twice a day is often needed to prevent constipation
        7. Use equianalgesic doses

8.   Use appropriate route of administration
   a.   Use oral medications, if possible, because of ease of administration and cost effectiveness
   b.   NSAID, ketorolac (Toradol), is available in IM preparation
   c.   Fentanyl (Duragesic) is available as a transdermal patch
   d.   Morphine and hydromorphone are available as rectal suppositories
   e.   Subcutaneous or intravenous administration of morphine and hydromorphone is sometimes needed; patient-controlled analgesia pumps can provide individualized pain relief

9.   Watch for development of tolerance

C.   The Three-Step Analgesic Ladder of the World Health Organization (see table that follows)
   1.   Designed for chronic, cancer pain but can be used as a guide for all types of pain management

THREE-STEP ANALGESIC LADDER OF THE WORLD HEALTH ORGANIZATION		
Step	**Oral Medications**	**Regimen**
Step 1	Acetaminophen 324-650mg Q 4-6° Salicylates: aspirin 325-650 mg Q 4° NSAIDS (dosage in next table) Tramadol 50-100mg Q 4-6°	Nonopioid ± adjuvant
If pain persists, maximize nonopioid and add step 2 opioid		
Step 2	Codeine 30-90 mg Q 4° Dihydrocodeine 32 mg Q 4° Hydrocodone 5-10 mg Q 4-6° Oxycodone 5 mg Q 6°	Opioid: mild-to-moderate pain +nonopioid ±adjuvant therapy
If pain persists at step 2, increase dose of opioid or change to step 3 opioid		
Step 3	Morphine IR 15-30 mg Q 4-6° Oxycodone 7.5-10 mg Q 4-6° Hydromorphone 4 mg Q 4° Fentanyl 50μg/hr Q 72°	Opioid: moderate-to-severe pain ±nonopioid ±adjuvant therapy

Adapted from WHO (1990). Cancer pain relief and palliative care: Report of WHO Expert Committee. WHO Technological Report Service, 804, 1-73.

D.   Acetaminophen (Tylenol - APAP) is a nonnarcotic agent with antipyretic, analgesic effects; minimal anti-inflammatory effects
   1.   Onset of 0.5-1 hour; duration 3-6 hours
   2.   "Ceiling effect" exists, but many patients have greater pain relief from a single 1000 mg dose compared to single 560 mg dose
   3.   Do not exceed 4 to 6 g per day to prevent liver damage
   4.   Few adverse reactions; hepatotoxicity in overdose or in chronic alcoholics following therapeutic dosage

E.   Acetylsalicylic acid (Aspirin - ASA) is a nonnarcotic agent with antipyretic, analgesic, and anti-inflammatory effects (see table on NSAIDs which follows)
   1.   Onset within 0.5 hours; duration 3-6 hours
   2.   "Ceiling effect" exists such that single doses greater than 650 mg do not result in greater degree of pain relief
   3.   Stop taking drug at least one week before surgery; single therapeutic dose irreversibly inhibits platelet function for the 7-day lifetime of platelet
   4.   Adverse reactions include Reye syndrome, hypersensitivity reactions (asthmatic patients particularly), dyspepsia, indigestion, gastric ulcers, irreversible inhibition of platelet aggregation, tinnitus, renal effects, anemia

5.   Monitor hematocrit, stool guaiac periodically; order plasma salicylate level determinations when patient is prescribed high dosages

6.   Avoid in patients with asthma, thrombocytopenia, GI disorders

F.   Other salicylic acid derivatives have a slower onset and longer duration than ASA, but are just as potent and cause fewer gastrointestinal and central nervous system side effects (See table on NSAIDs which follows)

G.   Nonsteroidal anti-inflammatory drugs (NSAIDs), nonnarcotic agents, used for mild to moderate pain and have antipyretic, analgesic, and anti-inflammatory effects (see table which follows for dosing recommendations); new Cox-2 inhibitors such as celecoxib (Celebrex) are also helpful and may have less GI side effects than NSAIDS

    1.   Useful for dental pain, rheumatoid arthritis, headaches, musculoskeletal pain, menstrual cramps, and bone pain with cancer

    2.   Major pathway of metabolism is hepatic

    3.   Patients have large variability in response to individual agents; switch to another NSAID/class if one agent is ineffective in an adequate trial

    4.   Before switching to another class of NSAIDs give an adequate trial of efficacy (1-2 weeks depending on half-life of drugs); instruct patient to continue to take drug at prescribed times even if pain stops

    5.   Always prescribe an adequate dosage (start with low dose and gradually increase to maximum dosage for patients in moderate pain)

    6.   Do not use combination of different NSAIDs

    7.   Side effects can occur: GI distress (take with meals to lessen this effect), fluid retention, peripheral edema, hepatic problems, renal disorders, and central nervous system effects such as dizziness and depression.

    8.   Be careful in prescribing if patient is on other drugs; NSAIDs may enhance oral hypoglycemic agents and coumarin

    9.   May impair diuretic function and antagonize the effects of antihypertensive medications by inhibiting renal prostaglandins

    10.   Baseline tests for long-term therapy include hematocrit, liver function tests, urinalysis, blood urea nitrogen (BUN), serum creatinine; often these diagnostic tests are rechecked in first month after initiation and then at 6-month intervals

NONSTEROIDAL ANTI-INFLAMMATORY DRUGS (NSAIDS)

Class & Agent	Half Life (hrs)	Tablet Size	Dose
FENAMATES			
Meclofenamate Sodium (Meclomen)	2	50, 100	50-100 mg Q 4-6 hrs; max 400 mg
Mefenamic Acid (Ponstel)	2-4	250	Initial: 500 mg, then 250 mg QID; max use 1 week
INDOLES			
Indomethacin (Indocin)	4.5	25, 50	25 mg BID or TID; max 200 mg daily
Sulindac (Clinoril)	7.8	150, 200	150 mg BID; max 400 mg/day
Tolmetin sodium (Tolectin)	1-1.5	200, 400, 600	400 mg TID; max 1800 mg/day
NAPHTHYLKANONE			
Nabumetone (Relafen)	20-30	500, 750	1 g/day QD or BID; max 2 g/day
OXICAMS			
Piroxicam (Feldene)	30-86	10, 20	20 mg QD
PHENYLACETIC ACID			
Diclofenac sodium (Voltaren)	2	25, 50, 75, 100 ext. rel.	50-75 mg BID; max 200 mg/day 100 mg ext. rel. QD

(continued)

NONSTEROIDAL ANTI-INFLAMMATORY DRUGS (NSAIDS) (CONTINUED)

Class & Agent	Half Life (hrs)	Tablet Size	Dose
PROPIONIC ACIDS			
Fenoprofen calcium (Nalfon)	2-3	200	200 mg Q 4-6 hrs
Flurbiprofen (Ansaid)	5.7	50, 100	50-100 mg TID
Ibuprofen (Motrin)	1.8-2.5	200, 400, 600, 800	400-600 mg Q 4-6 hrs; max 3.2 g/day
Ketoprofen (Orudis)	2-4	12.5, 25, 50, 75	50-75 mg TID or QID; max 300 mg/day
Naproxen (Naprosyn)	12-15	250, 375, 500	500 mg initially, followed by 250 mg Q 6-8 hrs
Naproxen sodium (Anaprox)	12-13	275, 550	550 mg initially, followed by 275 mg Q 6-8 hrs
Oxaprozin (Daypro)	20-30	600	1.2 g QD; low body weight or mild Sx 600 mg QD
PYRANOCARBOXYLIC ACID			
Etodolac (Lodine)	6-7	200, 300	200-400 mg Q 6-8 hrs; max 1200 mg/day
SALICYLATES			
Acetylsalicylic acid (ASA)	0.25	varies	325-650 mg Q 4-6 hrs; max 5200 mg/day
Diflunisal (Dolobid)	8-12	250, 500	500-1000 mg initially, followed by 250-500 mg q 8-12 hrs
Choline magnesium trisalicylate (Trilisate)	8-12	500, 750, 1000	500-1500 mg BID

11. The adult patient has a wide range of choices. In deciding which NSAID agent to prescribe consider the following:
    a. NSAIDS vary in their inflammatory and analgesic properties
       (1) For a strong anti-inflammatory effect use indomethacin (Indocin) which has a weak analgesic effect
       (2) Flurbiprofen (Ansaid), ibuprofen (Motrin), and etodolac (Lodine) are good analgesics
       (3) Ketoprofen (Orudis), naproxen (Naprosyn), and diclofenac (Voltaren) are well-balanced in their abilities to reduce inflammation and pain
    b. Drugs such as ibuprofen (Motrin), tolmetin sodium (Tolectin), and ketoprofen (Orudis), have short half-lives
       (1) May be safer and better for elderly patients
       (2) Beneficial for acute pain, particularly postoperative pain and pain from dental procedures
    c. Certain agents such as ketorolac (Toradol) are only indicated for acute to moderate short-term pain relief and should not be prescribed for chronic pain; injectable ketorolac (IM) has a longer duration, less drug abuse potential, less CNS side effects than morphine but similar potency of analgesia
    d. Consider drugs with long half lives such as oxaprozin (Daypro), nabumetone (Relafen), piroxicam (Feldene), and sulindac (Clinoril) in the following situations:
       (1) Patients who have trouble adhering to medication regimes
       (2) Patients who have conditions such as osteoarthritis and rheumatoid arthritis and need chronic medications
    e. For patients with gastritis and alcohol use, prescribe etodolac (Lodine) and possibly prophylaxis with misoprostol (Cytotec), omeprazole (Prilosec) or sucralfate (Carafate); avoid piroxicam (Feldene)
    f. Sulindac (Clinoril) or nonacetylated salicylate may be best with patients with renal disease and hypertension; ketorolac (Toradol) has profound detrimental effects on kidneys and is never used longer than 5 days and total dose should be no more than 40 mg by mouth
    g. Avoid using diclofenac sodium (Voltaren) with liver dysfunction; fenamates cause less hepatotoxicity
    h. Ketoprofen (Orudis) and diclofenac (Voltaren) may be safer with patients who have pulmonary problems (i.e., asthma)
    i. Mefenamic acid (Ponstel) is approved for primary dysmenorrhea

j. Consider type of dosing form
(1) Liquids: ibuprofen, indomethacin, naproxen
(2) Sustained release: diclofenac, indomethacin, ketoprofen, naproxen

H. Tramadol (Ultram), a central-acting analgesic, is sometimes used for treatment of mild-to-moderate pain; Particularly well suited when pain is not relieved by acetaminophen and the patient who cannot tolerate NSAIDS and wishes to defer opioid therapy

I. Step 2 should be initiated when the patient continues to have mild-to-moderate pain despite taking a nonopioid analgesia; the following should occur at this step:
1. Maximize the dose of the nonopioid analgesia -
2. And, add a step 2 opioid analgesia
3. Step 2 opioids are restricted for the treatment of moderate pain because of their dose-limiting side effects or because they are prepared with fixed combinations of nonopioid analgesics (see table that follows for classification of controlled drugs)
   a. Value of codeine (CIII) is limited because of increasing risk of side effects at doses above 1.5 mg per kg
   b. Hydrocodone (Lorcet, Lortab) (CIII) and oxycodone (Percocet) (CII) are limited because of their combinations with acetaminophen; for example, to not exceed 6 g of acetaminophen per day, patients cannot take more than 15 mg of these opioids

CONTROLLED DRUGS
CII: High potential for abuse which may lead to severe psychological or physical dependence. (Prescriptions must be written in ink or typewritten and signed by practitioner. Verbal prescriptions cannot be made.)
CIII: Use of these products may lead to moderate or low physical dependence or high psychological dependence. Prescriptions can be oral or written and may be redispensed.
CIV: These drugs have a low abuse potential, use may lead to limited physical or psychological dependence. Prescriptions may be oral or written and may be redispensed up to 5 times within 6 months.
CV: These drugs have a low abuse potential, may or may not require a prescription, and are subject to state and local regulation.

J. Step 3: If pain persists even when taking highest, safe dose of step 2 opioid, add a step 3 opioid to treat moderate to severe pain
1. Morphine is first line agent; Available in immediate release tablets, sustained release tablets (MS Contin) (CII), rectal suppository (Roxanol) (CII), liquid, injection, and intravenous
2. Other choices
   a. Oxycodone (Oxycontin) (CII)
   b. Hydromorphone (Dilaudid) (CII)
   c. Fentanyl (Duragesic) (CII) transdermal patches can control pain for 72 hours
3. Methadone (Dolophine) (CII) and levorphanol (Levo-Dromoran) are useful for severe pain, but because of long half-lives are not recommended for initial therapy

K. The following opioids are not recommended
1. Meperidine (Demerol) has a short half-life and its metabolite, normeperidine, is toxic
2. Propoxyphene (Darvon) has a long half-life and there is risk of accumulation of norpropoxyphene, a toxic metabolite,
3. Mixed narcotic agonist-antagonists such as pentazocine (Talwin) (CIV), butorphanol (Stadol) (CIV), and buprenorphine (Buprenex) (CIV) cause less constipation and biliary spasmodic activity but have the tendency to cause psychotomimetic responses

L. Adjuvant analgesics
1. Tricyclic antidepressants (TCAs) such as amitriptyline (Elavil) (most frequently used, but has most side effect) imipramine (Tofranil), desipramine (Norpramin), doxepin (Sinequan) are beneficial in certain circumstances:
   a. Have direct analgesic effects and may potentiate opiate analgesia
   b. Useful in treatment of pain due to nerve injury such as diabetic neuropathy

       c.   Starting dose for TCA in elderly is 10mg; in other adults 25 mg; upwardly titrate; effective dose is 75 mg but some patients require maximum of 150mg

2. Selective serotonin reuptake inhibitors (SSRIs) such as fluoxetine (Prozac) or sertraline (Zoloft) have fewer adverse effects than TCAs and may be beneficial

3. Caffeine may increase analgesic when given with other pain medications

4. Phenothiazines such as prochlorperazine (Compazine) 5-10 mg TID or QID or promethazine (Phenergan) 25 mg BID are useful as antiemetics when used in combination with other pain medications

5. Anticonvulsants are useful for management of brief lancinating pain in chronic neuralgia such as trigeminal neuralgia and postherpetic neuralgia; use one of following:

    a.   Carbamazepine (Tegretol) 400-800 mg/day in two divided doses (begin with 100 mg BID) for pain in trigeminal neuralgia

    b.   Gabapentin (Neurontin) 900-1800 mg/day in three divided doses (begin 300 mg HS for one day, then 300 mg BID for one, then 300 mg TID for one day and continue)

6. Mexiletine (Mexitil) 150-300 mg TID is beneficial for neuropathic pain

7. Corticosteroids are beneficial in patients with acute nerve compression, visceral distention, increased intracranial pressure and soft-tissue infiltration

8. Topical local anesthetics can help reduce pain of the affected dermatome; prescribe capsaicin cream 0.025% (Zostrix), particularly for osteoarthritis and diabetic neuropathy. Apply 3-4 times daily

M. Nonpharmacologic modalities to treat pain include meditation, relaxation, distraction, exercise, massage, acupuncture, surgery (cordotomy), neuroablative blocks (chemical destruction of nerves), and nervous system stimulaters such as dorsal column stimulaters (DCS) and transcutaneous electrical nerve simulators (TENS)

N. Interdisciplinary pain management

1. Specialists in the fields of anesthesia, neurology, physical therapy, internal medicine, nursing, psychology, and physical therapy can combine their efforts in chronic pain centers

2. Goals of interdisciplinary pain management are to ease suffering and reduce patient's reliance on opiates through nonpharmacological methods such as biofeedback, visual imagery, and stress management

O. Follow up is variable depending on source of pain

WEIGHT LOSS IN ADULTS (INVOLUNTARY)

I. Definition: Process that occurs when the number of calories available for utilization is below the patient's daily needs; the range of daily caloric intake for a moderately active adult is 2200-2800 calories for males and 1800-2100 calories for females who are not pregnant or lactating

II. Pathogenesis

A. Reduced food intake and/or anorexia can result in a calorie deficit from the following causes:

1. Psychological problems such as anorexia nervosa, depression, and anxiety

2. Physical and financial factors that limit purchasing, preparing, or eating food

    a.   Poor dentition

    b.   Immobility problems

    c.   Dysphagia

3. Drug-related problems such as digitalis excess or amphetamine abuse

4. Esophageal disease

5. Infections such as human immunodeficiency virus (HIV) infection, tuberculosis, fungal disease

6. Malignancy

7. Uremia

8.   Hepatitis
9.   Vitamin B deficiencies

B.   Calorie loss can occur because of malabsorption from the following conditions:
1.   Crohn's disease
2.   Pancreatic insufficiency
3.   Cholestasis
4.   Parasitic disease such as giardiasis
5.   Blind loop syndrome

C.   Calories can be lost in the urine or stool from the following illnesses:
1.   Uncontrolled diabetes mellitus
2.   Diarrhea

D.   Accelerated metabolism can contribute to weight loss in the following conditions:
1.   Hyperthyroidism
2.   Pheochromocytoma
3.   Fever
4.   Malignancy

III.   Clinical presentation of common causes of weight loss

A.   Anorexia nervosa and bulimia nervosa occur mainly in adolescent and young adult females who have a body image disturbance and an intense fear of becoming obese (see EATING DISORDERS section)

B.   Patients with HIV infection often have chronic anorexia, nausea, vomiting, and diarrhea due to drugs or to infections of the hepatobiliary system

C.   Malignancies, particularly of the gastrointestinal tract, pancreas, and liver are a common cause of weight loss and may be present without major signs and symptoms

D.   Uremia often presents initially with anorexia and subsequent weight loss

E.   Uncontrolled diabetes mellitus has weight loss and increased food intake

F.   Hyperthyroidism or thyrotoxicosis is the most common endocrine disease:
1.   Patients often have increased appetite, food intake, and motor activity
2.   In the elderly, "apathetic" hyperthyroidism may be present; weight loss and weakness may predominate with little evidence of the typical symptoms of thyroid hormone excess (SEE section on HYPERTHYROIDISM)

G.   In malabsorption syndrome, foul-smelling, bulky, greasy stools are typical

H.   Dramatic, rapid weight loss accompanied by aversion to food and later jaundice and abdominal pain characterizes pancreatic cancer

I.   In the elderly population, cancer, depression, drugs, neurologic disease (Alzheimer's Disease, stroke), and apathetic hyperthyroidism are common causes of weight loss

J.   Signs and symptoms of malnutrition may occur with any illness if there is a loss of 10 to 20% of normal body weight
1.   Typical complaints include fatigue, depressed immune function, increased susceptibility to infection, tendency for breakdown of skin, and changes in emotional stability such as irritability and apathy
2.   Laboratory tests: serum albumin <3.4g/dL and lymphocyte count <1,500

IV. Diagnosis/Evaluation

    A.   History
1. Carefully ascertain amount of weight loss; ask about change in clothing size if unable to elicit number of pounds lost
2. Validate amount of weight loss from a family member or significant other
3. Obtain a 24 hour daily food intake
4. Determine whether patient has loss of appetite, normal appetite, or increased appetite; unappealing thought, appearance and/or odor of food occurs with malignancy, drugs, depression
5. Ask about abnormal or bad taste in mouth (occurs in hepatitis, drugs, sinusitis, vitamin B deficiencies, zinc deficiency, psychological disorders)
6. If decreased food intake is suspected, explore symptoms of depression, poor dentition, dysphagia, alcohol and drug use, pain, nausea, vomiting, fatigue, and symptoms of heart failure
7. Question about chewing or swallowing difficulties (occurs in neurologic, dental, oral, esophageal or pulmonary diseases)
8. If anorexia nervosa is suspected ask about eating habits, self-image and attitudes about weight control
9. If malabsorption is suspected determine character of stools, signs of jaundice, easy bruising, sore tongue, and paresthesias
10. If calories lost in stool or urine is suspected, inquire about polyuria, polydipsia, nausea, and character of the stools
11. If accelerated metabolism is suspected inquire about fever, fatigue, melena, cough that has changed in character, and symptoms of hyperthyroidism such as tachycardia, nervousness, heat intolerance, menstrual disturbances, and palpitations
12. Obtain history of tobacco dependence
13. Question about alcohol and drug use
14. Inquire about previous history of hepatitis exposure, renal disease, endocrine problems
15. Determine family history, particularly noting any history of cancer in first-degree relatives

    B.   Physical Examination; assessment should focus on nutritional status as well as identification of the underlying cause of weight loss
1. Measure height and weight, comparing with previous measurements (see OBESITY section for determining optimal weights for adults)
    a. Unexplained losses of more than 5% of usual body weight over 6 months needs a systematic investigation
    b. Body weight measurement is not always a good indicator of weight loss; occasionally loss of body tissue is accompanied by equal gain in extracellular fluid such as ascites or edema; thus, it is important to observe face and limbs for loss of soft-tissue mass
2. Observe general appearance for wasting and signs of depression such as inappropriate dress and dull affect
3. Observe skin for pallor, ecchymosis, and jaundice
4. Examine mouth for poor dentition, glossitis, and lesions
5. Palpate neck for thyromegaly and lymphadenopathy
6. Perform a complete cardiovascular examination
7. Auscultate the lungs
8. Inspect abdomen for shape, scars, and masses
9. Auscultate abdomen for bowel sounds
10. Palpate and percuss abdomen for tenderness, ascites, masses, and organomegaly
11. Perform a rectal examination
12. Assess extremities for edema, muscle wasting, and skin turgor
13. Assess position and vibratory senses
14. Assess deep tendon reflexes; check for prolonged relaxation phase of reflexes that often occurs with thyroid disorders

C. Differential Diagnosis
    1. When weight loss occurs with increased food intake, consider diabetes, thyrotoxicosis, malabsorption, or possibly leukemia and lymphoma as the likely diagnosis
    2. When food intake is normal or decreased, consider psychological problems, malignancy, infection, renal disease, or endocrine problems as the likely diagnosis

D. Diagnostic Tests
    1. Diagnostic tests should be ordered based on the history and physical; an initial, recommended battery of tests includes three stool specimens for occult blood, CBC with differential, urinalysis, serum glucose, creatinine, albumin, and liver function tests and possibly chest x-ray and sedimentation rate
    2. Order thyroid stimulating hormone and T_4 in elderly patients because of the high incidence of thyroid disorders in this population; also order thyroid tests in patients who have not had reduced food intake with weight loss
    3. For patients with decreased intake consider ordering a serum calcium, potassium, and blood urea nitrogen
    4. If malnutrition is suspected, especially in the older patient, also order serum iron, transferrin, total iron-binding capacity, RBCs folate, B_{12}, and zinc levels
    5. For patients with impaired absorption, a quantitative stool fat examination by means of a 72-hour stool collection or a breath test is definitive test; but screening for malabsorption can be performed with Sudan stain of stool for fat and serum tests for carotenoids and folic acid
    6. Consider colonoscopy or flexible sigmoidoscopy, barium enema, upper endoscopy or upper gastrointestinal series with small bowel follow-through, abdominal ultrasonography, computerized tomography of the abdomen, or magnetic resonance imaging if concerns of abdominal malignancy exist
    7. Erythrocyte sedimentation rate, chest x-ray, and mammogram are recommended if concerns of other types of cancer exist
    8. Consider serum amylase and lipase if pancreatic disorder is suspected
    9. Stool for ova and parasites is ordered when giardia is suspected
    10. To assess nutritional status consider the following: serum albumin concentration, grip strength, triceps skin-fold thickness, arm muscle circumference, total lymphocyte count, serum transferrin and transthyretin (prealbumin) concentrations

V. Plan/Management

    A. Treat underlying cause of weight loss (i.e., treat depression with antidepressant medications or pancreatic insufficiency with oral pancreatic enzyme preparations)

    B. Patient with weight loss of more than 10-20% is often hospitalized and has extensive diagnostic evaluation; referral to specialist is needed

    C. Consultation with a dietician/nutritionist is beneficial

    D. Symptomatic therapy includes the following:
        1. Suggest patient eat small, frequent feedings (6 times per day) of foods with high-calorie density
        2. Encourage consumption of foods with high calorie density
        3. Suggest dietary supplements such as Ensure (see section on HIV INFECTION for other supplements)
        4. Consider ordering vitamin supplementation
        5. Recommend community resources such as Meals on Wheels/senior center lunch programs for elders
        6. For nausea, suggest salty foods, cool clear beverages, gelatin, popsickles; avoid sweet, greasy or high fat foods

E.   Follow Up
    1.   Scheduling of subsequent visits will depend on underlying cause of weight loss
    2.   If the cause of weight loss is not evident, weight loss is not severe, and patient is without psychological and physical abnormalities, schedule return visit in 2 to 4 weeks; encourage patient to keep daily record of food intake, activity level, and symptoms

REFERENCES

Agency for Health Care Policy and Research, Public Health Service, US Department of Health and Human Services (1993). Acute pain management in adults: Operative procedures. (AHCPR Pub. No. 92-0019). Rockville, MD: US Government Printing Office.

Amadio, P., Cummings, D.M., & Amadio, P. (1993). Nonsteroidal anti-inflammatory drugs: Tailoring therapy to achieve results and avoid toxicity. Postgraduate Medicine, 93, 73-96.

Baumann, T.J. (1993). Pain management. In J.T. DiPiro, R.L. Talbert, P.E. Hayes, G.C. Yee, Gary R. Matzke, & L.M. Posey (Eds.), Pharmacotherapy: A pathophysiologic approach (2nd ed.). Norwalk, CT: Appleton & Lange.

Davis, A.E. (1996). Primary care management of chronic musculoskeletal pain. Nurse Practitioner, 21(8), 72-82.

Dellasega, C., & Keiser, C.L. (1997). Pharmacologic approaches to chronic pain in the older adult. Nurse Practitioner, 22(5), 20-35.

Dowd, T.R., & Stewart, F.M. (1994). Primary care approach to lymphadenopathy. Nurse Practitioner, 19(12), 36-44.

Fletcher, R. H. (1997). Lymphadenopathy. In L. Dornbrand, A.J. Hoole, & R.H. Fletcher (Eds.), Manual of clinical problems in adult ambulatory care (3rd ed.). Philadelphia: Lippincott-Raven.

Foster, D.W. (1991). Gain and loss in weight. In J.D. Wilson, E. Braunwald, K.J. Isselbacher, R.G. Petersdorf, J.B. Martin, A.S. Fauci., & R.K. Root (Eds.). Harrison's principles of internal medicine (12th ed.). New York: McGraw-Hill.

Goroll, A.H., May, L.A., & Mulley, A.G. Jr. (1995). Evaluation of weight loss. In A.H Goroll, L.A. May & A.G. Mulley, Jr. (Eds.), Primary care medicine. Philadelphia: Lippincott.

Heizer, W.D. (1997). Weight loss. In L. Dornbrand, A.J. Hoole, & R.H. Fletcher (Eds.), Manual of clinical problems in adult ambulatory care. Philadelphia: Lippincott-Raven.

Levy, M.H. (1996). Pharmacologic treatment of cancer pain. New England Journal of Medicine, 335, 1124-1131.

Lipsky, M.S. (1996). Lymphadenopathy. In M.B. Mengel & L.P. Schwiebert (Eds.), Ambulatory medicine: The primary care of families (2nd ed.). Stamford, Conneticut: Appleton-Lange.

Mackowiak, P.A., Bartlett, J.G., Borden, E.C., Goldblum, S.E., Hasday, J.D., Munford, R.S., Nasraway, S.A., Stolley, P.d., & Woodward, T.E. (1997). Concepts of fever: Recent advances and lingering dogma. Clinical Infectious Disease, 25, 119-138.

Mauskop, A. (1998). Symptomatic care pending diagnosis: Pain. In R.E. Rakel (Ed.), Conn's current therapy 1998. Philadelphia: Saunders.

Polisson, R. (1996). Nonsteroidal anti-inflammatory drugs: practical and theoretical considerations in their selection. American Journal of Medicine, 100 (suppl 2A), 2A-31S-2A-36S.

Simon, H.B. (1995). Evaluation of fever. In A.H. Goroll, L.A. May & A.G. Mulley, Jr. (Eds.), Primary care medicine. Philadelphia: Lippincott.

Simon, H.B. (1995). Evaluation of lymphadenopathy. In A.H. Goroll, L.A. May & A.G. Mulley, Jr. (Eds.), Primary care medicine. Philadelphia: Lippincott.

Verdery, R.B. (1997). Clinical evaluation of failure to thrive in older people. Clinics in Geriatric Medicine, 13, 769-778.

WHO (1990). Cancer pain relief and palliative care: Report of WHO expert committee. WHO Technological Report Service, 804, 1-73.

Behavioral Problems

Alcohol Problems

Attention Deficit Hyperactivity Disorder

Eating Disorders

Obesity

Tobacco Use and Smoking Cessation

ALCOHOL PROBLEMS

I.   Definition: Problems caused by alcohol that may be acute or chronic, may range from mild to severe and vary in their response to treatment; problems exist on a continuum of increasing severity ranging from at-risk use to alcohol abuse to alcohol dependence

II. Pathogenesis

  A.   Causes of alcohol problems are incompletely understood

  B.   Male gender is associated with a higher prevalence; heavy drinking may be inversely associated with age, income, and educational level

III. Clinical Presentation

  A.   At-risk use is a pattern of alcohol consumption that places person at risk for adverse consequences (level of consumption exceeds **general norms** for moderate use). See CRITERIA FOR AT-RISK DRINKING and WHAT IS MODERATE USE? in the tables below

CRITERIA FOR AT-RISK DRINKING	
Men	> 14 drinks/ week or > 4 drinks/occasion
Women	> 7 drinks/week or > 3 drinks/occasion

Source: National Institute on Alcohol Abuse and Alcoholism (1995)

WHAT IS MODERATE USE OF ALCOHOL?	
Although there is some inconsistency in definitions, the definitions used by the National Institute on Alcohol Abuse and Alcoholism (1995) are as follows:	
Moderate Drinking	No more than 2 drinks a day for men and 1 drink a day for women No more than 1 drink a day for all persons over age 65
Exceptions	Persons in the following categories must abstain from alcohol use entirely: Pregnant women, those under 21, those who take medications that interact with alcohol or who have medical conditions such as liver disease

  B.   Alcohol abuse is the continued use of alcohol in spite of adverse consequences (UCR mnemonic--*U*se, followed by adverse *C*onsequences, followed by *R*epetition). Consequences may be physical, social, or psychological (see CRITERIA FOR ALCOHOL ABUSE table)

CRITERIA FOR ALCOHOL ABUSE	
Pattern of alcohol use in which 1 (or more) of the following 4 criteria are present within a 12-month period	
Recurrent alcohol use resulting in	✔ Failure to fulfill major role obligations (home, work, school) ✔ Placing self and others in potentially hazardous situations (DUI) ✔ Legal problems (e.g., arrest for DUI)
Continued alcohol use despite	✔ Persistent or recurrent social/interpersonal problems due to effects of alcohol

Adapted from the American Psychiatric Association. (1994). Diagnostic and statistical manual of mental disorders (4th ed.). Washington, DC: Author.

  C.   Alcohol dependence is a chronic disease characterized by impaired control over drinking, preoccupation with the drug alcohol, use of alcohol in spite of adverse consequences, and distortions in thinking, primarily denial (see CRITERIA FOR ALCOHOL DEPENDENCE table)

CRITERIA FOR ALCOHOL DEPENDENCE
Pattern of alcohol use in which 3 (or more) of the following 7 criteria are present within a 12 month period ✔ Physical tolerance (increased amounts are required for desired effect) ✔ Withdrawal symptoms when substance is discontinued ✔ Larger amounts of alcohol are used than intended ✔ Unsuccessful efforts to control use ✔ Much time and energy are spent in obtaining, using, and recovering from effects of alcohol ✔ Many social, work-related, and recreational activities are reduced because of alcohol use ✔ Continued use in spite of knowledge that alcohol causes physical and/or psychological problems

Adapted from the American Psychiatric Association. (1994). Diagnostic and statistical manual of mental disorders (4th ed.). Washington, DC: Author.

D. Alcohol use in US is associated with numerous health and social problems, 100,000 annual deaths and an economic cost of $100 billion

E. Motor vehicle accidents resulting from driving under the influence of alcohol are the leading cause of death in the 15-24 year old age group

F. Over 60% of all adults consume alcohol, and an estimated 10% of the adult population abuses alcohol

G. Alcohol abuse is more prevalent in men than in women; 10% of the drinking population consumes 50% of all alcohol

H. About 5-10% of the elderly population are heavy alcohol users

I. Alcohol problems among the elderly go largely unrecognized in that psychosocial factors (spouse, job, and legal pressures, e.g., DUI) are not likely to be present as the elder frequently lives alone, is retired, and no longer drives

IV. Diagnosis/Evaluation

    A. History
        1. Keep in mind that the history (including interview and use of questionnaires) is by far more sensitive and specific than are physical exam and laboratory findings
        2. All patients should be screened for alcohol problems. **Ask "Do you ever drink alcohol?"**
        3. If patient **ever** drinks, ask quantity-frequency questions which deal with level of consumption, which can help distinguish moderate from at-risk drinking and identify binge drinking (see LEVEL OF CONSUMPTION and GENERAL EQUIVALENCIES OF ALCOHOLIC BEVERAGES tables)

LEVEL OF CONSUMPTION	
Frequency	How many days in a week do you usually have something to drink?
Quantity	On days that you drink, how many drinks do you have?
Maximum	What is the most you had to drink on any one day during the past month?
Last drink	When was your last drink? (Persons with a problem know exactly)
Scoring and Interpretation	If quantity x frequency >7 drinks a week for women and >14 drinks for men, or if maximum per occasion is >3 for women and >4 for men, then patient exceeds criteria for low-risk drinking

Adapted from Bower, K.T., & Severin, J.D. (1997). Alcohol and other drug-related problems. In D.J. Knesper, M.B. Riba, & T.L. Schwenk (Eds.), Primary care psychiatry. Philadelphia: Saunders.

GENERAL EQUIVALENCIES OF ALCOHOLIC BEVERAGES*		
Hard liquor (80 proof spirits)		
1 shot or highball ((1.5 ounces)	=	1 drink
1/2 pint of liquor	=	~5 drinks
1 pint of liquor	=	~10 drinks
Wine (11% to 12% alcohol)		
1 glass of wine (5 ounces)	=	1 drink
1 bottle of wine (750 mL)	=	5 drinks
Beer (4% to 5% alcohol)		
1 12-ounce bottle or can	=	1 drink
1 40-ounce container	=	~3 drinks
1 6-pack of beer	=	6 drinks
Wine Coolers (5% alcohol)		
1 wine cooler (12 ounces)	=	1 drink

* One drink contains approximately 12 g of alcohol

4. Follow quantity-frequency questions with the CAGE questions. See THE CAGE QUESTIONNAIRE table

THE CAGE QUESTIONNAIRE	
C	Have you ever felt you ought to **C**ut down on your drinking?
A	Have people **A**nnoyed you by criticizing your drinking?
G	Have you ever felt bad or **G**uilty about your drinking?
E	Have you ever had a drink the first thing in the morning (**E**ye opener) to steady your nerves or get rid of a hangover?
Scoring and Interpretation	Person receives one point for each positive answer. One "yes" answer indicates hazardous drinking and two or more "yes" answers indicates alcohol abuse or dependence

Source: Bush, B., Shaw, S., Cleary, P., Delbanco, T.L., & Aronson, M.D. (1987). Screening for alcohol abuse using the CAGE questionnaire. American Journal of Medicine, 82, 231-235.

5. If patient answers "yes" to a CAGE question, prompt for more details
6. Patients who become angry and defensive with the CAGE questions have already responded positively to the second item in the questionnaire ("Have people Annoyed you by criticizing your drinking?")
7. If screening using quantity-frequency questions and CAGE questions indicates problems with alcohol, ask more specific questions based on criteria for alcohol abuse and criteria for alcohol dependence
8. Finally, carefully screen for use of other substances (high concomitant use of tobacco and other drugs by persons with alcohol problems)
9. Alternatives to the CAGE questionnaire are listed in SCREENING TESTS FOR ALCOHOL PROBLEMS table

SCREENING TESTS FOR ALCOHOL PROBLEMS		
Test	**Description**	**Source**
AUDIT (Alcohol Use Disorders Identification Test)	Excellent and simple 10-question, self-administered questionnaire that assesses both levels of consumption and related problems	Saunders, J.B., Aasland, O.G., Babor, T.F., & Unreal, N. (1993). Development of the Alcohol Use Disorders Identification Test (AUDIT): WHO collaborative project on early detection of persons with harmful alcohol consumption. Addiction: 88, 791-804
MAST (Michigan Alcoholism Screening Test)	Contains 24 items and there are several versions and scoring protocols available, including the simpler 13-item Short MAST	Hedlund, J.L., & Vieweg, B.W. (1984). The Michigan Alcoholism Screening Test (MAST): A comprehensive review. J. Operational Psychiatry: 15, 55-65
MAST-G (MAST-Geriatric Version)	Also contains 24 items and is for use in older adults ≥55. Unlike the regular MAST, questions about fights, arrests, and work difficulties have been eliminated	Blow, F.C., Brower, K.J., Schulenberg, J.E., Demo-Dananberg, L.A., Young, J.P., & Beresford, T.P. (1992). The Michigan Alcoholism Screening Test--Geriatric Version (MAST-G): A new elderly-specific screening instrument. Alcohol Clin Exp Res: 16, 372. Available from the University of Michigan Alcohol Research Center, 400 E. Eisenhower Pkwy, Suite 2A, Ann Arbor, MI 48108. Telephone: 313/998-7952
TACE	Contains 4 items and is based on the CAGE; for use with pregnant women	Russel, M., Martier, S.S., & Sokol, R.J., et al. (1994). Screening for pregnancy risk-drinking. Alcohol Clin Exp Res: 18, 1156-1161
TWEAK	Contains 5 items and is also for use with pregnant women	Ibid.

Adapted from Bower, K.T., & Severin, J.D. (1997). Alcohol and other drug-related problems. In D.J. Knesper, M.B. Riba, & T.L. Schwenk (Eds.), Primary care psychiatry. Philadelphia: Saunders.

B. Physical Examination
1. Note that an absence of findings on physical exam does not indicate that the patient is free of alcohol problems (Most early manifestations of alcohol abuse/dependence are psychosocial, not physical)
2. Assess general appearance: weight loss, emaciated appearance are late findings in chronic alcoholism
3. Examine skin for signs of chronic alcoholism (abnormal vascularization of the facial skin [spider angiomas] and jaundice when liver disease is present)
4. Perform abdominal exam for hepatomegaly and right upper quadrant tenderness
5. Male patients should be evaluated for gynecomastia, loss of axillary and pubic hair, and testicular atrophy
6. Perform complete neurologic exam, including mental status exam, cranial nerves, gait, sensory, motor, reflexes, Romberg test
7. During exam, note if patient smells of alcohol as alcohol on breath during primary care visit indicates that there is impaired control over drinking

C. Differential Diagnosis: Other mental disorders such as mood and anxiety disorders, psychosis, delirium, dementia; abuse of other psychoactive substances such as opiods, marijuana, hallucinogens, PCP, inhalants, and sedatives

D. Diagnostic Tests
1. CBC (elevated mean corpuscular volume is a marker of excessive alcohol consumption; may be elevated due to other causes such as dietary deficiencies--B_{12}, folate--liver disease, smoking)
2. Liver enzyme tests
   a. Gamma-glutamyl transpeptidase (GGT) is the most sensitive blood test for screening for detection of long-term heavy drinking; test lacks specificity as other causes of elevated GGT are such things as use of anticonvulsants, barbiturates, and from nonalcoholic liver disease

b. Aspartate aminotransferase (AST) and alanine aminotransferase (ALT) have a low sensitivity for detecting alcohol problems; if elevations are suspected to be due to liver problems, advise abstinence and monitor over time to see if they decline. The enzymes are also released by muscle tissue and can be elevated by such events as intensive weight training; AST:ALT ratio can be helpful with a ratio of 2:1 suggestive of alcohol-induced liver disease

3. Carbohydrate-deficient transferrin can detect heavy drinking and may be useful for monitoring alcohol-dependent patients

V. Plan/Management

A. Plan is determined by the **identification** and **confirmation** that the patient has problems with alcohol and by his/her **willingness to change** behavior

B. **Identification** of problem-drinking is determined primarily from screening using the CAGE and the Level of Consumption questions; the physical examination and the laboratory testing may provide additional evidence that a problem exists

C. **Confirming** the problem is based on the extent to which the patient meets the criteria for at-risk drinking, or for alcohol abuse or dependence and involves two important diagnostic issues
1. What happens when the patient uses alcohol? (adverse consequences), and
2. What happens when the patient tries to stop? (impaired control, tolerance and withdrawal)

D. Diagnostic Issues
1. **First diagnostic issue**. Assess problem areas first (adverse consequences) then link them to substance use. (Example: How are things going at home? At work? In your social life? and so on. As problems are introduced by the patient, be empathic, but ask patient "How do you think your use of alcohol fits in with this?")
2. **Second diagnostic issue**. Determine degree of **impaired control** by asking questions such as "Do you drink more than you intend to?" "Why do you think that happens?" "Do you ever make rules for your drinking?" "Are you able to follow those rules?" Assess **tolerance**. "Do you need more to get the same effect?" Ask about **withdrawal**. "Do you ever feel bad or sick when you try to stop drinking?"

E. **Motivation** for change on the patient's part is crucial to the success of any treatment plan. Appropriate questions to assess motivation are the following: "Are you concerned about your use of alcohol?" "Are you interested in changing?"; success of any intervention is dependent on the patient's willingness to participate in treatment goals

F. **Brief interventions have been demonstrated through research to be highly effective**
1. Can be conducted in the office for the following groups of patients: At-risk and problem drinkers who are not alcohol-dependent
2. Use the *FRAMES* acronym to guide the intervention

FRAMES FOR BRIEF INTERVENTIONS	
Feedback	related to screening tests, history, physical examination and laboratory findings should be provided as well as the implications of the findings (e.g., your liver enzyme GGT is increased to 128. The normal range for this enzyme is zero to 30 [show patient the lab report])
Responsibility	for changing alcohol use should be placed on the patient; success of treatment is up to patient
Advise	patient to cut down or abstain
Menu	of options should be presented to the patient in order to make the patient a partner in the decision-making process: Can attempt to stop on own; can attend AA meetings; can use self-help books
Empathic	approach is helpful
Self-efficacy	of the patient is encouraged by clinician's optimism relating to behavior change. Advise the patient to make a change--stop drinking altogether or if controlled drinking is an option in your opinion, to limit drinking to no more than 2 drinks a day

Adapted from Miller, W.R., & Rollnick, S. (1991). <u>Motivational interviewing: Preparing people to change addictive behavior</u>. New York: Guilford Press.

G. For all patients with alcohol problems regardless of their pattern (at-risk to dependent), abstinence for a minimum of two weeks is recommended at the beginning of the treatment regimen
    1. Initial period of abstinence allows provider/patient to assess impact of alcohol on patient's overall health and functioning
    2. Attainment of a two week period of abstinence appears to be related to patients reaching their ultimate goal, whether complete sobriety or controlled drinking
    3. More intensive treatments are indicated for patients with alcohol dependence

H. Refer patient and family to self-help groups such as Alcoholics Anonymous (AA) for patients, Al-Anon for families. These groups are extremely effective in maintaining sobriety and helping patients and families to cope. Refer family even if patient declines to attend
    1. Alcoholics Anonymous, PO Box 459, Grand Central Station, New York, NY 10163, 212/686-1100
    2. Al-Anon Family Group Headquarters, Inc., 1600 Corporate Landing Parkway, Virginia Beach, VA 23454-5616, 1-800-356-9996

I. Familiarize yourself with AA in your community by attending an open meeting
    1. With patient's permission, ask for an AA volunteer who is willing to act as sponsor to meet with patient in your office
    2. Sponsor should be same gender as patient

J. Recommend self-help books for both patients and family members (see table below)

SELF-HELP BOOKS FOR ALCOHOL PROBLEMS	
For the patient (author of book is a woman, so particularly useful for women patients)	Knapp, C. (1991). Drinking: A love story. New York: Doubleday Delacorte Press
For the patient (emphasis is on lifestyle as well as behavioral change)	Washington, A., & Boundy, D. (1990). Willpower is not enough: Understanding and recovering from addictions of every kind. New York: Harper-Perennial
For the school-aged child (8-12) whose father has an alcohol problem	Black, C. (1982). My dad loves me: My dad has a disease. Denver: Mac Publishing
For parents of a patient with alcohol problems (written by former US Senator George McGovern)	McGovern, G. (1996). Terry: My daughter's life and death struggle with alcoholism. New York: Villard
For adult children of alcoholics and their risk issues	Black, C. (1981). It will never happen to me: Children of alcoholics as youngsters-adolescents-adults. New York: Ballantine

K. Some patients may benefit from treatment initiated in an inpatient or residential setting; criteria for treatment in this setting include presence of severe coexisting medical/psychiatric conditions, risk of harm to self or others, failure to respond to less intensive therapy

L. Be familiar with at least one specialized treatment facility in your area
    1. Feedback from patients will help you learn which programs in your area are most effective
    2. Referral for family therapy may be indicated when complex problems are present

M. Pharmacologic adjuncts: Medications must be viewed as an adjunct to the process of recovery which is very time-consuming and difficult
    1. Disulfiram (Antabuse), 125-500 mg/day (available in 250 and 500 mg tabs)
    This medication may be used in patients who are motivated and who are involved with other modalities related to recovery. Must not be used until blood alcohol level is zero which is usually reached 24 hours after patient's last drink
        a. As with all medications, consult PDR regarding dosing and contraindications
        b. Liver function should be monitored at baseline, in 2-4 weeks, and then monthly for two months
        c. Counsel about avoidance of alcohol including OTCs with alcohol content while drug is being taken; must abstain from alcohol for 14 days after stopping disulfiram therapy
        d. Potentially severe interactions with alcohol limit its widespread use

2. Naltrexone (ReVia), 50 mg/day (available in 50 mg scored tabs). Believed to blunt the pleasurable effects of alcohol
   a. Indicated as adjunctive therapy for patients enrolled in residential alcohol treatment programs **only**
   b. Drug is not used on an out-patient basis and is contraindicated in patients with hepatitis or liver failure

N. Follow up is variable depending on type of treatment
   1. Patients for whom brief intervention is conducted: Follow up for two or more visits to monitor the patient's progress and assess need for additional approaches
   2. Patients who have been referred to alcohol treatment (either self-help groups or residential) should be followed for ongoing support; the natural course of alcohol problems includes remission as well as relapse

ATTENTION DEFICIT HYPERACTIVITY DISORDER

I. Definition: Descriptive category for cluster of symptoms that include inattention, impulsivity, and motor hyperactivity that are more frequent and severe than seen in persons of the same developmental level; this disorder is usually first diagnosed in childhood but can persist into adulthood

II. Pathogenesis: Causes are unknown but probably represent the interaction of a number of factors

   A. Persistence into adulthood suggests a biological basis

   B. Association between a mutant thyroid receptor beta gene (producing condition called resistance to thyroid hormone, RTH), suggests an endocrine relationship [70% of children and 42% of adults with RTH have ADHD]

   C. Clinical efficacy of anti-ADHD medications suggests that there is a neurochemical imbalance (dopamine is underactive)

   D. Defects in the frontal lobes have also been suggested

   E. Prenatal, natal, and perinatal factors have also been implicated as possible causative factors

III. Clinical Presentation

   A. Prevalence of ADHD in adulthood is unknown because of lack of epidemiologic studies in this age group; however, prevalence in adults has been estimated to range between 1% and 6%

   B. ADHD was once believed to largely resolve in childhood/adolescence but evidence now exists that the condition often persists into adulthood. **Important**: Not an acquired disorder of adulthood

   C. The gender distribution of ADHD is about even in adulthood which represents a dramatic shift from the childhood distribution of a male-to-female ratio of 10:1
   1. Discrepancy may be due to tendency of women to rate themselves much higher for presence of ADHD-assocated problems such as decreased concentration, restlessness, loss of self-control, anger, and lack of confidence
   2. May also be due to the fact that women tend to be more willing than men to seek help for psychological problems

   D. Many adults do not exhibit the full triad of inattention, impulsivity, and hyperactivity; either inattention or hyperactivity/impulsivity may predominate or patient may exhibit a combined type with all three behavioral characteristics present

E. Patients with inattention and distractibility seem unable to modulate their attention, often missing important information, overlooking details, and making mistakes in their social and family life and in the work-place; generally unable to complete started projects
   1. Inattention is a defining feature in both adult and childhood ADHD
   2. The social and occupational consequences of inattention in adults are especially disabling as the individual (via inattention to the somewhat ambiguous nature of interpersonal conduct) fails to acquire the subtle but fundamental social skills that allow for appropriate and productive interpersonal behavior
   3. On the other hand, adults with ADHD are often able to concentrate well on activities at which they excel and from which they derive pleasure; the inattention is thus selective
   4. ADHD adults have difficulty planning, prioritizing, and executing activities leading family, friends, and co-workers to judge them as unreliable and inconsiderate
   5. Impaired functioning often leads to failure in both family life and occupational pursuits leading to feelings of guilt, shame, and adoption of self-defeating behaviors which further compromise functioning

F. Impulsivity is expressed by low tolerance for passive waiting (in lines, in traffic), by inability to wait turn in conversations (interrupting or finishing another's sentences)
   1. Impulsivity is the symptom most likely to persist into adulthood
   2. This characteristic can leave the patient feeling immature, helpless, and guilty about impulse actions

G. **Hyperactivity is no longer a required diagnostic criterion for ADHD at any age**, and this is the most likely symptom to remit with age so that this characteristic is **often absent** in ADHD adults
   1. Motor hyperactivity is often more subtle in adults and the examiner must be very observant in order to detect this sign
   2. Signs of excess kinesis that suggest the patient is struggling against impulses to move are frequent shifts in position, frequent scratching, and exaggerated gesticulations

H. Diagnostic criteria for ADHD according to the American Psychiatric Associaton (1994) are contained in the following table
   1. Age-neutral wording for the criteria have been adopted in recognition of the potential lifelong persistence of ADHD
   2. There are no criteria specifically designed for adults; thus the criteria remain essentially unchanged from previous editions of the Diagnostic and Statistical Manual of Mental Disorders. Note there are **two** dimensions, inattention and hyperactivity/impulsivity, with behaviors specific to each dimension
   3. From these two dimensions, three subtypes are derived
      a. Predominantly inattentive type (criteria are met on inattention dimension, but **not** on the hyperactivity/impulsivity dimension)
      b. Predominantly hyperactive/impulsive type (criteria are met on hyperactive/ impulsive dimension but **not** on the inattention dimension)
      c. Combined type (criteria are met for both dimensions)

ADHD DIAGNOSTIC CRITERIA TABLE

Either 1 or 2

1. Six or more symptoms of inattention have persisted for at least a 6 month period to the degree that is maladaptive and inconsistent with developmental level:

Inattention-- The person **often**	➡ Fails to pay close attention to details resulting in careless mistakes
	➡ Has difficulty sustaining attention in activities (whether play or other tasks)
	➡ Does not seem to listen when being spoken to
	➡ Does not follow through on instructions and fails to complete schoolwork, chores, or duties in the workplace (not due to oppositional behavior or inability to understand directions)
	➡ Has difficulty with organization
	➡ Avoids, dislikes, or is reluctant to undertake activities that require sustained mental effort (such as schoolwork or homework)
	➡ Loses items necessary for tasks or activities
	➡ Becomes easily distracted by extraneous stimuli. Is forgetful in daily activities

(continued)

2. Six or more symptoms of hyperactivity-impulsivity have persisted for at least a 6 month period to a degree that is maladaptive and inconsistent with developmental level:

Hyperactivity-- The person **often**	➡ Fidgets with hands or feet or squirms in seat ➡ Leaves seat in situations where remaining in seat is expected ➡ Runs or climbs excessively in situations in which it is inappropriate to do so (in adolescents or adults, this may be limited to subjective feelings of restlessness) ➡ Has difficulty engaging in quiet play or leisure activities ➡ Is "on the go" or seems driven by a motor ➡ Talks excessively
Impulsivity-- The person **often**	➡ Blurts out answers before question has been asked ➡ Has difficulty waiting turn ➡ Interrupts or intrudes on others (butts into conversations or games)
In addition, the following must be true	➡ Some hyperactive-impulsive or inattentive behaviors were present **before** age 7 years ➡ Some impairment from the symptoms is present in two or more settings (home, school or work) ➡ Clear evidence of clinically significant impairment in social, academic, or work-related functioning must exist ➡ Symptoms may not better be accounted for by another mental disorder (e.g., mood, anxiety, personality, psychoses)

Adapted from American Psychiatric Association. (1994). <u>Diagnostic and statistical manual of mental disorders</u> (4th ed.) Washington, DC: Author

IV.   Diagnosis/Evaluation

    A.   History

        1.   Focus of history taking is to determine whether patient meets the diagnostic criteria for ADHD as outlined above. (**Note:** In adults, ADHD symptoms should not be the sole focus of the history as other psychiatric and behavioral disorders may result in similar clinical presentations)

        2.   History must come from multiple sources including spouse/significant other, parents, adult children (old report cards can be helpful in documenting problems during childhood)

        3.   Confirm that impairments were present in childhood (retrospective confirmation is required for the diagnosis)

        4.   Determine if symptoms persistent since childhood; symptoms do not wax and wane, nor are they episodic. **Important:** Patients who report long periods in which they were symptom-free are unlikely to have ADHD

        5.   Establish that the impairments in function are global (impacting all areas of his/her life-- family, social, work/school--rather than selective)

        6.   Use questionnaires developed for adults such as Wender Utah Rating Scale and Brown Attention-Activation Disorder Scale (see ADHD RATING SCALES table) [Consider referral of adults in whom ADHD is suspected to experts for diagnosis as this is a highly specialized area]

        7.   Determine if significant anxiety, depression, or substance abuse is present (see sections on ANXIETYDISORDERS, DEPRESSION, and ALCOHOL PROBLEMS)

        8.   Obtain social history, development history, family history, past and present medical history including psychiatric history, history of head trauma, seizure disorder, thyroid disease, and **current medications**

ADHD RATING SCALES FOR ADULTS

Wender Utah Rating Scale

Source: Ward, M.F., Wender, P.H., & Reimherr, F.W. (1993). The Wender Utah rating scale: An aid in the retrospective diagnosis of childhood attention deficit hyperactivity disorder. <u>American Journal of Psychiatry</u>, 150, 885-890.

Brown Attention-Activation Disorder Scale

Source: Brown, T.E. (1992). The Brown attention-activation disorder scale (BAADS). New Haven, CN: Yale U Press.

B. Physical Examination
  1. Complete neurologic exam including mental status exam [see ALZHEIMER'S DISEASE for an overview of the Mini-Mental State Examination (MMSE)], gait, muscular strength and tone, deep tendon reflexes, sensory responses
  2. Measure vision and hearing to rule out sensory impairment
  3. Results of the PE are usually negative

C. Differential Diagnosis
  1. Anxiety (suspect if symptoms present in only one setting, e.g., home, but not at work or school)
  2. Substance abuse (suspect if patient exhibits symptoms uncharacteristic of previous behavior)
  3. Depression (See DEPRESSION section)
  4. Sensory impairment
  5. **Note:** Most experts believe that adult ADHD is overdiagnosed and that anxiety, depression, or alcohol abuse are frequently the problem

D. Diagnostic Tests
  1. CBC with differential and thyroid panel
  2. No single neuropsychological test is diagnostic of ADHD; rating scales such as the ones listed in ADHD RATING SCALES FOR ADULTS table on the previous page can provide important data
  3. Use of rating scales for depression (Beck Depression Inventory) and anxiety (Beck Anxiety Inventory) can help in detection or exclusion of these disorders

> For information about obtaining these scales, complete with scoring instructions, write to The Psychological Corporation, 555 Academic Court, San Antonio, TX 78204-2498 or telephone at 210/ 299-1061.

V. Plan/Management

A. Adult patients who present with a pattern of symptoms consistent with ADHD should be referred to an expert for further evaluation and management
  1. There is an extremely high incidence of coexisting psychiatric disorders in patients with ADHD requiring expertise in diagnosis often beyond that of most primary care providers
  2. Further, the best approach to management of these patients is often unclear and is always very time consuming

B. Management that is typically provided by specialist to whom patient is referred is summarized in the following table

MANAGEMENT OF ADULTS WITH ADHD
Management for all patients usually involves nonpharmacologic therapies including group psychotherapy, educational programs, and cognitive-behavioral therapy Pharmacologic therapy is also an important treatment option for most patients ✦ Research studies relating to use of medications in the adult with ADHD are lacking; thus the mental health specialist must rely on his/her own experience in treatment and knowledge of this particular patient to guide therapeutic decisions ✦ The risk/benefit ratios of treatment with pharmacologic therapy should be discussed with the patient so that there is a full understanding of the side effects as well as the potential benefits (continued)

Medications Commonly Used to Treat ADHD in Adults

Drug	Dosage	Comments
Stimulants Methylphenidate HCL (Ritalin) [Supplied as 5, 10, 20 mg tabs]	10-60 mg/day in 2-3 divided doses, preferably 30-45 minutes before meals	Consult PDR for contraindications, precautions, and drug interactions which are numerous Adverse reactions include abuse potential, insomnia, anorexia, hypertension, arrythmias, Tourette's syndrome, seizures and blood dyscrasias
Dextroamphetamine sulfate (Dexedrine) [Supplied as 5 mg tabs]	5-40 mg/day in divided doses (Avoid late day dosing)	Consult PDR for contraindications, precautions, and drug interactions which are numerous Adverse reactions include **high** abuse potential, hypertension, tachycardia, CNS overstimulation, dry mouth, GI disorders, urticaria
Antidepressants Bupropion (Wellbutrin) [supplied as 75, 100 mg tabs]	Consult PDR for dosing recommendations	Considered a second-line drug Consult PDR for contraindications, precautions, and drug interactions Adverse reaction include agitation, CNS stimulation, seizures, dry mouth, insomnia, headache, GI disorders
TCAs: Desipramine (Norpramin), Imipramine (Tofranil), Nortriptyline (Pamelor) [see PDR for how specific drug is supplied]	Consult PDR for dosing recommendations for each drug	These medications typically produce more significant improvement in behavior than in cognition, relieving symptoms of anxiety, depression, and tics Onset of action is more rapid than in depression with some patients responding for relatively low doses Must obtain baseline and follow-up ECGs due to quinidine-like effects of drugs Consult PDR for contraindications, precautions, and drug interactions Adverse reactions include anticholinergic effects, CNS overstimulation, arrythmias, hypo and hypertension, and lethality in overdose

C.   Recommend resources for patients from the following table

RESOURCES FOR PATIENTS WITH ADHD

<u>Organizations</u>:	Children and Adults with Attention Deficit Disorders (CHADD), National Headquarters, Suite 185, 1859 North Pine Island Road, Plantation, FL 33322, 1/800-233-4050 Attention Deficit Disorder Association, 4300 West Park Blvd., Plano, TX 75093 National Institute of Mental Health/IRIB, 5600 Fishers Lane, Room 7C-02, Rockville, MD 20857
<u>Books</u>:	Driven to Distraction: Recognizing and Coping with Attention Deficit Disorder from Childhood Through Adulthood by E. Hallowell & J. Ratey. Published by Pantheon Books, New York, 1994 Especially good reference for diagnosis and treatment of ADHD in adults

D.   Follow Up

    1.   Keep in mind that evaluation and management of adult patients suspected of having ADHD is a very time-consuming process. Therefore, these patients are best managed in a specialized treatment center if one is available

    2.   Follow-up schedule is variable depending on whether patient is being managed in a specialty treatment center or in a primary care setting

    3.   For all patients on medications, very frequent monitoring for efficacy and for adverse events is essential

EATING DISORDERS

I.   Definition: Symptomatic disturbances of eating behavior unique to the developed world with anorexia nervosa (AN) and bulimia nervosa (BN) being the two major types

II.   Pathogenesis

  A.   Eating disorders are best understood using a multidimensional model that encompasses biologic vulnerability, family issues, and societal pressure

  B.   Eating behavior is a complex integration of a person's attitude toward food and internal physiology resulting in individual concepts of hunger and satiety

  C.   Persons with AN tend to have perfectionistic, rigid, inflexible and conforming personalities

  D.   Impact of family functioning on persons with AN and BN is difficult to determine, but family dynamics can influence both the development and the persistence of the disorder

  E.   A thin, unrealistic body size is idealized in today's society and concepts of beauty are highly related to body size in the media

III. Clinical Presentation

  A.   Disordered eating represents a spectrum of behavior that is unique to the developed world and is overwhelmingly a disease of young women

  B.   Female-to-male ratio of eating disorders is approximately 10:1; of the two disorders, males are much more likely to have BN and overexercise is quite common

  C.   Because of the infrequency of this diagnosis in males, diagnosis and treatment may be more difficult

  D.   Using strict diagnostic criteria, the prevalence in the young female population, the group most often affected, is approximately 1% for AN and about 3% for bulimia

  E.   Using less stringent criteria, a much higher percentage of young women regularly engage in disordered eating including rigid dieting, binging, and purging, all behaviors that place them at risk for a number of sequelae

  F.   Increasing prevalence over the past few decades, particularly for BN due to both increased diagnosing and because of increased emphasis on thinness in the US

  G.   Diagnostic criteria for AN according to DSM-IV (1994) are contained in the following table

---

DIAGNOSTIC CRITERIA FOR ANOREXIA NERVOSA

➡ Refusal to maintain weight at or above a minimally normal weight for age and height (body weight is less than 85% of expected)

➡ Intense fear of weight gain even though underweight

➡ Amenorrhea (in postmenarcheal females)

➡ Severe body-image disturbance in which weight has undue influence on feelings of self-worth; denial that current low body weight is problematic

➡ Types of Anorexia Nervosa:

  ✱ Restricting Type: During current episode of AN, person has not regularly engaged in binge eating or purging behavior

  ✱ Binge-Eating/Purging Type: During current episode of AN, person has regularly engaged in binge eating or purging behavior

---

Adapted from American Psychiatric Association. (1994). Diagnostic and statistical manual of mental disorders (4th ed.) Washington, DC: Author

H. Diagnostic criteria for BN according to DSM-IV (1994) are contained in the following table

DIAGNOSTIC CRITERIA FOR BULIMIA NERVOSA

➡ Recurrent episodes of binge eating which includes **both** of the following

  ✳ Eating, in a discrete time period, an amount of food substantially larger than most people would consume in the same time period

  ✳ A sense of lack of control over eating during episode

➡ Recurrent inappropriate compensatory behavior to prevent weight gain such as laxative, diuretic, enema use, induced vomiting, fasting, excessive exercise

➡ The above two behaviors occur, on average, at least 2 times/week for 3 months

➡ Feelings of self-worth unduly influenced by weight

➡ Disturbance does not occur exclusively during episodes of AN

➡ Types of Bulimia Nervosa:

  ✳ Purging Type: During the current episode of BN, person has engaged in self-induced vomiting, laxative, diuretic, or enema use on a regular basis

  ✳ Nonpurging Type: During the current episode of BN, person has used compensatory behaviors such as fasting or excessive exercise, but has not regularly engaged in self-induced vomiting, laxative, diuretic, or enema use

Adapted from American Psychiatric Association. (1994). Diagnostic and statistical manual of mental disorders (4th ed.) Washington, DC: Author

IV. Diagnosis/Evaluation

  A. History
    1. Obtain weight history including highest and lowest weights as adult (or adolescent), methods of losing weight, and how patient defines "ideal" weight
    2. Through appropriate questioning, establish the presence or absence of criteria for eating disorders (see DIAGNOSTIC CRITERIA FOR ANOREXIA AND BULIMIA NERVOSA in the preceding tables)
    3. If possible, obtain additional information from family/friends as patient may lack the capacity to accurately describe own behavior
    4. Inquire about other behaviors that can support the presence of an eating disorder such as preference for eating alone, severely limited food preferences, unusual eating habits (ritualistic patterns)
    5. Obtain a careful diet history, with a focus on overall caloric intake and intake of specific nutrients such as calcium
    6. In women, obtain a complete menstrual history
    7. Question about exercise patterns (overexercise believed to be especially prevalent in males with eating disorders)
    8. Ask what medications have been used or are currently being used to induce weight loss

  B. Physical Examination
    1. Measure weight with the patient undressed and gowned; measure height and calculate BMI (See OBESITY section for calculation of BMI)
    2. Measure blood pressure (resting and orthostatic hypotension are common) [see SYNCOPE section for DETERMINING ORTHOSTATIC HYPOTENSION table for details on assessment]
    3. Perform complete physical examination observing for the stigmata of vomiting which includes parotid enlargement, soft palate lesions, dental erosions, calluses of the knuckles
    4. Neurologic exam should include mental status, cranial nerves, motor and sensory systems, and cerebellar system

  C. Differential Diagnosis
    1. Numerous **medical conditions** can mimic presentation of eating disorders; however, persons with medical conditions that cause loss of appetite, weight loss, unexplained vomiting **lack the attitudinal features** of a primary eating disorder (obsession with thinness and body image distortion)

a. Inflammatory bowel diseases (stool is often positive for blood, and erythrocyte sedimentation rate is increased in IBD, and usually subnormal in eating disorders)

b. Thyroid disease (physical findings of hyperthyroidism are usually present and laboratory findings confirm the diagnosis)

c. Diabetes mellitus (laboratory findings confirm the diagnosis)

d. Central nervous system lesions and occult malignancies anywhere in the body (appropriate imaging studies)

e. Chronic infections such as tuberculosis and acquired immunodeficiency

2. Psychiatric disorders can also present with decreased appetite and weight loss

a. Mood disorders

b. Obsessive-compulsive disorder

c. Substance abuse

d. Psychotic disorders

D. Diagnostic Tests

1. Initial laboratory evaluation should include CBC, serum electrolytes, calcium, magnesium, and phosphorous levels; electrocardiogram

2. Patients with atypical presentations should have laboratory evaluation based on history and physical in order to rule out other diagnoses

3. Serum amylase levels are elevated during active vomiting and return to normal within 72 hours after vomiting ceases (may be helpful in documenting presence of bulimia)

V. Plan/Treatment

A. Goals of treatment including restoring and maintaining normal weight, and management of physiologic and psychologic abnormalities; treatment at a speciality center is ideal

B. In-patient versus out-patient management depends on the severity of the condition as well as availability of local resources and insurance status of the patient

1. Patients with hemodynamic instability, significant hypovolemia, arrhythmias, congestive heart failure, cardiomyopathy must be hospitalized

2. Failure of appropriate out-patient treatment is also a criterion for hospitalization

C. Most out-patient treatment for patients with eating disorders is managed by a decentralized team, with patients seeing a variety of providers (including a psychotherapist and nutritionist) who communicate with each other about the progress of the patient

D. Cognitive behavioral treatment is the treatment of choice for eating disorders

1. Objective of cognitive techniques is to change faulty thought processes such as all-or-none thinking, judgmental thinking, and catastrophizing

2. Objectives of behavioral techniques are to break patterns of disordered eating through the use of food monitoring, thought monitoring, meal regularity, and nutritional monitoring

3. Family therapy is often an important component of treatment

E. Role of the primary care provider is to monitor the medical aspects of the condition (weekly weigh-ins and periodic laboratory testing [CBC, serum electrolytes, and serum amylase levels]); and to coordinate the efforts of the other professionals involved in care

F. Refer patients to the following resources

❖ The National Eating Disorders Organization, 6655 South Yale Avenue, Tulsa, OK 74136; 918/481-4044; http://www.laureate.com

❖ The American Anorexia/Bulimia Association, 293 Central Park West, Suite 1R, New York, NY 10024; 212/501-8351; http://members.aol.com/amanbu

❖ National Association of Anorexia Nervosa and Associated Disorders, Box 7, Highland Park, IL 60035; 847/831-3438

G. Follow Up: Management of eating disorders requires concerted efforts over a long time period

1. In early stages of treatment, visits must be frequent in order to form therapeutic relationship and to provide close supervision of health status

2.   As patient becomes more stable, less frequent visits are appropriate; however, relapse is common

3.   Imperative that close communication between all professionals involved in care is maintained

OBESITY

I.   Definition: Excessive accumulation of body fat

II. Pathogenesis

A.   The simplistic view that obesity is caused when energy intake exceeds expenditure fails to take into account other factors such as chronic stress which can affect metabolism through increasing cortisol secretion

B.   Multiple factors interact and contribute to development of obesity: a genetic predisposition combines with environmental factors to produce the disorder

C.   In adults, a body mass index (BMI) between 18.5 and 24.9 (for all ages of both genders) is considered a healthy weight

D.   Persons with a BMI ≥25 are classified as overweight, and those with a BMI ≥30 are classified as obese

E.   Regional distribution of fat also plays a role in determining the risk of a given level of obesity
1.   Abdominal *apple-shaped* obesity is more common in men and associated with an increased risk of metabolic and cardiovascular complications
2.   Excess weight in the hips and thighs, described as *pear-shaped* obesity is more common in women and poses less risk of complications than *apple-shaped* obesity
3.   Men with waist measurements of >40 inches and women with waists >35 inches face an increased risk for health problems

III. Clinical Presentation

A.   Approximately one third of adult Americans are estimated to be overweight (about 58 million people)

B.   Prevalence of overweight has increased greatly over past 15 years in both genders of all ages and ethnic groups

C.   Prevalence rates are disproportionately high among black and Hispanic women as well as among Asian and Pacific Islanders, Native Americans, Alaska natives, and Native Hawaiians

D.   Risk for various cardiovascular and other diseases begins to rise at a BMI of 25 and risk of death increases as BMI reaches and surpasses 30

IV. Diagnosis/Evaluation

A.   History
1.   Determine weight milestones, including weight at birth, during early and late childhood, upon graduation from high school, college, and at marriage
2.   Obtain diet history, including usual number of meals per day; type and number of snacks
3.   Obtain psychosocial history, to detect emotional stresses at home or work/school which may be aggravating problem
4.   Ask about amount and type of physical activity engaged in each week

5. Motivation for weight loss and types and results of past dieting
6. Obtain past medical history for cardiovascular disease, diabetes mellitus, thyroid disease, hypertension, gout, emotional problems, orthopedic problems and dermatitis
7. Question about current medications

B. Physical Examination
1. Measure blood pressure taking care to use the correct size cuff
2. To determine degree of obesity, calculate body mass index as follows:
    a. Obtain patient's weight in kilograms and height in meters
    b. Divide weight by square of height ($W \div H^2$)
    c. For quick calculation for selected heights and weights, consult BMI table (KNOW YOUR BMI) on page 62
    d. As an alternative, plot the patient's height and weight on the chart HEALTHY WEIGHT OR OVERWEIGHT? to determine degree of obesity (moderate or severe overweight)
    e. To estimate fat distribution using the waist-to-hip ratio:
        (1) Measure person's waist at navel; measure hips at greatest circumference.
        (2) Divide waist measurement by hip measurement to get ratio. ($W \div H$)
        (3) See HEALTH RISK FOR MEN and HEALTH RISK FOR WOMEN in tables on page 63
3. Examination of the severely obese patient may be difficult (auscultation of the lungs and heart is compromised as is exam of the abdomen)
4. Skin over the neck may be hyperpigmented, thicker, and have a velvet appearance (acanthosis nigricans)
5. In women, observe for intertriginous dermatitis under breasts and abdominal panniculus
6. In men, examination of the genitalia may require that the prepubic fat tissue be lifted upward in order to visualize the penis which may be hidden by surrounding fat

C. Differential Diagnosis
1. Most obesity is the result of overeating
2. Major endocrine disorders that may manifest with obesity are the following:
    a. Pituitary and adrenal dysfunction
    b. Thyroid disease
    c. Polycystic ovarian disease
    d. Hypothalamic disease

Know Your BMI (Body Mass Index)

Weight (lb)	Height (ft, in)																
	4'10"	4'11"	5'0"	5'1"	5'2"	5'3"	5'4"	5'5"	5'6"	5'7"	5'8"	5'9"	5'10"	5'11"	6'0"	6'1"	6'2"
125	26	25	24	24	23	22	22	21	20	20	19	18	18	17	17	17	16
130	27	26	25	25	24	23	22	22	21	20	20	19	19	18	18	17	17
135	28	27	26	26	25	24	23	23	22	21	21	20	19	19	18	18	17
140	29	28	27	27	26	25	24	23	23	22	21	21	20	20	19	19	18
145	30	29	28	27	27	26	25	24	23	23	22	21	21	20	20	19	19
150	31	30	29	28	27	27	26	25	24	24	23	22	22	21	20	20	19
155	32	31	30	29	28	28	27	26	25	24	24	23	22	22	21	20	20
160	34	32	31	30	29	28	28	27	26	25	24	24	23	22	22	21	21
165	35	33	32	31	30	29	28	28	27	26	25	24	24	23	22	22	21
170	36	34	33	32	31	30	29	28	28	27	26	25	24	24	23	22	22
175	37	35	34	33	32	31	30	29	28	27	27	26	25	24	24	23	23
180	38	36	35	34	33	32	31	30	29	28	27	27	26	25	25	24	23
185	39	37	36	35	34	33	32	31	30	29	28	27	27	26	25	24	24
190	40	38	37	36	35	34	33	32	31	30	29	28	27	27	26	25	24
195	41	39	38	37	36	35	34	33	32	31	30	29	28	27	27	26	25
200	42	40	39	38	37	36	34	33	32	31	30	30	29	28	27	26	26
205	43	41	40	39	38	36	35	34	33	32	31	30	29	29	28	27	26
210	44	43	41	40	38	37	36	35	34	33	32	31	30	29	29	28	27
215	45	44	42	41	39	38	37	36	35	34	33	32	31	30	29	28	28
220	46	45	43	42	40	39	38	37	36	35	34	33	32	31	30	29	28
225	47	46	44	43	41	40	39	38	36	35	34	33	32	31	31	30	29
230	48	47	45	44	42	41	40	38	37	36	35	34	33	32	31	30	30

BMI: **What it means to your health (adults aged 20-65 years)**

BMI	What it means to your health
18.5-24.9	Good weight for most people
≥25	Risk for cardiovascular and other diseases increases
≥30	Risk of death increases

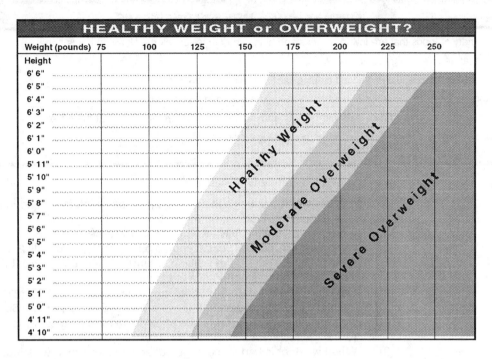

Figure 3.1. Healthy Weight Range for Adults.

Source: US Department of Agriculture, Department of Health and Human Services. (1995). <u>Nutrition and your health: Dietary guidelines for Americans</u>. Washington, DC: Author, p. 20.

HEALTH RISK FOR MEN				
Low Risk (Pears)		Moderate Risk		High Risk (Apples)
<.80	.85	.90	.95	1.00+
		Waist-to-hip ratio		

HEALTH RISK FOR WOMEN				
Low Risk (Pears)		Moderate Risk		High Risk (Apples)
<.70	.75	.80	.85	.90+
		Waist-to-hip ratio		

    D.   Diagnostic Tests: None are indicated unless history and physical examination suggest that obesity is secondary to a medical condition such as the ones listed under DIFFERENTIAL DIAGNOSIS in IV.C.

V.   Plan/Management

    A.   Overweight is a chronic condition which can only be controlled with long-term changes

    B.   All weight management programs should include the three components of dietary control, physical exercise, and psychosocial and eating behavior modification
        1.   Dietary control. Advise patient to decrease calorie intake by following the guidelines in the DIETARY GUIDELINES FOR AMERICANS in the following table

DIETARY GUIDELINES FOR AMERICANS

* Eat a variety of foods that are low in calories and high in nutrients--check the Nutrition Facts Label

* Eat less fat and fewer high-fat foods

* Eat smaller portions and limit second helpings of foods high in fat and calories

* Eat more vegetables and fruits without fats and sugars added in preparation or at the table

* Eat pasta, rice, breads, and cereals without fats and sugars added in preparation or at the table

* Eat less sugars and fewer sweets (like candy, cookies, cakes, soda)

* Drink less or no alcohol

2. Physical exercise
   a. Most desirable type of exercise is aerobic, progressive-intensity, endurance-type exercise (e.g., walking, jogging, swimming)
   b. Walking programs should follow these general guidelines
     (1) Over a 6-week period, patient should be encouraged to walk 2 miles at speeds faster than leisure walking, interrupted as needed with brief spurts of slower walking until endurance is attained
     (2) Objective is to exercise at 70% of maximum heart rate [0.7 x (220 - age)] for a minimum of 30 minutes four times a week. Example: For a 50 year old woman, the target heart rate she should aim for during exercise is 119 (0.7 x 170 [subtract 50 from 220] = 119)
     (3) When weather is bad, encourage patients to move their walk indoors-- shopping malls are a popular alternative, and many have walking clubs. For the nearest club, write the
        National Organization of Mall Walkers
        Post Office Box 191
        Hermann, MO 65041.
     (4) For patients who want to design their own walking program, tell them to send a self-addressed stamped envelop to
        Walking Test
        The Rockport Walking Institute
        220 Donald Lynch Boulevard
        Post Office Box 480
        Marlboro, MA 01752
3. Psychosocial and behavioral management
   a. Emphasize that all family members, fat and thin, will benefit from healthy foods and exercise
   b. Environmental cues may contribute to overeating; therefore, alterations of the environment may be helpful
   c. Examples include eating only at the table with dishes and silverware, use of small dishes, pacing self, eating slowly, not eating in front of the TV or reading while eating
   d. Self-help groups may be helpful. See COMMON WEIGHT REDUCTION PROGRAMS

COMMON WEIGHT REDUCTION PROGRAMS

Program	Telephone Number	Brief Description
TOPS (Take Off Pounds Sensibly)	800/932-8677	Diet plan based on food exchanges; all food can be purchased at grocery store. Weekly support group.
Overeaters Anonymous	515/891-2664	No special diet. Follows 12 step program patterned after Alcoholics Anonymous. Self-help group as needed.
Weight Watchers	516/939-0400	Patients choose from various calorie levels based on desired rate of loss. Many *Weight Watcher* brand products in grocery stores. Weekly support group meetings.

4. Pharmacologic management of obesity
    a. Sibutramine (Meridia), a neurotransmitter reuptake inhibitor that enhances the body's ability to regulate appetite, has been approved for the management of obesity in adults for weight loss and the maintenance of weight loss
    b. Must be used in conjunction with a reduced-calorie diet
    c. Recommended for use in adults with a BMI ≥30
    d. Dosing is 10 mg daily without regard to meals; available in 5, 10, 15 mg caps
    e. Regular monitoring of blood pressure is **absolutely** essential for all persons taking the drug; consult PDR for information regarding indications, contraindications, drug interactions, and adverse events
    f. Resources on nutrition and weight management are in the table below

RESOURCES ON NUTRITION AND WEIGHT MANAGEMENT
EatRight Lose Weight: Seven Simple Steps. Available from Oxmoor House, Inc., 800/884-3935
University of Alabama at Birmingham EatRight Nutrition Information Service Hot Line, 800/231-DIET for answers to nutrition questions

C. Optimally, all patients should be referred to a nutritionist for counseling

D. Follow Up: Plan a regular schedule of follow up to monitor and reinforce progress

TOBACCO USE AND SMOKING CESSATION

I. Definition: Destructive health behavior involving use of tobacco (cigarettes, chewing tobacco, and snuff)

II. Pathogenesis

    A. Tobacco smoke contains numerous substances which are toxic, mutagenic, or carcinogenic

    B. In addition to harmful volatile substances such as carbon monoxide, the particulate phase of cigarette smoke contains nicotine and tars

    C. The consequences of a product of combustion (smoke) being drawn into close contact with delicate pulmonary tissues are devastating

    D. The etiology of tobacco dependence is multidimensional with physiological, psychological, and social/behavioral factors
        1. Physiological factors include activation of the mesolimbic dopaminergic system ("reward circuit") and locus ceruleus (vigilance and arousal)
        2. Psychological factors evolve from positive feedback provided by pleasurable sensations
        3. Social/behavioral factors include the following: smoking becomes a habit or an automatic and intrinsic part of daily activities, and smoking can be used as a self-medication to reduce unpleasant sensations that occur with tobacco withdrawal or stress

III. Clinical Presentation

    A. Tobacco use is the most important cause of premature mortality, accounting for one out of every five deaths in the US
        1. Approximately 80-85% of lung cancer deaths are due to smoking (risk of lung cancer is 40% less after 5 years of smoking cessation)
        2. Majority (80-90%) of deaths from chronic obstructive lung disease are attributable to smoking
        3. About 30-40% of deaths from coronary heart disease are due to cigarettes (after 2-3 years of smoking cessation, this risk is almost back to baseline)

4. There is increased risk of stroke mortality for smokers
5. Other related conditions include peripheral arterial occlusive disease, head and neck cancer, esophageal cancer, pancreatic cancer, bladder cancer, periodontal disease, bronchitis, pneumonia, otitis media with effusion, and premature aging of the skin

B. Smoking affects heath of nonsmokers
1. Children exposed to environmental tobacco have increased risk of premature births, low birth weights, growth disorders, sudden infant death syndrome, and upper respiratory tract infections
2. Each year about 3,000 nonsmoking adults die of lung cancer as a result of breathing second-hand smoke

C. Physiological tolerance develops gradually with an increase of a few cigarettes a day initially to several packs a day in several years

D. Withdrawal from nicotine includes symptoms of anxiety, irritability, craving, hunger, restlessness, decreased concentration, drowsiness, sleep disturbances, tremors, sweating, dizziness, headaches, and gastrointestinal disturbances such as constipation

E. Smokeless tobacco is regularly used by 3% of adults and about 20% of male high school seniors

IV. Diagnosis/Evaluation

A. History
1. Inquire about smoking pattern such as number of years of smoking, how much tobacco is used, and depth of inhalation
2. Ask how long after awakening the first cigarette is smoked
3. Ask about past attempts at quitting including length of cigarette cessation, problems encountered, and reasons for relapse
4. Explore smoke-related symptoms such as cough, sputum production, shortness of breath, recurrent respiratory infections
5. Review family history and past medical history of tobacco-related diseases such as coronary heart disease, chronic obstructive pulmonary disease, and cancer

B. Physical Examination: Use the examination as an intervention, highlighting the damage that smoking can do to each body system which is assessed
1. Monitor vital signs, particularly blood pressure which adds an additional risk of heart disease if elevated
2. Examine ears, nose, sinuses, mouth, and pharynx, noting signs of inflammation due to irritation from tobacco
3. Perform complete exam of lungs
4. Perform complete exam of heart and peripheral vascular system

C. Diagnostic Tests
1. Consider spirometry
   a. If normal, stress the benefits of smoking cessation before damage occurs
   b. If abnormal, stress the importance of cessation before further damage occurs
2. Consider blood cholesterol levels to determine additional risk factors for heart disease

D. Differential Diagnosis: Tobacco use is a behavioral problem without a differential diagnosis

V. Plan/Management

A. Advise all smokers to stop
1. **Be clear**. In a straightforward manner tell the patient to stop smoking now
2. **Speak strongly**. Emphasize that quitting smoking is the single most important thing that patient can do for future health
3. **Personalize advice**: Point out reasons that smoking cessation will improve the personal health as well as the health of loved ones exposed to second-hand smoke. See GOOD REASONS FOR YOUR PATIENT TO QUIT SMOKING in the table that follows

GOOD REASONS FOR YOUR PATIENTS TO QUIT SMOKING	
Teenagers	Bad breath, stained teeth, cost, potential decrease in athletic prowess, frequent respiratory infections
Pregnant Women	Increased rate of spontaneous abortion, fetal death, low birth weight
Parents	Increased respiratory infections among children of smokers, poor role model for children
New Smokers	Easier to stop now
Asymptomatic Adults	Twice the risk of heart disease, six times the risk of emphysema, 10 times the risk of lung cancer, 5-8 year shorter life span, wrinkles
Symptomatic Adults	Upper respiratory infection, gum disease, dyspnea, ulcers, angina, claudication, osteoporosis, esophagitis, may not live long enough to enjoy retirement and grandchildren

Adapted from Glynn T, & Manley M. (1991). How to help your patients stop smoking: A national cancer institute manual for physicians. Bethesda, MD: National Institutes of Health.

4. If patient unwilling to quit, **record plans** to manage the smoking status in the progress notes and list tobacco use in the problem list. For children who reside in households with smokers, **always** list "Exposure to passive smoke" in the problem list in child's chart. See following table, SOURCE FOR MATERIALS FOR SMOKING CESSATION INTERVENTIONS to obtain chart markers, stamps, labels, and educational/motivational materials

SOURCE FOR MATERIALS FOR SMOKING CESSATION INTERVENTIONS	
American Academy of Family Physicians Ask for "AAFP Stop Smoking Kit" 1-800-274-2237	National Cancer Institute Ask for "Quit for Good Kit" and the manual for providers entitled, "How to Help Your Patients Stop Smoking"
American Cancer Society Ask for "Tobacco-Free Young America: A Kit for the Busy Practitioner" 1-800-ACS-2345	1-800-4-CANCER

B. Refer the patient for intensive smoking cessation programs
1. Intensive programs are strongly correlated with success
2. Intensive programs should consist of 4-7 sessions, each at least 20-30 minutes in length, lasting at least 2 weeks
3. Counseling should offer problem solving and skills training as well as social support

C. For patients who are unable/unwilling to enroll in an intensive program, assist patient with a quit plan (see ASSISTING THE PATIENT WITH A QUIT PLAN in table below)

ASSISTING THE PATIENT WITH A QUIT PLAN
Advise the smoker to:
➡ Set a quit date, ideally within 2 weeks ➡ Inform friends, family, and coworkers of plans to quit, and ask for support ➡ Remove cigarettes from home, car, and workplace and avoid smoking in these places ➡ Review previous quit attempts--what helped, what led to relapse ➡ Anticipate challenges, particularly during the critical first few weeks, including nicotine withdrawal
Give advice on successful quitting:
➡ Total abstinence is essential--not even a single puff ➡ Drinking alcohol is strongly associated with relapse ➡ Having other smokers in the household hinders successful quitting
Encourage use of nicotine replacement therapy:
➡ Both the nicotine patch and nicotine gum are effective pharmacotherapies for smoking cessation ➡ The nicotine patch may be easier to use than the gum in most clinical settings
Make culturally and educationally appropriate materials on cessation techniques readily available in your office

Source: Fiore, M.C., Bailey, W.C., Cohen, S.J., et al. (1996). Smoking cessation: Information for specialists. Clinical Practice Guideline. Quick Reference Guide for Smoking Cessation Specialists, No. 18. Rockville, MD: USDHHS, Public Health Service, Agency for Health Care Policy and Research and Centers for Disease Control and Prevention.

D. Success is also enhanced by clinician-provided social support which communicates caring and concern by being open to the patient's fears and difficulties

E. Clinician counseling even as brief as 3 minutes is effective; however, the more intense the treatment, the more effective it is in producing long-term abstinence

F. Pharmacologic support for smoking cessation
    1. Every smoker should be offered nicotine replacement therapy (patch or gum) except when medically contraindicated (see SUGGESTIONS FOR THE CLINICAL USE OF THE NICOTINE PATCH/GUM in the tables that follow)
        a. Use of nicotine replacement therapy with light smokers (10-15 cigarettes/day or less) has not been studied
        b. If used with light smokers, or smokers weighing less than 100 pounds, a lower starting dose should be considered
    2. Nicotine nasal spray (Nicotrol NS) is also available and appears to be safe and effective for highly nicotine-dependent smokers (smoke > 20 cigarettes/day, smoke immediately upon awakening and report history of severe nicotine withdrawal symptoms)
        a. Aqueous nasal spray containing 0.5 mg/spray
        b. Usually 1-2 doses/hr with a maximum of 5 sprays/hr, 40 doses/day
        c. May discontinue abruptly or tapered
        d. Use for maximum of 3 months
        e. Supplied as 1 bottle containing 10 mL (200 sprays) with metered spray pump
    3. Bupropion (Zyban) is a recent pharmacologic option for smoking cessation and is the only drug for this indication that is not nicotine based
        a. Mechanism of action is unclear, but believed to affect noradrenergic and dopaminergic mechanisms in the brain which have been implicated as pathways of nicotine addiction
        b. Available as a sustained-release tablet; dosage is 150 mg QD for 3 days and then BID (at least 8 hours between doses) for 7 to 12 weeks
        c. Patient should be advised to stop smoking during the 2nd week of therapy
        d. May be used with transdermal nicotine (**Patient must quit smoking when using transdermal nicotine**)

SUGGESTIONS FOR THE CLINICAL USE OF THE NICOTINE PATCH	
Patient Selection	Appropriate as a primary pharmacotherapy for smoking cessation Behavioral/educational support is recommended with this therapy
Precautions	***Pregnancy.*** Pregnant smokers should first be encouraged to attempt cessation without pharmacologic treatment. The nicotine patch should be used during pregnancy only if the benefits outweigh the risks. Similar factors should be considered in lactating women ***Cardiovascular Diseases.*** Nicotine patch should be used only after consideration of risks and benefits among particular cardiovascular patient groups: Those who are within 4 weeks of being post MI, who have arrhythmias, or who have worsening angina pectoris ***Skin Reactions.*** Up to 50% of patients using the nicotine patch have a local skin reaction. Less than 5% have a serious enough reaction to discontinue use
Dosage	Treatment of 8 weeks or less has been shown to be as efficacious as longer treatment periods. The following treatment schedules are suggested as reasonable for most smokers **Brand** — **Duration** — **Dosage** Nicoderm CQ (OTC), Habitrol — 4 weeks — 21 mg/24 hrs then 2 weeks — 14 mg/24 hrs then 2 weeks — 7 mg/24 hrs Prostep — 4 weeks — 22 mg/24 hrs then 4 weeks — 11 mg/24 hrs Nicotrol (OTC) — 6 weeks — 15 mg/16 hrs
Prescribing Instructions	**No smoking** while on the patch. *Location.* At the start of each day, the patient should place a new patch on a relatively hairless location between the neck and the waist *Activities.* No restrictions while using the patch *Time.* Patches should be applied as soon as patients waken on their quit day

Brand	Duration	Dosage
Nicoderm CQ (OTC), Habitrol	4 weeks	21 mg/24 hrs
	then 2 weeks	14 mg/24 hrs
	then 2 weeks	7 mg/24 hrs
Prostep	4 weeks	22 mg/24 hrs
	then 4 weeks	11 mg/24 hrs
Nicotrol (OTC)	6 weeks	15 mg/16 hrs

Adapted from Fiore, M.C., Bailey, W.C., Cohen, S.J., et al. (1996). Smoking cessation: Information for specialists. Clinical Practice Guideline. Quick Reference Guide for Smoking Cessation Specialists, No. 18. Rockville, MD: USDHHS, Public Health Service, Agency for Health Care Policy and Research and Centers for Disease Control and Prevention.

SUGGESTIONS FOR THE CLINICAL USE OF NICOTINE GUM	
Patient Selection	Appropriate as a primary pharmacotherapy for smoking cessation. Behavioral/educational support is recommended with this therapy
Precautions	***Pregnancy.*** Pregnant smokers should first be encouraged to attempt cessation without pharmacologic treatment. Nicotine gum should be used during pregnancy only if the benefits outweigh the risks. Similar factors should be considered in lactating women ***Cardiovascular Diseases.*** Nicotine gum should be used only after consideration of risks and benefits among particular cardiovascular patient groups: Those who are within 4 weeks of being post MI, who have arrhythmias, or who have worsening angina pectoris ***Side Effects.*** Common side effects of nicotine chewing gum include mouth soreness, hiccups, dyspepsia and jaw ache. These effects can often be alleviated by correcting chewing technique

Dosage	Nicotine gum (Nicorette) is available in 2-mg and 4-mg (per piece) doses and is OTC
	Patients should be advised to use the 2-mg gum except in special circumstances
	    2-mg strength limit: 30 pieces per day
	    4-mg strength limit: 20 pieces per day

Prescribing Instructions	**No smoking** while on the gum *Chewing Technique.* Gum should be chewed slowly until a "peppery" taste emerges, then "parked" between the cheek and gum to facilitate nicotine absorption. Gum should be intermittently "chewed and parked" for about 30 minutes *Absorption.* Acidic beverages (e.g., coffee, juices, soft drinks) interfere with the buccal absorption of nicotine, so eating and drinking anything except water should be avoided for 15 minutes before and during chewing *Scheduling of Dose.* Instructions to chew the gum on a fixed schedule (at least one piece every one to two hours) for one to three months may be more beneficial than ad lib use *Duration of Therapy.* Should be tailored to fit the needs of each patient. Generally prescribed for several months (1-3)

Adapted from Fiore, M.C., Bailey, W.C., Cohen, S.J., et al. (1996). Smoking cessation: Information for specialists. Clinical Practice Guideline. Quick Reference Guide for Smoking Cessation Specialists, No. 18. Rockville, MD: USDHHS, Public Health Service, Agency for Health Care Policy and Research and Centers for Disease Control and Prevention.

G. Follow Up
    1. Schedule followup contact either in person or by telephone
    2. Timing
        a. First followup contact within 2 weeks of quit date, preferably during first week
        b. Second contact within the first month
        c. Further followup contacts as needed
    3. Actions during followup visits
        a. Congratulate success
        b. If a relapse occurred, obtain recommitment to abstinence
        c. Remind patient that lapse can be used as learning experience
        d. Identify problems encountered and anticipate challenges in the immediate future
    4. Preventing relapse
        a. Congratulate, encourage, and stress importance of abstinence at every opportunity
        b. Review benefits derived from cessation
        c. Inquire about problems encountered and offer possible solutions
        d. Anticipate problems or threats to maintaining abstinence

REFERENCES

American Psychiatric Association. (1994). Diagnostic and statistical manual of mental disorders (4th ed.). Washington, DC: Author.

Aronne, L.J. (1998). Obesity. Medical Clinics of North America, 82, 161-182.

Barnes, H.N., & Samet, J.H. (1997). Brief interventions with substance-abusing patients. Medical Clinics of North America, 81, 867-880.

Brower, K.J., & Severin, J.D. (1997). Alcohol and other drug-related problems. In D.J. Knesper, N.B. Riba, & T.L. Schwenk (Eds.), Primary care psychiatry. Philadelphia: Saunders.

Brownwell, K.D. (1998). Obesity management: A comprehensive plan. American Journal of Managed Care, 4(3), 126-132.

Bush, B., Shaw, S., Cleary, P.,Delbanco, T.L., & Aronson, M.D. (1987). Screening for alcohol abuse using the CAGE questionnaire. American Journal of Medicine, 82, 231-235.

Bussey, B.F., & Morgan, S.L. (1997). Obesity: Is there effective treatment now? Consultant, 2945-2957.

Carek, P.J., Sherer, J.T., & Carson, D.S. (1997). Management of obesity: Medical treatment options. American Family Physician, 55, 551-558.

Feifel, D. (1996). Attention-deficit hyperactivity disorder in adults. Postgraduate Medicine, 100, 207-216.

Fiore, M.C., Bailey, W.C., & Cohen, S.J., et al. (1996). Smoking cessation: Information for specialists. Clinical Practice Guideline. Quick Reference Guide for Smoking Cessation Specialists. Rockville, MD: USDHHS, Public health Service, Agency for Health Care Policy and Research and Centers for Disease Control and Prevention.

Glynn, T.J., & Manley, M.W. (1991). How to help your patients stop smoking: A National Cancer Institute manual for physicians. Bethesda, MD: NIH Publication No. 92-3064.

Khouzam, H.R. (1997, August). Attention deficit hyperactivity disorder in adults: Guidelines for evaluation and treatment. Consultant, 2159-2165.

Larson, D. (1997). Smoking cessation: Counseling your patients. Clinician Reviews, 7, 57-80.

Miller, W.R., & Rollnick, S. (1991). Motivational interviewing: Preparing people to change addictive behavior. New York: Guilford Press.

National Institute on Alcohol Abuse and Alcoholism. (1995). The physicians' guide to helping patients with alcohol problems (NIH Publication No. 95-3769). Washington, DC: US Government Printing Office.

Nemethy, M. (1997). Attention deficit/hyperactivity disorder. Advance for Nurse Practitioners, 22-29.

O'Connor, P.G., & Schottenfeld, R.S. (1998). Patients with alcohol problems. New England Journal of Medicine, 338, 592-602.

Reid, M.C., & Anderson, P.A. (1997). Geriatric substance use disorders. Medical Clinics of North American, 81, 999-1016.

Rexrode, K.M., Hennekens, C.H., Willett, W.C., Colditz, G.A., et al. (1997). A prospective study of body mass index, weight change, and risk of stroke in women. JAMA, 277, 1539-1545.

Rosen, D.S., & Demitrack, M.A. (1997). Eating disorders and disordered eating. In D.J. Knesper, N.B. Riba, & T.L. Schwenk (Eds.), Primary care psychiatry. Philadelphia: Saunders

Rosenbaum, M., Leibel, R.L., & Hirsch, J. (1997). Obesity. New England Journal of Medicine, 337, 396-405.

Schteingart, D.E., Edwards, G.J., & Starkman, M.N. (1997). Obesity. In D.J. Knesper, N.B. Riba, & T.L. Schwenk (Eds.), Primary care psychiatry. Philadelphia: Saunders

Smith, T.A, House, R.F., Croghan, I.T., Gauvin, T.R. (1996). Nicotine patch therapy in adolescent smokers. Pediatrics, 98, 659-667.

Smith, M., Pomerlau, O.F., & Wadland, W. (1997). Nicotine and smoking. In D.J. Knesper, N.B. Riba, & T.L. Schwenk (Eds.), Primary care psychiatry. Philadelphia: Saunders.

Taylor, M.E. (1997). Evaluation and management of attention-deficit hyperactivity disorder. American Family Physician, 55, 887-901.

Tan, G., & Schneider, S.C. (1997). Attention-deficit hyperactivity disorder: Pharmacotherapy and beyond. Postgraduate Medicine, 101, 201-210.

US Department of Health & Human Services. (1995). Nutrition and your health: Dietary guidelines for Americans. Washington, DC: Author.

Wiseman, C.V., Harris, W.A., & Halmi, K.A. (1998). Eating disorders. Medical Clinics of North America, 82, 145-160.

Mental Health

ANXIETY DISORDERS

I.   Definition: Symptoms of physiological arousal (e.g., palpitations, sweating) accompanied by a psychological mood of excessive worry that interferes with normal functioning and persists over time

II.   Pathogenesis

    A.   Several hypotheses have been formulated regarding pathophysiological processes involved in anxiety with the same systems appearing to be invoked in "normal" and "disordered" anxiety

    B.   Role of neurochemical systems (norepinephrine, serotonin, and gamma-aminobutyric acid [GABA]) has been uncovered through observations of the effects of pharmacologic agents, principally benzodiazepines, on anxiety
        1.   Benzodiazepines appear to modulate anxiety by potentiating the action of GABA, the most prevalent inhibitory CNS neurotransmitter
        2.   Receptors for benzodiazepine are coupled with receptors for GABA in the brain, in both normal and disordered anxiety

    C.   The central noradrenergic system, specifically norepinephrine-producing neurons located in the nucleus locus ceruleus play an important role in anxiety dysregulation

III. Clinical Presentation

    A.   **Primary** anxiety disorders are psychiatric disorders with specific diagnostic categories and criteria as set forth by the American Psychiatric Association in the Diagnostic and Statistical Manual of Mental Disorders (DSM-IV) (1994)
        1.   Using DSM-IV nomenclature, the nine primary anxiety disorders are panic disorder without agoraphobia; panic disorder with agoraphobia; agoraphobia without a history of panic disorder; specific phobia; social phobia; obsessive-compulsive disorder; post-traumatic stress disorder; acute stress disorder and generalized anxiety disorder
        2.   Clinical presentations for primary anxiety disorders are briefly summarized in the table on page 73 (ANXIETY DISORDERS: ANXIETY AS A PRIMARY PSYCHIATRIC DISORDER) with several of the classifications **grouped together** to conserve space. **Note:** It is beyond the scope of this book to list all diagnostic criteria for all 9 classifications; thus, please consult the DSM-IV for a complete explication of the diagnostic classifications of anxiety, keeping in mind that most people with anxiety do not have a primary anxiety disorder

    B.   The majority of patients with anxiety **do not meet the criteria** for a **primary** anxiety disorder but fall into one of the other four categories useful for categorizing anxiety in a primary care setting. These four categories are the following: (1) adjustment disorder with anxious mood; (2) anxiety due to a general medical condition; (3) substance-induced anxiety disorder; (4) anxiety associated with another psychiatric condition
        1.   Many patients have anxiety as a response to psychosocial or physical stressors (adjustment disorder with anxious mood); patient is anxious for good reason, but anxiety is excessive
            a.   Highly prevalent among patients in outpatients settings
            b.   Should be suspected in patients who are experiencing a major psychosocial stressor (divorce or serious physical illness)

ANXIETY DISORDERS: ANXIETY AS A PRIMARY PSYCHIATRIC DISORDER

Disorder Category	Characteristics	Diagnostic Criteria
Panic Attacks (With or Without Agoraphobia) and Agoraphobia	**Panic attacks:** Sudden onset of intense fear or terror, with feelings of impending doom **Agoraphobia:** Anxiety about, or avoidance of, places/situations from which escape may be difficult in the event of a panic-attack	Must have had 4 attacks within 4 weeks with at least 4 of the following symptoms present: shortness of breath, dizziness, faintness, palpitations, tachycardia, trembling, sweating, choking, nausea or abdominal distress, derealization, numbness or tingling sensations, hot flashes or chills, chest pain or discomfort, fear of dying, fear of going crazy or losing control
Phobias (both Specific and Social)	**Specific Phobia:** Excessive and persistent fear of certain objects/ situations so that exposure to the stimulus provokes an immediate anxiety approach leading person to avoid the object/ situation or endure great anxiety when avoidance is not possible **Social Phobia:** Excessive anxiety provoked by certain types of performance/social situations such as giving a speech or dining in public places	Must have avoidant behavior that substantially interferes with occupational functioning, social and personal relationships
Generalized Anxiety Disorder	Excessive worry about several areas of life associated with a number of physical or psychological symptoms of anxiety; causes person great distress or impairment in social/occupational functioning	Must occur nearly every day and have persisted for at least 6 months. Three or more of the following six symptoms are predominant: restlessness/ feeling keyed up, easily fatigued, difficulty concentrating, irritability, muscle tension, sleep disturbance
Obsessive-Compulsive Disorder	Characterized by distressing, consuming obsessions (recurrent or persistent intrusive thoughts), and/or compulsions which are repetitive behaviors or mental acts that person feels compelled to perform	Either obsessions or compulsions must be present *Obsessions* ✓ Recurrent and persistent thoughts that are intrusive and inappropriate (not excessive worries about real-life problems) ✓ Person tries to ignore or suppress thoughts ✓ Person recognizes that thoughts are product of own mind (not imposed from without) *Compulsions* ✓ Repetitive behaviors (hand washing, ordering) or mental acts (praying, counting) that person feels driven to perform ✓ Behaviors or mental acts are aimed at preventing or reducing distress or preventing some dreaded event (no realistic relationship between behaviors/acts and events they are intended to prevent) At some point, the person has recognized that obsessions/compulsions are excessive or unreasonable; cause marked distress, are time consuming (>1 hour/day) or interfere with person's normal routine, functioning, or usual social activities or relationships
Posttraumatic Stress Disorder and Acute Stress Disorder	In both disorders, there is a re-experiencing of a traumatic event in the form of dreams, images, or feelings of reliving the event, often with intense psychological distress and physiological reactivity; there is avoidance of stimuli associated with the trauma and numbing of normal responsivity	Posttraumatic Stress Disorder: Duration of disturbance must be longer than 1 month Acute Stress Disorder: Symptoms occur within 1 month of the traumatic stressor

2. Anxiety due to a medical condition commonly occurs in patients with certain conditions
   a. Essential feature is that anxiety is direct physiological consequence of medical condition
   b. Examples of conditions that may cause symptoms are listed on page 75 (see MEDICAL CONDITIONS THAT MAY CAUSE ANXIETY table)
3. Substance-induced anxiety can be due to the direct physiological effects of certain medications or toxins
   a. Medications that have been implicated in causing anxiety symptoms include anesthetics and analgesics; stimulants such as amphetamines, bronchodilators, anticholinergics, insulin, thyroid preparations, antihistamines, corticosteroids, antihypertensives, anticonvulsants, antipsychotics, antidepressants
   b. Use of the following can also produce anxiety: alcohol, caffeine, cannabis, cocaine, hallucinogens, inhalants. Accidental (or purposeful) exposure to volatile substances such as gasoline, paint, insecticides, and carbon monoxide can also produce anxiety
   c. Anxiety can also occur as part of the withdrawal from the following: alcohol, cocaine, sedatives, hypnotics, anxiolytics
4. Anxiety associated with other psychiatric disorders (depression and alcohol dependence) is not uncommon
   a. Discriminating between an anxiety disorder and a depressive illness is quite difficult because of the overlap in symptoms (e.g., sleep, appetite disturbances, difficulty concentrating, irritability, fatigue are characteristic of both anxiety and depression). See DEPRESSION section for more information on this disorder
   b. High comorbidity of alcohol and anxiety problems; thus, all patients who present with symptoms of anxiety should be screened for alcohol abuse/dependence. See section on ALCOHOL USE, ABUSE, AND DEPENDENCE for details on screening and evaluation

IV. Diagnosis/Evaluation

A. History
   1. Inquire about onset and duration of symptoms (acute or chronic)
   2. Determine what specific events or situations are producing anxiety
   3. Determine extent to which feelings of anxiety are interfering with daily functioning (home, work/school, leisure activities)
   4. Patients who volunteer 1-2 symptoms of anxiety should be asked about presence of physiological and psychological symptoms of anxiety listed in the SYMPTOMS OF ANXIETY table below

SYMPTOMS OF ANXIETY	
Physiological	Palpitations, Shortness of breath, Sweating, Dry mouth, Light-headedness, Diarrhea, Nausea, Flushes or chills, Feeling shaky, Restless
Psychological	Excessive worry, Disordered sleep, Difficulty concentrating, Irritable

   5. Ask about caffeine intake, alcohol and other drug use
   6. Obtain complete medication history including prescription, OTC drugs, as well as any supplements/herbal/complementary medicine remedies
   7. Obtain complete past medical history, presence of any coexisting medical problems
   8. Inquire about history of psychiatric illness

B. Physical Examination: Exam should be directed toward ruling out diseases that may present as anxiety conditions (see C below).

C. Differential Diagnosis:
   1. Anxiety as a primary psychiatric disorder: Does the patient meet criteria for one of the primary anxiety disorders (see ANXIETY DISORDERS: ANXIETY AS A PRIMARY PSYCHIATRIC DISORDER table)

2. Anxiety as a response to psychological or physical stressors (adjustment disorder with anxious mood): Is the patient experiencing a major stressor such as divorce, financial ruin, or a serious physical illness that might explain symptoms?

3. Anxiety due to a medical condition: Does the patient have a medical condition that produces anxiety as a symptom? See MEDICAL CONDITIONS THAT MAY CAUSE ANXIETY table below

MEDICAL CONDITIONS THAT MAY CAUSE ANXIETY	
Cardiovascular	Congestive heart failure Coronary artery disease Pulmonary embolism Arrhythmia
Endocrine	Hyper/hypothyroidism Hypoglycemia Cushing's syndrome
Metabolic conditions	Vitamin B_{12} deficiency Porphyria
Neurological disorders	Neoplasms Temporal lobe epilepsy Encephalitis
Respiratory conditions	COPD Asthma Pneumonia

4. Substance-induced anxiety: Is the anxiety due to the direct physiological effects of medications or toxins that the patient is taking/or being exposed to? See III. B.3 above for list of substances that may be involved

5. Anxiety associated with other psychiatric disorders: Does the patient have a history of depression, alcohol dependence, or psychosis? The condition diagnosed as the primary disorder should be treated first. See sections on DEPRESSION and ALCOHOL USE, ABUSE, AND DEPENDENCE to assist in discriminating between anxiety disorder and depressive illness or alcohol dependence

D. Diagnostic Tests: None indicated except to determine if anxiety is secondary to an underlying medical condition

V. Plan/Treatment

A. General considerations in the treatment of anxiety disorders
1. Once a diagnosis has been made, determine if the disorder is appropriately treatable in a primary care setting
   a. In general, primary anxiety disorders that meet the <u>DSM-IV</u> criteria are best referred to a specialist for treatment, although the treatment is outlined here in recognition that not all patients can access or afford such services
   b. In most cases, patients in the other four categories (adjustment disorder with anxious mood; anxiety due to a general medical condition; substance-induced anxiety disorder; and anxiety associated with another psychiatric condition) can be managed by the primary care provider. Patients in the fourth category, however, are usually **very difficult** to treat and **referral** may be the best option
2. Educating the patient and family about the disorder and the availability of effective therapies should be provided whether or not the patient is referred to a specialist
3. A supportive, caring approach should be used as this can have a calming effect and reassure the patient that he/she is not "crazy"
4. If pharmacotherapy is initiated, the patient must be closely monitored until stable dosage and relief of symptoms are achieved

B. Patients with primary anxiety disorders are most responsive to a combination of cognitive and behavioral therapies (CBT) and medications
    1. Referral is indicated for these patients as the interventions (CBT) are beyond the expertise of most primary care providers. For more information on CBT, see WHAT ARE COGNITIVE AND BEHAVIORAL THERAPIES? table below

WHAT ARE COGNITIVE AND BEHAVIORAL THERAPIES?		
Therapy	**Central Concept**	**Therapeutic Techniques**
Cognitive	Psychological distress arises in part from self-defeating, irrational thoughts and beliefs; changing these thoughts and beliefs can reduce anxiety	➡ Helping patient see the link between the thoughts and the anxiety response ➡ Assisting patient to use "self-talk" to help deal with anxiety-provoking stressors ➡ Showing patient how to apply appropriate responses during stressful times, beginning with less stressful triggers and moving to more challenging ones ➡ Involves goal setting, activity assignments, and careful monitoring
Behavioral	Responses to certain cues are irrational; anxiety can be controlled through altering the behavioral response to anxiety provoking cues; most modern behavior therapy uses *exposure* as the central principle of treatment	➡ Exposure-based interventions involve the use of continuous exposure to the anxiety-provoking cue as the way to relieve anxiety (desensitization) ➡ Other techniques are the teaching of relaxation techniques and slow-breathing so that these become conditioned responses to cues ➡ Therapists also use participant modeling, or enacting a behavior then encouraging patient to repeat the behavior ➡ Involves goal setting, activity assignments, and careful monitoring

    2. Panic attack (with or without agoraphobia) and agoraphobia
        a. In most cases, CBT is the treatment of choice, but this approach may not be effective, available, or accessible
        b. First-line pharmacologic treatment is use of the antidepressant medications SSRIs and tricyclics (TCAs); SSRIs are usually better tolerated and safer but are more costly than TCAs
    3. Specific phobia
        a. CBT is the treatment of choice, with exposure therapy being the approach that is used most reliably
        b. Medications have no role in the management of specific phobias, although an occasional use of a benzodiazepine (BZ) may be justified (patient with fear of large crowds wants to attend son's graduation ceremony)
        c. Suggest that patients contact the Phobia Society of America, Post Office Box 2066, Rockville, MD 20852-2066 for information on support groups
    4. Social phobia
        a. CBT is the treatment of choice, again with exposure therapy being the most reliable approach
        b. Pharmacologic management is with SSRIs and MAOIs, with more patients responding to treatment with MAOI therapy **Note:** MAOIs have potentially serious hypertensive drug-food and drug-drug interactions and must be used with caution
        c. Beta blockers can also be used
        d. Recommend books for patients such as "Social Phobias: From Shyness to Stage Fright." New York: Basic Books, 1994.
    5. Generalized anxiety disorder (GAD)
        a. Pharmacologic therapy is the first-line treatment for patients with GAD a disorder that is very difficult to diagnose and manage
            (1) Antidepressants are effective for most patients with GAD, with about 70% of patients receiving benefit from this therapy
            (2) SSRIs and TCAs are all effective with agent selection based on safety, side effect profile, contraindications, and cautions, as well as cost
            (3) Benzodiazepines (BZs) are also effective for GAD but clinicians should be cautious in the use of this class of drugs because of problems with long-term therapy

          (4)   Buspirone is approved specifically for treatment of GAD and is a good choice for patients with true GAD. Side effects are common and the drug must be taken for many weeks before effectiveness can be determined; no withdrawal or dependence potential makes this a good choice

          (5)   Beta blockers are sometimes used to relieve the physiologic, but not the psychologic symptoms of anxiety

     b.   Traditional, insight-oriented psychotherapy (based on belief that self understanding leads to cure) as well as cognitive and behavioral therapy may be used

          (1)   Unfortunately, response to insight-oriented psychotherapy and CBT is often disappointing

          (2)   These modalities are not considered a principal therapy for GAD but may be supportive with drug therapy being the first-line treatment

     c.   Source of patient educations resources: National Institute of Mental Health, 5600 Fisher's Lane, Room 7C-02, Rockville, MD 20857, 301/443-4513; **Note:** Especially useful: "Anxiety Disorders," NIH-94-3879

6.   Obsessive-compulsive disorder

     a.   Difficult to treat, even for specialists, because of complexity of therapy and poor patient response characterized by frequent relapses

     b.   CBT is the mainstay, but this treatment is not as effective as it is for other anxiety disorders with only about 20% of patients completing treatment and remaining symptom free

     c.   Pharmacologic therapy is indicated for most patients with OCD, preferably as an adjunct to behavior therapy

          (1)   All of the SSRIs are effective and dosing is at the high end of the range

          (2)   Sexual difficulties (impotence, decreased libido, difficulty achieving orgasm) caused by the SSRIs are the reason many patients discontinue the medication even though OCD is improved

          (3)   Only about 60% of patients with OCD respond well to pharmacotherapy, and when the medication is stopped, almost all patients experience relapse

          (4)   The Obsessive-Compulsive Foundation (OCF) provides a forum for persons with OCD and for professionals: Obsessive-Compulsive Foundation, PO Box 70, Milford, CT 06460-0070, 203/878-5669

          (5)   Recommend self-help books such as "Too Perfect: When Being in Control Gets Out of Control" by A.E. Mallinger & J. DeWyze. New York: Clarkson Potter, 1992.

7.   Post-traumatic stress disorder (PTSD) and acute stress disorder

     a.   Patients with PTSD seem to have less benefit from treatment than do patients with other anxiety disorders; psychotherapy may be helpful but pharmacologic treatment with antidepressants is <u>not usually effective</u>. Use of benzodiazepines in PTSD patients <u>is not recommended</u>. Support groups may offer the most hope for helping patients manage the disorder

     b.   Patients with acute stress disorder are usually helped by supportive counseling; short-term (<1 week) use of benzodiazepines may also be effective

     c.   Victims of rape, incest, or abuse may be referred to the Rape, Incest, and Abuse National Network at 800/656-HOPE, which automatically connects the caller to a support agency

C.   Patients with adjustment disorders with anxious mood may be appropriately managed in primary care settings rather than speciality settings

     1.   Pharmacologic therapy using benzodiazepines for short-term can be very effective

     2.   For more chronic anxiety symptoms, a TCA can be used; Buspirone is also an alternative for patients who require chronic use of anti-anxiety medication

     3.   Supportive counseling (by primary care provider or clergy) or in-depth therapy by a mental health specialist can be helpful; relaxation therapy may also be helpful

D.   Medications useful in the treatment of anxiety disorders are summarized in the table on the next page

Medications Useful in the Treatment of Anxiety Disorders

Medications by Category	Usual Starting Dose*	Typical Therapeutic Dose*	Contra-indications	Important Class Side Effects	General Comments Relating to Medications Based on Category
Tricyclic antidepressants (TCAs)			Glaucoma, cardiac conduction abnormalities, high suicide risk	Anticholinergic: Dry mouth, constipation, blurred vision, orthostatic hypotension, weight gain, somnolence	Have largely been supplanted by SSRIs as first line treatment for anxiety disorders
Imipramine (Tofranil)	10 mg HS	100-200 mg/d			Initiation of treatment with TCAs may be associated with worsening of anxiety, so treatment is started low and titrated up as tolerated over first few weeks of treatment
Desipramine (Norpramin)	10 mg HS	100-200 mg/d			Effective for panic disorder, GAD
Amitriptyline (Elavil)	10 mg HS	100-200 mg/d			Less effective for social phobia
Nortriptyline (Pamelor)	10 mg HS	50-100 mg/d			Ineffective for OCD
					May be fatal in overdose; provide prescription for smallest amount feasible
Serotonin-specific reuptake inhibitors (SSRIs) and newer agents			Use of MAOI within prior 21 days	Somnolence, agitation, sweating, nausea, anorexia, sexual dysfunction	First line therapy for most anxiety disorders
Fluoxetine (Prozac)	10 mg Q AM	20-80 mg/d			Greater tolerability and safety than TCAs
Paroxetine (Paxil)	10 mg QD	20-50 mg/d			Lower potential for dependence as compared with the BZs
Sertraline (Zoloft)	25 mg QD	50-200 mg/d			Treatment of anxiety is usually begun with half usual starting dose for depression to reduce anxiety often associated with initiation of therapy
Fluvoxamine (Luvox)	25 HS	50-300 mg/d			Doses should be raised after one week to therapeutic levels
Nefazodone (Serzone) (Serotonin-reuptake effect; also regulates serotonin type 2 (5-HT$_2$) receptors)	50 mg QD	150-300 mg/d			Patients with OCD and PTSD may require higher doses than patients with other disorders
Venlafaxine (Effexor) (Mixed neurotransmitter reuptake inhibitor)	18.75-25 mg QD	75-150 mg/d			Onset of benefit usually occurs within 2-3 weeks of treatment
					Nefazodone is contraindicated with terfenadine, astemazole, triazolom, and cisapride
Benzodiazepines			History of substance abuse	Sedation, dizziness, incoordination, amnesia, headache	All are effective and are drug of choice for GAD
Alprazolam (Xanax)	0.25 mg TID	0.5-6 mg/d			High-potency BZs (Alprazolam and Clonazepam) are best for panic disorder
Clonazepam (Klonopin)	0.5 mg BID	1-4 mg/d			Clonazepam is a long-acting agent and permits less frequent dosing
Chlorazepate (Tranxene)	3.75 mg BID	7.5-60 mg/d			Alprazolam and Diazepam have rapid onset and can provide rapid relief, Alprazolam and Lorazepam are short-acting and can minimize drug accumulation
Diazepam (Valium)	2 mg BID	4-40 mg/d			Patients with drug or alcohol abuse history are at risk for abuse of BZs
Lorazepam (Ativan)	1 mg BID	2-6 mg/d			Advantages of BZs are their rapid onset of effect
Buspirone (BuSpar)	7.5 mg BID	20-30 mg/d		Nervousness, insomnia, weakness, dizziness, paresthesia, nausea, diarrhea	Onset of antianxiety effects may require 4 weeks or more
					As efficacious as BZs after 4 weeks of therapy
					Maximum therapeutic effect may not be evident for 4-6 weeks
					Not useful in situations requiring immediate therapy or as-needed therapy

*Elderly/debilitated patients are usually treated with approximately one-half of dose listed.

E.   Patients with anxiety due to a medical condition require treatment of the underlying cause

F.   For patients with anxiety that is substance-induced
1.   If medication that is being taken for another condition is the cause, consider switching to another class that may not produce anxiety
2.   If licit or illicit drugs (e.g., cannabis, cocaine, hallucinogens, inhalants, or caffeine) are causing the anxiety, provide patient with counseling/referral to drug detoxification program

G.   Patients with anxiety associated with another psychiatric condition, most often depression, should be treated for the primary problem. See sections on DEPRESSION and ALCOHOL USE, ABUSE, AND DEPENDENCE for assistance in dealing with patients who have either of these problems. As stated above under V.A.1.b., most patients in this category should be referred to a specialist if possible

H.   Follow Up
1.   Variable depending on diagnosis and involvement in treatment (e.g., If in-office counseling is being provided for an adjustment disorder, may need to be weekly for several weeks)
2.   When pharmacotherapy is used, monitor the patient closely (every 2-3 weeks) until a stable dosage and relief of symptoms are achieved
3.   Long-term use of antidepressants and BZs is often required

DEPRESSION

I.   Definition: Unipolar mood disorders characterized by physical and psychological symptoms that cause significant distress and impairment in functioning and occur in the absence of elevated mood (mania or hypomania)

II.   Pathogenesis

A.   Theories related to a biologic etiology of depression include the following:
1.   Biogenic amine hypothesis: Occurs as result of depletion of levels of serotonin
2.   Receptor suprasensitivity hypothesis: Results from suprasensitive catecholamine receptors in response to decreased levels of catecholamine in brain

B.   Theories related to a psychosocial etiology of depression include the following:
1.   Psychoanalytic: Mourning of symbolic object loss with rigid superego that leads one to feel worthless
2.   Cognitive: Cognitive triad of (a) automatic negative thoughts and negative self-view (b) negative interpretation of experience and pessimistic view of the world, and (c) negative view of future

III.   Clinical Presentation

A.   Unipolar depressive disorders are psychiatric disorders with specific diagnostic categories and criteria as set forth by the American Psychiatric Association in the Diagnostic and Statistical Manual of Mental Disorders (DSM-IV) (1994)
1.   Using DSM-IV nomenclature, the three unipolar depressive disorders are major depressive disorder (MDD), dysthymic disorder, and minor depressive disorder (**Note:** Minor depressive disorder is the most common form of a diagnostic category called "depressive disorder, not otherwise specified," a category that includes several disorders)
a.   Major depressive disorder (MDD) is the most severe form of unipolar depression and consists of history of one or more major depressive episodes
b.   Dysthymic disorder is a milder and chronic form of depression
c.   Minor depressive disorder is characterized by fewer than five symptoms of MDD

B.   Diagnostic criteria for each of the three disorders are summarized in the following tables

---

DIAGNOSTIC CRITERIA FOR MAJOR DEPRESSIVE DISORDER

Depressed mood (can be irritable mood in children/adolescents) or markedly decreased pleasure in most activities. Duration ≥ 2 weeks

At least five of the following symptoms are present nearly every day
  ✓ Depressed mood (can be irritable mood in children/adolescents)
  ✓ Loss of interest or pleasure in most activities
  ✓ Significant weight loss/gain or decreased/increased appetite
  ✓ Insomnia or hypersomnia
  ✓ Psychomotor agitation or retardation
  ✓ Loss of energy or fatigue
  ✓ Feelings of worthlessness or excessive/inappropriate guilt
  ✓ Diminished ability to think/concentrate or indecisiveness
  ✓ Recurrent thoughts of suicide or death

Symptoms cause clinically significant distress or psychosocial impairment

Symptoms are not better accounted for by bereavement or are not due to a general medical condition or psychotropic substance

Presence of a single or multiple major depressive episodes

No history of mania or hypomania

The major depressive episode is not superimposed upon psychotic disorders and is not better accounted for by schizoaffective disorder

Adapted from American Psychiatric Association. (1994). Diagnostic and statistical manual of mental disorders (4th ed.). Washington, DC: Author.

DIAGNOSTIC CRITERIA FOR DYSTHYMIC DISORDER

Depressed mood (can be irritable mood in children/adolescents present for at least **one year**), for most of the day, for more days than not, for at least 2 years

Presence, when depressed, of at least two of the following symptoms:
  ✓ Poor appetite or overeating   ✓ Low self-esteem
  ✓ Insomnia or hyposomnia   ✓ Poor concentration or difficulty making decisions
  ✓ Low energy or fatigue   ✓ Feelings of hopelessness

During a two-year period (**one year**, children/adolescents), never without a depressed mood (irritable mood, children/adolescents) for more than 2 months at a time

No evidence of major depressive episode during the first 2 years of disturbance (1 year, children/adolescents)

No history of mania, hypomania, or cyclothymia

Symptoms not caused by general medical condition or psychotropic substance

Symptoms cause clinically significant distress or psychosocial impairment

Adapted from American Psychiatric Association. (1994). Diagnostic and statistical manual of mental disorders (4th ed.). Washington, DC: Author.

DIAGNOSTIC CRITERIA FOR MINOR DEPRESSIVE DISORDER

Presence of fewer than five symptoms of MDD

Duration of symptoms at least 2 weeks

Disturbance does not occur exclusively during course of psychotic disorders

Adapted from American Psychiatric Association. (1994). Diagnostic and statistical manual of mental disorders (4th ed.). Washington, DC: Author.

C.   Lifetime risk of MDD ranges from 7 to 12% in men and 20 to 25% in women, with fewer than 50% of patients receiving treatment for their condition

D.   Slightly over half of patients treated for MDD receive their care from non-psychiatrists with primary care providers having a substantial role in management of this disorder

E. MDD accounts for total costs of about $40 billion per year and is associated with high levels of impairment in work, social, and physical activities

F. Dysthymic disorder has a prevalence rate among primary care patients of about 4% and a female-to-male ratio of 1:7

G. By far, most patients who present to primary care providers with significant depressive symptoms do not meet the criteria for major depression, but instead have a minor depressive disorder

H. Depression in the elderly may be difficult to distinguish from dementia as some symptoms of depression (e.g., disorientation, memory loss, and distractibility) may suggest dementia

I. Three observations may help distinguish between depression and dementia in the elderly:
1. Whereas the onset of a major depressive disorder occurs over a period of days to weeks, the onset of dementia is slow and insidious
2. Whereas depressed persons can answer questions correctly if given enough time, those with dementia cannot
3. Finally, a therapeutic trial of antidepressant medication produces improvement/recovery in depression but not in dementia

J. Elderly may not present with feelings of sadness but instead present with somatic complaints and depression may be "masked"

K. Presently, only about 10% of older adults who suffer from depression receive treatment, largely because of the misguided belief on the part of some health care providers (and elderly patients) that depression is an inevitable, untreatable part of aging caused by illness, bereavement, and other events that require difficult life adjustments

IV. Diagnosis/Evaluation

A. History
1. Ask about onset, duration, and description of symptoms. Ask about symptoms that characteristically occur by referring to tables above that contain diagnostic criteria for MDD, dysthymic disorder, and minor depressive disorder
2. Ask if these symptoms are new of if they have occurred before (current and past psychiatric history)
3. Ask about the impact of these symptoms or level of impairment
    a. Does the patient have difficulty functioning at home/school/work?
    b. How are interpersonal relationships affected?
4. Ask about presence of identifiable stressors using these three categories:
    a. Major discrete stressors: Ask about deaths, divorces, job losses
    b. Chronic stressors: Ask about marital conflict, abuse, on-going chronic illness of patient or family member
    c. Minor daily stressors: Ask about demands at work, home, that may be causing patient to feel overwhelmed
5. Ask about mood swings (if present, consider bipolar disorder)
6. Ask about alcohol/drug use
7. Obtain past medical history and medication history (Medications that may cause depression include steroids, antihypertensives, estrogen, NSAIDs, digoxin, and anti-Parkinson drugs)
8. Always ask patients with depressive symptoms about suicidal thinking, impulses, and personal history of suicide attempts. (Suicidal risk factors are hopelessness, caucasian race, male gender, age over 65, living alone, personal and family history of suicide attempts, personal and family history of alcohol/substance abuse)

B. Physical Examination
1. While completing history, part of mental status exam should be obtained:
    a. Observe general appearance and behavior (usual to see inattention to personal appearance, tearful, downcast, poor eye contact)

b.   Pay attention to affect (usually constricted, intense) mood (one of frustration, sadness), and speech (usually soft, low with little spontaneity)

c.   If inattention occurs during history taking, it should be documented during exam by testing ability to recall series of random numbers

2.   Physical exam should be directed toward ruling out an infectious, neoplastic, metabolic, or neurologic disorder

C.   Differential Diagnosis
1.   Bipolar depression
2.   Psychotic disorders, particularly schizophrenia
3.   Bereavement
4.   Substance abuse
5.   Dementia
6.   Anxiety disorder
7.   Medical conditions such as thyroid, other endocrine disorders, neurological problems, as well as medications that treat those disorders

D.   Diagnostic Tests
1.   Consider use of screening questionnaires that are self-administered

a.   The Beck Depression Inventory and the Zung Self-Rating Depression Scale have been used extensively in primary care research

b.   The Geriatric Depression Scale (GDS) is an appropriate screening tool for assessing depression in the elderly (**Note:** Not valid in patients with cognitive impairment) [see BRIEF DESCRIPTION AND SOURCE--BDI, ZUNG, and GDS in the following table]

BRIEF DESCRIPTION AND SOURCE--BDI, ZUNG, & GDS		
Scale	**Description**	**Source**
Beck Depression Inventory	21 items with 4 statements each Emphasis is on cognitive symptoms of depression All items apply to "the past week, including today"	For information about obtaining this scale, complete with scoring instructions, write to: The Psychological Corporation 555 Academic Court San Antonio, Texas 78204-2498 (210)299-1061
Zung Self-Rating Depression Scale	20 items, rated by how much of the time each depressive symptom is present Zung describes scale as "depression thermometer"	For more information about this scale, consult the following publications: Zung, W.W.K. (1965). A self-rating depression scale. Archives of General Psychiatry, 12, 63-70. Zung, W.W.K. (1990). The role of rating scales in the identification and management of the depressed patient in the primary care setting. Journal of Clinical Psychiatry, 51 (Suppl), 72-76.
Geriatric Depression Scale	15 yes/no questions Takes 5-7 minutes to complete, is one page long, and easy to understand	For more information about this scale, consult the following publication: Sheikh, J.I., & Yesavage, J.A. (1986). Geriatric depression scale (GDS): Recent evidence and development of a shorter version. In T.L. Brink (Ed.), Clinical Gerontology: A Guide to Assessment and Intervention. Binghamptom, NY: Haworth Press.

2.   Consider the following screening tests to rule out an organic cause and substance use
a.   CBC, sedimentation rate, VDRL, chemistry profile, thyroid profile
b.   Drug screen

V. Plan/Treatment

    A. The following categories of patients should be referred to a specialist for treatment:
1. Those with high suicide risk (Patients who admit to suicidal thinking, have a realistic plan, and have access to weapons, particularly guns)
2. Women who are pregnant or plan to become pregnant
3. Patients with no evidence of social support
4. Patients who are disabled by the depression (unable to function at work/school, unable to take care of day-to-day responsibilities)
5. Patients with comorbid conditions (primary anxiety disorder, substance abuse, dementia)
6. Patients who fail to respond to one or two adequate trials of antidepressants

    B. Patients who are **not** in the above categories and who have (1) moderate or severe depression that has persisted for 1 month or longer, or (2) mild-to-moderate depression that is chronic and interferes with routine functions of family/work/school life are candidates for treatment with both pharmacologic and nonpharmacologic therapies
1. Pharmacotherapy: Mainstay of treatment by primary care providers is pharmacologic therapy with two classes of drugs most commonly used--selective serotonin reuptake inhibitors (SSRIs) and tricyclic antidepressants (TCAs)
2. Nonpharmacologic therapies: Includes psychotherapy/counseling as well as other modalities such as exercise and behavior change
    a. May be considered an alternative to medications in patients who are very reluctant to take medications
    b. A more accurate concept of the role of this treatment modality is to support/augment medications rather than replace them

    C. Pharmacotherapy with antidepressants
1. Selective serotonin reuptake inhibitors (SSRIs) are **first-line treatment** for depression based on excellent safety record and safety during overdose
    a. Table below lists their usual starting dose and target dose
    b. Most common side effects of this class of drugs are nausea, anorexia, weight loss, excessive sweating, nervousness, insomnia, sexual dysfunction, sedation, headache, and dizziness

TREATMENT FOR DEPRESSION: **SELECTIVE SEROTONIN REUPTAKE INHIBITORS (SSRIs)**			
Medication	**Available As**	**Initial Dose***	**Titrate Dose Up To Target Dose***
Fluoxetine (Prozac)	10, 20 mg caps	20 mg/day	20-40 mg/day in AM
Sertraline (Zoloft)	25, 50, 100 mg scored tabs	50 mg/day	75-150 mg/day in AM
Paroxetine (Paxil)	10, 20, 30, 40 mg tabs	10-20 mg/day	20-40 mg/day in AM
Fluvoxamine (Luvox)	25, 50, 100 mg tabs	50 mg/day	150-200 mg/day (given in 2-3 divided doses with largest dose at HS)
Citalopram HBr (Celexa)	20, 40 mg tabs	20 mg/day	40 mg/day any time of day
Venlafaxine (Effexor) (mixed neurotransmitter reuptake inhibitor)	25, 37.5, 50, 75, 100 mg scored tabs	75 mg/day (given in 2 divided doses)	150-300 mg/day (given in 2-3 divided doses)
Note: Extended-release venlafaxine (Effexor XR) has been approved for once-daily dosing. Effexor XR is available in 37.5, 75, and 150 mg caps. The single dose should be taken in AM. The same total daily dose can be given in a single dose			

*Elderly/debilitated patients are usually treated with approximately one-half of dose listed.

2. Tricyclic antidepressants (TCAs) are also effective but cause many side effects that reduce patient compliance
    a. Because they block cholinergic muscarinic receptors, TCAs can cause dry mouth, constipation, urinary retention, blurred vision, and sinus tachycardia

b. Because they block histamine H_1 receptors, TCAs can cause sedation, increased appetite, weight gain, hypotension, and potentiation of central depressant drugs

c. Because they block α_1 adrenergic receptors, TCAs can cause postural hypotension, dizziness, reflex tachycardia, and potentiation of the antihypertensive effect of some drugs

d. TCAs can have a significant effect on cardiac conduction through a quinidine-like effect and are **contraindicated** in patients with cardiac conduction disorders

e. TCAs are also **contraindicated** in patients with narrow-angle glaucoma and prostatic hypertrophy (See PDR for a full discussion of contraindications and precautions; **overdoses can be lethal!**)

f. With gradual dosage escalation, most bothersome side effects of TCAs subside after a few weeks; persistence of anticholinergic side effects can be minimized by adding cholinergic smooth-muscle stimulants (e.g., bethanecol)

g. Obtain an EKG **before** prescribing these drugs and **after four weeks** of TCA treatment

h. Tables below list usual starting dose and target dose of TCAs and tips for selecting a TCA

TREATMENT FOR DEPRESSION: TRICYCLIC ANTIDEPRESSANTS (TCAs)			
Medication	Available As	Initial Dose*	Titrate Dose Up To Target Dose*
Amitriptyline (Elavil)	10, 25, 50, 75, 100, 150 mg tabs	25 mg QHS	100-150 mg QHS
Amoxapine (Asendin)	25, 50, 100, 150 mg	50 mg BID	100-200 mg BID
Clomipramine (Anafranil)	25, 50, 75 mg caps	25 mg QHS	150-200 mg QHS
Desipramine (Norpramin)	10, 25, 50, 75, 100, 150 mg tabs	25-50 mg QHS or QAM	50-300 mg QHS or in divided doses
Doxepin (Adapin or Sinequan)	10, 25, 50, 75, 100, 150 mg caps	25-50 mg QHS	150-200 mg QHS
Imipramine (Tofranil)	10, 25, 50, 75, 100, 125, 150 mg caps	50 mg QHS	150-200 mg QHS or in divided doses
Nortriptyline (Pamelor)	10, 25, 50, 75 mg caps	25 mg QHS	75-100 mg QHS or in divided doses
Protriptyline (Vivactil)	5, 10 mg tabs	10 mg QAM	15-40 mg QAM
Trimipramine (Surmontil)	25, 50, 100 mg caps	75 mg/day in 2-3 divided doses	100-150 mg QHS or in divided doses

*Elderly/debilitated patients are usually treated with approximately one-half of dose listed.

TIPS FOR SELECTING A TCA
Drugs from the secondary amine group which includes desipramine, nortriptyline, and protriptyline cause fewer anticholinergic side effects and sedation, and are generally better tolerated than TCAs from the tertiary amine group

✦ Amitriptyline (Elavil), a tertiary amine, is considered to be the **most** anticholinergic and **most** sedating TCA

✦ Desipramine (Norpramin), a secondary amine, is considered to be the **least** anticholinergic and **least** sedating TCA

✦ Nortriptyline (Pamelor), also a secondary amine, is somewhere in the middle of the two above TCAs in terms of anticholinergic effects and sedation

3. Atypical antidepressants (bupropion, mitrazapine, nefazodone, and trazodone) have chemical structures different from both TCAs and SSRIs and are also used to treat depression
   a. Table below lists their usual starting dose and target dose

Medication	Available As	Initial Dose*	Titrate Dose Up To Target Dose*
Bupropion (Wellbutrin)	75, 100 mg tabs	200 mg/day in 2 divided doses	300-400 mg/day in 3-4 divided doses with at least 8 hrs between. Avoid HS
Mirtazapine (Remeron)	15, 30 mg scored tabs	15 mg/day at HS	15-45 mg/day at HS
Nefazodone (Serzone)	100, 150 mg scored tabs 200, 250 mg tabs	200 mg/day in 2 divided doses	300-600 mg/day in 2 divided doses
Trazodone (Desyrel)	50, 100, 150, 300 scored tabs	150 mg/day in divided doses	300-400 mg/day in divided doses

TREATMENT FOR DEPRESSION: ATYPICAL ANTIDEPRESSANTS

*Elderly/debilitated patients are usually treated with approximately one-half of dose listed.

   b. Lack significant cardiac effects and are relatively safe in overdose
   c. Side-effect profile is variable, depending on particular agent
   d. **Bupropion**: Most common side effects are agitation, dry mouth, insominia, headache, nausea, vomiting, constipation, tremor; **contraindicated** in persons with seizure disorder or bulimia
   e. **Mirtazapine**: Most common side effects are related to H_1-receptor blocking activity and include sedation, increased appetite, weight gain, dizziness, dry mouth, constipation; good candidate for **combination strategies** as drug-drug interactions with other antidepresssants are relatively uncommon
   f. **Nefazodone**: Most common side effects are headache, fatigue, orthostatic hypotension (caused by blockage of α_1-adrenergic receptors), dry mouth, constipation, sedation
   g. **Trazodone**: Most common side effects are drowsiness, dizziness, headache, nausea, and orthostatic hypotension, priapism in men (extremely rare but serious and is not dose related) [**Note**: Trazodone is an effective antidepressant but it is most often used in the management of insomnia associated with SSRI use. Dosing for this indication is 25-50 mg at HS]
4. Monoamine Oxidase Inhibitors (MAOIs) are used primarily in treatment-resistant patients; patients should be referred to a specialist for initiation of this class of antidepressants. Many serious and lethal side effects associated with the MAOIs

D. Provide education regarding side effects **prior** to prescribing any antidepressant
   1. Emphasize that all antidepressants produce some side effects
   2. Inform patient about the most commonly occurring adverse effects and emphasize that most side effects are manageable
   3. Encourage patient by informing him/her that most side effects resolve with time
   4. Help the patient to remember that most side effects are better than depression

E. Evaluate treatment response to pharmacologic therapy at 4-6 weeks
   1. Many patients will respond to an **adequate trial** (usually 8 weeks, but at least six weeks at therapeutic doses) of the first medication tried
   2. If there is not an adequate response, consider the following steps:
      a. Inquire about compliance (**Remember!** Preparation of the patient with education increases likelihood of compliance)
      b. Determine need for increased dosing (52% of primary care providers use lower than recommended doses)
      c. Continue current medication, at full dose for an additional 2-4 weeks, to give the medication an adequate trial

F.   Evaluate treatment response to pharmacologic therapy at 8 weeks
      1.   Patients who are not significantly improved on full dose should be switched to another medication or placed on a combination therapy
      2.   Switching antidepressants usually follows the sequence below:
            a.   Switch to agent in same class (change from one SSRI to another)
            b.   Switch to agent in different class (change from an SSRI to a TCA)
            c.   Switch to an atypical agent
      3.   Combination therapies usually follow the pattern below:
            a.   Combine an SSRI at full dose and a low-dose TCA (e.g., 25 mg/day)
            b.   Combine an SSRI at full dose and buspirone at full dose (e.g., 10-20 mg/BID)
      4.   The National Institutes of Health estimates that as many as 70% of older adults do not take antidepressants as prescribed for two reasons:
            a.   They fear side effects
            b.   They do not experience immediate improvement, and so discontinue the medication

G.   See TIPS FOR DEALING WITH SIDE EFFECTS table

TIPS FOR DEALING WITH SIDE EFFECTS		
Problem	Solution	Consider
Dry eyes	Dry eye agents such as Cellufresh or Naturale Free	Prescribing medication with few or no anticholinergic effects (SSRIs) **Note:** Avoid Paroxetine, the most anticholinergic of the SSRIs
Constipation	Increase fluids and activity Increase fiber intake/use bulking agents	As above
Sedation	If sedation occurs with AM dosing, change dosing to PM	As above
Insomnia	If insomnia occurs with PM dosing, change dosing to AM	Prescribing trazodone, 25-50 mg at HS for patients with SSRI-related insomnia OR Consider switching to nefazodone which preserves sleep architecture and is an excellent choice for patients with insomnia
Dizziness, headache	Many patients develop tolerance for common side effects (that are annoying but not dangerous) over several weeks	Continuing with present regimen
Gastrointestinal complaints	Assure patients problems diminish over time; advise to take with food	If using sertraline which is highly associated with GI discomfort, consider switching to another SSRI such as fluoxetine
Weight gain	Use SSRIs which are appetite suppressants	

H.   **Nonpharmacologic therapies:** Cognitive and interpersonal therapies are probably the most efficacious forms of psychotherapy for patients with depressive disorders
      1.   Cognitive therapy is aimed at correcting the negative views of self, world, and future that many depressed persons hold
            a.   Focus is on helping patient gain new skills, enhance confidence, and broaden social circle
            b.   Homework assignments are typically provided to help patient meet goals
      2.   Interpersonal therapy focuses on resolution of problematic interpersonal relationships or stressful events in patient's life
            a.   Providing patient with opportunities to talk about conflicts and ways to problem-solve can be very therapeutic
            b.   A common interpersonal deficit is social isolation; practical suggestions such as joining a social, religious group, or taking a class, or becoming a volunteer can help decrease isolation and promote feelings of being connected in the patient
      3.   Patients should be referred for cognitive and interpersonal therapies as most primary care providers lack the time and expertise for these approaches

I.   **Nonpharmacologic therapies:** Exercise Programs are low cost alternatives to psychotherapy and may be combined with antidepressants to potentiate the medication effects
1.   Exercise appears to have both direct and indirect effects on relief of depression
2.   Prescribe a 10-minute daily walk with a gradual increase in walking time to 30 minutes/day; write the exercise prescription on a prescription pad to demonstrate the value of the daily walk
3.   An organized exercise class may be helpful as it increases the likelihood that the patient will interact with others on a regular basis

J.   **Nonpharmacologic therapies:** Recognize the value of helping the patient find pleasure in daily living
1.   "Doing better" may be a prerequisite to "feeling better"
2.   Prescribe a single pleasurable activity each day (e.g., buying self flowers, going to a movie)
3.   Encourage patient to continue in activity even though it may initially fail to elicit feelings of pleasure
4.   Have patient keep a log of activities to discuss at periodic visits, again as a way of demonstrating provider confidence in the therapeutic approach
5.   Suggest self-help books such as "Feeling Good: The New Mood Therapy" by David Burns. New York: Avon Books, 1980.

K.   **Nonpharmacologic therapies:** Support groups are another low-cost option for patients with depression
1.   Many no-cost support groups are available for depressed patients
2.   Groups that meet in many communities include Adult Children of Alcoholics, Overeaters Anonymous, bereavement groups, and incest survivors groups

L.   Special concern: Treatment of depression in elders
1.   Initiation of treatment in older persons can have dramatic improvement on quality of life through helping to maintain optimal level of functioning and independence
2.   As in younger adults, the elderly tend to tolerate SSRIs better than TCAs
3.   Although TCAs and SSRIs appear to have comparable efficacy in elderly patients, the effectiveness of SSRIs may be greater than that of TCAs because of fewer and more acceptable adverse effects
4.   Psychotherapy, including cognitive and interpersonal therapies may have particular utility in elders who are depressed
       a.   Most elders have to deal with very stressful situations such as loss of family members, friends, and functional ability
       b.   Role disputes and interpersonal conflicts are common occurrences for many elders as they deal with declining independence
       c.   In many cases, there are low degrees of social support for elders
5.   Research supports the need for long-term treatment of depression that occurs in late life
       a.   For patients with first onset of depression in late life, at least six months of treatment beyond recovery is recommended
       b.   For patients with recurrent illness, at least 12 months of treatment beyond recovery is recommended
6.   Older patients with recurrent depression may need antidepressant treatment indefinitely to remain well
       a.   Long-term treatment should be of the same type and intensity as that which was successful in the initial, acute phase
       b.   In practice, the intensity of antidepressant therapy is frequently prematurely decreased

M.   Follow Up
1.   During **acute therapy** (first 8-12 weeks) phase, patient should return for weekly visits for the first 4 weeks; then at 8 weeks after treatment is initiated
       a.   One purpose of visits during the acute phase is to evaluate response to non-pharmacologic therapies

        b.   A second purpose for weekly visits for the first 4 weeks is for titrating dose of antidepressants up to therapeutic levels; at 4 weeks after treatment is initiated, to evaluate response, then at 8 weeks after treatment is initiated, to again evaluate response

2.   During continuation therapy (5-6 months after acute therapy phase), administration of the medication is continued to maintain control over the depression and the patient is encouraged to continue the nonpharmacologic therapies; patient should be seen every 2 months during this period

        a.   Patients may be tempted to discontinue the medication as well as the nonpharmacologic therapies after the acute phase has abated, because they are significantly improved

        b.   Fewer relapses occur when antidepressant is continued at least 4-6 months after clinical response is obtained

3.   Maintenance therapy is important to prevent a recurrence; risk factors for recurrent depression are history of frequent/multiple episodes of depression, and duration of the initial episode of >2 years; patient may be seen every 3-6 months during this period

DOMESTIC VIOLENCE: ELDER AND DISABLED ADULT ABUSE AND NEGLECT

I.   Definition: The infliction of physical pain, injury, or mental anguish, unreasonable confinement, or willful deprivation of services which are necessary to maintain mental and physical health of a disabled adult or elderly person

II.   Pathogenesis

    A.   Etiology is unclear, but a number of recurrent theories emerge:

        1.   Dependency of the adult/elder arising from multiple medical illnesses or mental impairment is frequently encountered

        2.   Financial conditions also appear to play a role in the occurrence of abuse, with the abused person having limited resources and imposing a financial burden on the abuser

    B.   Alcoholism and drug dependency in a caregiver enhance the likelihood of abuse

III.   Clinical Presentation

    A.   Almost 2 million older adults (>60) are abused annually

    B.   Victims of abuse are likely to be among the old-old, the mean age being 84

    C.   Victim is usually a woman and perpetrator most often is spouse, adult child, but paid and informal caregivers may also be responsible

    D.   Almost 50% of abused have moderate to severe mental impairment

    E.   Physical indicators of abuse:

        1.   Unexplained fractures, burns, bruises, welts, bald spots, human bite marks

        2.   Bruises or bleeding in external genitalia

    F.   Behavioral indicators of abuse:

        1.   Withdrawn, lethargic, wears clothes inappropriate to season to cover body

        2.   Sleep disorders, poor appetite, depressed mood

G. Physical indicators of neglect:
    1. Inappropriate dress, poor hygiene
    2. Unattended medical needs (lacking hearing aids, dentures, eyeglasses)

IV. Diagnosis/Evaluation

    A. History
        1. Obtain social history including information about living arrangements, primary caregiver, and family functioning
        2. Screening for violence (with only the patient present) should be made a **routine part** of preventive care for elderly and disabled persons. One approach is to ask the SAFE questions

SAFE QUESTIONS	
Stress/Safety	What stresses do you have in your relationships? Do you feel safe in your relationship with (name family member/friend)?
Afraid	Are there situations in which you feel afraid? Have you ever been threatened or abused?
Friends/Family	✓ If positive responses to items above: Ask "Are your friends/family aware that this is happening?" ✓ If negative responses to items above: Ask "Do you think you could tell them if it did happen?" "Would they help you?"
Emergency Plan	✓ Do you have a safe place to go in an emergency situation? ✓ Would you like to talk with a social worker/counselor to help you develop a plan?
Any questions answered affirmatively should be followed with additional questions in order to determine the following: ✓ How and when mistreatment occurs ✓ Who perpetrates it ✓ How the patient copes with it	

Adapted from Ashur, M.L. (1993). Asking about domestic violence: SAFE questions (Letter to the editor). JAMA 269, 2367.

        3. If physical injury is present, ask detailed questions relating to time or occurrence and how it occurred
            a. Long interval between injury and seeking help is red flag
            b. Story that is inconsistent, contradictory, or fails to adequately explain injury is red flag
        4. If behavioral problems are evident, ask appropriate questions to determine etiology by asking direct questions such as the following:
            a. Are you alone a lot?
            b. Has anyone ever failed to help you take care of yourself when you needed help?
            c. Has anyone ever made you do things you did not want to do?
            d. Any positive responses should prompt asking how and when this occurs, who the perpetrator is, and how the patient copes with the mistreatment
        5. Question about past or present medical problems, current medications
        6. Interview patient and complete a mental status exam
            a. Determine if the patient is cognitively impaired and unable to provide reliable information
            b. Patients who are cognitively impaired my require other data sources such as family members, neighbors, clergy, friends (in addition to the caregiver who may also be the perpetrator)
        7. History should be carefully recorded as it may be part of a court case; stories that change over time are suggestive of abuse -- thus, statements made as part of the initial disclosure take on added significance

    B. Physical Examination
        1. Record height, weight, and blood pressure, noting any decline in weight that may indicate poor nutritional status
        2. Observe behavior during exam for fearfulness, listlessness, and withdrawn behavior

3. Inspect skin for hydration status, burns, bruises, bites, and lacerations
   a. Use measuring tape and record on anatomic diagrams on chart
   b. Accidental injuries usually occur on extensor surfaces; bruises or lacerations on other areas require more careful evaluation
4. Examine head focusing on any patchy hair loss, battle's sign (bruising over mastoid process behind ears) raccoon eyes, and blood behind the tympanic membranes. **Note:** Serious intracranial injuries caused by direct blows may have few or no external signs
5. Examine abdomen for signs of injury. **Note:** Cutaneous signs of abdominal injury are rare: Blunt trauma to abdomen can cause serious injury difficult to detect with physical exam alone

C. Differential Diagnosis
1. Unintended injury
2. Poverty resulting in poor clothing/hygiene
3. Self-neglect due to cognitive/physical impairment

D. Diagnostic Tests: History and physical exam dictate tests

V. Plan/Treatment

A. Because of the associated trauma and pain, adult abuse is a health care issue; because it involves disturbed family relationships, it is a social service agencies issue; because assault and abuse are involved, it is a criminal justice system issue

B. Once a case of adult abuse is identified, a multidimensional approach at intervention is important

C. While the intervention must be individualized, some generalizations can be made:
1. If the life of the adult is in jeopardy, Adult Protective Services (APS) must be notified; the patient must be removed from hostile environment and placed in safe place (this is the minority of cases)
   a. APS in each sate has the legal responsibility for investigation/intervention when adult abuse/neglect suspected
   b. Mandatory reporting laws vary from state to state; know your responsibility as a health care provider in your state
2. If the adult is not in immediate danger, more comprehensive assessment can take place and implementation of supportive services aimed at alleviating some of the factors can be put into effect
   a. If risk factors for adult abuse or neglect are dealt with at an early stage, and if the caregiver is open to receiving assistance and support, prevention of abuse (or more severe abuse) may be possible
   b. Maintaining the independence and functional capabilities of both the abused person and the support system is the focus
   c. Institutionalization of the abused adult may be the best solution when needs for care outstrip the care-person's ability to provide care
   d. Providing support in the abused adult's home in terms of homemaker services and Meals-On-Wheels may relieve tension
   e. Psychiatric/alcohol abuse counseling referral, and treatment for the perpetrator may be indicated

D. Follow Up: Primary care providers have a responsibility to monitor the outcomes of all cases of adult abuse and neglect which have come to their attention

DOMESTIC VIOLENCE: PARTNER ABUSE

I.   Definition: Physical or emotional intimidation or violation of one member of a presently or previously intimate couple by the other; may involve physical battering, sexual coercion, or assault, psychological intimidation, physical restraint, or financial exploitation

II.   Pathogenesis

A.   Men who commit domestic violence have no common set of traits and no consistent predictive personality characteristics

B.   Alcohol and drug use can worsen violence, but has not been found to cause it

C.   The major issue in all abusive relationships is control

D.   Many abusive partnerships are characterized by cycles of violence in which abuse occurs, the perpetrator repents, the couple reconciles and then the whole cycle repeats

III. Clinical Presentation

A.   About 30% of women who present to emergency departments for injuries of any kind have been injured by a partner

B.   The major risk factor for being the victim of abuse is female gender; actions by men against women tend to be much more aggressive, more numerous, and more severe than actions by women against men

C.   Data regarding partner violence against heterosexual men, gay men, and lesbians is largely lacking but clinical experience confirms that such violence does exist, but on a much smaller scale than violence against women that is perpetrated by men

D.   Physical indicators of abuse:
      1.   Injuries to victims can be of many types, but most commonly involve the head, neck, and torso
      2.   Complaints such as chronic pain, headaches, sleep disturbances may be the presenting complaint when there has been an injury

E.   Behavioral indicators of abuse:
      1.   Most primary care visits by victims of abuse are for stress-related conditions rather than for physical trauma
      2.   Psychological symptoms that derive from abuse include depression, anxiety, and suicide attempts
      3.   Alcohol or drug abuse may also be present
      4.   Many times abuse begins or escalates during pregnancy

IV.   Diagnosis/Evaluation

A.   History
      1.   Obtain social history including current living arrangements and significant relationships
      2.   Screening for domestic violence should be incorporated into every health maintenance visit (or visit for acute care if patient presents with a stress-related illness); patient should be interviewed alone without partner present.   One approach is to ask the SAFE questions (see SAFE QUESTIONS table)

SAFE QUESTIONS	
Stress/Safety	What stresses do you have in your relationship with your partner? How do you handle disagreements? Do you feel safe in your relationship with (name spouse/partner)? Should I be concerned for your safety?
Afraid	Are there situations in which you feel afraid? Have you ever been threatened or abused? Has your partner forced you to have sexual intercourse that you did not want?
Friends/Family	✓ If positive responses to items above: Ask "Are your friends/family aware that this is happening?" ✓ If negative responses to items above: Ask "Do you think you could tell them if it did happen?" "Would they help you?"
Emergency Plan	✓ Do you have a safe place to go in an emergency situation? ✓ If you are in danger now, would you like me to help you find a shelter? ✓ Would you like to talk with a social worker/counselor to help you develop a plan?

Any questions answered affirmatively should be followed with additional questions in order to determine the following:
- ✓ How and when mistreatment occurs
- ✓ Who perpetrates it
- ✓ How the patient copes with it
- ✓ What she plans to do to protect herself (and children)

Adapted from Ashur, M.L. (1993). Asking about domestic violence: SAFE questions (Letter to the editor). JAMA 269, 2367.

3. If physical injury is present, ask detailed questions relating to time or occurrence and how it occurred
   a. Long interval between injury and seeking help is red flag
   b. Story that is inconsistent, contradictory, or fails to adequately explain injury is red flag
   c. Maintain a high index of suspicion when there is a discrepancy between injury and its explained mechanism
   d. Injuries sustained from battering are often attributed to household injuries, such as "I fell." In such case, ask for a more detailed description of how accident occurred
4. Question about past or present medical problems, current medications
5. History should be carefully recorded; stories that change over time are suggestive of abuse -- thus, statements made as part of the initial disclosure take on added significance

B. Physical Examination
   1. Record height, weight, and blood pressure
   2. Observe behavior during exam for fearfulness, listlessness, and withdrawn behavior
   3. Inspect skin for burns, bruises, bites, and lacerations
      a. Use measuring tape and record on anatomic diagrams on chart
      b. Accidental injuries usually occur on extensor surfaces; bruises or lacerations on other areas require more careful evaluation
   4. Examine head focusing on any patchy hair loss, battle's sign (bruising over mastoid process behind ears) raccoon eyes, and blood behind the tympanic membranes. **Note:** Serious intracranial injuries caused by direct blows may have few or no external signs
   5. Examine abdomen for signs of injury. **Note:** Cutaneous signs of abdominal injury are rare: Blunt trauma to abdomen can cause serious injury difficult to detect with physical exam alone

C. Differential Diagnosis
   1. Unintended injury
   2. Self-inflicted injury

D. Diagnostic Tests: History and physical examination dictate tests

V.   Plan/Treatment

    A.   Competent adults who are experiencing abusive treatment may present for health care, but may refuse to leave their living situation or take legal action
        1.   Victims of long term abuse may not be psychologically or practically able to change their situation
        2.   It is not helpful to insist that they do so, or to suggest that they "must like" the abuse

    B.   Whereas state laws require health care professionals to report suspected abuse or neglect involving children and elderly and disabled adults, no such reporting requirement apply to competent adults who choose to stay in abusive relationships; health care providers, however, must report to law enforcement agencies injuries inflicted by dangerous weapons such as firearms and knives

    C.   Referral to community resources is important because it gives the abused person a sense of hope; important telephone numbers of agencies should be given on plain paper (**Important**: Become familiar with local resources/reporting procedures and keep the information readily available!)

    D.   National family violence resources are listed in the following table

NATIONAL FAMILY VIOLENCE RESOURCES
✦ National Domestic Violence Hot Line: 800/799-SAFE (TDD hearing impaired: 800/787-3224)
✦ National Resource Center on Domestic Violence: 800/537-2238
✦ Department of Justice Response Center: 800/421-6770
✦ Division of violence prevention of the Centers for Disease Control and Prevention: 770/488-4646
✦ Family Violence and Sexual Assault Institute: 903/534-5100
✦ National Center for Assault Prevention: 908/369-8972
✦ National Coalition Against Domestic Violence: 303/839-1852
✦ National Council on Child Abuse and Family Violence: 800/222-2000
✦ National Institute for Violence Prevention: 508/833-0731

    E.   Encouraging the victim to involve family members or friends who are sympathetic can help decrease the isolation that victims of abuse often experience

    F.   A nonjudgmental, supportive attitude toward the victim must be maintained; such concern may eventually be pivotal in the patient's decision to take definitive action against the abusive partner

    G.   Follow Up
        1.   Confidentiality must be assured
        2.   Arrange for a safe way to follow up by telephone until situation has stabilized (at least for the present)
        3.   Ask for name of friend or family member who could be contacted if telephone contact with the patient is not possible

GRIEF

I.   Definition: A variable but normal response to loss, deprivation, injury, illness, or disenfranchisement

II.   Pathogenesis

      A.   A full depressive syndrome that is a normal reaction to loss

      B.   Persons with uncomplicated bereavement regard the feeling of depressed mood as normal and transitory

III. Clinical Presentation

      A.   Feelings of depression and associated symptoms of poor appetite, weight loss, and insomnia following loss

      B.   Feelings of guilt, if present, are usually related to things done or not done at time of death by the survivor (if the loss is via death)

      C.   Approximately 80% of persons are markedly improved in 10 weeks after the loss

      D.   Morbid preoccupation with feelings of worthlessness and prolonged functional impairment indicate abnormal grieving and the development of major depression

IV.   Diagnosis/Evaluation

      A.   History
            1.   Determine when loss occurred, how person is accepting and coping with loss
            2.   Prior experience with patient/family is crucial in making an assessment of adjustment
            3.   Ask about functional status (if able to carry out usual activities)
            4.   Ask about presence of support system
            5.   Determine if patient is able to mourn
            6.   Determine if patient is experiencing despair to the level of self-harm

      B.   Physical Examination: Not indicated

      C.   Differential Diagnosis: Major depressive disorder

      D.   Diagnostic Tests: None indicated

V.   Plan/Management

      A.   Interventions for acute grief
            1.   Encourage patient to mourn, and to express grief in ways that are consistent with the person's particular personality (people mourn differently). Message to patient should be "You have the right to mourn"
            2.   Encourage family and small group of people who knew deceased to talk about him/her in presence of the grieving patient
            3.   Emphasize that grief is normal, and the goal is not to get rid of it as quickly as possible
            4.   Recognize that your presence is the most important comfort you have to offer. Avoid the pressure to provide your own philosophy of death and loss (or to talk about your own losses). Don't worry about what to say; being present and listening are what the patient needs, not your advice. Message should be, "I care"
            5.   Provide patient tranquility but not sedation via medication (low dose lorazepam for 1-2 days may help with sleep which is always very disrupted during acute grief). Patients need to get some rest in order to cope with demands of dealing with arrangements which frequently must be made

6.   Don't use medications to interfere with the right to mourn, but to soothe, promote sleep, and relieve anxiety during the first hours after the loss

7.   Accept patient's grief for loss that conventional society may not acknowledge as very important (such as loss of pet)

8.   Recognize that providers are not equally capable of intervening effectively in situations of acute loss

B.   Return to routines: Encourage mourner to return to normal routines as soon as is practical (no more than 2 weeks between death and return to work/school)

C.   Physical exercise: Recommend daily exercise which can be very beneficial in dealing with depression

D.   Support groups: Some families benefit from sharing with a group; others do not; prior knowledge about family functioning should guide referral

E.   Patient or family with significant preexistent psychopathology cannot be expected to adjust in the same way as healthy persons and should be referred for counseling

F.   Discourage use of psychotropic drugs except for the first 1-2 days after loss; most often, pressure to treat the primary mourner with medications comes from secondary mourners (those for whom the death causes far less grief, but who also suffer)

I.   Follow Up: Frequently by telephone/mail over the period of acute grief during first few weeks; can offer checkup during the first nine months, depending on mourner's wishes or needs. Be alert for delayed grief reaction. These reactions may occur close to anniversary of a death (anniversary reaction)

INSOMNIA

I.   Definition: Sleep that is unrefreshing or nonrestorative as well as a persistent difficulty in falling or staying asleep

II.   Pathogenesis

A.   Sleep disorders have been given the acronym DIMS (*d*isorders of *i*nitiating and *m*aintaining *s*leep)

B.   Insomnia is classified according to duration: transient or chronic insomnia
1.   Transient insomnia lasts only a few days and is generally due to situational stress, acute medical illness, jet lag, or self-medication
2.   Chronic insomnia lasts for >4 weeks and the etiology is multifactorial

C.   Generally, causes of insomnia can be categorized as follows:
1.   Drug-induced insomnia from both nonprescription drugs (alcohol, decongestants, caffeine) and prescription drugs (for example, thyroid hormones, β-agonists, β-blockers, stimulating tricyclics)
2.   Psychiatric disorders such as mood or anxiety disorders
3.   Acute or chronic stress such as associated with loss
4.   Medical conditions including gastrointestinal, cardiac, genitourinary, respiratory, endocrine, CNS, MSK conditions, as well as pain from any cause
5.   Disordered circadian rhythms, such as from jet lag, shift work
6.   Sleep disordered breathing, as may occur in obesity or obstructed breathing
7.   Nocturnal myoclonus, associated with restlessness of the legs
8.   Primary sleep disorder with difficulty initiating or maintaining sleep with no apparent underlying cause

III.   Clinical Presentation

A.   Approximately 30 percent of adults in the US experience either transient or chronic insomnia, and about 20 percent of that group consult a clinician for the problem

B.   Divorced, separated, and widowed persons have insomnia more often than married persons

C.   Complaints about insomnia increase with age, so that up to 65% of the elderly suffer from insomnia at some point
1.   Alterations in the stages of sleep occur as a normal part of the aging process; older persons get less deep delta sleep and more lighter stage 1 sleep, and frequently return to consciousness during the night
2.   Elderly people spend more time in bed, take longer to fall asleep, have increased nocturnal wakefulness, and experience more sleepiness during the day than do younger adults

D.   Persons who abuse alcohol often have no difficulty in falling asleep but have early morning insomnia

E.   Patients with an underlying psychiatric disorder may complain about feeling irritable, having difficulty falling asleep, and being tired all the time; insomnia may be chief complaint in many psychiatric disorders

F.   Diagnosis of chronic primary insomnia requires that the following be present:
1.   Difficulty in initiating or maintaining sleep or the presence (for at least one month) of nonrestorative sleep that results in marked impairment in social or occupational functioning
2.   Disturbance is not due to another sleep or mental disorder, or the effects of a drug or medical condition
3.   A diagnosis of exclusion that is reached after more specific medical and psychiatric diagnoses have been ruled out

IV.   Diagnosis/Evaluation

A.   History
1.   Ask about onset, duration of problem, and whether onset is linked with a specific event/situation. (Transient insomnia may be related to recent change in person's life; search for any recent changes at home or work, use of medications, use of substances such as caffeine, nicotine, or alcohol)
2.   Inquire about number of hours in bed each night; pattern of insomnia (is falling asleep or staying asleep, or both, the problem)
3.   Ask about daytime napping, occupation (shift work) and travel patterns
4.   Obtain past medical and psychiatric history
5.   With patient permission, interview appropriate family members for additional data (ask whether the patient snores loudly, behaves abnormally during sleep [e.g., confused, combative] or is excessively sleepy during day)

B.   Physical Examination: Should be focused based on history

C.   Differential Diagnosis: Causes of insomnia listed under II.C. above should be ruled out Remember: Chronic primary insomnia is a diagnosis of exclusion!

D.   Diagnostic Tests: None indicated unless dictated by history and physical examination

V.   Plan/Management

A.   Treat underlying causes when present
1.   When an underlying cause such as major depression, alcohol or drug abuse, or a medical condition such as osteoarthritis causing pain is found, the underlying cause should be treated with referrals as necessary

2. When insomnia is suspected of being drug-induced, treatment by eliminating the drug (if possible), reducing the dosage, or changing the timing of the dosing may be attempted (for example, caffeine intake might be limited to the early morning)

3. When sleep-disordered breathing is suspected, refer for an evaluation that includes electroencephalographic sleep staging and simultaneous electrocardiography and monitoring of respiration and limb movements (sleep laboratory evaluation is expensive and may not be an option)

B. When no underlying cause can be found, institute educational and behavioral interventions
   1. Instruct patient to keep a log or diary for 2 weeks which includes the following:
      a. Bedtime, hours spent in bed
      b. Hours slept, number of awakenings, time of arising
      c. Estimate of sleep quality
      d. Timing and quantity of meals
      e. Use of alcohol, medications
   2. Examine sleep log or diary after 2 weeks to assess sleep patterns and problems; as appropriate and based on sleep diary, implement a behavioral intervention called stimulus-control therapy, described in the following table

---

STIMULUS-CONTROL THERAPY

Instruct patient as follows

- ✓ Go to bed only when sleepy
- ✓ Use bed only for sleeping (sex is the one exception)
- ✓ Do not read, eat, work, or watch television in bed
- ✓ If unable to go to sleep after 15-20 minutes in bed, get up, go into another room, and read with a dim light; do not watch television because the full-spectrum light produced by the TV has an arousing effect
- ✓ Do not return to bed until sleepy (goal is to reestablish the connection between the bed and sleep, rather than the bed and lying awake)
- ✓ Get out of bed at the same time each day, regardless of total hours of sleep
- ✓ Establishing a wake-up time helps to stabilize the sleep-wake schedule
- ✓ Minimize daytime napping; if absolutely necessary, a brief early-afternoon nap may be taken
- ✓ Instruct patient to avoid caffeine, nicotine, alcohol, and stimulating medications such as decongestants
- ✓ Continue to keep sleep diary

Adapted from Bootzin, R.R., & Perlis, M.L. (1992). Nonpharmacologic treatments of insomnia. Journal of Clinical Psychiatry, 53(6) suppl, 37-41.

C. Sleep restriction therapy is another behavioral intervention that may be helpful
   1. Based on limiting time in bed to the actual time spent sleeping (sleep efficiency)
   2. To use this method, first determine patient's present level of sleep efficiency, which is the percentage of time in bed that is spent sleeping (Example: patient who is in bed for 8 hours, 4 hours of which are spent in actual sleep has a sleep efficiency of 50%)

SLEEP RESTRICTION THERAPY

Advise patient to do the following:

- ✓ Go to bed much later than usual
- ✓ Stay in bed only as long as sleeping, even if it is only 4-5 hours, then get up
- ✓ This allows a "sleep debit" to accrue which increases ability to fall asleep and stay asleep
- ✓ Incrementally, increase the amount of time spent in bed, by adding 15 minutes per week to start of each night's bed time
- ✓ Instruct the patient to continue to rise at the same time (when he/she awakes)
- ✓ The goal should be that at least 85% of the time spent in bed is spent sleeping
- ✓ A sleep debit must occur so that falling asleep and staying asleep will be likely

Adapted from Speilman, A.J., Saskin, P., & Thorpy, M.J. (1987). Treatment of insomnia by restricting time in bed. Sleep, 10(1), 45-55.

D. Supplement both Stimulus-Control and Sleep-Restriction Therapies with education about good health practices such as eating a healthy diet, avoiding substance use (nicotine, caffeine, alcohol), the benefits of exercise, and the role of environmental factors such as light, noise, and temperature that can be detrimental to sleep

E.   Recommend the following book for self-help:

<table>
<tr><td colspan="1">SELF-HELP FOR SLEEP DISORDERS</td></tr>
<tr><td>Karvey, N.B. (1995). <u>Practical book of remedies: 50 ways to sleep better.</u> Lincolnwood, IL: Publication International. To order, call (800) 745-9299</td></tr>
</table>

F.   Consider prescribing medications which have a limited role in insomnia treatment

G.   General principles can guide the rational use of pharmacotherapeutic management of chronic insomnia
1.   Use the lowest effective dose
2.   Prescribe for short-term use only (3-4 weeks)
3.   Use every other night or every third night rather than nightly
4.   Discontinue gradually and be alert for rebound insomnia
5.   Agents with shorter half lives are preferred in order to decrease daytime sedation

H.   Commonly prescribed sedative agents are contained in the following table

AGENTS COMMONLY PRESCRIBED TO TREAT INSOMNIA

Medication	Usual Therapeutic Dose (mg/day)		Time Until Onset in Minutes	Elimination Half Life	Comments
	Adult	Elderly >65			
Benzodiazepines					
Triazolam (Halcion)	0.125-0.250	0.125	15-30	1.5-5	Short acting and good for onset insomnia; withdrawal may occur
Temazepam (Restoril)	15 - 30	7.5 - 15	45-60	3-20	Intermediate acting and good for frequent wakening; less effective for sleep onset problems
Flurazepam (Dalmane)	15 - 30	Avoid using in elderly	45-60	40-250	Accumulation and daytime sedation are common
Estazolam (ProSom)	1- 2	0.5 - 1	30-45	8-24	Newer agent with acceptable efficacy; daytime sedation is a problem
Quazepam (Doral)	7.5 - 15	7.5	45-60	40-75	Newer agent with acceptable efficacy; daytime sedation is a problem
Nonbendodiazepines					
Zolpidem (Ambien)	5 - 10	5	30	1.5 - 4.5	Low abuse potential and does not encourage tolerance or disturb sleep architecture
Trazodone (Desyrel)	50 - 150	25 - 100	30 - 60	5 - 9	Good for antidepressant-induced insomnia (e.g., fluoxetine) Use of this drug as a hypnotic agent is not an indication approved by FDA

I.   In prescribing these drugs, adhere to the basic principles for rational pharmacotherapy for insomnia listed above

J.   Caution: Do not prescribe these medications for use by pregnant women, persons with possible sleep apnea, and patients with renal and hepatic insufficiency

K.   As with all medications, consult the PDR for specific prescribing recommendations, contraindications, and adverse reactions

L.   Follow Up
    1.   In 2 weeks to examine sleep diary and in 1 month to re-evaluate usefulness of whichever behavioral recommendation was prescribed first (either stimulus-control or sleep-restriction therapy)
    2.   If stimulus-control therapy was implemented and failed, recommend sleep-restriction therapy next, and re-evaluate in 1 month
    3.   If no improvement, and other underlying causes have been ruled out, refer to sleep laboratory for evaluation if that is an option

REFERENCES

American Academy of Child and Adolescent Psychiatry. (1997). Practice parameters for the assessment and treatment of children and adolescents with anxiety disorders. Journal of American Academy of Child and Adolescent Psychiatry, 36(10 Suppl), 69s-84s.

American Psychiatric Association. (1994). Diagnostic and statistical manual of mental disorders (4th ed.). Washington, DC: Author.

Bhatia, S.C., & Bhatia, S.K. (1997). Major depression: Selecting safe and effective treatment. American Family Physician, 55, 1683-1694.

Blazer, D.G., Grossberg, GT., & Pollock, B.G. (1998, May). Managing depression in the elderly. Patient Care, 73-97.

Block, M., Gelenberg, A.J., & Malone, D.A. (1997, March). Rational use of the newer antidepressants. Patient Care, 49-77.

Bootzin, R.R., & Perlis, M.L. (1992). Nonpharmacologic treatment of insomnia. Journal of Clinical Psychiatry, 536 (Suppl), 37-41.

Brummel-Smith, K., Rubenstein, L.Z., & Whitehouse, P.J. (1998, May). A practical guide to screening and assessment. Patient Care, 31-67.

Buckman, R., Lipkin, M., Dourkes, B.M., & Tolle, S.W. (1997, June). Strategies and skills for breaking bad news. Patient Care, 61-72.

Cole, S., & Raju, M. (1996). Making the diagnosis of depression in the primary care setting. American Journal of Medicine, 101 (Suppl. 6A), 10s-25s.

Douglass, A.B., & Aldrich, M.S. (1997). Insomnia and sleep disorders. In D.J. Knesper, M.B. Riba, & T.L. Schwenk (Eds.), Primary care psychiatry. Philadelphia: Saunders.

Eyler, A.E., Cohen, M., & Kershaw, M.O. (1997). Domestic violence and abuse. In D.J. Knesper, M.B. Riba, & T.L. Schwenk (Eds.), Primary care psychiatry. Philadelphia: Saunders.

Greden, J.F., & Schwenk, T.L. (1997). Major mood disorders. In D.J. Knesper, M.B. Riba, & T.L. Schwenk (Eds.), Primary care psychiatry. Philadelphia: Saunders.

Hooberman, R.E. (1998). Psychotherapy in the context of primary care. The Female Patient, 23, 23-28.

Kaplan, H.I., & Sadock, B.J. (1996). Pocket handbook of clinical psychiatry (2nd ed.). Baltimore: Williams & Wilkins.

Katerndahl, D.A. (1997). Panic disorder. Postgraduate Medicine, 10, 147-166.

Kupfer, D.J., & Reynolds, C.F. (1997). Management of insomnia. New England Journal of Medicine, 336, 341-345.

Lebowitz, B.D., Pearson, J.L., Schneider, L.S., Reynold, C.F., Bruce, M.L., Conwell, Y., & Katz, T.R. (1997). Diagnosis and treatment of depression in late life: Consensus statement update. Journal of the American Medical Association, 278, 1186-1190.

Marshall, J.R. (1997). Panic disorder: A treatment update. Journal of Clinical Psychiatry, 58(1), 36-42.

Monane, M. (1992). Insomnia in the elderly. Journal of Clinical Psychiatry, 536 (suppl), 45-55.

Morgan, C. (1997). Anxiety. In L. M. Rucker (Ed.), Practice of adult ambulatory medicine. Baltimore: Williams & Wilkins.

Neese., R.M., & Zamorski, M.A. (1997). Anxiety disorders in primary care. In D.J. Knesper, M.B. Riba, & T.L. Schwenk (Eds.), Primary care psychiatry. Philadelphia: Saunders.

Neufeld, B. (1996). SAFE questions: Overcoming barriers to the detection of domestic violence. <u>American Family Physician, 53</u> (8), 2575-2580.

Pelayo, R., & Yuen, K.M. (1997). Insomnia. In L. M. Rucker (Ed.), <u>Practice of adult ambulatory medicine</u>. Baltimore: Williams & Wilkins.

Pollack, M.H., Smoller, J.W., & Lee, D.K. (1998). Approach to the anxious patient. In T.A. Stern, J.B. Herman, & P.L. Slavin (Eds.), <u>The MGH guide to psychiatry in primary care</u>. New York: McGraw-Hill.

Reade, J. (1998). Approach to domestic violence. In T.A. Stern, J.B. Herman, & P.L. Slavin (Eds.), <u>The MGH guide to psychiatry in primary care</u>. New York: McGraw-Hill.

Redmond, G. (1997). Mood disorders in the female patient. <u>International Journal of Fertility, 42</u>(2), 67-72.

Rosenbaum, J.F., & Fava, M. (1998). Approach to the patient with depression. In T.A. Stern, J.B. Herman, & P.L. Slavin (Eds.), <u>The MGH guide to psychiatry in primary care</u>. New York: McGraw-Hill.

Shua-haim, J.R., Sabo, M.R., Comsti, E., & Gross, J.S. (1997). Depression in the elderly. <u>Hospital Medicine, 33</u>(7), 45-58.

Spielman, A.J., Saskin, P., & Thorpy, M.J. (1987). Treatment of insomnia by restriction of time in bed. <u>Sleep, 10</u>(1), 45-55.

Valenstein, M.V., & Klinkman, M.S. (1997). Minor depression. In D.J. Knesper, M.B. Riba, & T.L. Schwenk (Eds.), <u>Primary care psychiatry</u>. Philadelphia: Saunders.

Vanderhoff, B.T., & Miller, K.L. (1997). Major depression: Assessing the role of new antidepressants. <u>American Family Physician, 55</u>(1), 249-254.

VanDerPol, C.A., Setter, S.M., & Hunter, K.A. (1996). Depression in community dwelling elders. <u>Postgraduate Medicine, 103</u>(3), 165-174.

Vasquez, L.S. (1997). Depression. In L. M. Rucker (Ed.), <u>Practice of adult ambulatory medicine</u>. Baltimore: Williams & Wilkins.

Weilburg, J.B., & Richter, J.M. (1998). Approach to the patient with disordered sleep. In T.A. Stern, J.B. Herman, & P.L. Slavin (Eds.), <u>The MGH guide to psychiatry in primary care</u>. New York: McGraw-Hill.

Weisman, A. (1998). The patient with acute grief. In T.A. Stern, J.B. Herman, & P.L. Slavin (Eds.), <u>The MGH guide to psychiatry in primary care</u>. New York: McGraw-Hill.

Wells, B.G., DiPiro, J.T., Schwinghammer, T.L., & Hamilton, C.W. (1998). <u>Pharmacotherapy handbook</u>. Stanford, CT: Appleton & Lange.

CHAPTER 5

Metabolic and Endocrine Problems

DIABETES MELLITUS

I. Definition: Group of metabolic diseases characterized by hyperglycemia from defects in insulin secretion, insulin action, or both

II. Pathogenesis; etiologic classification of diabetes mellitus (DM)

A. Type 1 [formerly known as insulin-dependent (IDDM), or juvenile-onset diabetes] due to β-cell destruction which usually results in absolute insulin deficiency; can be either of the following forms:
    1. Immune-mediated
    2. Idiopathic

B. Type 2 [formerly known as non-insulin dependent type (NIDDM) or adult-onset diabetes]
    1. Characterized by resistance to the action of insulin; also, may have impairment of insulin secretion
    2. Risk factors include the following:
        a. Family history of diabetes
        b. >20% over ideal body weight
        c. Race (American Indian, Hispanic, or African American)
        d. Age >45 years
        e. Plus any of the following factors: previously diagnosed impaired glucose tolerance (IGT), hypertension or hyperlipidemia, women with a history of gestational diabetes mellitus or who have delivered babies >9 pounds
    3. Some obese adolescents may have this type

C. Other specific types of diabetes
    1. Genetic defects in β-cell function
    2. Genetic defects in insulin action
    3. Diseases of the exocrine pancreas (pancreatitis, trauma, infection, pancreatectomy, and pancreatic carcinoma)
    4. Endocrinopathies such as acromegaly, Cushing's syndrome, pheochromocytoma
    5. Drug or chemical-induced diabetes (thiazide diuretics, steroids, phenytoin, nicotinic acid, thyroid hormones, α-interferon)
    6. Infections such as congenital rubella or cytomegalovirus
    7. Uncommon forms of immune-mediated diabetes ("stiff man" syndrome and anti-insulin receptor antibodies)
    8. Other genetic syndromes such as Down's syndrome, Klinefelter's syndrome and Turner's syndrome

D. Gestational diabetes mellitus (GDM): Glucose intolerance with onset during pregnancy (will not be discussed further in this section)

E. Impaired glucose tolerance (IGT): Plasma glucose levels are higher than normal but not diagnostic of diabetes mellitus; intermediate stage between glucose homeostasis and diabetes

III. Clinical Presentation

A. Criteria for diagnosing diabetes mellitus (see following table)

DIAGNOSTIC CRITERIA FOR DIABETES MELLITUS*
✔ Symptoms of diabetes (polydipsia, polyuria, and weight loss) plus casual plasma glucose concentration ≥200 mg/dl (11.1 mmol/l); "casual" is any time of day without regard to time since last meal   **OR**   ✔ Fasting plasma glucose (FPG) ≥126 mg/dl (7.0 mmol/l); "fasting" is no caloric intake for at least 8 hours   **OR**   ✔ 2 hour plasma glucose ≥200 mg/dl during a oral glucose tolerance tests (OGTT); OGTT should be performed using a glucose load containing the equivalent of 75-g anhydrous glucose

*These criteria should be confirmed by repeat testing on a different day except in the case of unequivocal hyperglycemia with acute metabolic decompensation

Adapted from American Diabetes Association. (1998). Report of the Expert Committee on the diagnosis and classification of diabetes mellitus. Diabetes Care, 21,(Supp. 1), S5-S19

B. Criteria for diagnosing impaired fasting glucose (IFG) or IGT, respectively: FBG ≥110 mg/dL (6.1 mmol/l) and < 126 mg/dl (7.0 mmol/l) or 2-hour glucose ≥140 (7.8 mmol/l) and <200 mg/dL (11.1 mmol/l)

C. Type 1 diabetes
 1. Occurs in approximately 10% of all persons diagnosed with diabetes
 2. Usually appears with acute onset of symptoms: polydipsia, polyphagia, polyuria, weight loss, blurred vision, and frequent infections such as dermatologic fungal infections
 3. After the initial presentation of symptoms, the newly diagnosed patient often undergoes a "honeymoon" period or remission phase which may last from several months to 2 years
 4. Ketoacidosis rarely occurs today due to good diagnostic testing; symptoms in severe cases include dehydration, Kussmaul respirations, fruity or acetone odor to breath, and impaired consciousness
 5. Can occur at any age (rarely after age 30) with highest incidence between ages 10-14 years

D. Type 2 diabetes
 1. Occurs mainly in adults >30 years of age
 2. Gradual onset and slow progression of symptoms
  a. Many patients are asymptomatic and have diabetes for numerous years before they are diagnosed
  b. Frequently, these patients already have complications when they are diagnosed
 3. Fatigue is a common symptom
 4. Initially, these patients do not need insulin to survive, but approximately 50% of patients will eventually require insulin
 5. Ketoacidosis rarely occurs except in times of stress, illness or infection
 6. Hyperglycemic hyperosmolar nonketotic coma occurs predominantly in type 2 diabetics
  a. Characterized by blood glucose >600 mg/dl, minimal ketosis, serum osmolality >340 and profound dehydration
  b. Often precipitated by hyperglycemic-inducing drugs (steroids, diuretics), therapeutic procedures (surgery, dialysis, hyperalimentation), chronic disease, and acute stress
 7. Patients with undiagnosed Type 2 diabetes are at risk for coronary heart disease, stroke, peripheral vascular disease, dyslipidemia, and hypertension

E. Impaired glucose tolerance (IGT)
 1. Patients are asymptomatic and are at risk for developing coronary heart disease and diabetes
 2. IGT is associated with insulin resistance syndrome which is also known at syndrome X or the metabolic syndrome

F. Macrovascular and microvascular complications occur in Type 1 and Type 2 diabetes of sufficient duration
   1. Retinopathy is the leading cause of new adult blindness in U.S.
      a. Background retinopathy or nonproliferative retinopathy involves microaneurysms and dot hemorrhages but does not impair vision unless it involves the macula
      b. Retinopathy often develops 7 years before clinical diagnosis is made
      c. Occurs in almost every patient who has had diabetes for 10-20 years or more
      d. Proliferative retinopathy can lead to blindness and involves neovascularization (new vessels develop) with retinal detachment and vitreous hemorrhages; occurs in 60-70%% of patients with Type 1 and 30% of patients with Type 2 diabetes
   2. Nephropathy
      a. Develops in 35-45% of patients with Type 1 and 20% with Type 2
      b. Progresses from the development of microalbuminuria to overt proteinuria and finally to end-stage renal disease(ESRD) (this process may take as long as 23 years); diabetes is the most common single cause of ESRD in U.S.
   3. Neuropathy
      a. Most common manifestation is a peripheral, symmetric sensorimotor neuropathy which is usually only minimally uncomfortable
      b. A minority of patients have painful peripheral neuropathy with lancinating or burning pain
      c. Autonomic neuropathy may affect gastric or intestinal motility, erectile function, bladder function, cardiac function, and vascular tone
   4. Cardiovascular Disease: Diabetes is a major risk factor
   5. Other complications include an increased prevalence of infections, cognitive impairment, and contractures of digits (Hammer toes)

IV. Diagnosis/Evaluation

A. History
   1. To establish the diagnosis, explore the following:
      a. Symptoms such as fatigue and complications associated with diabetes
      b. Explore family history of diabetes and other endocrine problems
      c. With adult females, ask about gestational history including the weight and condition of all babies, and whether complications occurred during pregnancy or at the time of labor and delivery
   2. In patients who are already diagnosed, inquire about the following:
      a. Frequency, severity, and cause of hypoglycemia or ketoacidosis
      b. Symptoms and treatments of chronic eye, kidney, nerve, genitourinary (including sexual), bladder, gastrointestinal function, heart, peripheral vascular, foot, and cerebrovascular complications
      c. Prior or current infections
      d. Previous and current pharmacological, nutritional, and self-management treatment plans
      e. Patterns and results of glucose monitoring
      f. Dietary habits (especially amount of carbohydrates such as juices), nutritional status, and weight history
      g. Amount, intensity, and frequency of exercise
      h. Risk factors for atherosclerosis such as smoking, hypertension, obesity
      i. Psychological, sociological and economic factors that may impact on management plan

B. Physical Examination
   1. Measure height and weight (and compare to norms)
   2. Determine vital signs including orthostatic blood pressure measurements
   3. Examine skin including sites of previous insulin administration if applicable
   4. Complete a thorough ophthalmoscopic examination (best done with dilation)
   5. Perform a thorough mouth and dental examination
   6. Palpate thyroid

7. Perform complete cardiac examination
8. Palpate and auscultate pulses
9. Perform abdominal examination; check for liver enlargement
10. Assess hand and wrist mobility, checking for contractures
11. Carefully examine feet
12. Perform complete neurological exam
13. May need to do a complete physical exam to exclude any sources of occult infection

C. Differential Diagnosis
1. Glucosuria without hyperglycemia occurs in benign renal glucosuria or in renal tubular disease
2. Diabetes insipidus presents with polyuria and polydipsia but not hyperglycemia
3. Transient hyperglycemia is present when patients have severe stress from trauma, burns or infection or are on glucocorticoids

D. Diagnostic Tests
1. Screening tests to detect diabetes in asymptomatic, undiagnosed individuals (see table); American Diabetic Association recommends the following:

SCREENING CRITERIA
✦ Testing should be considered in all individuals ≥45 years and, if normal, it should be repeated at 3-year intervals
✦ Testing should be considered at a younger age or be performed more frequently in individuals who
• are obese (≥120% desirable body weight or a BMI ≥ 27 kg/m²)
• have a first-degree relative with diabetes
• are members of a high-risk ethnic population (e.g., African-American, Hispanic-American, Native American, Asian-American, Pacific Islander)
• have delivered a baby weighing >9 lb or have been diagnosed with GDM
• are hypertensive (≥140/90)
• have an HDL cholesterol level ≤ 35 mg/dl (0.90 mmol/l) and/or a triglyceride level ≥250 mg/dl (2.82 mmol/l)
• on previous testing, had IGT or IFG
✦ Fasting Plasma Glucose (FPG) is test of choice (fast for 8 hours prior to test)
✦ If FPG is ≥126 mg/dl, repeat test on different day to confirm diagnosis

Adapted from American Diabetes Association. (1998). Report of the Expert Committee on the diagnosis and classification of diabetes mellitus. Diabetes Care, 21,(Supp. 1), S5-S19

a. Random plasma glucose measurements can be made when food or drink has been ingested within 3 hours preceding test; ≥200 mg/dL is considered a positive screening test and the diagnosis of diabetes should be confirmed with an additional test, preferably a fasting plasma glucose (FPG) test
b. Screening for autoantibodies related to type 1 diabetes is not recommended outside the context of research studies
c. Consider screening lean new-onset diabetic patients for type 1 diabetes by measuring postprandial serum C peptide
2. Tests to determine the degree of glycemic control
a. Glycosylated hemoglobin (HbA₁ or HbA₁C)
(1) Reflects mean glucose levels for the preceding 2-3 months
(2) Order at least every 6 months for well-controlled patients
(3) Order more often (every 3 months) in diabetics with poor control or when beginning new therapies
(4) Levels <7.5% indicate good diabetic control
(5) Falsely elevated levels may occur in presence of uremia, alcoholism, and aspirin use
b. Glycated serum protein indicates glycemic control in a short period of time and needs to be performed monthly; currently this test is not recommended
3. Tests helpful in defining associated complications and risk factors:
a. Order fasting lipid profile: total cholesterol, high-density lipoprotein (HDL) cholesterol, low density lipoprotein (LDL) cholesterol, and triglycerides
(1) Order when diabetes is first diagnosed
(2) Order annually; patients with borderline or abnormal values require additional testing

b.　Order annual serum creatinine
c.　Order annual urinalysis: ketones, glucose, protein, sediment
　　(1)　If protein is positive, a quantitative measure should be performed
　　(2)　If protein is negative a test for the presence of microalbuminuria is necessary (see IV.D.3.d), which immediately follows
d.　Testing for microalbuminuria
　　(1)　In adults with Type 2 diabetes, test at the time of diagnosis
　　(2)　Because microalbuminuria rarely occurs with short duration of type 1 diabetes or before puberty, individuals with type 1 diabetes should begin testing with puberty and after 5 years duration
　　(3)　Because of marked day-to-day variability in albumin excretion, at least two of three collections measured in a 3- to 6-month period should show elevated levels before arriving at a diagnosis of microalbuminuria
　　(4)　Testing for microalbuminuria can be performed by 3 methods
　　　　(a)　Measurement of the albumin-to-creatinine ratio in a random, spot collection
　　　　(b)　24 hour collection with serum creatinine which allows for simultaneous measurement of creatinine clearance
　　　　(c)　Timed collection such as 4 hours or overnight
　　(5)　Microalbuminuria and clinical albuminuria is defined in following table

DEFINITIONS OF ABNORMALITIES IN ALBUMIN EXCRETION			
Category	24-h Collection	Timed Collection	Spot Collection
Normal	<30 mg/24 h	<20 μg/min	< 30 μg/mg creatinine
Microalbuminuria	30-300 mg/24 h	20-200 μg/min	30-300 μg/mg creatinine
Clinical albuminuria	>300 mg/24 h	>200 μg/min	>300 μg/mg creatinine
Two of three specimens collected within a 3- to 6-month period should be abnormal before considering a patient to have crossed one of these diagnostic threshholds. Exercise within 24 hours of infection, fever, congestive heart failure, marked hyperglycemia, and marked hypertension may elevate urinary albumin excretion over baseline values			

Adapted from American Diabetes Association. (1998). Diabetic nephropathy. Diabetes Care, 21, (Supp. 1), S50-S53.

e.　In type 1 patients, order T_4 and thyroid stimulating hormone; order in type 2 patients if clinical presentation indicates a need
f.　Order ECG when diagnosed and then periodically depending on risk factors and symptomatology
g.　Some, but not all authorities, also suggest regular serum BUN and CBC tests
4.　Diabetic ketoacidosis presents with reduced plasma bicarbonate, reduced blood pH, increased anion gap, and hyperlipidemia; hyperkalemia often occurs with significant metabolic acidosis

V.　Plan/Management

A.　The Diabetes Control and Complications Trial (DCCT), a long-term, multi-center trial, found that type 1 diabetics with tight glycemic control of their plasma glucose had a significant reduction in their risk for developing diabetic retinopathy, nephropathy, and neuropathy when compared with the standard treatment groups; the U.K. Prospective Diabetes Study found that tight glycemic control reduced diabetes-related (particularly macrovascular) events in type 2 diabetics
1.　Degree of tight glycemic control must be individualized and balanced with the risk of developing hypoglycemia; be cautious in advising tight control to elderly patients with significant atherosclerosis who may be particularly vulnerable to permanent damage from hypoglycemia
2.　Goals of glycemic control are shown in the following the table

GLYCEMIC CONTROL			
Measurement	Nondiabetic	Goal	Additional action suggested*
Preprandial glucose (mg/dl)**	<110	80-120	<80 or >140
Bedtime glucose (mg/dl)**	<120	100-140	<100 or >160
Glycosylated hemoglobin	<6	<7	>8

*Additional action must be individualized. Actions may be referral to endocrinologist, change in medications, self-management education, etc.
**Measurement of capillary blood glucose

Adapted from American Diabetes Association. (1998). Standards of medical care for patients with diabetes mellitus. Diabetes Care, 21,(Supp. 1), S23-S31.

B. Hospitalization is recommended for patients with ketoacidosis or hyperosmolar nonketotic coma

C. All diabetic patients benefit from medical nutritional therapy (MNT), exercise, and extensive patient education
  1. Type 1 diabetics also require insulin therapy
  2. Type 2 diabetics may be controlled with diet and exercise alone, however, oral antidiabetic agents and, in some cases, insulin may be needed for blood glucose control

D. Patient education is essential; education must be integrated with all aspects of the plan (also, see patient education in each of the following sections)
  1. Discuss basic pathophysiology of diabetes
  2. Explain long-term complications of diabetes, emphasizing that recent research indicates that these complications can be prevented or delayed when blood glucose is well controlled
  3. Encourage patient to wear Medic-Alert tags

E. Nutritional recommendations: Diet is an important aspect of the treatment plan and collaboration or referral to a dietician is beneficial
  1. Currently, there is no one "diabetic" diet or meal plan; medical nutrition therapy (MNT) should be individualized
  2. Patients with Type 1 diabetes:
    a. Cannot be treated with diet alone
    b. Monitor blood glucose levels and adjust insulin based on the amount of food usually consumed; individuals on intensified insulin programs can make adjustments in rapid or lispro insulin to cover carbohydrate content of meals and/or snacks and for deviations from typical eating and exercising habits
    c. Plan meals to provide the amount of calories and nutrients that are expected to be metabolized when insulin is administered
      (1) Keep timing and amount of calories and nutrients in meals the same each day
      (2) Have a consistent, daily pattern of exercise and physical activity (may need supplemental snacks before and after exercise; may need to alter insulin dosage before activity)
    d. Carbohydrate counting in which the patient takes insulin based on the amount of insulin consumed for a meal may be effective; approximately 1 unit of insulin will cover 10-15 grams of carbohydrate consumed
    e. Patients of various ages have different caloric needs (see following table)

GUIDELINES FOR CALCULATING CALORIE REQUIREMENTS		
Age	**Gender**	**Calories**
15-20 years	Female	13-15 calories/pound desired body weight
	Male	15-18 calories/pound desired body weight
Adults:	Male & Female	
Physically Active		14-16 calories/pound desired body weight
Moderately Active		12-14 calories/pound desired body weight
Sedentary		10-12 calories/pound desired body weight

Adapted from Bode, B.W., Davidson, P.C., & Steed, R.D. (1997). In J.S. Skyler. <u>Diabetes Dek: Professional Edition.</u> Infodek: Atlanta.

3. Patients with type 2 diabetes can often improve blood glucose levels by moderate weight loss (5-9 kg or 10-20 lb) and hypocaloric diets (250-500 calories less than average daily intake as calculated from diet history) **alone**; spacing of meals throughout day and regular exercise can also improve control

4. Dietary recommendations for both types of diabetics include the following:
   a. Carbohydrates should make up approximately 50-60% of the total calories; unrefined carbohydrates and fiber should be eaten whenever possible
   b. Protein intake should be the recommended dietary allowance for Americans or about 10-20% of daily calories
   c. Total fat should comprise <30% of total calories with saturated fats restricted to <10% of total calories and cholesterol <300 mg/day; unsaturated fats should replace saturated fats
   d. Patients can use nutritive and nonnutritive sweeteners
   e. Balance in salt is needed with upper limit of 3000 mg/day but recognizing that sodium restriction may lead to electrolyte imbalance

F. Exercise recommendations: Exercise positively affects the levels of blood glucose by increasing metabolism and over an extended period can reduce insulin resistance
   1. Exercise program should be started after an appropriate health exam which focuses on heart, blood vessels, eyes, kidneys and nervous system
   2. A graded exercise test should be performed on patients at high risk for cardiovascular disease
   3. Patients who have complications of the eye, kidney, and autonomic neuropathy should avoid strenuous exercise
   4. Patients with peripheral neuropathy or problems with their feet should take precautionary measures such as proper footware
   5. For patients on insulin therapy, the following guidelines are helpful
      a. Avoid exercising at times when insulin is at its peak action
      b. Monitor blood glucose before and after exercise to identify when changes in insulin or food intake are necessary and to learn glycemic response to different exercise conditions
      c. Avoid exercise if FPG levels are <80 mg/dl or >250 mg/dl and ketosis is present or if glucose levels are >300 mg/dl, regardless of whether ketosis is present
      d. Ingest added carbohydrates if glucose levels are <100 mg/dl
      e. Eat added carbohydrates as needed to avoid hypoglycemia; keep carbohydrate-based food readily available during and after exercise; in general, one serving of carbohydrates increases plasma glucose about 40 points
      f. Avoid exercising extremities in which insulin has recently been injected
      g. For patient's with type 2 diabetes, exercise should be a high priority; benefit is probably greatest when it begun early in course of disease

G. Insulin therapy: Goals of normalized glycohemoglobin must be balanced with risks of hypoglycemia; insulin is required for management of type 1 diabetes and in some patients with type 2 diabetes
   1. Consider type of insulin to use
      a. If patients are on beef or pork insulin, do not switch if they are well-controlled
      b. Newly diagnosed diabetics should be on human insulin because of its lower incidence of insulin allergy, resistance, and lipoatrophy (see following table for brand names of human insulin)
   2. Use U-100 insulin
   3. Consider onset, peak, and duration of various insulin preparations (see following table)

VARIOUS HUMAN INSULIN PREPARATIONS			
Type	Onset (hours)	Peak (hours)	Duration (hours)
Rapid acting analog			
Humalog (Lispro)	<0.25	1	3.5-4.5
Short acting			
Humulin R	0.5	2.4	6-8
Novolin R	0.5	2.5-5	8
Velosulin BR	0.5	1-3	8
Intermediate acting			
Humulin N (NPH)	1-2	6-12	18-24
Novolin N (NPH)	1.5	4-12	24
Humulin L (Lente)	1-3	6-12	18-24
Novolin L (Lente)	2.5	7-15	22
Long acting			
Humulin U (Ultralente)	4-6	8-20	24-48
Premixed: Insulin isophane suspension (NPH)/regular insulin (R)*			
Humulin 70/30	0.5	2-12	24
Humulin 50/50	0.5	3-5	24
Novolin 70/30	0.5	2-12	24

*Do Not use premixed with Type 1 diabetics as it severely limits flexibility

   4. Initiating insulin therapy
      a. Give a total daily dose of 0.6 units per kg (others recommend 0.5-1.0 units)
      b. Give 2/3s of total dose in AM and 1/3 in evening
         (1) The morning (AM) dose should be 2/3s of intermediate insulin and 1/3 of regular insulin
         (2) The evening (PM) dose should include 50% of intermediate insulin and 50% of regular insulin
   5. Honeymoon phase: after initial therapy is instituted this phase occurs and may last 12-18 months; insulins dosages may be reduced to 0.2-0.5 units/kg/day (important to tell patients about this phase to prevent false beliefs that the diabetes is partially cured)
   6. Long-term insulin therapy
      a. Dosage: 0.6-0.8 units/kg/day; adolescents may need 1.0-1.5 units/kg/day
      b. Determine the pattern or regimen of insulin therapy (see following table)

COMMON INSULIN REGIMENS

Regimen	Dosing	Comments
2-Injection -or- Split/Mix	2/3s of total daily dosing in am 1/3 of total daily dosing in pm - then - AM - 2/3 NPH + 1/3 regular or lispro† PM - 1/2 NPH + 1/2 regular or lispro†	✦Best in Type 2 and early Type 1 ✦Disadvantages: poor peaking of noon insulin & excess insulin at night (to resolve this problem, limit noon meal and eat a bedtime snack)
3-Injection	Of total daily dose: AM* -40% NPH & 15% regular or lispro† PM** -15% regular or lispro† Bedtime -30% NPH	✦Advantage: Less risk of nighttime hypoglycemia & better control of dawn phenomenon or persistent AM hyperglycemia ✦Disadvantages: poor peaking of insulin at noon (to resolve, limit noon meal)
4-Injection or Prandial/Basal	Of total daily dose: Before each meal (Prandial insulin) -20-25% regular or lispro† At bedtime (Basal insulin) - 25-40% NPH, lente, or ultralente	✦Requires committed patient and care-provider, with frequent self-blood-glucose monitoring ✦Disadvantage: No more than 5 hours can transpire between meals ✦Advantage: Clear relationship between insulin dose and glucose level
Continuous Subcutaneous Insulin Infusion -or- Insulin Pump Therapy	-Continually delivers regular insulin or lispro -Provides both basal insulin release and adjustable pre-meal bolus release	✦Indications: Inability to control glucose with 2 or more injections; recurrent, major hypoglycemia due to hypoglycemic unawareness, loss of counter-regulatory mechanisms or variable absorption of modified insulins ✦Prerequisites: Patient must have intellectual & emotional abilities for self-care ✦Advantages: Closely resembles endogenous insulin release; results in more predictable insulin absorption and fewer dosage errors ✦Disadvantages: Expensive; blood glucose must be monitored 4 times/day

* AM is before breakfast: regular insulin should be taken 30-45 minutes before breakfast and lispro should be taken 15 minutes before breakfast
**PM is before evening meal or supper
†Lispro is often more convenient for patients because it can be injected immediately before meals and can lessen the likelihood of late post-prandial hypoglycemia and nocturnal hypoglycemia but is more expensive and needs more intensive monitoring than regular insulin

Adapted from Mengel, M.B. (1996). Diabetes mellitus. In M.B. Mengel & L.P. Schwiebert (Eds.), Ambulatory medicine (2nd ed.), pp. 412-419. Stamford, CT: Appleton & Lange.

7.   Adjusting insulin is based on daily blood glucose levels and on peak effect of a given insulin dose (patients should record their blood glucose and insulin doses with comments on a flow sheet)
   a.   Calculating adjustments: Adjustments should be made by 20% increments or decrements; for example, 1 unit for doses of 5 units or 2 units for doses of 10 units
   b.   Downward adjustments should be made the day following a "below range blood glucose" to avoid repeat hypoglycemia
   c.   Upward adjustments should be delayed for 2 days to establish a pattern
   d.   Consider timing and type of insulin when making adjustments (see following table):

ADJUSTING INSULIN THERAPY

Insulin	Affected Blood Glucose Value
AM* Intermediate	Post-lunch Pre-supper
AM* Regular	Post-breakfast Pre-lunch
PM** Intermediate	Early morning
PM** Regular	Bedtime
Bedtime Intermediate	Early morning

*AM is before breakfast
**PM is before evening meal or supper

8. In patients who have high postprandial blood glucose, acarbose therapy in combination with insulin may be beneficial (acarbose is currently the only oral antidiabetic agent that is approved for use in type 1 diabetes)
   a. Beginning dose is 25 mg QD taken with first bite of breakfast
   b. Slowly increase dosage to maximum daily dose of 100 mg with each meal
   c. Do not use with patients who are taking lispro
9. Tips on administering insulin therapy (see following table)

TIPS ON INSULIN THERAPY

★ Insulin should approximate the natural release of insulin by the beta cell
★ Administer Insulin to provide a basal amount in 40-50% of total daily dose as well as peaks after each meal
★ One time a day insulin therapy is **not** sufficient for patients with Type 1 diabetes
★ Be careful in adjusting insulin with type 1 diabetics; they are very sensitive to adjustments because they have no endogenous insulin secretion
★ Consider giving PM NPH at bedtime to reduce early morning hyperglycemia
★ Use NPH when there is a need to mix with another type of insulin
★ Consider the following when blood glucose is not controlled with insulin: malignant insulin resistance, occult infection, noncompliance, poor coping skills

---

10. Patient education concerning the administering, storage, and disposal of insulin is essential (see following table)

PATIENT EDUCATION - INSULIN THERAPY

• Insulin in use can be kept at room temperature, for one month only, to limit local irritation at injection site; unopened insulin should be refrigerated
• When mixing insulins, the clear, short-acting insulin should be drawn into syringe first
• Syringes can be prefilled and stored in a vertical position in the refrigerator for 3 weeks (do not allow if using Lispro)
• Usually, the insulin should be given 30-60 minutes before eating; lispro should be taken 15 minutes before eating
• Subcutaneously inject insulin into upper arm, anterior and lateral aspects of thigh, the buttocks and abdomen (with exception of a circle with a 2-inch radius around the navel); Do not rotate to different anatomical sites, but do make injections in different areas of one anatomical site
• Dispose syringes in resistant disposal container and contact local public health unit or local trash-disposal authority for appropriate disposal provisions
• Proper procedure of syringe reuse involves cleaning needle after use and putting in refrigerator (only teach patients who have good cognitive and psychomotor functioning)
• Syringe alternatives such as jet injectors, pen-like devices, and insulin-containing cartridges are usually expensive but may be more convenient and improve technique of insulin injection

---

H. Treatment of type 2 diabetes is based on a step-wise plan
   1. **Patients with fasting blood glucose <250 mg/dl**: initiate medical nutrition therapy (MNT) and exercise; if patient's glucose is not controlled within 3 months, advance to next step
   2. **Patients with fasting blood glucose ≥250 mg/dl and <400 mg/dl who do not have signs of dehydration, acidosis, or marked ketosis**: in addition to MNT and exercise, they should begin monotherapy with an oral antidiabetic agent (see following table); approximately 30-40% of patients do not satisfactorily respond to oral agents
      a. Precautions and contraindications for oral antidiabetic agents
         (1) Sulfonylureas: use cautiously in persons allergic to sulfa drugs, those with liver damage, renal impairment, alcohol abuse problems; contraindicated in pregnant women
         (2) Metformin: contraindicated in persons prone to acidosis, those with renal disease and those with congestive heart failure (CHF) who require drug treatment to manage their CHF; use cautiously in persons with liver dysfunction, sepsis, alcohol abuse problems, adrenal or pituitary insufficiency
         (3) α-glucosidase inhibitors: contraindicated in persons with cirrhosis and significant gastrointestinal problems; use cautiously in persons with renal dysfunction
         (4) Troglitazone: use cautiously in persons with hepatic disease (monitor ALT values regularly)

(5) Repaglinide: titrate carefully in renal and hepatic dysfunction; older age, debilitation, malnutrition, stress, adrenal or pituitary insufficiency increase the risk of hypoglycemia

		ORAL HYPOGLYCEMIC AGENTS	
Drug	**Mechanism of Action**	**Usual Maintenance Range** (doses/day)	**Major Adverse Reactions**
SULFONYLUREAS	⇑ Endogenous insulin		Hypoglycemia & Weight Gain
Long acting			
Glyburide (Micronase/Diaβeta)		1.25-20 mg (1-2)	
Glyburide micronized (Glynase PresTabs)		0.75-12 mg (1-2)	
Glipizide (Glucotrol XL)		5-10 mg (1-2)	
Intermediate			
Glipizide (Glucotrol)		2.5-25 mg (1-2)	
Glimepiride (Amaryl)		1-4 (1-2)	
METFORMIN (Glucophage)	⇓Hepatic glucose production ⇑Insulin action on muscle glucose uptake (may cause small weight loss & ⇓ serum low density lipoprotein cholesterol and triglycerides)	500-2500 mg (2-3)	-Diarrhea -⇓Serum Vit. B$_{12}$ -Lactic acidosis with incorrect dosing
α-GLUCOSIDASE INHIBITORS	Delays carbohydrate digestion & ⇓ postprandial glucose		-Flatulence & -Abdominal Discomfort
Acarbose (Precose)		25-100 (3)	
Miglitol (Glyset)		25-50 (?)	
TROGLITAZONE (Rezulin)	⇑ Insulin action on muscle and fat glucose uptake	200-400 mg (1)	-Slight ⇓ in RBCs -⇓ in estrogen & progesterone in women taking contraceptives and possibly postmenopausal women on HRT -Increased serum transaminase levels
MEGLITINIDE Repaglinide (Prandin)	⇑ Endogenous insulin	0.5-16 mg (3)	Hypoglycemia, weight gain, cold-like and flu-like symptoms

b. Selection of best oral antidiabetic agent for monotherapy
(1) Sulfonylureas are most effective when blood glucose is severely elevated; also may be first choice for lean, older persons
(a) Glyburide is agent of choice for fasting hyperglycemia
(b) Glipizide is agent of choice for postprandial hyperglycemia (take 30 minutes pre-meal for best effects)
(2) Acarbose, troglitazone, and metformin are effective for diabetics with recent onset
(3) Metformin and troglitazone may be most effective in persons who are insulin resistant (Syndrome X) (obese persons with FBG <240 mg/dl)
(4) Acarbose or miglitol may be most effective in persons with mild fasting hyperglycemia and who have predominantly postprandial hyperglycemia
(5) Repaglinide (Prandin) lowers blood glucose by stimulating the release of insulin from the pancreas (non-sulfonylurea beta-cell stimulator); has a quick onset of action and a short duration of action; take with meals
c. Begin slowly and increase dose every 1-2 weeks on the basis of self glucose monitoring until glucose is controlled

d. When glucose is controlled with a low dose, once a day dosing is recommended; when larger doses of oral agent are needed to control glucose, doses are split and given twice a day
    (1) Dosage given in morning and evening (before dinner) will depend on results of self glucose monitoring
    (2) Increase morning dose when the evening blood glucose is elevated; increase evening dose when the morning glucose is elevated
e. Treatment should continue for one month before changing to another therapy (generally takes 3-6 weeks of drug therapy to attain normoglycemia)

3. **When patient fails to respond to first antidiabetic agent**, switch to second agent of if increasing dose results in only a minimal response, consider switching to second agent

4. **If second agent also fails,** try a combination of antidiabetic agents; a logical approach is to add a drug which decreases insulin requirements with a drug that increases insulin availability; possible combinations include:
a. Sulfonylureas plus metformin
b. Sulfonylureas plus acarbose
c. Sulfonylureas plus troglitazone
d. Metformin and repaglinide

5. **If combination oral antidiabetic agent therapy fails**, replace one of oral agents with insulin
a. Continue one antidiabetic agent at current dose
b. Add 10 units of intermediate acting human insulin at bedtime or calculate .25 units/kg of ideal body weight
c. Self blood glucose monitoring is needed
d. Increase insulin 3-5 units every 3-4 days until desired fasting blood glucose is achieved
e. In elderly, use insulin as last resort because of dangers of hypoglycemia
    (1) Keep insulin patterns simple
    (2) Use premix insulins if possible to avoid errors
    (3) Consider use of prefilled insulin pens
f. It is controversial, whether oral antidiabetic agents should be continued indefinitely with insulin therapy or whether they should be slowly titrated downward and stopped
g. There also is no consensus when to discontinue insulin therapy; some authorities suggest that when blood glucose levels are controlled at acceptable targets, the insulin dosage may be tapered down and patient can be treated with no drugs or oral agent

6. **In patients with blood glucose ≥400 mg/dl or patients who have signs of dehydration, acidosis, or marked ketosis,** begin insulin therapy

I. Self-monitoring of blood glucose has replaced urine testing as a method to assess glucose control; however, Type 1 patients need to check urine for ketones whenever their blood glucose level is >300 mg/dL, during illness, stress, pregnancy or when symptoms of ketoacidosis such as nausea, vomiting, or abdominal pain are present
1. Frequent monitoring is essential when patients are on intensive insulin therapy or insulin pump therapy; monitor blood glucose before meals, at bedtime and occasionally in the middle of night
2. Less frequent monitoring may be appropriate for some patients, but even these patients should adhere to the following recommendations:
a. When medications are altered:
    (1) Patient should check blood glucose before each meal, at bedtime, and 2-4 in AM for 3 days
    (2) Next 7 days, blood glucose can be checked before breakfast and dinner
b. After glucose is initially controlled, monitoring can be once a day at different times
c. When glucose is stabilized, check 2-4 times per week at different times

J. Contingency plan for managing hypoglycemia episodes
1. Teach patient and family the signs and symptoms of hypoglycemia such as shakiness, sweating, restlessness, hunger, headache, confusion, or seizures

2. Instruct patient to carry 10-15 g of oral glucose (2 glucose tablets, 5 lifesavers, or 4 oz. of orange juice) to eat in case of a hypoglycemic reaction
3. Family or friends should be instructed in administering a subcutaneous or intramuscular injection of glucagon if patient is unresponsive or unable to swallow; dose is 1 mg
4. After consciousness is regained, patient should ingest oral carbohydrates to prevent further hypoglycemia
5. Encourage patient to carry medical identification

K. Managing diabetes when the patient is ill; difficult to predict if blood glucose will increase or decrease during sickness; teach patients the following:
1. Continue to take usual dose of insulin or oral agent
2. Perform self-blood-glucose monitoring several times a day as well as check urine for ketones (twice a day)
3. If patients are able to drink, increase intake of non-caloric fluids
4. Drink small continuous amounts of sugar-containing liquids such as Gatorade or Coke in conjunction with the readings from their self-monitoring if they are vomiting or nauseated
5. Call health care provider in following circumstances
   a. Inability to drink fluids
   b. Blood glucose is >240 mg/dl and urine is positive for ketones

L. Management of associated problems and complications. Growing recognition that tight glycemic control prevents or delays many of the following problems
1. Diabetic ketoacidosis and hyperosmolar coma usually require referral to an endocrinologist
   a. Encourage fluid intake to prevent dehydration
   b. Initial workup: electrolytes, urinalysis, serum ketones, CBC, ECG, chest x-ray
   c. Treatment is usually insulin, fluids, and potassium replacement
2. Diabetic retinopathy: Refer to ophthalmologist; laser therapy and vitrectomy have been effective
3. Nephropathy
   a. Annually screen for microalbuminuria to detect early nephropathy
   b. Patients with microalbuminuria will likely progress to clinical albuminuria (≥300 mg/24 hours) and decreasing glomerular filtration rate (GFR) over a period of years; once clinical albuminuria appears, the risk of end-stage renal failure is high in type 1 diabetes and significant in type 2 diabetes
   c. Achieving normoglycemia and lowering blood pressure have proven to delay progression of nephropathy
      (1) Prescribe a angiotensin-converting enzyme (ACE) inhibitor to all type 1 patients with microalbuminuria even if they are normotensive;
         (a) Periodically monitor potassium levels to detect an adverse drug reaction of hyperkalemia
         (b) Periodic monitor urine albumin to document the effect of treatment and to detect the rare case of adverse effects of drug therapy
      (2) Normotensive type 2 patients with microalbuminuria must be assessed individually to determine their need for an ACE inhibitor; however, if these patients develop hypertension or show progression of microalbuminuria, an ACE inhibitor should be ordered
   d. Protein intake should be approximately the adult Recommended Dietary Allowance (RDA); protein restriction should be initiated when GFR starts to fall; meal plans should be developed by a registered dietician
   e. Refer to a subspecialist in diabetic renal disease when GFR falls to <70 ml • min^{-1} • 1.73 m^{-2}, when serum creatinine is greater than 2.0 mg/dl, or there is hypertension or hyperkalemia
   f. Phosphate lowering therapies may be helpful
4. Cardiovascular disease: Needs careful monitoring and intensive efforts to reduce risk factors and delay further progression of the disease.
   a. Lipid abnormalities: most common pattern of dyslipidemia in type 2 diabetics is elevated triglycerides and decreased HDL cholesterol levels

      (1)   Behavioral interventions, diet therapy, and education should be initiated first (see section DYSLIPIDEMIA); patients with coronary vascular disease or very high LDL cholesterol levels ($\geq$200 mg/dl [5.15 mmol/l]) should be started on drug therapy simultaneously with behavioral therapy

      (2)   Begin drug therapy after behavioral interventions, diet therapy, and glucose interventions in following patients:

           (a)   Diabetic patients with coronary heart disease (CHD) and an LDL cholesterol >100 mg/dl (2.60 mmol/l)

           (b)   Diabetic patients without preexisting CHD and an LDL cholesterol $\geq$130 mg/dl (3.35 mmol/l)

           (c)   Diabetic patients with triglyceride levels >400 mg/dl (4.50 mmol/l); clinical judgement should be used in patients with triglycerides between 200 (2.30 mmol/l) and 400 mg/dl (4.50 mmol/l)

      (3)   Treatment of LDL cholesterol is first priority for drug therapy (see following table)

ORDER OF PRIORITIES FOR TREATMENT OF ADULT DIABETIC DYSLIPIDEMIA

LDL cholesterol lowering*
    First choice: HMG CoA reductase inhibitor (statin)
    Second choice: Bile acid binding resin (resin)

HDL cholesterol raising
    Behavioral interventions such as weight loss, increased physical activity and smoking cessation
    Difficult except with nicotinic acid, which is relatively contraindicated

Triglyceride lowering
    Glycemic control first priority
    Fibric acid derivative (gemfibrozil)[†]
    Statins are moderately effective at high dose in hypertriglyceridemic patients who also have high LDL

Combined hyperlipidemia
    First choice: Improved glycemic control plus high dose statin
    Second choice: Improved glycemic control plus statin[††] plus gemfibrozil[††]
    Third choice: Improved glycemic control plus resin plus gemfibrozil
                    Improved glycemic control plus statin[††] plus nicotinic acid (glycemic control must be monitored carefully)

*Decision for treatment of high LDL before elevated triglyceride is based on clinical trial data indicating safety as well as efficacy of the available agents.

[†]Gemfribrozil should not be started alone in patients with both elevated triglycerides and elevated LDL cholesterol.

[††]The combination of statins with nicotinic acid and especially with gemfribrozil may carry an increased risk of myositis.

Adapted from American Diabetes Association. (1998). Management of dyslipidemia in adults with diabetes. Diabetes Care, 21, (Supp. 1), S36-S39.

---

      b.   <u>Post myocardial infarction care</u>: cardioselective beta blockers such as atenolol or metoprolol may decrease mortality even more in diabetics than in nondiabetics; new evidence is showing that these beta blockers do not increase risk of serious hypoglycemia

      c.   Daily intake of aspirin (81-325 mg/day of enteric coated) is recommended for secondary prevention in patients with large vessel disease and as primary prevention in high-risk patients

5.   <u>Hypertension</u> should be treated aggressively with goal to reduce arterial blood pressure to below 130/85 mm Hg

      a.   In patients with type 1 diabetes, persistent hypertension is often a manifestation of diabetic nephropathy; in type 2 patients, hypertension is often part of Syndrome X

      b.   As for other hypertensive patients, lifestyle modification should be initially employed

      c.   ACE inhibitors, alpha-blockers, calcium antagonists and diuretics are preferred because they have less adverse effects on glucose homeostasis, lipid profiles, and renal function

      d.   ACE inhibitor is preferred for patients with diabetic nephropathy; angiotensin II receptor blockers are alternative medications

6.   <u>Neuropathy</u>

      a.   Distal, sensorimotor type requires no treatment except to teach client about foot care to prevent ulcer formation

      b.   Painful neuropathy may respond to tricyclic antidepressants such as amitriptyline (Elavil) 25 to 75 mg at bedtime, phenytoin (Dilantin) 100 mg TID (maximum dose 200 mg TID), carbamazepine (Tegretol) 400-800 mg/day in two divided doses, topical capsaicin 0.025% cream (Zostrix) TID or QID (also available in 0.075% cream), or mexiletine (Mexitil) 75 mg (initial dosing) to 225 mg TID; avoid narcotics

7. Autonomic nervous system problems
   a. Gastroparesis may respond to metoclopramide (Reglan) 10 mg given 30 minutes before meals; diabetic diarrhea may respond to clonidine
   b. Impotence may respond to oral medications [sildenafil (Viagra)], penile injections (papaverine, phentolamine or prostaglandin), or intraurethral drug suppositories (see section on ERECTILE DYSFUNCTION)
   c. Overflow incontinence (see section on INCONTINENCE) may respond to bethanechol
8. Diabetic foot ulcers: A comprehensive foot examination and sensorimotor examination is needed on all patients; patients with high risk for ulcers should have these exams performed at every visit
   a. Patient education and prevention
      (1) High-risk patients should perform daily foot inspections
      (2) Teach prevention of foot problems such as how to maintain good foot hygiene, avoidance of injury or infection to feet (never go barefoot, wear sandals, wear well-fitting shoes, clean white socks), avoidance of factors that decrease circulation to feet (tight socks), necessity of smoking cessation and care when problems arise
   b. Diagnosis and treatment of foot ulcers
      (1) Consider ordering x-rays and possibly other imaging studies to exclude subcutaneous gas, presence of foreign body, osteomyelitis and Charcot's foot (presents with acutely swollen foot and no radiographic abnormalities; treatment is observation, rest, elevation, and immobilization as well as referral to specialist)
      (2) Consider obtaining a culture: Irrigate necrotic tissue with sterile saline, followed by curettage of base of ulcer
      (3) Abscesses should be incised and drained. Debride wound as needed
      (4) Minimize weight bearing on ulcer with bed rest, special shoes, casts
      (5) Adequate nutrition is essential for healing
      (6) May need surgical treatment
      (7) If ulcer is infected, order Augmentin 500 mg PO TID
      (8) Patients with slow healing ulcers may have decreased pulses and need Doppler studies to demonstrate that they are candidates for vascular reconstruction

M. Referrals and health maintenance plan
   1. Eye examination: Patients >9 years who have had diagnosis for 3-5 years, all patients diagnosed after age 30 years, and any patient with visual problems should have annual comprehensive examinations by an ophthalmologist or optometrist
   2. Consult with podiatry services as needed
   3. Referral to dentist and dental hygienist is often indicated
   4. Discuss contraception and emphasize the importance of glucose control before conception and during pregnancy in women of childbearing age

N. Current research
   1. Prophylactic therapies to prevent the development of clinical type 1 diabetes
   2. Use of metformin for prevention of type 2 diabetes for persons who have impaired glucose tolerance
   3. Administration of humalog (lispro) after meals to enable patients to adjust insulin requirements based on how much food was eaten

O. Follow Up: Scheduling of return visits will depend on type of diabetes, degree of glucose control, changes in therapeutic plan, and presence of illnesses or complications of diabetes
   1. Patients beginning insulin or who are making a major change in their insulin program need frequent contact with the health team, possibly daily, until control is achieved and risk of hypoglycemia is low
   2. Patients beginning treatment with medical nutrition therapy or oral glucose-lowering agents may need weekly visits until control is achieved

3. Most patients should be seen at least quarterly until their treatment goals have been achieved; thereafter, the frequency of visits can be decreased such as every 6 months to a year
4. Increase visits if patients are involved in intensive insulin therapy, not meeting glycemic or blood pressure goals, or there is evidence of progression in microvascular or macrovascular complications

DYSLIPIDEMIA

I. Definition: Elevation of one of or more of the following: cholesterol, cholesterol esters, phospholipids, or triglycerides

II. Pathogenesis

    A. Pathophysiology
        1. An elevated cholesterol level is an independent and significant risk factor for coronary heart disease (CHD)
        2. Blood cholesterol levels are regulated by lipoproteins or "carriers" which are a combination of lipids (fats) and proteins.
        3. High-density lipoproteins (HDL), major carriers, are thought to prevent or delay atherogenesis because of their low fat content and their probable role in carrying lipids away from blood vessels to the liver for degradation
        4. The other major carrier, low density lipoproteins (LDL), are considered harmful lipoproteins because they help to keep cholesterol in the blood vessels, forming fatty deposits.

    B. Etiology
        1. Primary hyperlipidemia occurs in individuals with specific inherited traits that result in defects in lipid metabolism or transport
        2. Several secondary factors can contribute to hyperlipidemia
            a. Obesity
            b. Low activity levels
            c. High dietary fat, cholesterol, and calorie intake
            d. Endocrine disorders such as diabetes mellitus, Cushing's syndrome, hypothyroidism, lipodystrophies, anorexia nervosa, acute intermittent porphyria
            e. Renal disorders such as uremia and nephrotic syndrome,
            f. Hepatic disorders such as primary biliary cirrhosis, acute hepatitis, hepatoma
            g. Immunologic disorders such as systemic lupus erythematosus
            h. Stress
            i. Alcohol
            j. Medications (see following table)

DRUGS THAT ALTER PLASMA LIPIDS			
Drug	Cholesterol	Triglycerides	HDL-Cholesterol	Comment
α-AGONISTS AND ANTAGONISTS (e.g., prazosin, doxazosin, clonidine)	⇓	⇓	⇑	
β-BLOCKERS				
non-selective	No change	⇑	⇓	transient effects; cardio-selective agents affect lipids less; α-blocking agents are lipid neutral
selective	No change	⇑	⇓	
alpha blocking	No change	No change	No change	
				(continued)

DRUGS THAT ALTER PLASMA LIPIDS (CONTINUED)				
Drug	**Cholesterol**	**Triglycerides**	**HDL-Cholesterol**	**Comment**
DIURETICS thiazides	⇑	⇑	⇑	• effects may be transient
ESTROGENS Hormone Replacement Therapy (HRT)	-------	⇑	⇑	HRT may ⇓ LDL by 10-15%.

Oral Contraceptive Pills (OCP)
  Monophasics
  Triphasics
	
	⇑
	⇑
		
		⇑
		⇑
			
			⇑
			⇑
				OCP can ⇑ CHOL and TRIG, mainly
				due to progestin component

Cyclosporine	⇑	No change	No change	• LDL-C ⇑ by 30%

Ethanol	No Change	⇑	⇑	• Marked elevations may occur in
				  hypertriglyceridemic patients
				• modest intake of ethanol (2 oz/day)
				  may ⇑ HDL-C

Glucocorticoids	⇑	⇑	-------	
Isotretinoin	⇑	⇑	⇓	• reversible changes seen 8 weeks after stopping the drug

Adapted from McKenney, J.M. (1995). Hyperlipidemia. In M.A. Koda-Kimble & L.Y. Young (Eds.). Applied therapeutics: The clinical use of drugs (6th ed.). Vancouver: Applied Therapeutics.

III. Clinical Presentation: Most patients are asymptomatic, but some individuals may have the following:

   A. Vascular problems are the most frequent adverse clinical sequelae
       1. In the most severe forms of hyperlipidemia which are due to specific inherited traits, cholesterol levels can reach as high as 1200 mg/dL and these patients develop coronary heart disease (CHD) in childhood and usually die before age 30
       2. In contrast, many patients with other types of hyperlipidemia, do not develop symptoms of CHD until they are in their 60s or 70s
       3. No research has documented that expensive, lengthy interventions to lower cholesterol levels in children are more efficacious in lowering coronary artery disease than shorter, less-costly interventions which are begun during adulthood

   B. Dermatological manifestations can occur: Xanthomas which are cutaneous or subcutaneous papules, plagues or nodules may develop in the tendons, extensor surfaces of the extremities, buttocks, knees, skin folds, scars, and eyelids

   C. Gastrointestinal problems may develop, particularly with hypertriglyceridemia
       1. Severe abdominal pain which is often associated with pancreatitis can occur
       2. Hepatomegaly or splenomegaly may be present
       3. Less severe symptoms include mild pain, nausea, vomiting and diarrhea

   D. Other clinical manifestations include premature arcus cornea, aortic stenosis, Achilles tendinitis, hyperinsulinemia, hyperuricemia, arthritis, and possibly cholelithiasis

IV. Diagnosis/Evaluation

   A. History
       1. Ask about previous or present cardiovascular disease
       2. Inquire about presence or absence of CHD risk factors (see list of risk factors in the following table)

CORONARY HEART DISEASE RISK FACTORS OTHER THAN LOW-DENSITY LIPOPROTEIN CHOLESTEROL

Positive
- Age, years
    Men ≥45
    Women ≥55 or premature menopause without estrogen replacement therapy
- Family history of premature CHD
- Smoking
- Hypertension
- HDL cholesterol <35 mg/dL (0.9 mmol/L)
- Diabetes

Negative
- HDL Cholesterol ≥60 mg/dL (1.6 mmol/L)

3. Explore past medical history including pancreatitis, renal disease, liver disease, vascular disease, diabetes mellitus, and hypothyroidism
4. Inquire about family history of premature cardiovascular disease or lipid disorders
5. Complete a medication history particularly asking about anabolic steroids, oral contraceptives, and anticonvulsants which can elevate cholesterol levels
6. Explore amount of alcohol consumption
7. Inquire about typical diet over a 24-hour period
8. Determine amount and intensity of physical activity
9. Ask about occurrence of xanthomas and abdominal pain
10. If female, ask about menstrual history and type of hormone replacement therapy if applicable

B. Physical Examination
1. Measure blood pressure
2. Measure height and weight
3. Observe skin for cutaneous xanthomas
4. Palpate thyroid
5. Perform a complete heart and vascular exam
6. Perform a complete abdominal exam; assess for hepatomegaly and splenomegaly

C. Differential Diagnosis: Rule out all secondary causes listed under pathogenesis

D. Diagnostic Tests (plan/management describes these screening tests again); all adults ≥20 years of age should have total cholesterol measured every 5 years
1. High density lipid (HDL) levels should be measured at same time if accurate laboratory testing procedures are available (nonfasting measurement is acceptable)
2. Based on screening tests, some adults will need subsequent lipoprotein analysis (see plan/management)

V. Plan/Management

A. Initial management of adults **without** coronary heart disease (CHD) is a 2-step process (see table):
1. Step 1: Measure total cholesterol and HDL cholesterol
2. Step 2: Based on these results in Step 1 and presence or absence of risk factors, determine management plan or proceed to lipoprotein analysis
3. Diet (see V.C), exercise, and education are first line therapies and drug intervention is reserved for high risk patients

STEP 1 AND STEP 2 OF INITIAL MANAGEMENT IN ADULTS WITHOUT CHD

Total Serum Cholesterol (mg/dL)	HDL (mg/dL)	Risk Factors	Actions
Desirable cholesterol			
<200	≥35	+/-	Educational materials*; repeat HDL and cholesterol levels in 5 years.
<200	<35	+/-	Lipoprotein analysis**
Borderline high blood cholesterol			
200-239	≥35	<2	Educational materials*; repeat HDL and cholesterol in 1-2 years.
200-239	<35 OR	≥2	Lipoprotein analysis**
High blood cholesterol			
≥240	Regardless of HDL and risk factors		Lipoprotein analysis**

Lipoprotein Analysis[†]	Risk Factors	Actions
Desirable LDL		
<130	+/-	Educational material*; reevaluate in 5 years.
Borderline high risk LDL		
130-159	<2	Educational material*; reevaluate in 1 year.
130-159[†]	AND ≥2	Evaluate clinically[‡] and begin Step 1 Diet, Assess at 4-6 weeks and at 3 months **Goal** for patients with ≥2 risk factors is LDL <130mg/dl
High risk LDL		**Goal** for patients with <2 risk factors is LDL <160mg/dl
≥160	+/-	- If goals met, begin long-term monitoring program of total cholesterol & teaching (q 3-4 months for year one and q 6 months thereafter) If goal **not** met, refer to dietician and begin Step II diet - Consider drug therapy if diet therapy fails (**need a minimum of 6 months of intensive diet therapy before beginning drug therapy**)

*Educational materials consist of information on dietary modification, physical activity, and other risk-reduction activities.
**Lipoprotein analysis: Measurement of fasting levels of total cholesterol, total triglyceride, and HDL cholesterol. LDL cholesterol is calculated as follows: LDL cholesterol = (Total cholesterol - HDL Cholesterol) - (Triglyceride/5).
[†]Assignment to categories is done on the following basis: Average of 2 lipoprotein analysis; if first 2 LDL tests differ by >30 mg/dL, order third test within 1-8 weeks and take average value of 3 tests.
[‡]Clinical evaluation should include complete history, physical exam, and basic laboratory tests.

Adapted from the National Cholesterol Education Program. (1993). Summary of the second report of the National Cholesterol Education Program (NCEP) Expert Panel on Detection, Evaluation, and Treatment of High Blood Cholesterol in Adults (Adult Treatment Panel II). Journal of American Medical Association, 269, 3015-3023.

B.   Initial management of adults **with** CHD (see following table)

INITIAL MANAGEMENT OF PATIENTS WITH CHD

*Lipoprotein analysis is required on all patients; all patients should begin Step II diet
Goal: Reduce LDL to ≤100 mg/dl
          If LDL cholesterol >100 mg/dL: evaluate clinically and consider drug therapy
          If LDL cholesterol ≤100 mg/dL: continue on diet therapy & physical activity, annual lipoprotein analysis
Dietary therapy is an ongoing process and should be continued when patients are prescribed drug treatment

Adapted from National Cholesterol Education Program. (1997). Cholesterol lowering in the patient with coronary heart disease. National Institutes of Health, National Heart, Lung, and Blood Institute, NIH Publication No. 97-3794.

C. Dietary therapy occurs in 2 steps, Step I and Step II diets, and is aimed at reducing intake of saturated fatty acids, cholesterol and at promoting weight loss in overweight patients by eliminating excess total calories and increasing physical activity (see following table on foods to eat and avoid in diet therapy)

1. Step I Diet should be prescribed and explained; involves intake of the following:
   a. Saturated fat: 8-10% of total calories
   b. Total fat: 30% or less of total calories
   c. <300 mg of cholesterol per day
2. Step II Diet or intensive dietary therapy (often dietician is consulted or implements the diet therapy); involves intake of the following:
   a. Saturated fat intake: <7% of calories
   b. Cholesterol: <200 mg per day
   c. Weight reduction of overweight patients and increased physical activity should be encouraged

EXAMPLE OF FOODS IN STEP I AND STEP II DIETS		
Food group	Foods to eat	Foods to avoid
Lean meat, poultry and fish (≤6 oz a day)	Beef, pork, lamb–lean cuts, well-trimmed Poultry, without skin Fish, shellfish	Beef–regular, ground beef, fatty cuts, spare ribs, organ meats Fried fish and chicken Regular luncheon meat
Eggs (step 1: ≤4 yolks per week; step II: ≤2 yolks per week)	Egg whites, cholesterol-free egg substitute	Egg yolks
Low-fat dairy products (2 to 3 servings a day)	Milk–skim, 1/2% or 1% low-fat milk Nonfat or low-fat yogurt, cottage cheese, coffee creamer, sour cream	Whole milk, 2% low-fat milk, imitation milk Whole-milk yogurt Regular cheese & cottage cheese Ice cream Cream, half & half
Fats and oils (≤6 to 8 teaspoons a day)	Unsaturated oils–safflower, sunflower, corn, soybean, canola, olive, peanut Soft margarine Salad dressings–made from unsaturated oils, fat-free or low-fat Seeds and nuts, peanut butter Cocoa powder	Coconut oil, palm oil Butter, lard, shortening, bacon fat, hard margarine Salad dressings–made with egg yolk, cheese, whole milk, sour cream Coconuts Milk chocolate
Breads and cereals (≤6 servings a day)	Whole grain breads, English muffins, bagels Oat, wheat, corn, and multigrain cereals, pasta, rice, dry beans and peas Low-fat crackers Homemade baked goods containing unsatu- rated oils, skim or 1% milk, egg substitute	Croissants, breads in which eggs, fat, or butter are major ingredients Most granolas High-fat crackers
Soups	Low-fat and reduced-sodium varieties	Soups containing whole milk, cream, meat fat, poultry fat
Vegetables (3 to 5 servings a day)	Fresh, frozen, or canned vegetables without added fat or sauce	Fried vegetables or those with butter, cheese, or cream sauce
Fruits (2 to 4 servings a day)	Fresh, frozen, canned, or dried fruits	Fried fruit or fruit with cream sauce
Sweets and modified-fat desserts	Frozen yogurt, sherbet, sorbet, ice milk, popsicles Cookies, cake, pie, pudding prepared with egg substitute, skim, or 1% milk, unsaturated oils	Commercially baked goods.

Adapted from National Cholesterol Education Program. (1993). Second report for the Expert Panel on Detection, Evaluation, and Treatment of High Blood Cholesterol in Adults (adult treatment panel II). Bethesda, MD: National Cholesterol Education Program, National Institutes of Health, National Heart, Lung, and Blood Institute.

D. Determine whether a patient is a candidate for drug therapy (see table that follows for a summary of these guidelines)

CANDIDATES FOR DRUG THERAPY**			
Patient	**LDL (mg/dL)**	**Goal LDL (mg/dL)**	**Action**
*Without CHD + <2 risk factors	≥190	<160	Begins drugs after at least 6 months of dietary therapy.
*Without CHD + ≥2 risk factors	≥160	<130	Begin drugs after at least 6 months of dietary therapy.
With CHD	≥130	≤100	Begin drugs. Period for observing diet results may be short.
With CHD	100-129	≤100	Use clinical judgment about need for drugs.

*Patients with severe hypercholesterolemia, multiple risk factors, and certain diseases should also have drug therapy.
**Drug therapy can be delayed in young men (<35 years of age) and premenopausal women with <220 mg/dL LDL.

Adapted from Expert Panel on Detection, Evaluation, and Treatment of High Blood Cholesterol in Adults. (1993). JAMA, 269(23), 3015-3023.

E. Prescribe drug therapy according to the following guidelines:
1. Statins or the HMG-CoA reductase inhibitors produce the greatest LDL cholesterol lowering, are well-tolerated, and decrease mortality from coronary artery disease; considered drugs of choice for most patients (see following tables); atorvastatin results in best clinical outcomes of all the statins

SUMMARY OF STATINS (HMG CoA REDUCTASE INHIBITORS)	
Doses of available drugs	
Atorvastatin (Lipitor)	Start 10 mg QD; max. 80 mg QD
Lovastatin (Mevacor)	Start 20 mg QD with evening meal; max. 80 mg in one or 2 divided doses
Simvastatin (Zocor)	Start 5-10 mg QD with evening meal; max 40 mg QD
Pravastatin (Pravachol)	Start 10-20 mg HS; max. 40 mg HS
Fluvastatin (Lescol)	Start 20-40 mg HS; max. 80 mg in 2 divided doses
Major use	To lower LDL cholesterol
Contraindications	Active or chronic liver disease
Use with caution	Concomitant use of cyclosporine, gemfibrozil or niacin
Major adverse effects	Elevated hepatic transaminase, myopathy, upper and lower gastrointestinal complaints; use with anticoagulant may increase prothrombin time
Comments	Dosages should be adjusted at 4-week intervals Order liver function tests every 4-6 weeks during first 15 months of therapy and then, periodically Order creatine kinase if patient reports muscle discomfort & weakness or brown urine

Adapted from National Cholesterol Education Program. (1997). Cholesterol lowering in the patient with coronary heart disease. National Institutes of Health, National Heart, Lung, and Blood Institute, NIH Publication No. 97-3794.

2. Bile acid sequestrants; valuable in patients with moderately elevated LDL cholesterol, in patients with hepatic disease, and when medications are needed in young adult men and premenopausal women (see following table)

SUMMARY OF BILE ACID SEQUESTRANTS	
Doses of available drugs	
Cholestyramine (Questran Light)	Start 1 packet mixed with fluid or food 1-2 times/day; max. 4-6 packets in 2-3 divided doses
Colestipol (Colestid tablets)	Start 2 g with adequate fluids 1-2 times/day; increase by 2 g 1-2 times/day at 1-2 months intervals; max. 16 g/day
Major use	To lower LDL cholesterol
Contraindications	Familial dysbetalipoproteinemia Triglycerides >500 mg/dL
Use with caution	Triglycerides >200 mg/dL
Major adverse effects	Gastrointestinal complaints Decreased absorption of other drugs (take other meds at least one hour before or four to six hours after the sequestrants) Pancreatitis in patients with hypertriglyceridemia
Comments	To reduce GI complaints suggest the following: *Take medicine slowly, reducing amount of swallowed air *Increase fluid and fiber intake and drink with pulpier liquids such as orange juice *May combine with psyllium hydrophilic mucilloid such as Metamucil

Adapted from National Cholesterol Education Program. (1997). Cholesterol lowering in the patient with coronary heart disease. National Institutes of Health, National Heart, Lung, and Blood Institute, NIH Publication No. 97-3794.

3. Nicotinic acid is especially useful in patients with moderately elevated LDL cholesterol, elevated triglycerides, and low HDL cholesterol (see following table)

SUMMARY OF NICOTINIC ACID	
Doses of available drugs	
Nicotinic acid derivative* (Niaspan)	>16 years: 375 mg QD for 1st week, then 500 mg QD for 2nd week, then 750 mg QD for 3rd week, then 1 g QD for weeks 4-7; may increase by 500 mg every 4 weeks; max is 2g/day
Nicotinic acid derivative (Nicolar)	Start with 1 g with food TID; adjust in increments of 500 mg at 2-4 week intervals; max. 6 g/day
Major use	Useful in most lipid and lipoprotein abnormalities
Contraindications	Chronic liver disease
Use with caution	Type 2 diabetes mellitus, gout, or hyperuricemia
Major adverse effects	Flushing (less with Niaspan) and itching of skin, gastrointestinal distress, hepatotoxicity (especially sustained-release form), hyperglycemia, hyperuricemia or gout limit its use
Comments	- Take enteric-coated aspirin before dose to lessen adverse effects - Liver function, blood glucose, and uric acid should be evaluated before beginning niacin and after reaching therapeutic dosage or increasing the dose level

*Swallow whole; take at bedtime with low-fat meal or snack. Avoid concomitant alcohol and hot beverage.

Adapted from National Cholesterol Education Program. (1997). Cholesterol lowering in the patient with coronary heart disease. National Institutes of Health, National Heart, Lung, and Blood Institute, NIH Publication No. 97-3794.

4. Fibric acids are not listed as major drugs because they do not substantially reduce LDL cholesterol; not FDA recommended as single drug for patients with CHD
   a. Beneficial for treatment of very high triglyceride levels
   b. Valuable in treating clients with familial dysbetalipoproteinemia (familial hyperlipoproteinemia, type III)

  c. Prescribe gemfibrozil (Lopid) 1.2 g/day in 2 divided doses 30 minutes before morning and evening meals; new agent, fenofibrate (TriCor), is also available in micronized 67 mg caps

  d. Usually well tolerated, but some patients have gastrointestinal complaints

  e. Monitor liver function tests at baseline and then periodically

  f. Increase likelihood of developing gallstones

  g. Potentiate the effects of anticoagulants

 5. Estrogen, hormone replacement therapies, and raloxifene may be considered for postmenopausal women with high serum cholesterol

  a. Estrogen and combined estrogen-progestin therapies lower LDL cholesterol and raise HDL cholesterol; all hormone replacement therapies slightly increase triglycerides

  b. Raloxifene has favorable effects on lipid profiles but not as marked overall as with estrogen-progestin therapies

F. When response to initial drug therapy is not adequate (check LDL level at 6-8 weeks except for patients on nicotinic acid who should be checked after maximum niacin dose has been reached, typically at 4-6 weeks) consider the following:

 1. Ascertain that patient is adhering to therapy

 2. Titrate drugs to find optimum dose; statins, nicotinic acid, and the bile acid sequestrants must be titrated to maximum efficacy

 3. Consider adding a second agent after discussing potential adverse effects with the patient

  a. Drawbacks of combination therapy can be reduced by using low doses of each drug

  b. Combination of a bile acid sequestrant with either nicotinic acid or a statin has the potential of lowering LDL cholesterol levels by 40- 50% or more

  c. Although most drugs can be used in combination, some combinations should be used cautiously (see following table for selecting combination therapy)

DRUG SELECTION FOR COMBINATION THERAPY		
Lipid Levels	**Single Drug**	**Combination Drug**
Elevated LDL-cholesterol and triglycerides <200 mg/dL	Statin Nicotinic acid (NA) Bile acid sequestrant (BAS)	Statin + BAS Statin + NA* NA + BAS
Elevated LDL-cholesterol and triglycerides 200-400 mg/dL	Statin Nicotinic acid	Statin + NA* Statin + Gemfibrozil[†] NA + BAS NA + Gemfibrozil

*Possible increased risk of myopathy and hepatitis.
[†]Increased risk of myopathy. Must be used with caution.

Source: National Cholesterol Education Program. (1997). Cholesterol lowering in the patient with coronary heart disease. National Institutes of Health, National Heart, Lung, and Blood Institute, NIH Publication No. 97-3794.

G. Appropriate treatment of elderly patient with dyslipidemia is controversial because few previous studies have included large number of older patients

 1. Use of cholesterol-lowering medications leads to more adverse effects and drug interactions in the elderly than in younger patients, but there is a high number of elderly patients with CHD and drugs could have substantial reduction in morbidity and mortality in this group of patients

 2. Discuss risks and benefits with patients and collaboratively decide on plan

H. Future therapeutic modalities

 1. Lifibrol is a lipid-lowering agent under investigation

 2. Gene therapy may be a future modality for patients with genetic disorders such as familial hypercholesterolemia

 3. Plasmapharesis in which the patient's plasma is replaced with salt-free human albumin is a potential therapy for patients with severe dyslipidemia

 4. Surgery such as partial ileal bypass, portacaval shunt, or liver transplantation shows promise for patients with severe dyslipidemia who do not respond to other treatments

I. Treatment of hypertriglyceridemia
    1. Classification of triglyceride levels
        a. Normal: <200 mg/dL
        b. Borderline-high: 200-400 mg/dL
        c. High: 400-1000 mg/dL
        d. Very high: >1000 mg/dL (patients with this level are at high risk for acute pancreatitis)
    2. Nonpharmacologic therapies such as weight reduction in overweight patients, alcohol restriction and increased physical activity are recommended
    3. Patients who have high triglyceride levels in association with "atherogenic" dyslipidemias (e.g., familial combined hyperlipidemia), and patients with very high triglycerides (to prevent acute pancreatitis) may need drug therapy: consider nicotinic acid, fibric acids, and atorvastatin

J. Treatment of dyslipidemia in patients with diabetes mellitus (See management of associated problems of diabetes in section on DIABETES MELLITUS)
    1. Diabetic patients (men and women) should be managed aggressively, similar to recommendations for secondary prevention with the patient with established CHD
    2. Type 2 diabetes is associated with a two- to fourfold excess risk of coronary heart disease

K. In patients with chronic nephrotic syndrome, treat hypercholesterolemia (major lipid condition in this disease) with the statins

L. Non-perscription agents: insufficient research to recommend their use (see following table for possible lipid lowering benefits)

NON-PRESCRIPTION AGENTS FOR LOWERING LIPIDS		
Drug	**Effect on Cholesterol**	**Comment**
Antioxidants Vitamin E & C, beta carotene	Vitamin E may ⇑ TG* and ⇑ LDL-C*	• Although antioxidants may protect LDL-C* from oxidation, they increase serum LDL-C* levels. Can ⇓ Vitamin K
Fish Oil-omega-3-polyunsaturated fatty acids	May ⇓ TG* 30-50% (9-12 caps/day) May ⇑ LDL-C*	• Can cause thrombocytopenia, glucose intolerance, and bleeding disorders
Water soluble fibers (Oat bran 56g or Psyllium 2 oz)	⇓ LDL-C* 5-20%	• Can combine with resins to decrease constipation and possibly improve lipids
Garlic	⇓ TC* 10% and ⇓ TG* 13%, May ⇓ LDL-C* and ⇑ HDL-C*	• May inhibit HMGCoA reductase • Also may inhibit platelet aggregation

*TG = Triglyceride; LDL-C = low density lipid cholesterol; TC = total cholesterol; HDL-C = high density lipid cholesterol

Adapted from the VA Medical Advisory Panel. (1996). Pharmacologic management of hyperlipidemia. PBM Publication No. 96-0002.

M. Follow Up
    1. Patients without CHD who were placed on cholesterol-lowering diet therapy need total cholesterol levels drawn at 4-6 weeks and 3 months after beginning diets
        a. If these total cholesterol levels meet the goals, an LDL level should be drawn to confirm
        b. Long-term monitoring, after meeting goals of diet therapy:
            (1) Every 3 months for the first year
            (2) Then every 6 months in subsequent years
    2. Patients with CHD and LDL <100 mg/dL and those patients with CHD and LDL 100-129 mg/dL who were not started on drug treatment should have lipoprotein analysis yearly
    3. After starting drug therapy, all patients should have the LDL cholesterol level measured at 6-8 weeks except those on nicotinic acid who should have LDL cholesterol measured after they have reached maximum dose of niacin, typically at 4-6 weeks.

a. If the LDL goal has been achieved, the patient should be seen at 2-3 month intervals through first year or more frequently when drugs requiring closer follow up are used to assess the cholesterol response and possible drug adverse effects
b. Long-term monitoring can consist of serum total cholesterol at follow-up visits with lipoprotein analysis done annually

HYPERTHYROIDISM

I. Definition: Condition that results when tissues are exposed to an excess of thyroid hormone; clinical manifestation is termed thyrotoxicosis

II. Pathogenesis

   A. Typically, results from the uncontrolled secretion or release of thyroid hormones, thyroxine (T_4) and triiodothyronine (T_3) into the blood stream

   B. Etiology of hyperthyroidism in the general population
      1. Most common cause is Graves' disease
         a. It is an autoimmune condition also referred to as diffuse toxic goiter
         b. Heredity also plays a role in the development of this disease
      2. The second most common cause is toxic nodular goiter which is due to a hyperfunctioning multinodular goiter
      3. Subacute thyroiditis is another cause and has an unknown etiology (possibly viral)
      4. Silent thyroiditis also has an unknown etiology; 50% of the cases involve pregnant women
      5. Solitary, hyperfunctioning adenoma is a less common thyroid abnormality of unknown etiology
      6. Ingestion of iodide-containing drugs and contrast media are associated with hyperthyroidism
      7. Less commonly, other factors stimulate the thyroid to produce thyroid hormone:
         a. Thyroid-stimulating hormone (TSH) from a pituitary TSH-secreting tumor
         b. Human chorionic gonadotropin (hCG) from a choriocarcinoma

III. Clinical Presentation (see table under III.I. to differentiate conditions causing thyrotoxicosis); elderly patients may have few symptoms and signs except for weight loss and cardiac abnormalities

   A. Graves' Disease
      1. Condition is 8 times more common in females than males
      2. Often has a insidious onset; patients may be asymptomatic for months
      3. Elderly patients often present with only unexplained weight loss or weakness
      4. Disease is often self-limited, lasting 1-2 years
      5. Patients typically have one or more of the following complaints:
         a. Nervousness which manifests as irritability, inability to concentrate, emotional lability, or insomnia
         b. Weight loss may be present even though appetite is often increased
         c. Bowel movements tend to increase
         d. Heat intolerance is a common symptom
         e. Palpitations may be a troublesome, intermittent complaint
      6. The following are signs:
         a. Hair may be fine and silky; thinning of hair may occur
         b. Nails may develop onycholysis (irregular separation of the nail plate from the nail bed near its distal end), psoriasis (ridges in nail), or onychomycosis (thickening and yellowing of nail)
         c. Skin may have diffuse hyperpigmentation, particularly over the extensor surfaces of the elbows, knees, and small joints
         d. Dermopathy may occur and is thickening of the skin on the legs (pretibial area) or less frequently on the foot, back, hands or face

e. Eye changes include the following:
(1) Ophthalmopathy and exophthalmus is caused by the hypertrophy of the eye muscles coupled with increased connective tissue in the orbit; may cause diplopia, difficulty converging eyes, trouble in preforming extreme movements of gaze, and in rare cases, blindness
(2) Lid lag may be present
(3) Lid retraction with increased scleral visibility above and below the iris often gives the patient the appearance of "staring"
f. Thyroid may be visibly or palpably enlarged; thrill can sometimes be palpated or bruit can sometimes be auscultated
g. May have widespread lymphadenopathy and at times, splenomegaly
h. Postural tremor, particularly of the hands, is commonly found
i. Skeletal muscle wasting with proximal myopathy develops as the disease progresses
j. Long-standing conditions may lead to osteoporosis and back pain
k. In severe cases, signs of heart failure may be present

B. Thyroid storm is a life-threatening syndrome that may occur with decompensated hyperthyroidism
1. Stressful events such as trauma and infection often precipitate an episode
2. Symptoms such as nausea, vomiting, and abdominal pain may precede the storm
3. Patient often is agitated, confused, delirious, psychotic, or comatose with high fever and diaphoresis
4. Tachycardia is always present; tachyarrhythmias may occur

C. Multinodular goiters (see section on THYROID NODULE)
1. Usually affects older individuals who have long-standing goiters
2. Often presents with only subtle signs of hyperthyroidism such as weight loss, depression, anxiety and insomnia

D. Subacute thyroiditis (also called painful thyroiditis or de Quervain's thyroiditis)
1. Affected persons are usually aged 40 to 50; female to male ratio is 4:1
2. Patients often complain of severe pain in thyroid area which may extend to ear on same side
3. Low grade fever is often present
4. Thyroid gland is firm and tender
5. Signs and symptoms mentioned under Graves' disease are often present with exception of exophthalmus and pretibial myxedema
6. Symptoms frequently develop after a respiratory or viral prodrome
7. As the disease progresses, the patient may become mildly hypothyroid and then eventually return to a euthyroid state with complete recovery within approximately 2-6 months

E. Silent thyroiditis (also called painless thyroiditis or subacute lymphocytic thyroiditis)
1. Approximately 90% of reported U.S. cases occur in the Great Lakes region
2. Occurs between ages 30-40 years; female to male ratio is 4:1
3. Thyroid gland becomes swollen and nonfunctional
4. Neck is not tender
5. Half of all patients eventually develop hypothyroidism

F. Solitary hyperfunctioning adenoma (see section on THYROID NODULE)
1. Elderly individuals are more likely to become thyrotoxic from the adenoma
2. Extent of patient's condition is positively related to mass of the nodule; nodules >4 cm in diameter often produce signs and symptoms of thyrotoxicosis as mentioned under Graves' disease with exception of exophthalmus and pretibial myxedema

G. Patients with Hashimoto's thyroiditis may experience transient hyperthyroidism, but later become euthyroid or hypothyroid

H. Subclinical hyperthyroidism
1. Consistently low TSH with normal free T_4 and T_3 levels
2. Some patients may be symptomatic
3. Often develops into hyperthyroidism

I. Consider a rare TSH-secreting pituitary tumor if the patient has signs and symptoms of thyrotoxicosis with a TSH that is normal or high

DIFFERENTIATING FEATURES OF CONDITIONS CAUSING THYROTOXICOSIS				
Cause	**Thyroid Gland**	**FT₄I**	**TSH**	**RAIU**
Graves' disease	Diffusely enlarged	⇑	Suppressed	⇑
Multinodular goiter	Nodular	⇑	Suppressed	⇑
Subacute thyroiditis	Tender, firm	⇑	Suppressed	⇓
Silent thyroiditis	Nontender, enlarged	⇑	Suppressed	⇓
Hyperfunctioning adenoma	Firm, enlarged	⇑	Suppressed	⇑
TSH-secreting pituitary tumor	Enlarged	⇑	Normal or high	⇑

FT₄I: free thyroxine index; TSH: thyroid stimulating hormone; RAIU: radioactive iodine uptake

IV. Diagnosis/Evaluation

A. History
1. A complete review of systems is needed because symptoms may be subtle and involve every system of the body
2. Inquire about changes in weight
3. Obtain a complete medication history
4. Inquire about previous endocrine problems and autoimmune diseases in patient's past medical history or family history

B. Physical Examination
1. Observe general appearance, paying particular attention to signs of nervousness or hyperactivity
2. Measure blood pressure, resting pulse, temperature and weight
3. Inspect and palpate skin, noting pigmentation pattern, moistness, and turgor
4. Inspect hair for texture and thickness, nails for ridges, discoloration or splitting
5. Examine fingers and toes for thickening or acropachy
6. Examine eyes, noting exophthalmos, lid lag, and/or extraocular movements
7. Test visual acuity
8. Assess for lymphadenopathy
9. Observe the neck and palpate the thyroid, noting thrills, nodules, diffuse enlargement, firmness, and tenderness; measure size (see section on HYPOTHYROIDISM)
10. Auscultate thyroid for bruits
11. Palpate for lymphadenopathy and splenomegaly
12. Auscultate the heart, noting murmurs and rate and rhythm
13. Assess the abdomen for splenomegaly
14. Do a complete neuromuscular exam, noting fast relaxation of tendon reflexes
15. Evaluate for tremor (can place piece of paper on outstretched hand to observe for movement of paper with slight tremors)
16. Test muscular strength; focusing on signs of proximal muscle weakness
17. Assess lower extremities, noting pretibial myxedema

C. Differential Diagnosis
1. Neoplasm is often suspected due to weight loss and weakness that typically accompanies hyperthyroidism
2. Congestive heart failure and atrial fibrillation
3. Psychological problems such as panic disorder and depression
4. Tremors such as essential, physiological, cerebellar, and senile

5. Suppressed TSH and elevated T_4 levels occur in conditions not associated with hyperthyroidism
   a. Estrogen administration or pregnancy raises thyroid binding globulin resulting in high T_4 levels but normal free T_4 and sensitive TSH
   b. Glucocorticoids, amiodarone therapy, dopamine therapy, severe illness, and pituitary dysfunction may result in suppressed TSH in the absence of hyperthyroidism

D. Diagnostic Tests (see table under III.I for typical test results with various types of hyperthyroidism)
   1. Order sensitive assay for thyroid-stimulating hormone (TSH) (expected value should be lower than normal or undetectable); with widespread availability of third-generation ultra-sensitive TSH assays, this test is the most important
   2. Usual recommendation is to also order a free T_4, which measures unbound thyroxine in serum, to confirm diagnosis (expected values should be higher than normal); the alternative, second-line test, a total T_4, can be altered with estrogen and pregnancy
   3. If free T_4 levels are normal, order T_3 level because approximately 5% of hyperthyroid patients have normal T_4 levels
   4. Consider ordering 24-hour radioiodine uptake (RAIU) test in two situations
      a. To determine the correct dosage of radioactive iodine to treat Graves' disease or toxic multinodular goiter
      b. To differentiate Graves' disease and multinodular goiter from subacute thyroiditis and silent thyroiditis (in both types of thyroiditis the RAIU test will be low; whereas in Graves' disease and multinodular goiter it is elevated). However, the RAI uptake test may not be necessary to confirm diagnosis of Graves' disease if the patient has ophthalmopathy, clinical hyperthyroidism and a diffusely enlarged gland
   5. Thyroid autoantibodies including TSH receptor antibody (TSI or TRab): not ordered routinely except in selected cases such as pregnancy
   6. Thyroid scan [either ^{123}I (first choice) or technetium-99m], particularly useful in assessing the functional status of palpable thyroid irregularities or nodules related to a toxic goiter
   7. In females, perform a urine pregnancy test
   8. Computed axial tomography (CAT scan) or magnetic resonance imaging (MRI) of the orbit is often recommended for patients with exophthalmos, particularly those patients with unilateral eye signs
   9. Consider electrocardiogram for elderly patient or those with cardiac arrhythmias
   10. Consider dual energy radiographic absorptiometry to determine osteoporosis

V. Plan/Management:

A. Three treatments (radioactive iodine, antithyroid drugs, and surgery) are available for acquired hyperthyroidism; patients and/or parents should be advised of risks and benefits of each treatment and collaborate in making decisions about their plan of care

B. Radioactive iodine (Sodium iodide, I^{131}, Iodotope) is treatment of choice for most adults who have Graves' disease and severe symptoms of thyrotoxicosis with multinodular goiter and single hyperfunctioning adenoma
   1. Many experts recommend an ablative dose of radioactive iodine whereas some prefer to try to render the patient euthyroid with smaller doses
   2. Radioactive iodine works slowly; most patients become euthyroid or hypothyroid in 8-26 weeks
      a. In the days or weeks after administration, increased release of thyroid hormone may worsen hyperthyroidism; one of the following may be helpful:
         (1) Adjunctive therapy with β-blockers (see V.D.)
         (2) Others prescribe antithyroid drugs (see V.C) before and sometimes after radioiodine therapy to deplete stores of thyroid hormone and prevent exacerbation of hyperthyroidism (particularly beneficial for elderly patients who are more at risk for serious heart disease); discontinue antithyroid drugs for at least 3 days before and three days after radioiodine therapy
      b. Monitor free T_4 and T_3 every 6-8 weeks; therapy with levothyroxine is started when patient becomes either euthyroid or hypothyroid (see section on HYPOTHYROIDISM)

3. Other complications include the following:
   a. Ophthalmopathy may worsen
   b. Therapy contraindicated in pregnant women; always order pregnancy testing in patients who are scheduled for this therapy
   c. Women should use birth control 6 months after therapy, even though studies have not found teratogenic effects from therapy
   d. Breastfeeding is contraindicated

C. Antithyroid drugs, propylthiouracil (PTU) and methimazole (Tapazole), were used extensively in the past; today these drugs are used temporarily to regress the thyroid sufficiently for thyroid ablation with either radioiodine or surgery or, less frequently, as a first-line treatment
   1. Drugs will control excessive production of thyroid hormone, but about half of patients will have a remission if no other treatment is instituted
   2. Often the preferred initial treatment pregnant women, patients scheduled for surgery, and patients with mild disease and small goiters
   3. Elderly and cardiac patients may be given antithyroid drugs before and after radioactive therapy is used (see V.B.2.a)
   4. One of the following drugs are usually prescribed:
      a. Methimazole (Tapazole) is often first choice because it is long-acting; initial adult dosage is 20-30 mg BID or TID (available in 5 and 10 mg tablets); when patient is euthyroid use maintenance therapy of 5-10 mg QD or BID
      b. Propylthiouracil (PTU) has the most rapid onset with initial adult dosage of 100-150 mg every 8 hours (available in 50 mg tablets); when patient is euthyroid use maintenance therapy of 50-100 mg BID
   5. May need to give both these drugs at higher dosages if patient is severely ill
   6. It takes 4-6 weeks for patients taking methimazole and 6-12 weeks for patients taking PTU to reach euthyroid state; monitor with thyroid tests every 6 weeks
   7. Patients usually remain on drugs for 1-2 years, then drug is gradually withdrawn with the hope of permanent remission
   8. Consider prescribing levothyroxine sodium (Synthroid) after the patient becomes euthryoid
   9. Instruct patient to call provider if severe sore mouth, sore throat or fever develop (signs of agranulocytosis, a rare side effect of both drugs)
   10. Order WBC count before initiating therapy and then periodically during the first 3 months of treatment; however, agranulocytosis occurs so rapidly that periodic monitoring is not considered cost-effective by some experts
   11. A transient rash may occur; symptomatically treat with an antihistamine

D. Adjunctive therapy:
   1. β-blockers may be initiated before or in conjunction with radioactive iodine therapy
      a. Provide symptomatic relief, stabilize the patient with all types of hyperthyroidism and reduce the signs and symptoms of thyrotoxicosis
      b. Propranolol (Inderal LA) 160 mg daily with maximum of 720 mg or atenolol (Tenormin) 50-100 mg daily with maximum of 200 mg may be prescribed.
   2. Patients who cannot tolerate β-blockers may be prescribed a calcium channel blocker such as diltiazem
   3. Gradually, discontinue adjunctive therapy as soon as patient is euthyroid

E. Patient education
   1. Recommend a supplemental multivitamin; additional calcium and vitamin D may rebuild bone density lost during period of hyperthyroidism; remind patients that increased thyroid hormone is a risk factor for osteoporosis
   2. Successful treatment of hyperthyroidism may be followed by serious depression; warn patient and family of this potential risk and frequently monitor mental health

F. Surgical therapy is a less frequently considered option due to potential complications such as hypoparathyroidism and vocal cord paralysis

G. Thyroid storm, a medical emergency, requires prompt therapy
   1. Antithyroid drugs are often recommended and coadministered with corticosteroids, beta-adrenergic blockers and iopanoic acid (Telepaque)
   2. Other supportive measures include fluids, nutritional support and electrolyte corrections

H. Ophthalmopathy
1. For mild cases prescribe eye lubricants such as petrolatum, mineral oil ocular ointment (Lucri-Lube), apply 1/4" as needed; local mechanical therapies such as sunglasses, elevation of head of bed, and eye protectors during sleep may also be helpful
2. When condition progresses, refer to specialist and consider use of high-dose prednisone, orbital irradiation, or surgical decompression of the orbit

I. Patients with multinodular goiter
1. If patient has elevated T_4 levels and symptoms, treatment of choice is radioactive iodine
2. Patients who are euthyroid do not require pharmacological treatment unless the gland is cosmetically disfiguring or causing obstruction

J. Subclinical hyperthyroidism
1. Defined as suppressed TSH with normal serum T_4 and T_3
2. Treatment is controversial but is usually recommended in the following cases:
    a. Subclinical hyperthyroidism associated with toxic goiter, toxic adenoma, and multi-nodular goiter
    b. Elderly patients at high risk for atrial fibrillation
    c. Menopausal women not taking estrogen replacement who are at high risk for bone loss
3. Treatment of choice is often antithyroid drugs, but radioactive iodine and surgery are sometimes recommended, especially in patients with goiters and adenomas

K. Subacute thyroiditis is a self-limiting condition and does not require permanent therapy
1. Nonsteroidal anti-inflammatory agents may be prescribed to relieve the pain; occasionally oral prednisone 20-40 mg per day in divided doses and tapered over two to four weeks is needed to control pain
2. May prescribe beta-adrenergic antagonists or anti-thyroid drugs when patient has thyrotoxic symptoms

L. Silent thyroiditis does not require pharmacological treatment, however patients' thyroid hormone levels must be monitored periodically as approximately 50% of these patients develop hypothyroidism

M. Treatment of single, hyperfunctioning adenoma is radioactive iodine

N. Immediate referral for patients with a pituitary tumor

O. Follow Up
1. Patients treated with radioactive iodine
    a. Order free T_4 levels every 4-8 weeks until patient becomes euthyroid or hypothyroid and thyroid hormone replacement is needed
    b. Once patients are stable, schedule visits at 3 months, then 6 months, and then annually
2. Patients on antithyroid drugs
    a. Free T_4 level should be measured after a month of treatment and every 2-3 months thereafter
    b. Order WBC after several weeks of therapy and after any changes in drug doses
    c. Order liver enzymes every 3-6 months when patient is stable
3. Patients on ß-adrenergic antagonists should be initially followed every 1-3 months, and then periodically depending on symptoms
4. Patients who are not treated with medications should be followed periodically based on their diagnosis and clinical presentation (i.e., every 3-12 months)

HYPOTHYROIDISM

I.   Definition: Condition in which serum thyroid hormone levels are not sufficient to maintain normal intracellular hormone levels

II.   Pathogenesis of acquired hypothyroidism

   A.   Primary hypothyroidism is the most common form
      1.   Most likely an autoimmune disease
      2.   Often occurs as sequel to Hashimoto's thyroiditis (also called chronic thyroiditis)

   B.   Post-therapeutic hypothyroidism is the second most common form and occurs after treatment with one of the following:
      1.   Radioactive iodine
      2.   Surgery or a thyroidectomy
      3.   Thioamide drugs

   C.   Transient hypothyroidism is often associated with acute or subacute thyroiditis which may have a viral etiology

   D.   Hypothyroidism can occur after hyperthyroidism in women following pregnancy (postpartum thyroiditis)

   E.   Less common causes include iodine ingestion, neck irradiation, and certain medications such as lithium or para-aminosalicylic acid

   F.   Hypothyroidism can occur with a malfunctioning of the hypothalamic-pituitary axis as a result of deficient secretion of thyroid releasing hormone (TRH) from the hypothalamus or lack of secretion of thyroid stimulating hormone (TSH) from the pituitary

III. Clinical Presentation

   A.   Severity of acquired hypothyroidism is contingent on the duration and extent of hormone deficiency; symptoms range from vague and subtle symptoms to severe, multisystem problems associated with myxedema
      1.   Early symptoms have an insidious onset and consist of fatigue, dry skin, slight weight gain, cold intolerance, constipation, and heavy menses
      2.   As disease progresses, following symptoms present: very dry skin, yellow skin, coarse hair, hair loss of lateral eyebrows, slight alopecia, hoarseness, continued weight gain, slight impairment in mental activity, depression, and hypersomnia
      3.   Myxedematous changes occur in later stage with thickened, scaly and "doughy" skin, enlarged tongue, muscle weakness, joint complaints, hearing impairment, bradycardia, possibly cardiac enlargement, pleural effusion and ascites
      4.   Signs and symptoms of hypothyroidism may be similar to normal aging changes, making it difficult to detect the disease in elderly patients
      5.   Myxedema coma is an infrequent sequelae of long-standing disease
         a.   Usually occurs in the elderly, and is precipitated by intercurrent illness
         b.   Symptoms, in addition to obtundation or coma, include hypothermia, bradycardia, respiratory failure, and possibly, cardiovascular collapse

   B.   Patients with Hashimoto's thyroiditis have variable symptoms
      1.   Frequently, the patient experiences transient hyperthyroidism and later becomes hypothyroid, but some may remain euthyroid; in rare cases, the patient may change from hypothyroid to euthyroid or hyperthyroid
      2.   Thyroid may be atrophic, normal-sized, or enlarged

C.	In "subclinical" hypothyroidism, patients have nonspecific complaints, normal levels of serum thyroid hormone but an elevation of TSH; may have an enlarged thyroid

D.	With malfunctioning of the hypothalamic-pituitary axis, there may be loss of axillary and pubic hair, amenorrhea, and postural hypotension; low levels of TSH and T_4 will be present

E.	Thyroid nodules are common in patients with hypothyroidism; sudden enlargement of thyroid gland raises concern of thyroid lymphoma (see section on THYROID NODULE)

F.	The following groups of individuals are at high risk for developing hypothyroidism
	1.	Patients with a strong family history of thyroid disease
	2.	New mothers in the postpartal period
	3.	Persons over the age of 65 years
	4.	Individuals with autoimmune diseases (e.g., Addison's disease)

IV.	Diagnosis/Evaluation

A.	History
	1.	A complete review of systems is needed because symptoms are subtle and may involve every system of the body
	2.	Ask about pain and swelling or enlargement in the neck
	3.	Ask about history of radiation to the neck
	4.	Inquire about previous endocrine problems in past or family medical history
	5.	Obtain a complete medication history
	6.	In women, determine date, characteristics, and duration of last menstrual period
	7.	If patient was previously diagnosed with thyroid disease, ascertain past symptoms, treatments, and responses; in past, patients were frequently treated with medications for reasons that are unacceptable by today's standards

B.	Physical Examination
	1.	Observe overall appearance, noting slow movements and dull facies
	2.	Measure height and weight
	3.	Measure blood pressure, resting pulse, temperature and weight
	4.	Inspect head for coarseness and thinning of hair, thinning of eyebrows, thickened tongue
	5.	Assess for lymphadenopathy
	6.	Inspect the neck; fully extend neck and observe from front and side; observe for prominences and scars (evidence of previous surgery)
	7.	Palpate neck and thyroid for the following:
		a.	Tenderness
		b.	Consistency (i.e., firmness, fluctuance)
		c.	Measure size of gland
		d.	Note whether there is a focal nodule or diffuse growth
	8.	Auscultate thyroid for bruits
	9.	Determine point of maximal impulse (PMI) as an indirect method for uncovering dilation and hypertrophy of the heart
	10.	Auscultate heart, noting rate, rhythm, and murmurs
	11.	Do a complete lung exam
	12.	Palpate for splenomegaly
	13.	Auscultate the abdomen, noting bowel sounds which may be diminished in hypothyroidism
	14.	Perform a complete neurological exam; tendon reflexes may have a brisk contraction and a prolonged relaxation period in hypothyroidism

C.	Differential Diagnosis: The following conditions mimic certain characteristics of hypothyroidism
	1.	Ischemic heart disease
	2.	Nephrotic syndrome
	3.	Cirrhosis

D. Diagnostic Tests
  1. Screen for thyroid disease in the following individuals:
     a. All symptomatic individuals
     b. Females >60 years because of the high prevalence of hypothyroidism
     c. Past history of medically or surgically treated thyroid disease (screen annually)
     d. Past history of receiving supervoltage x-ray therapy to neck for nonthyroid cancer
     e. Patients with other autoimmune diseases and those with cognitive dysfunction, unexplained depression and hypercholesterolemia
     f. Patients on lithium therapy
     g. Patients with type 1 diabetes; 10% of these patients develop hypothyroidism in their lifetime; obtain sensitive TSH levels at regular intervals particularly if a goiter develops
     h. Consider screening for patients with infertility problems, repeated pregnancy losses, menstrual irregularities, and a family history of thyroid disease
  2. Diagnostic testing for acquired hypothyroidism includes the following: (all tests may be normal in patients with chronic thyroiditis)
     a. Order a sensitive thyroid-stimulating hormone (TSH) assay (most labs now use the sensitive third-generation assay) which is the most cost-effective test for assessing thyroid function
        (1) TSH is elevated in hypothyroidism
        (2) If serum TSH is normal, there is no need for additional thyroid tests as 98% of the time T_4 is normal when TSH is normal
     b. Order free T_4 assay in following circumstances
        (1) When TSH is elevated, a low free T_4 level will confirm the diagnosis of acquired hypothyroidism
        (2) When hypothyroidism secondary to pituitary or hypothalamic failure is suspected
           (a) TSH may be normal, low, or mildly elevated with secondary hypothyroidism; (TSH does not rise proportionally to low T_4)
           (b) Further evaluation is needed with results suggesting secondary hypothyroidism: neuroradiologic studies, measurement of serum prolactin, and assessment of pituitary-adrenal and pituitary-gonadal function
     c. If autoimmune thyroiditis is suspected, order either antimicrosomal antibody (anti-TPO antibody) which is test or choice or antithyroglobulin antibody; positive in 95% of patients with Hashimoto's thyroiditis
     d. Thyroid scan or sonogram may be needed to evaluate suspicious structural thyroid abnormalities
     e. The free thyroxine index provides an indirect estimate of free T_4 and is rarely ordered today
  3. Consider ordering the following:
     a. Serum electrolytes, blood urea nitrogen, creatinine, glucose, calcium, PO_4, and albumin levels
     b. Urine pregnancy test
     c. Urinalysis to detect proteinuria
     d. Lipid studies for hyperlipidemia which often occurs with hypothyroidism
  4. During pregnancy, patients may need increases in their medication doses; check TSH each trimester

V. Plan/Management

A. Consult specialist when patient is myxedemic, has significant cardiac disease, has secondary hypothyroidism, or is chronically ill or hospitalized with abnormal thyroid function tests

B. Pharmacological treatment with levothyroxine (Levothroid, Levoxine, Synthroid, Euthyrox) is recommended first-line therapy for acquired hypothyroidism; do not switch brands as there may be variability in potency among brands

1. Full dose of brand Levothroid is 100-125 micrograms (0.1-0.125 mg) per day, which may be started in young, otherwise healthy adults; increase by 25 micrograms QD every 2-3 weeks based on clinical condition and laboratory values; average dose is 125 micrograms (0.125 mg) QD and maximum dose is 300 micrograms (0.30 mg)
2. In elderly patients and patients at risk for exacerbation of heart disease the starting dose should be 25-50 micrograms (0.025-0.050 mg); dose should be gradually increased every 2-6 weeks as tolerated until the optimal dose of 75-150 micrograms (0.075-0.150 mg) is reached
3. Continually monitor response to medication
    a. TSH assay should be ordered every 4-6 weeks until concentration is normalized (Keep in mind that TSH levels may remain elevated for several months despite effective treatment; rapid increase in medication based on TSH levels should be avoided because of the risk of thyrotoxicosis or excessive thyroid hormones)
    b. Ask patient about symptoms of thyrotoxicity such as tachycardia, nervousness, tremor and evaluate with diagnostic tests
        (1) If hyperthyroidism is confirmed the current dose of levothyroxine should be withheld for one week and restarted at a lower dose
        (2) Some patients remain asymptomatic even with elevated free T_4 and/or TSH abnormalities; these patients should have dose reduced until TSH concentration is normalized to prevent development of osteoporosis which may occur with levothyroxine overreplacement
    c. Signs and symptoms of hypothyroidism should improve within 2 weeks and resolve within 3-6 months
4. Maintenance treatment is lowest dosage required to maintain euthyroidism with a nonelevated serum TSH and a normal or slightly elevated T_4
5. Drug interactions
    a. Drugs such as cholestyramine, ferrous sulfate, sucralfate, and aluminum hydroxide antacids may interfere with levothyroxine absorption from the stomach; space levothyroxine at least 4 hours from these medications
    b. May need to increase dose of levothyroxine when used with phenytoin, carbamazepine, and rifampin

C. Liothyronine sodium (Cytomel) replaces T_3: used in only rare circumstances as an alternative medication

D. Treatment of subclinical hypothyroidism is controversial
    1. Levothyroxine therapy is usually recommended, particularly if thyroid autoantibodies are positive and TSH is >10 μU per mL
        a. The adverse effects of levothyroxine must be weighed against benefits
            (1) May improve subtle abnormalities, prevent goiter growth, forestall the development of frank hypothyroidism, and make the patient feel better
            (2) Therapy decreases LDL cholesterol and total cholesterol in some patients which may be an additional benefit
        b. Do not treat this condition with too high doses of levothyroxine which may cause subclinical hyperthyroidism and result in osteoporosis or cardiac dysfunction; important to decrease dosage if TSH is suppressed below the normal range
    2. Elderly or cardiac patient with only a slight TSH elevation may do better without levothyroxine treatment
    3. Patients who are not treated should be re-evaluated every 6-12 months

E. Transient, sub-acute hypothyroidism
    1. Usually condition is self-limited and symptoms resolve in 2-3 months
    2. Therapy is not needed if symptoms are minimal; pain can be treated with relatively large doses of non-steroidal anti-inflammatory drugs
    3. If symptoms are significant and hypothyroidism is prolonged, therapy should be started; re-evaluate these patients every 6-8 weeks

F. Follow Up: Acquired hypothyroidism
    1. When beginning medication therapy, patient's therapeutic response should be monitored every 4-6 weeks until TSH is normalized
    2. After medication dosage is stabilized, schedule visits every 6-12 months and order serum TSH assays
    3. If drug dosage is changed, patient should return to care provider in 2-3 months for repeat TSH
    4. Values within normal limits imply adequate treatment
    5. Undetectable TSH levels suggest overtreatment and medications should be decreased
    6. TSH >20 μU/L indicates undertreatment or noncompliance; after ascertaining that patient is taking medication, increase dose

THYROID NODULE

I.   Definition: Single thyroid nodule in an individual whose thyroid gland is otherwise normal

II. Pathogenesis

    A. Mechanism underlying thyroid nodule formation and growth is unknown

    B. Singular nodules more common in following individuals:
        1. Women
        2. Elderly individuals
        3. Persons exposed to ionizing radiation
        4. Persons living in areas endemic for iodine deficiency

    C. Types
        1. Most palpable solitary nodules are actually the largest of poorly demarcated, multiple colloid nodules that merge with surrounding tissue in a small, multinodular goiter
        2. Benign adenomas are common and usually grow slowly; most patients are euthyroid but those with large adenomas may be hyperthyroid
        3. Follicular adenomas arise spontaneously from follicular epithelium and have well-developed fibrous capsules
        4. Thyroid cysts
            a. About 15-25% of thyroid nodules are cystic
            b. May resolve after the diagnostic fine needle aspiration

III. Clinical Presentation

    A. Asymptomatic neck mass is the major clinical finding

    B. Patients who actually have multinodular goiters may present with symptoms of thyrotoxicosis; however, as the nodules age, there is gradual loss of glandular function and they eventually become hypothyroid

    C. Malignant nodules must be differentiated from other nodules
        1. Fewer than 5% of all nodules are malignant
        2. Death due to malignant nodules is uncommon
        3. Risk factors include extremes in age (< 30 years and > 60 years), male gender, history of head and neck irradiation, family history of medullary thyroid carcinoma, occurring either alone or with multiple endocrine neoplasia type II (MEN II)

4. Malignant nodules are usually large, fixed, nontender, firm, irregular and fail to move with swallowing
    a. Patients with malignant nodules do not usually have symptoms of hypothyroidism or hyperthyroidism
    b. Rapid tumor growth and symptoms of local invasion raise probability of cancer
5. Patients often have hoarseness and enlarged cervical lymph nodes

IV. Diagnosis/Evaluation

A. History
    1. Ask about symptoms suggesting local invasion such as hoarseness, dysphagia, and obstruction
    2. Ask whether neck is tender or painful
    3. Inquire about symptoms that typically accompany both hypothyroidism and hyperthyroidism
    4. Inquire about history of external irradiation to head, neck, chest or exposure to nuclear fallout
    5. Inquire about family history of thyroid problems
    6. Ask about medication history
    7. Ascertain that patient is not pregnant

B. Physician Examination
    1. Palpate nodule (see physical examination in section on HYPOTHYROIDISM)
        a. Determine whether it is a singular or multiple nodule
        b. Note tenderness, consistency, size, whether it is fixed or movable
    2. Check for cervical adenopathy
    3. Check for signs of hypothyroidism and hyperthyroidism which require a complete physical with emphasis on the skin, eyes, heart, and musculoskeletal and nervous systems (see sections on HYPERTHYROIDISM & HYPOTHYROIDISM)

C. Differential Diagnosis: essential to differentiate malignant from benign nodules (see clinical presentation)

D. Diagnostic Tests
    1. Fine-needle aspiration biopsy has become the initial test in most patients with palpable nodules larger than 1.5 cm because it is safe, inexpensive, and results in a better selection of patients who are in need of surgery than other tests
    2. Order serum thyroid-stimulating hormone concentration to determine whether patient is euthyroid, hypothyroid, or hyperthyroid; if TSH is low, order a free T_4 to determine the extent of thyroid hypersecretion
    3. Radionuclide scans are useful in patients with indeterminate cytologic results; hot nodules are benign in 98% of cases whereas 5-10% of cold nodules are malignant
    4. Ultrasonography
        a. Can determine if nodule is a cyst
        b. Cannot distinguish benign from malignant nodules but can be beneficial in determining rate of growth in subsequent visits
    5. Order serum calcitonin in patients who have a family history of medullary thyroid carcinoma or other components of MEN II

V. Plan/Management (Usually refer patient to endocrinologist)

A. Patient can be followed safely without pharmacological therapy if he/she has a negative fine needle biopsy and is euthyroid
    1. In past, asymptomatic patients with benign nodules were often treated with levothyroxine suppressive therapy to shrink the nodule
    2. Due to potential risks of osteoporosis and heart disease, today, most experts carefully follow patients without levothyroxine treatment
    3. Nodules which increase in size should be biopsied again or surgery should be performed

B. Patients who have abnormal thyroid hormone levels should be treated based on clinical guidelines presented in HYPOTHYROIDISM section and HYPERTHYROIDISM section

C. Main indications for surgery are malignancy, indeterminate cytologic features, disabling symptoms or neck disfigurement

D. Patient Education: Instruct patient to call provider if there is change in nodule size, development of lymphadenopathy, pain, dysphagia, hoarseness, or new or worsening symptoms of hypothyroidism and hyperthyroidism

E. Follow Up
   1. Patients who have benign nodules and who are euthyroid require annual office visits to determine nodule's size and hormonal output
   2. Patients with benign nodules but abnormal thyroid hormone levels and clinical manifestations need more frequent monitoring
   3. Follow up for patients with malignant nodules is variable

GYNECOMASTIA

I. Definition: Proliferation of glandular component of male breast

II. Pathogenesis: Due to an imbalance between serum estrogen and androgen levels with an excess of estrogens resulting in breast duct proliferation

A. Physiologic causes
   1. Breast enlargement in puberty is associated with lower free testosterone levels and excessive levels of estrogen created by peripheral conversion of adrenal androgens
   2. As a part of normal aging, older men may have breast enlargement due to normal or increased conversion of androgens to estrogens in extraglandular tissues (abnormal liver function or drug therapy may be contributing causes)

B. Pathological causes
   1. Tumor: testicular, adrenal, pituitary, breast, lung,
   2. Chronic diseases: liver disease, renal disease and dialysis, pulmonary disease, nervous system damage
   3. Malnutrition
   4. Hyperthyroidism or hypothyroidism
   5. Adrenal disorders
   6. Primary gonadal failure
   7. Secondary hypogonadism
   8. Enzymatic defects of testosterone production
   9. Androgen-insensitivity syndromes
   10. Drugs such as hormones, anti-infectives (e.g., isoniazid, ketoconazole, metronidazole), antiulcer drugs, cardiovascular drugs (e.g., digoxin, verapamil, captopril, spironolacone), psychoactive agents (e.g., diazepam, tricyclic antidepressants, phenothiazines), drugs of abuse (e.g., alcohol, amphetamines, heroin, marijuana), and phenytoin and penicillamine
   11. Idiopathic gynecomastia
   12. Familial gynecomastia

C. The most common causes are idiopathic gynecomastia (approximately 25%), gynecomastia due to puberty (approximately 25%), drugs (approximately 10-20%), cirrhosis or malnutrition (approximately 8%) and primary hypogonadism (8%).

D. The following are risk factors for developing gynecomastia: Klinefelter's syndrome, obesity, testicular failure, recovery from prolonged severe illness associated with malnutrition and weight loss, positive family history, Peutz-Jeghers syndrome, male pseudohermaphroditism, and alcoholism

III. Clinical Presentation

A. Physiological
   1. In puberty, gynecomastia is characterized by the following:
      a. High prevalence; occurs in approximately 38-65% of pubertal boys
      b. Average age at onset is between 12-14 years
      c. Usually occurs during Tanner stages II, III, or IV
      d. More common in obese boys due to excessive conversion of androgens to estrogens in the adipose tissue
      e. Has 3 different types
         (1) Type I is characterized by 1 or more subareolar nodules which are freely movable
         (2) Type II presents with nodules beneath areola but extending beyond areolar perimeter
         (3) Type III resembles breast development of sexual maturity rating 3 in the female
      f. Transitory tenderness is common in Types I and II
      g. Breasts are of a firm, rubbery consistency in Types I and II, whereas in Type III consistency is similar to female breast
      h. There is an absence of ulceration or nipple retraction
      i. Often unilateral but may progress to bilateral disease
      j. Enlargement resolves spontaneously in several months to 2 years except for breast development which has progressed beyond Tanner stage II (will never fully regress)
      k. Patients' testes are normal in size and volume for Tanner stage and no other physical abnormalities are present
   2. Occurs in about 40-60% of men 50 years of age and older

B. Pathological
   1. Tumors: Risk of breast cancer in males is proportional to the amount of breast tissue present; increased risk in patients with substantial gynecomastia
   2. Familial gynecomastia may be an X-linked recessive or sex-linked autosomal dominant trait
   3. Patients with other pathological causes present with variable signs and symptoms

IV. Diagnosis/Evaluation

A. History
   1. Carefully determine the age of onset of gynecomastia, and its course and duration
   2. Ask about pain and discharge from breast
   3. Ask whether the breast(s) is(are) growing or shrinking
   4. Inquire about medication history
   5. Inquire about alcohol use and illegal drug use
   6. Obtain a complete nutrition history
   7. Determine whether patient is active in athletics and/or lifts weights to identify breast enlargement due to pectoral muscle hypertrophy
   8. Inquire about family history of breast enlargement
   9. Inquire about previous medical history including liver, renal, pulmonary, nervous, adrenal, pituitary and endocrine disorders
   10. Inquire about any recent weight loss or gain
   11. Explore the impact of the gynecomastia on the patient's lifestyle and self-image

B. Physical Examination
   1. Obtain measurements of height, weight, and arm span
   2. Assess general health and observe for evidence of feminization such as lack of male hair distribution and a eunuchoid body habitus

3. With patient lying supine, grasp breast between thumb and forefinger and gently bring the 2 fingers toward the nipple; a disk-like mound of tissue is often felt with gynecomastia
   a. Measure dimensions of glandular tissue and areolae
   b. Note consistency, tenderness, and mobility of any lesion or mass; squeeze nipple and note any discharge
4. Palpate for axillary lymphadenopathy
5. Check for signs of thyroid hormone excess such as thyromegaly, tachycardia, and diaphoresis
6. Check for signs of liver dysfunction such as hepatomegaly, jaundice and skin changes
7. Deeply palpate upper abdomen for tumor of the adrenal glands or kidney
8. Perform complete testicular examination
   a. Measure size of testes (small, firm testes are characteristic of Klinefelter's syndrome)
   b. Palpate for masses or tumor

C. Differential Diagnosis: Gynecomastia in the adult male may be a normal physiologic phenomenon or a result of a pathologic condition
   1. Pseudogynecomastia presents with smooth, fatty enlargement of breasts without glandular proliferation; more common in obese males
   2. Breast cancer is characterized by a unilateral, hard or firm mass which is fixed to the underlying tissues and may be associated with dimpling of the skin, retraction or crusting of the nipple, nipple discharge or bleeding, or axillary lymphadenopathy.
   3. Neurofibromas, lipomas, and dermoid cysts are other breast masses that may present like gynecomastia

D. Diagnostic Tests: Ordered on the basis of patient's clinical presentation
   1. Laboratory tests are usually not needed if patient has signs and symptoms of pubertal gynecomastia (see preceding clinical presentation)
   2. When the following characteristics exist, there is a need for further evaluation:
      a. Males with genital abnormalities such as small testes with penile enlargement, hypospadias, or incomplete testicular descent
      b. Males >18 years with recent onset of enlarging and tender breasts
      c. Males who have physical abnormalities without a known etiology
      d. Breast masses which are large (>4 cm in diameter)
   3. Consider the following workup for the above mentioned group of males who need further evaluation (Consultation with a specialist is often recommended)
      a. Serum β-hCG level (may be elevated in carcinomas)
      b. Serum estradiol (may be elevated in interstitial-cell tumors and feminizing adrenal tumors)
      c. Luteinizing hormone (LH) and testosterone to detect testicular failure, increased primary estrogen production and carcinomas
      d. Dehydroepiandrosterone (may be abnormal in adrenal diseases)
      e. Prolactin (may be elevated in pituitary tumors)
      f. Thermography and testicular ultrasound should be considered when patient has a suspected testicular tumor
      g. Chest film to screen for pulmonary tumors and metastatic lesions
      h. Thyroid or liver function tests, if indicated
      i. BUN and creatinine, if indicated
      j. Chromosomal karyotype (if both testes small)
   4. Order mammogram or fine-needle aspiration biopsy if breast enlargement is not characteristic of typical gynecomastia

V. Plan/Management

A. Consider consultation with an endocrinologist in the following situations: any male with physical abnormalities, pubertal males whose breast development has occurred without genital changes, breast enlargement which persists (>2 years) or is >4 cm, males older than 18 years of age

B. If the patient has pubertal gynecomastia reassurance should be given that the condition is physiological and transient in nature

C. Postpubertal males who have had a thorough negative evaluation will also need assurance that the breast enlargement is not pathological

D. Males that have residual fibrous tissue may benefit from referral to a surgeon if they are embarrassed or emotionally distressed by the breast enlargement

E. Medical approaches to treating gynecomastia have included use of antiestrogens (i.e., clomiphene, tamoxifen), testosterone, nonaromatizable androgens, and danazol in pubertal boys, and diethylstilbestrol (DES) in elderly men

F. Follow Up
   1. Follow up will vary depending on patient's clinical diagnosis
   2. Males with pubertal gynecomastia should be re-evaluated every 3-6 months

REFERENCES

Adlin, V. (1998). Subclinical hypothyroidism: Deciding when to treat. American Family Physician, 57, 776-780.

Ahmed, S.M., Clasen, M.E., & Donnelly, J.F. (1998). Management of dyslipidemia in adults. American Family Physician, 57, 2192-2204.

American Association of Clinical Endocrinologist and the American College of Endocrinology. (1995). AACE clinical practice guidelines for the evaluation and treatment of hyperthyroidism and hypothyroidism. Endocrine Practice, 1, 56-62.

American Diabetes Association. (1993). Implications of the diabetes control and complications trial. Diabetes Care, 16(11), 1517-1520.

American Diabetes Association. (1995). Intensive diabetes management. Alexandria, VA.: Author.

American Diabetes Association. (1998). Diabetes mellitus and exercise. Diabetes Care, 21 (Supp. 1), S40-S44.

American Diabetes Association. (1998). Diabetic nephropathy. Diabetes Care, 21 (Supp. 1), S50-S53.

American Diabetes Association. (1998). Foot care in patient with diabetes mellitus. Diabetes Care, 21 (Supp. 1), S54-S59.

American Diabetes Association. (1998). Insulin Administration. Diabetes Care, 21 (Supp. 1), S72-S75.

American Diabetes Association. (1998). Management of dyslipidemia in adults with diabetes. Diabetes Care, 21 (Supp. 1), S36-S39.

American Diabetes Association. (1998). Nutrition recommendations and principles for people with diabetes mellitus. Diabetes Care, 21 (Supp. 1), S32-S35.

American Diabetes Association. (1998). Report of the Expert Committee on the diagnosis and classification of diabetes mellitus. Diabetes Care, 21 (Supp. 1), S5-S19..

American Diabetes Association. (1998). Screening for type 2 diabetes. Diabetes Care, 21 (Supp. 1), S20-S22.

American Diabetes Association. (1998). Standards of medical care for patients with diabetes mellitus. Diabetes Care, 21 (Supp. 1), S54-S55.

American Diabetes Association. (1998). Tests of glycemia in diabetes. Diabetes Care, 21 (Supp. 1), S69-S71.

Bakker-Arkema, R.G., Davidson, M.H., Goldstein, R.J., et al. (1996). Efficacy and safety of a new HMG-CoA reductase inhibitor, atorvastatin, in patients with hypertriglyceridemia. JAMA, 275, 128-133.

Baliga, B.S., & Fonseca, V.A. (1997). Recent advances in the treatment of type II diabetes mellitus. American Family Physician, 55, 817-824.

Bauer, D.C., & Brown, A.N. (1996). Sensitive thyrotropin and free thyroxine testing in outpatients. Archives of Internal Medicine, 156, 2333-2337.

Bode, B.W., Davidson, P.C., & Steed, R.D. (1997). In J.S. Skyler (Ed.), Diabetes Dek: Professional Edition. Atlanta: Infodek

Bantle, J.P. & Robertson, R.P. (1997). New approaches to the treatment of type II diabetes mellitus. Hospital Medicine, 19-34.

Begany, T., Braverman, L.E., Dworkin, H.J., & Macindoe II, J.H. (1998). When to screen, when to treat thyroid disease. JAAPA, 11 (4), 72-87.

Braunstein, G.D. (1993). Gynecomastia. The New England Journal of Medicine, 328, 490-495.

Darling, G.M., Johns, J.A., McCloud, P.I., et al. (1997). Estrogen and progestin compared with simvastatin for hypercholesterolemia in postmenopausal women. New England Journal of Medicine, 337, 595-601.

Einhorn, D. (1997). Advances in managing insulin-dependent diabetes. Family Practice Recertification, 19 (2), 13-34.

Gavin, J.R., Reasner, C.A., II, Weart, C.W., & Labson, L. (1998). Oral antidiabetic drugs: One size does not fit all. Patient Care, 32(3), 40-68.

Gharib, H., & Mazzaferri, E.L. (1998). Thyroxine suppressive therapy in patients with nodular thyroid disease. Annals of Internal Medicine, 128, 386-394.

Gotto, A.M. (1997). Cholesterol management in theory and practice. Circulation, 96, 4424-4430.

Grundy, S.M. (1997). Prevention of coronary heart disease through cholesterol reduction. American Family Physician, 55, 2250-2258.

Hennessey, J.V. (1996). Diagnosis and management of thyrotoxicosis. American Family Physician, 54, 1315-1324.

Hermus, A.R., & Huysmans, D.A. (1998). Treatment of benign nodular thyroid disease. New England Journal of Medicine, 338, 1438-1447.

Hoeg, J.M. (1994). Familial hypercholesterolemia: What the zebra can teach us about the horse? JAMA, 271, 543-546.

Inzucchi, S.E., et al. (1998). Efficacy and metabolic effects of metformin and troglitazone in type II diabetes mellitus. New England Journal of Medicine, 338, 867-872.

Jacobs, M.B. (1991). Gynecomastia: A bothersome but readily treatable problem. Postgraduate Medicine, 89, 191-193.

Krieger, D.R., Nathan, D.M., Schade, D.S., & Trubo, R. (1998). Insulin: Recent developments and common quandaries. Patient Care, 32 (3), 71-88.

Linder, B. (1997). Improving diabetic control with a new insulin analog. Contemporary Pediatrics, 14 (10), 52-73.

Massaferri, E.L. (1993). Management of a solitary thyroid nodule. The New England Journal of Medicine, 328, 553-559.

Massaferri, E.L. (1997). Evaluation and management of common thyroid disorders in women. American Journal of Obstetrics and Gynecology, 176, 507-514.

McKenney, J.M. (1995). Hyperlipidemia. In M.A. Koda-Kimble & L.Y. Young (Eds.). Applied therapeutics: The clinical use of drugs (6th ed.). Vancouver: Applied Therapeutics.

Mengel, M.B. (1996). Diabetes mellitus. In M.B. Mengel & L.P. Schwiebert (Eds.), Ambulatory medicine (2nd ed). Stamford, CT: Appleton & Lange.

Nathan, D.M. (1993). Long-term complications of diabetes mellitus. The New England Journal of Medicine, 328, 1676-1683.

National Cholesterol Education Program. (1993). Summary of the second report of the National Cholesterol Education Program (NCEP) Expert Panel on Detection, Evaluation, and Treatment of High Blood Cholesterol in Adults (Adult Treatment Panel II). Journal of American Medical Association, 269, 3015-3023.

National Cholesterol Education Program. (1997). Cholesterol lowering in the patient with coronary heart disease. National Institutes of Health. National Heart, Lung, and Blood Institute. NIH Publ. #97-3794.

National Institute of Health Consensus Development Panel on Triglyceride, High-Density Lipoprotein, and Coronary Heart Disease. (1993). Triglyceride, high-density lipoprotein, and coronary heart disease. Journal of American Medical Association, 269, 505-510.

Neuman, J.F. (1997). Evaluation and treatment of gynecomastia. American Family Physician, 55, 1835-1844.

Petrone, L.R. (1996). A primary care approach to the adult patient with nodular thyroid disease. Archives of Family Medicine, 5, 92-99.

Revak-Lutz, R. (1997). Diabetes mellitus. Class outline at College of Nursing, University of Florida.

Sadler, C., & Einhorn, D. (1998). Tailoring insulin regimens for type 2 diabetes mellitus. JAAPA, 11 (4), 55-71.

Schilling, J.S. (1997). Hyperthyroidism: Diagnosis and management of Graves' disease. Nurse Practitioner, 22, (6), 72-95,

Stone, N.J. (1996). Lipid management: Current diet and drug treatment options. <u>American Journal of Medicine, 101</u> (suppl 4A), 4A-40S-4A-48S.

Siminoski, K. (1995). Does this patient have a goiter? <u>JAMA, 273,</u> 813-817.

Singer, P.A., Cooper, D.S., Levy, E.G., Ladenson, P.W., Braverman, L.E., Daniels, G., Greenspan, F.S., McDougall, I.R., & Nicolai, T.F. (1995). Treatment guidelines for patients with hyperthyroidism and hypothyroidism. <u>JAMA, 273,</u> 808-812,

Tamborlane, W.V., & Ahern, J. (1997). Implications and results of the diabetes control and complications trial. <u>Pediatric Clinics of North America, 44,</u> 285-299.

UK Prospective Diabetes Study (UKPDS) Group. (1998). Intensive blood-glucose control with sulphonylureas or insulin compared with conventional treatment and risk of complications in patients with type 2 diabetes. <u>Lancet, 352,</u> 837-853.

VA Medical Advisory Panel. (1996). Pharmacologic management of hyperlipidemia. PBM Publication No. 96-0002.

Vijan, S., Hofer, T.P., & Hayward, R.A. (1997). Estimated benefits of glycemic control in microvascular complications in type 2 diabetes. <u>Annals of Internal Medicine, 127,</u> 788-795.

Wallace, K., & Hofmann, M.T. (1998). Thyroid dysfunction: How to manage overt and subclinical disease in older patients. <u>Geriatrics, 53</u> (4), 32-41.

Wiczyk, H.P. (1998). Recognizing thyroid disease. <u>The Female Patient, 23</u>(3), 9-22.

Wright, A., Cull, C., Holman, R., & Turner, R. (1998). United Kingdom prospective diabetes study 24: A 6-year, randomized, controlled trial comparing sulfonylurea, insulin and metformin therapy in patients with newly diagnosed type 2 diabetes that could not be controlled with diet therapy. <u>Annals of Internal Medicine, 128,</u> 165-175.

Infectious Disease

CAT SCRATCH DISEASE

I. Definition: Infection causing unilateral regional adenitis usually due to scratch of a cat

II. Pathogenesis

    A. *Bartonella henselae* (previously *Rochalimaea)* is the causative pathogen in most cases

    B. Pathogen enters the body through a break in the skin, usually caused by the scratch of a cat (usually cats are immature and not ill); dogs, monkeys, and fleas are other possible transmitters of infection

    C. Period of communicability unknown; not directly transmitted from person to person

III. Clinical Presentation

    A. Most cases (80%) are persons <20 years

    B. Clinical diagnosis of cat scratch disease (CSD) is based on the presence of 3 out of 4 of the following criteria:
        1. History of animal (usually cat) contact, with presence of a scratch or inoculation lesion of the eye, skin, or mucous membrane
        2. Positive cat scratch disease skin test
        3. Regional lymphadenopathy (predominant sign) with normal laboratory results for other causes of lymphadenopathy (see section on LYMPHADENOPATHY)
        4. Biopsied lymph node has characteristic histopathologic features

    C. Natural history:
        1. Cat scratch occurs and produces a primary cutaneous lesion 7-12 days later; lesion typically begins as a macule, progresses to a papule then to a vesicle
        2. Regional lymph node enlargement typically follows lesion in 1-2 weeks
            a. Node is usually singular, measuring between 1.5-5.0 cm
            b. Area around affected node is usually tender, warm, erythematous and indurated

    D. In most cases, the illness is self-limited with minimal malaise, headaches, and generalized aching; approximately 30% of cases have fever and mild systemic symptoms

    E. Lymphadenopathy usually regresses within 2-4 months, but may persist for more than a year

    F. Occasionally, Parinauds' oculoglandular syndrome develops
        1. Soft granuloma or polyp develops on palpebral conjunctiva
        2. Preauricular lymphadenopathy is usually present
        3. Patient typically does not recall cat scratch or bite; hypothesized that pathogen is transmitted in saliva left on cat's fur; patient pets cat, rubs eye, and transmits organism to conjunctiva

    G. Other rare complications include encephalitis, splenomegaly, and hepatic granulomata

IV. Diagnosis/Evaluation

    A. History
        1. Ask about onset and duration of all symptoms
        2. Determine whether patient lives in household with a cat (particularly kitten) or other animals
        3. Carefully determine whether patient saw scratch or bite of any animal
        4. Specifically ask whether any skin lesion was noticed within the last 2-3 months
        5. Ask about symptoms which typically accompany CSD such as low-grade fever and aching

6. Ask about symptoms which are related to other illnesses that present with lymphadenopathy such as pharyngitis (mononucleosis), weight loss and fatigue (malignancy), cough (tuberculosis), ear pain (otitis media), facial tenderness (sinusitis), mouth pain (dental abscess)
7. Inquire about symptoms which would denote complications of CSD such as abdominal pain, neurological complaints, conjunctivitis

B. Physical Examination
1. Obtain vital signs, noting temperature
2. Carefully examine skin for inoculation lesion which may be hidden in the interdigital webs of fingers, eyelids, or scalp
3. Observe skin for exanthem
4. Palpate all areas where lymph nodes are present, noting any node enlargement, erythema, or tenderness (see section on LYMPHADENOPATHY)
5. If a node is enlarged, assess the area that the node drains for signs of infection
6. Inspect eyes for signs of conjunctivitis
7. Do a complete head, ears, eyes, nose, and throat exam to rule out infection
8. Auscultate heart and lungs
9. Palpate abdomen for organomegaly, masses and tenderness
10. Perform a neurological examination to rule out complications

C. Diagnostic Tests: usually no tests are needed
1. Indirect fluorescent antibody test for detection of serum antibody to antigens of *Bartonella* species is sometimes helpful (available through the Centers for Disease Control and Prevention)
2. A newer test, enzyme immunoassay, may be more accurate in detecting the antibody
3. Polymerase chain reaction assays are available in some commercial laboratories
4. A cat scratch antigen skin test was used in past but is no longer recommended
5. A stain (Warthin-Starry silver impregnation stain) can be used to identify the pathogen if lymph node, skin, or conjunctival tissue is available
6. Biopsy of the node may be necessary when malignancy is suspected

D. Differential Diagnosis: Involved lymph node in CSD is usually tender whereas nodes are usually nontender in noninfectious diseases (see sections on LYMPHADENOPATHY and CERVICAL ADENITIS for further discussion)

V. Plan/Management

A. Management is usually symptomatic; complete resolution occurs without medications in 2-4 months
1. Prescribe analgesics for pain (see section on PAIN MANAGEMENT)
2. Recommend application of local heat to affected nodes
3. Limitation of vigorous activity is advised to prevent trauma to the node

B. Antibiotic therapy may be beneficial in immunosuppressed patients and other patients who are severely ill but is **NOT** recommended for healthy patients
1. Intramuscular gentamicin (Garamycin), oral trimethoprim-sulfamethoxazole (Bactrim), ciprofloxacin (Cipro) or rifampin (Rifadin) are possible choices
2. Therapy is discontinued when enlarged node has decreased in size (about 10 mm), the patient has no systemic symptoms and has been afebrile for at least one week

C. Node aspiration is done when nodes are tender and fluctuant; excision of the node is usually unnecessary but is curative and can relieve symptoms

D. Patient Education
1. Animals do not need to be destroyed or removed from the house
2. No person-to-person transmission so patients do not need to be isolated
3. Instruct patients to always thoroughly cleanse animal scratches and bites to prevent CSD

4. Persons with immune deficiencies should avoid contact with cats that scratch or bite
5. Recommend control of fleas as patients who own flea-infested kittens have greatly increased risk for disease

E. Follow Up: None needed if patient's condition remains stable

FIFTH DISEASE (ERYTHEMA INFECTIOSUM)

I. Definition: Mild viral disease with an erythematous eruption

II. Pathogenesis

A. Causal agent is human parvovirus B19

B. Mode of transmission probably is through contact with infected respiratory secretions or blood

C. Incubation period
1. 4-14 days from acquisition of infection to onset of initial symptoms
2. Rash and joint symptoms present 2-3 weeks after infection

D. Period of communicability: Greatest before onset of rash; probably not communicable after onset of rash; patients with aplastic crises are contagious from before the onset of symptoms and at least through the week after onset

III. Clinical Presentation

A. Parvovirus B19 infections are ubiquitous and cases can occur as a community outbreak or sporadically
1. Outbreaks frequently occur in elementary or junior high schools
2. Secondary spread to susceptible household members is common

B. >50% of adults have serologic evidence of past infection and are not susceptible to reinfection whereas only 5-10% of young children are immune

C. Approximately 20% of all persons with infection are asymptomatic

D. First manifestation is typically a rash which usually appears without fever or other symptoms; in some cases there may be a prodrome with fever, headache, conjunctivitis, coryza, and pharyngitis

E. Rash is characteristic
1. First erupts as a bright, erythematous rash on cheeks and forehead with circumoral pallor; adults often do not have rash on face
2. A maculopapular rash on the proximal extremities occurs the following day
3. Rash gradually spreads to trunk and distal extremities leaving a lacelike appearance as it clears; this stage lasts 2-4 days
4. In third stage, rash appears transiently when skin is traumatized by pressure, sunlight, or extremes of hot and cold

F. Adults may have complications such as arthritis and arthralgias which may last a few months to 4 years

G. Infection during pregnancy can result in fetal hydrops and death (risk of fetal death is <10% after proven maternal infection in first half of pregnancy and less in second half)

IV.   Diagnosis/Evaluation

   A.   History
      1.   Question about degree, onset and duration of fever or prodromal symptoms
      2.   Ask patient to describe progression of rash
      3.   Ask whether rash becomes more visible when patient is in sunlight or becomes overheated
      4.   Determine whether there are other accompanying symptoms
      5.   Determine whether other family or household members have similar symptoms
      6.   Inquire about symptoms which would denote complications such as joint pain and stiffness
      7.   Determine medication use
      8.   Inquire about present and past health history of patient and other household members; specifically question about immunosuppression and pregnancy in women

   B.   Physical Examination
      1.   Measure vital signs
      2.   Assess general appearance
      3.   Carefully inspect skin, apply pressure to skin noting whether rash becomes more visible
      4.   To rule out other viral exanthems may need to perform a complete head, eyes, ears, nose, throat and mouth exam
      5.   Assess neck for nuchal rigidity and adenopathy
      6.   Auscultate heart and lungs
      7.   Assess joints for tenderness, swelling, and range of motion

   C.   Differential Diagnosis: "Slapped cheek" appearance, lacy rash, and transient nature of rash with heat, cold and pressure are characteristic of fifth disease

   D.   Diagnostic Tests
      1.   No tests are needed unless diagnosis is uncertain or when treating immunosuppressed patients or pregnant women
      2.   Assay for serum B19-specific IgM antibody is available for confirming infection within the past several months; serum IgG antibody indicates previous infection and immunity
      3.   Other tests are investigational such as the nucleic acid hybridization assay or polymerase chain reaction assay

V.   Plan/Management

   A.   Treatment is symptomatic for healthy persons; usually the condition is benign and self-limited

   B.   Patients with aplastic crisis may need blood transfusions

   C.   For immunosuppressed patients with chronic infection, intravenous immunoglobulin therapy is effective

   D.   Control procedures
      1.   Precautions for pregnant women:
         a.   Routine exclusion from the workplace where disease is occurring is not recommended due to the high prevalence of B19, the low incidence of ill effects on fetus, and the fact that avoidance of child care or teaching classrooms can only reduce but not eliminate the risk of exposure
         b.   Explanation of the relatively low potential risk and option of serologic testing should be given to pregnant women who have been in contact with patients in the incubation period of disease or who were in aplastic crisis; fetal ultrasound can be offered to assess damage to the fetus
      2.   Children with fifth disease may attend child care or school as they are not contagious
      3.   Good hand washing and disposal of facial tissues containing respiratory secretions lessen transmission of infection

   E.   Follow Up: None needed unless complications develop

INFLUENZA

I.   Definition: Acute viral disease of the respiratory tract

II.   Pathogenesis

A.   Causal agent is influenza virus of 3 antigenic types (A, B, and C)

B.   Mode of transmission: Spread from person to person by direct contact, by large droplet infection, or by articles recently contaminated with nasopharyngeal secretions; during an outbreak, airborne transmission by small-particle aerosols may occur

C.   Incubation period: Short, ranges from 1-3 days

D.   Period of communicability is probably from 3-5 days from clinical onset; patients are most infectious in the first 24 hours before onset of symptoms and during the period of peak symptoms; viral shedding in nasal secretions usually stops within 7 days of onset of infection

III. Clinical Presentation

A.   Influenza virus infection occurs in epidemics which last approximately 5-6 weeks and may be associated with attack rates as high as 10-20% of the population

B.   Incidence in persons over 70 years of age is approximately four times that of persons under 40 years of age; individuals over age 65 years account for approximately 90% of the influenza-associated deaths in the U.S.

C.   Reason for continuing problems with epidemic influenza is the phenomenon of antigenic variation in which there are alterations in the structure of antigens, leading to variants which the general population has little or no resistance against

D.   Characterized by abrupt onset of fever, malaise, diffuse myalgia, headache, and nonproductive cough; later, sore throat, nasal congestion, and cough become more prominent
1.   Unlike other common respiratory infections, severe malaise may linger for several days
2.   Cough is usually the most frequent and troublesome symptom and may be associated with substernal discomfort
3.   Symptoms usually last about 3-4 days, but cough and malaise may persist for 1-2 weeks

E.   Gastrointestinal tract manifestations such as nausea, vomiting and diarrhea occur in children, but are less common in adults

F.   Influenza can affect metabolism of certain medications such as theophylline and result in toxicity from high serum concentrations

G.   Complications include primary influenza pneumonia, secondary bacterial pneumonia, myositis (calf tenderness), and central nervous system problems; Reye syndrome is associated primarily with influenza B

IV.   Diagnosis/Evaluation

A.   History
1.   Inquire about onset and duration of symptoms, specifically question about myalgia and malaise which occur with influenza, but may not be present in other respiratory infections
2.   To ascertain that patient does not have complications associated with influenza, ask about chest pain, hemoptysis, severe muscle pain, and central nervous system manifestations such as confusion
3.   Determine whether household members or close contacts of patient are ill

4. Determine when patient had last influenza vaccine
5. Obtain a medication history, especially ask about use of theophylline

B. Physical Examination
   1. Observe general appearance for lassitude and distress
   2. Measure vital signs
   3. Assess hydration status
   4. Perform complete eyes, ears, nose, and throat examination
   5. Palpate sinuses for tenderness
   6. Examine neck for nuchal rigidity and cervical adenopathy
   7. Auscultate heart
   8. Perform complete lung exam
   9. Abdominal exam and neurological exam should also be considered in severe cases

C. Differential Diagnosis
   1. Other viral illnesses
   2. Pneumonia

D. Diagnostic Tests
   1. Epidemiologic data are usually sufficient to make diagnosis in uncomplicated cases (in other words, when it is known that a certain influenza type is prevalent in a community, most persons with fever, respiratory symptoms and myalgia can safely be assumed to have influenza)
   2. Consider cultures of nasopharyngeal secretions; must collect within the first 72 hours of illness
   3. Change in antibody titers between acute and convalescent sera using complement fixation, hemagglutination inhibition, neutralization, or enzyme immunoassay tests can help confirm diagnosis retrospectively
   4. Consider CBC and urinalysis

V. Plan/Management

A. Two antiviral agents, amantadine and rimantadine, diminish the severity and shorten the course of influenza A but not influenza B (see following table on DOSAGE FOR AMANTADINE AND RIMANTADINE TREATMENT)
   1. Consider antiviral treatment for unvaccinated patients with severe disease or those with underlying medical problems which may increase their risk for severe or complicated influenza infection
   2. Start therapy as soon as possible after onset of symptoms
   3. Duration of therapy: 2-5 days or for 24-48 hours after patient becomes asymptomatic; immunocompromised patients may require longer course
   4. Prescribe either amantadine or rimantadine; choice of antiviral depends on the following two factors
      a. Incidence of CNS-related adverse effects is higher when amantadine is used; adverse effects more common in patients with seizure disorders, psychiatric disorders, elderly, and patients with renal insufficiency
      b. Some experts recommend rimantadine in patients with mild to moderate renal insufficiency

DOSAGE FOR AMANTADINE AND RIMANTADINE TREATMENTS		
Antiviral agent	14-64 years of age	≥65 years of age
Amantadine* (Symmetrel)	100 mg BID	≤100 mg/day
Rimantadine¶ (Flumadine)	100 mg BID	100-200¨ mg/day

* Check drug package insert when administering amantadine to persons with creatinine clearance ≤10 mL/min
¶ Reduce dose to 100 mg/day for persons with severe hepatic dysfunction or those with creatinine clearance ≤10 mL/min. Cautiously monitor persons with less severe hepatic or renal dysfunction taking >100 mg/day
¨ Elderly nursing home residents: prescribe only 100 mg/day of rimantadine; any person ≥65 years with possible side effects should have reduced dose

Adapted from CDC: Prevention and control of influenza: Recommendations of the Advisory Committee on Immunization Practices. MMWR, 46(No. RR-9), 1-25.

B. In clinical trials, a short course of ribavirin has been associated with a modest shortening of symptomatology in healthy young adults; currently ribavirin is not approved for treatment of influenza

C. Other supportive measures may be needed depending on clinical presentation
   1. Treatment of fever and myalgia: Recommend acetaminophen, ibuprofen, or aspirin in adults (see section on FEVER for doses)
   2. Treatment of cough if patient cannot sleep or rest (encourage patient to use only at bedtime)
      a. Suggest dextromethorphan polistrex (Delsym): Adults 10 mL every 12 hours
      b. Alternatively, prescribe cough suppressants which include codeine

D. Patient Education
   1. Recommend rest and increased fluids
   2. Encourage cessation of smoking in household
   3. Teach patient to return to clinic if chest pain, dyspnea, hemoptysis, wheezing, increased temperature, agitation, behavioral changes, or confusion occur
   4. Instruct patient who is taking amantadine to be cautious of concurrent medications that affect the central nervous system such as antihistamines and anticholinergic drugs

E. Control Measures
   1. Consider influenza vaccine for certain groups of individuals (see following table, TARGET GROUPS FOR INFLUENZA VACCINE)
   2. Administer influenza vaccine in the fall (optimal time is October to mid-November), before the start of the influenza season (see following table DOSE AND SCHEDULE OF INFLUENZA VACCINE for administration of vaccine)
      a. Elderly persons and persons with certain chronic diseases may develop lower postvaccination antibody titers than healthy, young adults; in elderly population vaccine is 80% effective in preventing death, but only 30-40% effective in preventing influenza illness
      b. Annual vaccination is recommended
      c. Do **not** administer vaccination to persons known to have anaphylactic hypersensitivity to eggs without consulting an expert in infectious disease
      d. Do **not** vaccinate adults with acute afebrile illnesses until their symptoms have abated

---

TARGET GROUPS FOR INFLUENZA VACCINE

Groups at Increased Risk for Influenza-Related Complications

- Persons greater than or equal to 65 years of age

- Residents of nursing homes or chronic-care facilities

- Adults and children with chronic disorders of the pulmonary or cardiovascular system, including children with asthma

- Adults and children who have chronic metabolic diseases, renal dysfunction, hemoglobinopathies or immunosuppression (including immunosuppression caused by medications)

- Children and adolescents (6 months-18 years) who are receiving long-term aspirin therapy and might be at risk for developing Reye syndrome after influenza

- Women who will be in the second or third trimester of pregnancy during the influenza season

Groups That Can Transmit Influenza to Persons at High Risk

- Health care providers in both hospitals and outpatient settings

- Employees of nursing homes and chronic-care facilities who have contact with residents

- Providers of home care to persons at high risk

- Household members (including children) of persons in high risk groups including high risk infants

Special Groups

- Persons with HIV infection: vaccine effective in persons with mild AIDS-related symptoms and high CD4+ T-lymphocyte counts

- Breast-feeding is not contraindicated for vaccination

- Persons traveling to foreign countries: risk of exposure to influenza varies depending on season and destination; if persons traveling were not vaccinated the previous fall or winter, encourage vaccine

- General population: administer to any person who wishes to receive; especially encourage persons who provide community services and students or other persons living in institutional settings

Adapted from American Academy of Pediatrics. (1997). Summaries of infectious diseases. In Peter, G. (Ed.). 1997 Red Book: Report of the Committee on Infectious Diseases (24th ed.). Elk Grove Village, IL: Author

DOSE AND SCHEDULE FOR INFLUENZA VACCINE *†			
Age Group	Product	Dosage	# Doses
6-35 months	Split virus only	0.25 mL	1-2§
3-8 years	Split virus only	0.50 mL	1-2§
9-12 years	Split virus only	0.50 mL	1
>12 years	Whole or split virus	0.50 mL	1

* The recommended site of vaccination is the deltoid muscle for adults and older children. The preferred site for infants and young children is the anterolateral aspect of the thigh

† Dosages are those recommended in recent years; refer to product circular each year for correct dosage

§Two doses given at least 1 month apart are recommended for children <9 years who are receiving vaccine for the first time

Adapted from American Academy of Pediatrics. (1997). Summaries of infectious diseases. In Peter, G. (Ed.). 1997 Red Book: Report of the committee on infectious diseases (24th ed.). Elk Grove Village, IL: Author

F. Chemoprophylaxis with rimantadine or amantadine is an alternative method of protecting patients against influenza (see following table for PERSONS FOR WHOM CHEMOPROPHYLAXIS IS INDICATED)
1. Chemoprophylaxis is not a substitute for vaccination; vaccination is preferred for prevention of influenza
2. Chemoprophylaxis in vaccinated persons may provide additional protection and does not interfere with the immune response
3. For maximal effectiveness of prophylaxis, drug must be taken each day for duration of influenza activity in community; to be cost effective, prophylaxis should only be prescribed during period of peak influenza activity

PERSONS FOR WHOM CHEMOPROPHYLAXIS IS INDICATED
➡ Persons at high risk who were vaccinated after circulation of influenza A in the community has begun; chemoprophylaxis is helpful during the interval before a vaccine response or 2 weeks after the recommended vaccine schedule has been completed
➡ Unimmunized persons who provide care to high-risk individuals
➡ Immunodeficient persons whose antibody response to vaccine is likely to be poor
➡ High-risk persons for whom vaccine is contraindicated
➡ May also administer chemoprophylaxis to any healthy person over age 1 year for whom the prevention of influenza is considered particularly desirable; these persons should also be immunized

Adapted from American Academy of Pediatrics. (1997). Summaries of infectious diseases. In Peter, G. (Ed.). 1997 Red Book: Report of the Committee on Infectious Diseases (24th ed.). Elk Grove Village, IL: Author

4. Prophylactic doses
a. Children 1-9 years and children <40 kg: Amantadine 5 mg/kg/day in 1-2 doses*
b. Children 10-13 years who weigh ≥40 kg: Amantadine 100 mg BID*
c. Children ≥14 years and adults <65 years: 100 mg BID of either amantadine or rimantadine**
d. Adults ≥65 years: ≤100 mg/day of amantadine or 100 or 200 mg/day of rimantadine** (reduce dose of amantadine in elderly who experience side effects when taking 200 mg/day)
e. *Alternative and acceptable dosage for children who weigh >40 kg and adults is 100 mg/day in 1 or 2 divided doses
f. **For persons with severe hepatic dysfunction or those with creatinine clearance ≤10 mL/min, reduce dose of rimantadine to 100 mg/day

G. Follow Up
1. No follow up needed if symptoms resolve within one week
2. Reevaluate if symptoms persist beyond 7-10 days

LYME DISEASE

I. Definition: Infection caused by *Borrelia burgdorferi*, a member of the family of spirochetes or corkscrew-shaped bacteria

II. Pathogenesis

    A. Ticks transmit disease to humans during the nymph stage when they are small in size and are likely to feed unnoticed on individuals for 2 or more days

    B. Small mammals, particularly rodents, are important hosts of ticks and critical for maintenance of *B. burgdorferi* in nature; deer are hosts for the adult tick

    C. Adult ticks are less likely to transmit disease because they are readily noticed and removed; transmission of the disease is unlikely if tick attachment is less than 48 hours.

    D. Incubation period is 3-31days (typically 7-14 days); late manifestations occur several months to more than one year later

III. Clinical Presentation

    A. Incidence of Lyme disease is increasing and there has been an expansion of the affected geographic area; leading vector-borne disease in U.S.

    B. Highest incidence in the US occurs in the northeast from Massachusetts to Maryland, north-central states, especially Wisconsin and Minnesota, and the west coast, particularly northern California

    C. Most human infections occur between the months of April and October in U.S.

    D. Less than 50% of all patients with Lyme disease remember receiving a tick bite

    E. Case definition for the national surveillance of Lyme disease
        1. Individual with erythema migrans
        2. Individual with at least one manifestation and laboratory confirmation of infection

    F. First stage is called early localized and is characterized by the following:
        1. Erythema migrans (EM) is a lesion that starts as a red macule or papule at the site of a recent tick bite and enlarges over days or weeks to form a large, round lesion, often with central clearing
            a. Lesion must measure at least 5 cm to be considered EM
            b. Lesion varies in size, shape and may be vesicular or necrotic in the center
        2. Fever, malaise, headache, neck stiffness and arthralgia may occur with rash; these symptoms may be intermittent over several weeks

    G. Second stage is called early disseminated disease and presents as the following:
        1. Characteristic rash, multiple erythema migrans, develops 3 to 5 weeks after tick bite and appears as annular erythematous lesions which are smaller but similar to primary lesion; occurs in about 50% of patients
        2. Other common manifestations: Palsies of cranial nerves, meningitis, conjunctivitis and systemic symptoms such as arthralgia, myalgia, headache, and fatigue; carditis is a rare occurrence

H.   Third stage is called late disease and signs and symptoms in this stage may not present until months or years after tick bite; characterized by following:
1.   Recurrent arthritis which is pauciarticular and affects large joints, particularly the knees
2.   Central nervous system manifestations such a encephalopathy and neuropathy may also occur

IV.   Diagnosis/Evaluation

A.   History
1.   Ask about possible exposure to tick bites such as recent camping trip, frequent yard work, pets who are outside in vegetation
2.   Ask patient to describe the duration, characteristics, and course of any skin lesion
3.   Question about fatigue, headache, fever, myalgias after outdoor exposure
4.   Inquire about late manifestations such as arthritis and nervous system and cardiac problems

B.   Physical Examination
1.   Carefully inspect the skin
2.   Palpate for lymphadenopathy
3.   Perform a thorough cardiac exam
4.   Inspect joints for swelling, tenderness or erythema
5.   Perform a neurological examination

C.   Differential Diagnosis
1.   Rheumatoid arthritis
2.   Meningitis/encephalitis
3.   Viral syndrome
4.   Tularemia
5.   Acute rheumatic fever
6.   Systemic lupus erythematosus
7.   Rocky Mountain spotted fever
8.   Bell's palsy
9.   Reiter syndrome

D.   Diagnostic Tests
1.   Patients presenting with rash resembling erythema migrans or with arthritis, or who have a history of characteristic rash, and a previous tick bite should have empiric antibiotic therapy; no diagnostic tests are needed
2.   For patients who do not meet the above criteria in IV.D.1, but who have objective clinical signs and who live in a community in which Lyme disease is present or who have a pre-test probability of 20% should undergo a two-test protocol:
a.   First, order an enzyme-linked immunosorbent assay (ELISA) or an immunofluorescence assay; these tests often have false positive results
b.   Follow with a Western blot for specimens found to be indeterminant; positive test increases likelihood that patient has Lyme disease whereas negative test rules out disease
3.   Patients with singular symptoms of arthralgias, myalgia, headache, fatigue or palpitations have a low chance of having Lyme disease and should not be tested
4.   Other diagnostic tests are not usually ordered but may be beneficial:
a.   In patients with suspected primary erythema migrans, skin culture with a saline-lavage needle aspiration and a 2-mm punch biopsy of the leading edge of lesion successfully obtains causative organism in 60%-80% of cases
b.   Changes in antibody levels in paired acute-phase and convalescent-phase serum samples may help diagnose disease, but published data are not yet available to determine the clinical utility of this approach

V. Plan/Management

    A. Treat the following patients with antibiotics (see following table on Recommended Therapy)
        1. Patients with erythema migrans or a history of this lesion and a positive history of tick bite
        2. Patients with pre-test probability of ≥20% who have positive results from two-test protocol (ELISA or immunofluorescence assay and Western blot)

    B. Do not treat patients whose only evidence of Lyme disease is a positive immunologic test; the risks of empiric antibiotic treatment outweigh the benefits

RECOMMENDED TREATMENT		
Disease Category	**Drug/Duration**	**Adult Dosage**
Early Localized Disease*	Doxycycline (Vibramycin) 14-21 days (drug of choice)	100 mg BID
	OR	
	Amoxicillin (Amoxil) 14-21 days	250-500 TID
Early Disseminated and Late Disease		
➡ Multiple erythema migrans	Same as early disease except duration is 21 days	
➡ Isolated facial palsy	Same as early disease, except duration is 21-28 days[††]	
➡ Arthritis	Same as early disease except duration is 28 days	
➡ Persistent or recurrent arthritis[§]	Ceftriaxone (Rocephin) IV or IM for 14-21 days	2 g QD or 1 g BID
➡ Carditis	OR	
➡ Meningitis or Encephalitis	Penicillin G IV for 14-21 days	20 million units in 4 divided doses

*Cefuroxime axetil and erythromycin are alternative drugs for patients allergic to penicillin
[†]Do not give corticosteroids
[‡]Antibiotics do not affect resolution of nerve palsy; purpose is to prevent late disease
[§]Considered persistent when there is objective evidence of synovitis for at least 2 months after treatment is initiated. Some experts use a second course of an oral agent before using an IV antibiotic

Adapted from American Academy of Pediatrics. (1997). Summaries of infectious diseases. In Peter, G. (Ed.). 1997 Red Book: Report of the committee on infectious diseases (24th ed.). Elk Grove Village, IL: Author

    C. For patients without objective clinical signs, antimicrobial prophylaxis after a tick bite is not recommended because of the low rate of transmission and fact that transmission requires 24-48 hours of tick attachment; consult specialist in certain cases such as when patient is pregnant or when patient has been exposed to long duration of feeding by tick as evidenced by removal of an engorged tick

    D. Prevention: Teach patient the following:
        1. Remove leaves and clear brush and tall grass from around houses and at the edges of gardens
        2. Avoid tick-infested areas in the late spring and summer months
        3. Always inspect body carefully after being outdoors
        4. Daily inspect pets and remove ticks
        5. Wear lightly colored clothing so that ticks can be seen more easily
        6. Prevent ticks from getting under clothing; tuck pant legs into socks or tape area where pants and socks meet, and tuck shirt into pants

7.   Wear a hat and long-sleeved shirt
8.   Avoid overhanging grass and brush by walking in the center of trails
9.   Spray permethrin on clothing or treat clothes with permethrin which kills ticks on contact and prevents tick attachment
10. Spray insect repellent containing N,N-diethyl-m-toluamide (DEET) on all exposed skin other than face, hands and abraded skin (must reapply every 1-2 hours); use DEET sparingly because of rare reports of serious neurologic complications after use (wash treated skin with soap and water after being outdoors)
11. Remove clothing and wash and dry it in high temperature after outdoor exposure
12. Remove attached ticks with tweezers; pull tick straight back with a slow steady force; disinfect skin before and after tick is removed; do not use nail polish, alcohol, or matches to remove

E.   Follow Up
1.   Patients treated with oral antibiotics should be reevaluated at the end of treatment
2.   Patients with more severe symptoms should be seen more frequently based on their clinical condition

INFECTIOUS MONONUCLEOSIS

I.   Definition: Acute viral syndrome with classic triad of fever, pharyngitis, and adenopathy

II. Pathogenesis

A.   Causal agent is the Epstein-Barr virus (EBV)

B.   Spread person-to-person by the oropharyngeal route (via saliva); rarely via blood transfusion

C.   Incubation period is from 30 to 50 days

D.   Period of communicability is indeterminant but may be prolonged
1.   Pharyngeal excretion may persist for many months or more after illness
2.   Asymptomatic carriage is common

III. Clinical Presentation

A.   Common infection in college-age adults and adolescents living in group settings such as educational institutions

B.   Spectrum of disease is variable; patients may be asymptomatic or suffer from fatal infection

C.   Common signs and symptoms include the classic triad of fever, exudative pharyngitis, adenopathy (particularly posterior cervical), as well as fatigue, eyelid edema, headache, pain behind eyes, and a palatal petechial rash

D.   Atypical lymphocytosis often accompanies disease and approximately 95% of adults will have abnormal liver function tests

E.   Splenic enlargement may occur; usually resolves within the first month of the illness

F.   Duration of the illness is variable with the average, uncomplicated illness lasting 3-4 weeks

G. Complications occur more often in patients under 10 or over 50 years of age and include central nervous system (CNS) disorders such as aseptic meningitis, encephalitis and the Guillain-Barré syndrome; rare complications include splenic rupture, thrombocytopenia, agranulocytosis, myocarditis, hemolytic anemia

H. The definition of "chronic" infectious mononucleosis is still controversial

IV. Diagnosis/Evaluation

    A. History
1. Ask about onset of symptoms
2. Ascertain that patient does not have trouble breathing or severe swallowing difficulty
3. Question about severe headaches, weakness, and confusion (CNS complications of mononucleosis)
4. Ask about fever, sore throat, malaise, rash
5. Question about recent history of exposure to others with mononucleosis

    B. Physical Examination
1. Observe general appearance
2. Measure vital signs
3. Observe skin for exanthems
4. Perform a complete ears, nose, and throat examination
5. Auscultate the heart
6. Auscultate the lungs, making certain that the patient does not have upper airway obstruction from enlarged tonsils and lymphoid tissue
7. Palpate abdomen for organomegaly
8. Perform a neurological examination to rule out CNS complications

    C. Differential Diagnosis
1. Streptococcal or viral pharyngitis (posterior cervical adenopathy and splenomegaly help distinguish pharyngitis of infectious mononucleosis from other types of pharyngitis)
2. Viral syndromes
3. Hepatitis
4. Cytomegalovirus infection
5. Toxoplasma infection
6. Secondary syphilis

    D. Diagnostic Tests
1. Order complete blood count with differential: Absolute lymphocytosis in which more than 10% of cells are atypical is characteristic
2. Order Mono test or nonspecific tests for heterophil antibody (Monospot, Paul-Bunnell test, and slide agglutination reaction are most widely available)
    a. Will identify 90% of cases in adults
    b. Early in the course of this illness, some patients who are infected may have a negative Mono test because the level of antibodies in the blood has not reached sufficient levels; if patient continues to have symptoms repeat Mono test in 7-10 days
    c. A positive result may remain positive for up to a year after the initial illness
3. Consider obtaining throat swab and perform rapid strep test. If the rapid strep test is negative (3-30% of patients with mononucleosis also have streptococcal infection) send a throat culture
4. Consider ordering liver function tests
5. EBV antibody seroconversion test is usually not performed in uncomplicated cases but may be needed in adults without heterophile antibodies or who have a negative monospot test and there is a suspicion of mononucleosis

V. Plan/Management

    A. Patients with uncomplicated acute mononucleosis require only symptomatic therapy
        1. Most authorities advise NOT to treat uncomplicated mononucleosis with corticosteroid therapy or acyclovir
        2. Pain medication and warm salt water gargles may help the discomfort of the sore throat

    B. If patient has concomitant streptococcal pharyngitis treat with erythromycin (E-Mycin): Prescribe 250 mg QID for 10 days. (Do not prescribe ampicillin or amoxicillin-containing agents because they frequently cause a rash; infrequently, penicillin can also cause a rash)

    C. For patients with more severe symptoms, consult specialist and consider the following:
        1. Corticosteroid therapy may be useful for treating some complications such as obstructive tonsillar enlargement, autoimmune hemolytic anemia, thrombocytopenia, aplastic anemia, encephalitis, myocarditis, pericarditis, and massive splenomegaly; prescribe prednisone 1mg/kg per day orally for 7 days and then taper
        2. Acyclovir in combination with corticosteroids has been recommended but the clinical benefits have not been demonstrated except in HIV-infected patients with oral hairy leukoplakia

    D. Patient Education
        1. Contact sports, heavy lifting, and strenuous activity should be avoided for at least one month or until resolution of splenomegaly because an enlarged spleen is susceptible to rupture
        2. Help patient plan a realistic schedule of rest with modification of work and/or school responsibilities depending on patient's condition
        3. Increased fluid intake may be beneficial
        4. Patient does not need to be isolated from others, but to prevent spread of disease teach the following: good hand washing technique, avoidance of sharing eating or drinking utensils with others, avoidance of kissing or sharing oral secretions
        5. Remind patient to avoid alcohol consumption for at least a month to decrease the work of the liver
        6. Instruct patient with a recent history of mononucleosis to avoid donating blood
        7. Tell patient to avoid ampicillin or amoxicillin during course of disease as a drug-related rash may develop
        8. Instruct patient to immediately report pain in left upper area of abdomen or in shoulder as this could be a sign of splenic rupture
        9. Inform patient that recovery is typically in 2 to 4 weeks, but that some patients have a slow recovery of 2 to 3 months

    E. Follow Up: Every 1-2 weeks until symptoms resolve

RHEUMATIC FEVER

I. Definition: Inflammatory, multisystem disease that occurs 1-5 weeks to 6 months after group A streptococcal pharyngitis

II. Pathogenesis

    A. One widely-held theory is that antibodies that react with *Streptococcus* cross-react with human cardiac myocytes (carditis), cartilage (arthritis), and thalamic and subthalamic nuclei of the central nervous system (chorea)

B. Another theory suggests that hereditary plays a role whereby individuals who develop acute rheumatic fever (ARF) have a particular immune response to *Streptococcus*

III. Clinical Presentation

A. Although the frequency and severity of acute rheumatic fever (ARF) cases have decreased in the U.S. in the last century, rheumatic heart disease remains the leading cause of cardiac death in individuals between 5 and 24 years of age

B. The initial, nonspecific group of symptoms is a gradual onset of fever, malaise, and weight loss

C. A history of pharyngitis within the preceding three months occurs in about 20% of the children diagnosed with ARF

D. Criteria for the diagnosis of rheumatic fever have been revised (see table that follows)

CHARACTERISTICS OF ACUTE RHEUMATIC FEVER (JONES CRITERIA, UPDATED 1992)

Two major manifestations or one major and 2 minor manifestations are required to make the diagnosis:

Major manifestations	*Minor manifestations*
Carditis	Clinical
Polyarthritis	Fever
Chorea	Arthralgias
Erythema marginatum	Previous acute rheumatic fever or evidence of preexisting rheumatic heart disease
Subcutaneous nodules	
	Laboratory
	Acute phase reaction
	Leukocytosis
	Elevated erythrocyte sedimentation rate
	Abnormal C-reactive protein
	Prolonged PR interval or other electrocardiographic changes

Plus

Evidence of a preceding streptococcal infection such as elevated or increasing antistreptolysin-O or other streptococcal antibodies, positive throat culture for group A streptococcus, recent scarlet fever

Adapted from Dajani, A.S., et al. (1993). Guidelines for the diagnosis of rheumatic fever: Jones criteria, updated 1992. Circulation, 87, 302-307.

E. Carditis, a major manifestation, is defined as a new or changed murmur, a pericardial friction rub or effusion, and a recent or worsening heart enlargement with or without heart failure

F. Polyarthritis, the most common major manifestation, is a benign condition
   1. The arthritis is migratory and usually involves the larger joints such as the knees, ankles, elbows and wrists
   2. If untreated, the arthritis lasts for about 4 weeks and almost never results in permanent joint deformity

G. Sydenham's chorea is a benign sign which presents as purposeless, involuntary, rapid movements of the trunk and/or extremities; often accompanied with muscle weakness and emotional lability

H. Erythema marginatum is a rare manifestation
   1. Presents as red, nonpruritic, macular lesions with rounded or serpiginous margins and pale centers
   2. The exanthem is transient and migratory and occurs mainly on trunk and proximal extremities; rash may be brought out by application of heat

I. Subcutaneous nodules are painless and freely movable nodules under the skin which are found over the extensor surfaces of certain joints, particularly the elbows, knees, and wrists

J. Arthralgias and fever are nonspecific, minor manifestations which support the diagnosis of ARF when only a single major manifestation is present

K. Other common symptoms not included in the Jones criteria are weight loss, fatigue, irritability, abdominal pain, and epistaxis

L. Diagnostic test abnormalities are often present
1. Prolonged P-R interval on the electrocardiogram and elevated erythrocyte sedimentation rate (ESR) and C-reactive protein are nonspecific findings but provide supporting data that ARF is present
2. Patients may have positive throat cultures or rapid antigen tests for group A streptococci; patients may have elevated or rising streptococcal antibody titers

M. ARF lasts an average of less than 3 months; fewer than 5% of the cases persist for more than 6 months

N. The major complications are chronic cardiac valve disease and mitral regurgitation; aortic and mitral stenosis murmurs are not heard acutely, but may be present in adults who had ARF as children

IV. Diagnosis/Evaluation:

A. History
1. Specifically, inquire about onset, duration, and severity of any sore throat within preceding 3 months
2. Ask about duration and presence of all major and manifestations of ARF as well as nonspecific complaints such as weight loss, fatigue, and abdominal pain
3. Question about history of heart murmur or previous cardiac diseases
4. Determine family history of ARF
5. Ask about medication use; use of aspirin can mask signs of inflammation and tends to prolong the course of ARF

B. Physical Examination
1. Measure vital signs, noting elevated temperature
2. Inspect skin for exanthems, lesions, and nodules
3. Perform a complete exam of the ears, nose, and throat
4. Palpate for lymph nodes
5. Perform a complete cardiac exam
6. Auscultate the lungs
7. Assess all joints for tenderness, erythema, warmth and swelling
8. Perform a complete, neuromuscular exam

C. Differential Diagnosis: Diagnosis of ARF must be differentiated from other immunologic and infectious diseases such as the following:
1. Juvenile rheumatoid arthritis
2. Kawasaki syndrome
3. Reiter's syndrome
4. Rheumatoid arthritis
5. Systemic lupus erythematosus
6. Lyme disease

D. Diagnostic Tests
1. Obtain specimens for rapid antigen test and throat culture on all patients with sore throats who are at high risk for ARF (children between 4 to 17 years old, individuals with previous ARF, and close contacts of patients with a history of ARF); if rapid test is negative, send throat culture
2. To document a recent streptococcal infection, obtain acute and convalescent serum samples at 2-4 week intervals; all samples should be tested simultaneously
   a. A rise in titer of two or more dilution increments between the acute-phase and convalescent-phase specimens is significant
   b. The most commonly used antibody assays are antistreptolysin O, antistreptokinase, and anti-deoxyribonuclease B
3. Order C-reactive protein and erythrocyte sedimentation rate

V. Plan/Management

A. Treatment of acute rheumatic fever varies depending on severity of attack; consultation with a specialist is recommended
  1. Because anti-inflammatory therapy such as aspirin may mask inflammation and prolong the duration of attacks, codeine is the analgesic of choice for mild attacks
  2. Corticosteroid therapy is reserved for patients with severe carditis; Dose is 1 mg/kg/day; once the disease is controlled, taper drug over 2-3 weeks
  3. Bed rest should be maintained until the C-reactive protein level has been normal for 2 weeks
  4. Carditis is treated with inotropic agents, diuretics, vasodilators and possibly corticosteroids
  5. Chorea is treated with sedatives and minor tranquilizers

B. Prevention of initial attacks or primary prevention of ARF involves adequate treatment of group A beta-hemolytic streptococcal infections of the upper respiratory tract
  1. Treatment of choice is penicillin oral or intramuscular:
    a. Adults: Penicillin V (Pen-Vee-K) 500 mg BID or TID for at least 10 days
    b. Children: Penicillin V (Pen-Vee-K) 250 mg BID or TID for 10 days. Available 125 mg/5 mL and 250 mg/5 mL liquid
    c. Benzathine penicillin 600,000 units for children <60 pounds;1,200,000 units (1.2 million units) for larger children and adults
      (1) Be familiar with signs, symptoms and treatment of anaphylaxis and observe patient for 30 minutes after injection.
      (2) Bring medication to room temperature before injecting to reduce discomfort
  2. Alternative antibiotics:
    a. Erythromycin: For adults prescribe erythromycin estolate (E-mycin): 20-40 mg/kg/day BID or TID for 10 days; for children prescribe erythromycin ethyl succinate (Eryped) 40mg/kg/day BID or TID for 10 days; available 200mg/5mL and 400mg/5mL susp
    b. Cefadroxil monohydrate (Duricef): For adults prescribe 500 mg capsules BID for 10 days; for children prescribe 30 mg/kg once a day or in 2 divided doses. Available formulations include 125 mg/5mL, 250 mg/5 mL, and 500 mg/5mL suspensions for 10 days; do not use in patients with allergies to penicillin

C. Prevention of recurrent attacks of ARF or secondary prevention
  1. Patients with history of ARF are at a high risk for recurrence of ARF if they develop a streptococcal group A upper respiratory tract infection
  2. Because both asymptomatic and symptomatic infections can trigger a recurrence, continuous prophylaxis is recommended for patients with a well-documented history of ARF
  3. Begin prophylaxis, after full course or antibiotics to eradicate residual Group A Beta-hemolytic streptococcus even if throat culture is negative; promptly treat family members who have current or previous rheumatic fever
  4. Prescribe one of the following medication regimens (see following table)

SECONDARY PROPHYLAXIS OF ACUTE RHEUMATIC FEVER		
Drug	Dose	Frequency
Benzathine penicillin G IM	>60 pound: 1,200,000 units. ≤60 pound: 600,000 units.	Every 3-4 weeks
Penicillin V PO	250 mg	BID
Sulfadiazine PO	>60 pound (27 kg): 1 gm ≤60 pound (27 kg): 500mg	QD QD
Erythromycin PO*	250 mg	BID

*For patients allergic to penicillin and sulfadiazine

*Adapted from Dajani, A., et al., 1995. Treatment of acute streptococcal pharyngitis and prevention of rheumatic fever: A statement for health professionals. Pediatrics, 96, 758-764.

5. The duration of continuous prophylaxis is controversial. Duration of treatment is dependent on risk of recurrence. Risk increases with multiple, previous attacks and in persons who have increased risk of exposure to streptococcal infections such as school teachers, health professionals, or military recruits; recommendations for therapy duration are as follows:
    a. Patients who have had rheumatic carditis need long-term antibiotic prophylaxis into adulthood or possibly for life
        (1) Patients with persistent valvular disease need prophylaxis for at least 10 years after the last episode of ARF and at least until age 40 (continue prophylaxis even after valve surgery)
        (2) Patients with carditis but no residual heart disease such as persistent valvular disease need prophylaxis for 10 years or well into adulthood whichever is longer
    b. Patients who have had ARF without carditis should be carefully assessed, but providers can consider discontinuing prophylaxis in 5 years or until age 21 whichever is longer

D. Prophylaxis for bacterial endocarditis prior to medical or surgical procedures is important; antibiotic regimens used to prevent the recurrence of ARF are inadequate for prevention of bacterial endocarditis (see two tables on RECOMMENDED STANDARD PROPHYLACTIC REGIMEN on the following page)
    1. Endocarditis prophylaxis is recommended for high and medium-risk patients:
        a. High risk patients: prosthetic cardiac valves, previous bacterial endocarditis, complex, cyanotic congenital heart disease, surgically constructed systemic pulmonary shunts or conduits
        b. Medium risk patients: ARF patients who have acquired valvular dysfunction but NOT for patients with previous ARF without valvular dysfunction; other moderate risk patients include those with uncorrected cardiac congenital defects, hypertrophic cardiomyopathy, mitral regurgitation, mitral valve prolapse with murmur, and possibly men >45 years with mitral valve prolapse without murmur
    2. Prophylaxis is recommended for procedures likely to cause bacteremia (see table that follows)

PROCEDURES IN WHICH ENDOCARDITIS PROPHYLAXIS IS RECOMMENDED			
Dental	**Respiratory Tract**	**Gastrointestinal Tract**	**Genitourinary Tract**
Periodontal surgery	Tonsillectomy	Sclerotherapy for esophageal varices	Prostatic surgery
Scaling	Adenoidectomy	Esophageal stricture dilation	Cystoscopy
Professional teeth cleaning	Surgery - resp. mucosa	Endoscopic retrograde cholangiography	Urethral dilation
	Bronchoscopy with bronchoscope	Biliary tract surgery	
		Surgery assoc. with intestinal mucosa	

Adapted from Dajani, A.S. et al. (1997). Prevention of bacterial endocarditis: Recommendations by the American Heart Association. JAMA, 277, 1794-1801.

RECOMMENDED STANDARD PROPHYLACTIC REGIMEN FOR DENTAL, ORAL, RESPIRATORY TRACT, AND ESOPHAGEAL PROCEDURES

Situation	Drug	Timing
Standard general prophylaxis	Amoxicillin Adult: 2 g Child: 50 mg per kg	One hour before procedure and not continued more than 6-8 hours
Patients unable to take PO medications	Ampicillin Adult: 2 g Child: 50 mg per kg	Given IM or IV 30 minutes before procedure
Patients allergic to penicillin	Clindamycin (Cleocin) Adult: 600 mg Child: 20 mg per kg -or-	One hour before procedure and not continued more than 6-8 hours
	Cefadroxil (Duricef) or Cephalexin (Keflex) Adult: 2 g Child: 50 mg per kg -or-	One hour before procedure and not continued more than 6-8 hours
	Azithromycin (Zithromax) or Clarithromycin (Biaxin) Adult: 500 mg Child: 15 mg per kg	One hour before procedure and not continued more than 6-8 hours
Patients allergic to penicillin and unable to take oral medication	Clindamycin (Cleocin) Adult: 600 mg Child: 20 mg per kg -or-	Given IM or IV within 30 minutes of procedure
	Cefazolin (Kefzol) Adult: 1 g Child: 25 mg per kg	Given IM or IV within 30 minutes of procedure

Adapted from Dajani, A.S. et al. (1997). Prevention of bacterial endocarditis: Recommendations by the American Heart Association. JAMA, 277, 1794-1801.

RECOMMENDED STANDARD PROPHYLACTIC REGIMEN FOR GENITOURINARY AND GASTROINTESTINAL PROCEDURES

Situation	Drug	Adults' Dose	Children's Dose
Standard general prophylaxis for patient with ARF and valvular dysfunction	Amoxicillin -or- Ampicillin	2 g PO one hour before procedure -or- 2 g IM or IV within 30 minutes of procedure	50 mg per kg PO one hour before procedure -or- 50 mg per kg IM or IV within 30 minutes of procedure
Patients with ARF and valvular dysfunction who are allergic to penicillin	Vancomycin	1 g IV over one to two hours; infusion should be completed within 30 minutes of procedure	20 mg per kg IV over one to two hours; infusion should be completed within 30 minutes of procedure

Adapted from Dajani, A.S. et al. (1997). Prevention of bacterial endocarditis: Recommendations by the American Heart Association. JAMA, 277, 1794-1801.

3. Patient Education for preventing bacterial endocarditis
   a. Teach patient to maintain good oral health with regular brushing, flossing, and visits to dentist to reduce sources of bacterial seeding
   b. Teach about the risks and sequella of bacterial endocarditis; emphasize that patients must take responsibility in communicating to health care providers about their cardiac condition and possible need for prophylaxis before procedures

E. Follow Up
1. For primary prevention or prevention of ARF with penicillin for Group A beta-hemolytic streptococcal pharyngitis no "test of cure" throat culture is needed unless the patient is at unusually high risk for developing ARF
2. For patients with ARF, return visits depend on their clinical condition
   a. Typically, patients can be reevaluated when they return for prophylaxis every 3-4 weeks if they receiving an intramuscular antibiotic, otherwise schedule visits for every 4-6 weeks
   b. C-reactive protein needs to be closely monitored until it returns to normal levels; after C-reactive protein is normalized, monitor periodically for 6-8 additional weeks

ROCKY MOUNTAIN SPOTTED FEVER

I. Definition: Systemic, febrile illness with characteristic rash that results from bite of infected tick

II. Pathogenesis

A. Infectious agent is *Rickettsia rickettsii*

B. Mode of transmission
1. Tick must attach and feed on blood for approximately 4-6 hours to become infectious in humans
2. No person-to-person transmission

C. Incubation period ranges from 2-14 days

III. Clinical Presentation

A. Most common arthropod-borne disease

B. Most cases are in south Atlantic, southeastern, and south central states; other areas include the upper Rocky Mountain states, Canada, Mexico and South and Central America

C. Patient typically presents with sudden onset of moderate to high fever (which persists if untreated for 2-3 weeks), severe headache, myalgia, conjunctival injection, nausea and vomiting

D. Characteristic maculopapular rash usually appears before the sixth day of illness
1. Rash spreads from wrists and ankles to trunk, neck and face
2. In untreated patients, the lesions become petechial in about 4 days, then purpuric and coalesced

E. Thrombocytopenia develops in most patients; anemia is present in about 30% of cases

F. Disease can persist for 3 weeks and can be severe with central nervous system, cardiac, pulmonary, gastrointestinal, and renal involvement as well as disseminated intravascular coagulation which can lead to shock and ultimately to death; case fatality rate is 15-20% in untreated individuals but death is uncommon when diagnosis and treatment are prompt

IV. Diagnosis/Evaluation

A. History
1. Inquire about onset, duration, and characteristics of all symptoms
2. Ask patient to describe characteristics and progression of any rashes or skin lesions
3. Inquire about possible exposure to tick bites such as recent camping trip or frequent yard work
4. May need to do a complete review of systems to detect complications from the infection

B. Physical Examination
1. Measure vital signs, noting fever
2. Observe general appearance for signs of distress and lethargy
3. Carefully inspect skin for rashes and lesions
4. Inspect eyes for conjunctival injection
5. Palpate for lymphadenopathy
6. Perform complete heart, lung, and neurological examinations to rule out complications

C. Differential Diagnosis
1. In early stage, disease resembles systemic viral infections
2. In advanced disease, bacterial sepsis, meningitis, and meningococcemia are part of differential diagnosis

D. Diagnostic Tests
1. Consider ordering acute and convalescent sera, group-specific serologic tests (a fourfold rise in antibody titer is diagnostic of the disease)
    a. Titers can be determined by indirect fluorescent antibody, complement fixation, latex agglutination, indirect hemagglutination, or microagglutination
    b. Never delay initiation of antimicrobial treatment to confirm clinical suspicion of the disease
2. Consider ordering a CBC with differential, BUN, serum albumin, serum electrolytes, and liver function studies

V. Plan/Management (consult specialist)

A. Important to treat patients with antimicrobial therapy early in the course of disease; mortality sharply increases when therapy is delayed until the sixth day of illness
1. Oral doxycycline (Vibramycin) is the drug of choice. Dose is 100 mg BID after a loading dose of 200 mg; therapy is continued until patient is afebrile for at least 2-3 days; usual course is 7-10 days
2. In patients with severe disease in whom meningococcemia is also in the differential diagnosis, chloramphenicol should be considered for use; prescribe chloramphenicol (Chloromycetin) 50-100 mg/kg/day orally or intravenously in 4 divided doses. Therapy is continued until patient is afebrile for at least 2-3 days; usual course is 7-10 days

B. Patients who have any signs of complications should have a specialist consult and probably be admitted to the hospital because of the dangers of vascular collapse

C. Prevention: Teach patient about measures to avoid tick bites (see section on LYME DISEASE)

D. Follow Up
1. Because of the possible dangerous complications of the disease, close monitoring is needed
    a. Teach patients to return to clinic if any danger signs such as alterations in mental status, stiff neck, severe headache, prolonged nausea and vomiting, shortness of breath, decreased urine output, high fever, severe weakness and dizziness occur
    b. Patients should return to clinic within 24-48 hours of initial visit; then patient should be reevaluated at the end of the antimicrobial therapy
2. Patients using chloramphenicol need frequent serum platelet counts and CBCs

RUBELLA (GERMAN MEASLES)

I.   Definition: Febrile viral disease with diffuse maculopapular rash; postnatal rubella is usually mild and congenital rubella is associated with high incidence of congenital anomalies

II.   Pathogenesis

    A.   Causal agent is rubella virus which is a RNA virus

    B.   Spread by direct contact with secretions of nose and throat

    C.   Incubation period ranges from 14-21 days

    D.   Period of communicability
        1.   One week before and 5-7 days after onset of rash
        2.   Infants with congenital rubella may shed virus for months after birth

III. Clinical Presentation

    A.   Importance of this viral illness is not the morbidity of the disease itself, but rather the consequences that can occur to a fetus during a maternal infection

    B.   Before the use of vaccines, rubella was a wide-spread disease; today the incidence of disease has declined by more than 99% from the prevaccine era

    C.   Most cases today occur in young, unvaccinated adults and outbreaks in colleges and occupational settings; approximately 10% of young adults are susceptible to rubella

IV.   Diagnosis/Evaluation

    A.   History
        1.   Inquire about duration and occurrence of rash, fever, and enlarged lymph nodes which indicate rubella as well as other symptoms such as cough, coryza, conjunctivitis, pharyngitis which are associated with other exanthematous diseases
        2.   Ask about recent exposure to persons with a rash
        3.   Ask about medication and drug use
        4.   Inquire about history of rubella illness and/or illnesses with exanthems (history of rubella illness is not a reliable indicator of immunity; identification of immune status is based on the presence of demonstrable antibodies)

    B.   Physical Examination
        1.   Measure vital signs
        2.   Inspect skin, noting characteristics of exanthem
        3.   To eliminate other exanthematous diseases as the diagnosis, examination of the following areas is often needed
            a.   Eyes, noting signs of conjunctivitis
            b.   Head, ears, nose, and throat
            c.   Mouth for signs of Koplik's spots which indicate measles, not rubella
            d.   Neck, noting nuchal rigidity and adenopathy
            e.   Heart, noting murmurs

    C.   Differential Diagnosis
        1.   Rubeola
        2.   Rocky Mountain spotted fever
        3.   Scarlet fever
        4.   Infectious mononucleosis
        5.   Enterovirus
        6.   Drug reaction

D. Diagnostic Tests
1. Order acute (within 7-10 days after onset of disease) and convalescent sera (2-3 weeks later); a fourfold or greater rise in titer or seroconversion is indicative of infection
2. Many virology laboratories can detect specific rubella IgM antibody
3. To determine immune status and presence of antibodies, order latex agglutination, fluorescence immunoassay, passive hemagglutination, hemolysis-in-gel or enzyme immunossay; the hemagglutination inhibition antibody test is not as sensitive and is no longer recommended
4. The virus may be isolated from the pharynx one week before until 2 weeks after exanthem; blood, urine, and cerebrospinal fluid can also yield virus

V. Plan/Management

A. Treatment: Patient's condition is usually mild and only symptomatic treatment is needed such as rest and increased fluid intake

B. Primary prevention of rubella; efforts should be made to vaccinate all postpubertal adolescent and adult males and females who have not been immunized or who have not been proven serologically to be immune to rubella
1. Females should be counseled to avoid pregnancy for 3 months after vaccination
2. Do not give vaccine in the 2 weeks before or 3 months after administration of immunoglobulin or blood
3. Serious illness is a contraindication for vaccine, but minor illness with or without fever should not preclude vaccination

C. Treatment of exposed persons
1. Pregnant women need blood specimens tested for rubella antibody; consult specialist for further treatment of exposed pregnant women; routine use of immune globulin is not recommended and only considered if termination of pregnancy is not an option
2. Live rubella vaccine given after exposure does not prevent the disease, but may be indicated in nonpregnant persons for protection against developing rubella in the future

D. Control procedures
1. All cases of rubella should be reported to the local health unit
2. In institutions such as hospitals, patients suspected of having rubella should be isolated
3. Patients should not go to work or school for 7 days after onset of rash
4. Efforts should be made to identify and counsel all pregnant females who had contact with patient with infection

E. Follow up is usually not needed unless the patient must return for convalescent titers after 2-3 weeks of initial illness

RUBEOLA (MEASLES)

I. Definition: Acute, highly communicable viral disease consisting of fever, rash, and presence of cough, coryza or conjunctivitis

II. Pathogenesis

A. Causal agent is the measles virus which is an RNA virus

B. Transmitted between individuals by direct contact with infectious droplets, or less frequently, by air-borne spread

C. Incubation period is 8-12 days from exposure to onset of symptoms

D. Period of communicability: Patient is infectious 1-2 days before onset of symptoms and 3-5 days prior to rash to approximately 4 days after rash

III. Clinical Presentation

    A. One of most serious exanthematous diseases

    B. Prior to widespread immunization, measles were common in childhood; effective immunization programs have reduced rate by 99%

    C. About 5% of all measles cases are due to vaccine failure

    D. Center for Disease Control's clinical case definition is as follows:
        1. Generalized rash lasting 3 or more days
        2. Fever greater than 38.3°C (100.9°F)
        3. At least one of the following symptoms: cough, coryza and conjunctivitis (sometimes referred to as the 3 "C"s)

    E. Typically, patients have a prodrome with fever and the 3 "C"s which lasts between 1-4 days; patients are usually very ill during this time

    F. As prodromal symptoms reach a peak, the exanthem appears and is characterized by the following:
        1. Deep, red macular rash which begins on face and neck and spreads down trunk and extremities
        2. Rash begins as discrete lesions but then becomes confluent and salmon-colored (referred to as a morbilliform rash)
        3. When fever subsides, around the sixth day, a faint brown stain on the skin remains and desquamation of the skin often begins

    G. Koplik's spots are pathognomonic for measles; this enanthem presents as tiny, bluish white spots on an erythematous base which cluster adjacent to the molars on the buccal mucosa

    H. Most patients recover rapidly after the first 3-4 days

    I. Complications include otitis media, pneumonia, croup, and encephalitis

IV. Diagnosis/Evaluation

    A. History
        1. Inquire about duration and occurrence of rash, cough, conjunctivitis, coryza and Koplik's spots
        2. Explore the presence of other symptoms which denote complications of measles such as chest pain, ear pain and confusion
        3. Ask about immunization status
        4. Ask about recent exposure to persons with a rash
        5. Inquire about medical history (immunosuppressed patients may need different treatment regimens; patients who are chronically ill often develop life-threatening symptoms)
        6. Ask about medication use

    B. Physical Examination
        1. Measure vital signs
        2. Inspect skin, noting characteristics of exanthem
        3. Examine eyes, noting signs of conjunctivitis
        4. Examine head, ears, nose, and throat because complications of measles often involve these parts of the body
        5. Examine mouth for signs of Koplik's spots
        6. Examine neck for adenopathy and nuchal rigidity
        7. Auscultate heart
        8. Patients need daily examination of chest to rule out complications such as pneumonia
        9. Perform a mental status examination and a neurological exam to rule out complications such as encephalitis

C.   Differential Diagnosis
1.   Rubella
2.   Rocky Mountain spotted fever
3.   Scarlet fever
4.   Infectious mononucleosis
5.   Secondary syphilis
6.   Enterovirus
7.   Drug reaction

D.   Diagnostic Tests: Order one of the following:
1.   Antibody titers when rash first appears and then at convalescence or 2-4 weeks later (significant rise in antibody concentrations between acute and convalescent sera is characteristic of measles)
2.   Serum IgM antibody levels (presence of measles-specific IgM antibodies is characteristic; IgM antibody peaks ten days after rash onset and disappears after 20 to 60 days)
3.   Measles virus can be detected by viral isolation in cell culture from nasopharyngeal secretions, conjunctiva, blood or urine during the febrile period of illness

V.   Plan/Management

A.   The following patients should be considered for Vitamin A supplementation:
1.   Patients with measles who live in communities where Vitamin A deficiency is a problem and where mortality related to measles is ≥1%
2.   Patients > 6 months with measles who have one of the following risk factors:
a.   Immunodeficiency
b.   Ophthalmologic evidence of vitamin A deficiency including night blindness, Bitot's spots, or evidence of xerophthalmia
c.   Impaired intestinal absorption
d.   Moderate to severe malnutrition, including that associated with eating disorders
e.   Recent immigrants from areas where high mortality rates from measles have occurred
3.   Recommended dose: single dose of 200 000 IU orally (Available in 50 000 IU/mL solution)

B.   Symptomatic Treatment
1.   Provide rest and fluids
2.   Instruct patient to avoid bright lights due to problems with photosensitivity
3.   Frequently monitor for signs and symptoms of complications of measles

C.   Treatment of exposed persons
1.   Give live measles vaccine if exposure was within 72 hours (may give to infants as young as 6 months). Recommended dose is 0.5 mL, given subcutaneously
2.   Give immune globulin to induce passive immunity and to prevent or modify symptoms within 6 days of exposure. Do not give immune globulin with the live measles vaccine
a.   Recommended dose of immune globulin is 0.25 mL/kg/dose IM (immunocompromised patients should receive 0.5 mL/kg). Maximum dose is 15 mL
b.   Immune globulin is especially indicated for susceptible household contacts of measles, particularly immunocompromised contacts, and contacts younger than 1 year of age, and pregnant women
c.   Live measles virus vaccine should be given approximately 5-6 months after immune globulin administration, provided patient is >12 months

D.   Control Procedures
1.   Infected patients should be isolated for at least 4 days after appearance of rash
2.   Persons exposed to measles who are susceptible to developing the infection should be isolated from 5th day post-exposure up to and including the 21st day
3.   All reports of measles cases should be reported to the local health unit and investigated promptly

4. All patients who cannot provide documentation of measles immunity should be vaccinated or excluded from school, work, or other public places
5. Investigate immune status of family members and other immediate contacts; prescribe vaccine if appropriate

E. Patient Education
1. Teach patient to take daily temperature readings; fever lasting more than 4 days suggests presence of complications
2. Teach patient and/or parents to monitor for signs of complications of measles such as how to count respirations and how to assess for changes in respiratory status and changes in level of consciousness

F. Follow Up
1. Patient with measles should be examined by health care provider (can be a nurse) every day during acute phase to rule out development of complications
2. Patient should be seen in the clinic office about 3-4 days after onset of exanthem

SCARLET FEVER (SCARLATINA)

I. Definition: Acute, infectious disease with vascular response to bacterial exotoxin and usually associated with streptococcal pharyngitis

II. Pathogenesis

A. Caused by circulating erythrogenic toxin that is produced by group A hemolytic *Streptococcus* and to a lesser extent, certain strains of staphylococci
1. If streptococcus is the source of the toxin, it usually has a pharyngeal focus
2. May rarely follow infection of wounds, burns or streptococcal or staphylococcal skin infections

B. Mode of transmission is usually via direct projection of large droplets or physical transfer of respiratory secretions
1. Rarely may be due to contaminated articles or ingestion of contaminated milk or other food
2. Prolonged carriage of streptococci may occur in the throat or upper respiratory tract for weeks to months

C. Incubation period usually ranges from 3-5 days

D. Period of communicability: During incubation period and clinical illness or approximately 10 days; person is no longer infectious after 24 hours of antibiotic therapy

III. Clinical Presentation

A. In the past, disease had a high morbidity and mortality from systemic toxicity and the sequella of rheumatic fever and glomerulonephritis; complications less common today due to use of antibiotics

B. Incidence highest in children 6-12 years of age but can occur in adulthood

C. Usually an abrupt onset of fever, pharyngitis, and headache; less common is abdominal pain

D. Exanthem appears 24-48 hours after infection and lasts 4-10 days
1. Presents as fine, pin-head sized eruptions, often confluent, on an erythematous base which blanches on pressure
2. Rash has the texture of sandpaper

3. Rash rapidly becomes generalized but is typically absent on the face which usually has a flushed appearance with circumoral pallor
4. Petechia may be present in a linear pattern along the major skin folds in the axillae and antecubital fossa (Pastia's sign)
5. Rash fades 3-4 days after onset
6. Desquamation of the skin usually occurs at the end of first week and usually disappears by end of 3 weeks

E. Patient may have enanthem of a "strawberry" tongue which presents as a thick white coat with hypertrophied red papillae

F. Staphylococcal scarlet fever can be differentiated from streptococcal scarlet fever in the following ways:
1. There is no circumoral pallor or strawberry tongue
2. The erythematous skin is often painful or tender
3. Desquamation of the superficial epidermis occurs as with the streptococcal illness; if the superficial skin separates and sloughs after only a few days, the patient should be classified as having scalded skin syndrome

G. Generalized lymphadenopathy is common in both streptococcal and staphylococcal scarlet fever

H. Complications include otitis media, sinusitis, bacteremia, rheumatic fever, glomerulonephritis; rarely occur with prompt diagnosis and treatment

IV. Diagnosis/Evaluation

A. History
1. Inquire about onset and duration of symptoms, particularly pharyngitis, rash, headache, fever, and abdominal pain
2. Ask about any associated symptoms such as ear pain, chest pain, edema which may be related to complications of scarlet fever
3. Inquire about the possibility of infected skin wounds
4. Question whether other members of the household, classmates, or work colleagues have been ill with streptococcal pharyngitis or other communicable diseases
5. Ask about medication history
6. Ask about previous medical history
7. Determine whether patient is allergic to penicillin

B. Physical Examination
1. Measure vital signs
2. Observe general appearance for signs of toxicity and respiratory distress
3. Inspect skin; noting exanthem, Pastia's lines, facial flushing with circumoral pallor
4. Palpate skin, noting any rough texture
5. Perform a complete eyes, ears, nose, and mouth exam
6. Perform a thorough examination of the pharynx, noting exudate, color, and swelling
7. Perform a complete cardiovascular and chest exam
8. Palpate abdomen for organomegaly

C. Differential Diagnosis
1. Rubeola
2. Rubella
3. Infectious mononucleosis
4. Toxic shock syndrome
5. Drug reactions (sulfonamides, penicillin, streptomycin, quinine, and atropine)

D. Diagnostic Tests
1. Obtain throat swab for rapid antigen test and a duplicate swab for a throat culture; if rapid test is positive, treat for streptococcal infection; if rapid test is negative, process throat culture

2. Household contacts of index patient who have symptoms should be cultured, but do not culture asymptomatic household contacts unless there is an outbreak

V. Plan/Management: Treatment of scarlet fever is no different from that of streptococcal pharyngitis (see section on PHARYNGITIS)

   A. Treatment of choice is penicillin oral or intramuscular:
      1. Adults: Penicillin V (Pen-Vee-K) 250 mg TID or QID for 10 days
      2. Benzathine penicillin 1.2 million units IM. Be familiar with signs, symptoms and treatment of anaphylaxis and observe patient for 30 minutes after injection

   B. Alternative antibiotics:
      1. Erythromycin: Adults prescribe (E-mycin): 250 mg q 6 hours for 10 days
      2. Cefadroxil monohydrate (Duricef): Adults prescribe 500 mg capsules BID for 10 days

   C. If staphylococcal scarlet fever is suspected, prescribe dicloxacillin (Dynapen) 15-20 mg/kg/day in divided doses every 6 hours for 10 days

   D. Patient Education
      1. Discuss communicability of disease; patient should not return to work or school until at least 24 hours after beginning antimicrobial therapy
      2. Warn patient that skin desquamation may occur
      3. Assure family that rheumatic fever does not occur with appropriate antimicrobial therapy

   E. Follow Up
      1. Posttreatment throat cultures are indicated only for patients who have a high risk for rheumatic fever or who are still symptomatic after treatment
      2. No follow up is needed for patients with uncomplicated illnesses

VARICELLA (CHICKENPOX)

I. Definition: Viral disease with a pruritic, vesicular exanthem that appears in crops

II. Pathogenesis

   A. Causal agent is varicella-zoster virus (VZV) which is a member of the herpesvirus family

   B. Transmission (highly contagious disease)
      1. Primarily, spread by respiratory secretions which become airborne
      2. Contact with fluid from vesicles can spread disease
      3. Direct contact with patient with shingles may also spread the virus and cause chickenpox in the susceptible host

   C. Incubation period is 10-21 days with an average of 14-16 days

   D. Patient is communicable one to two days before the rash is apparent until all the vesicles have crusted, typically 5 days after onset of rash

III. Clinical Presentation

   A. Commonly occurs in children between 5 and 10 years old, but is becoming more common in adolescents and young adults

   B. In adults the prodrome and illness are often severe and the course is prolonged; there also is a 25-fold increased risk of mortality

C. A few hours to days after the prodrome a macular rash, typically on the scalp, neck or upper trunk emerges:
1. Exanthem occurs in stages: begins as macules, then turns to papules, and then to vesicles all within 12-24 hours
2. When vesicles begin to resolve, crusts develop
3. Rash spreads centrifugally (away from center) and lesions may occur on mucous membranes of mouth, conjunctivae, esophagus, trachea, rectum and vagina
4. Usually patient has little scarring unless infection of skin occurs

D. Certain groups of patients have more severe cases
1. Patients with leukemia may suffer severe, prolonged or fatal chickenpox
2. Immunocompromised patients often have eruption of lesions and high fever for 2 weeks
3. AIDS patients may develop chronic chickenpox

E. Complications are uncommon but may include the following:
1. Secondary bacterial skin infection (*Group A Streptococcus* or *Staphylococcus aureus*), acute cerebellar ataxia, meningoencephalitis, thrombocytopenia, glomerulonephritis, and varicella pneumonia (which is rare in normal children, but the most common complication in older patients)
2. Reye syndrome was more common in the past due salicylate therapy

F. The virus remains in a latent form after the primary infection; zoster or shingles results with reactivation

IV. Diagnosis/Evaluation

A. History
1. Ask patient to specifically describe when and where the first lesion occurred
2. Ask about the spread and changes that have occurred in the characteristics of the lesions
3. Ask about prodromal symptoms
4. Question about associated symptoms or potential complications such as pulmonary and nervous problems
5. Inquire about recent exposure to chickenpox
6. Ask about any self-treatments
7. Determine whether patient is immunocompromised or has any other risk factors
8. Ask whether any household contacts lack immunity to varicella and if there are immunocompromised individuals who were exposed to infected patient

B. Physical Examination
1. Observe skin and describe types of lesions, location of lesions, arrangement of lesions
2. Palpate for adenopathy
3. Auscultate heart and lungs
4. Perform a focused neurological examination

C. Differential Diagnosis
1. Scabies
2. Herpes simplex
3. Folliculitis
4. Viral exanthems such as coxsackievirus and echovirus have vesicles, but these vesicles do not usually crust as occurs in chickenpox
5. Contact dermatitis
6. Insect bites
7. Drug eruptions
8. Impetigo
9. Hand-foot-and-mouth disease
10. Secondary syphilis

D. Diagnostic Tests
    1. Usually none needed
    2. Immunofluorescent staining of vesicular scrapings from skin lesion with monoclonal antibodies can detect virus
    3. To demonstrate a recent infection, can order acute and convalescent titers
    4. Serologic tests include enzyme immuno-assay, latex agglutination, indirect fluorescent antibody, and fluorescent antibody-to-membrane antigen

V. Plan/Management

A. Consider oral acyclovir therapy. Acyclovir (Zorvirax) therapy can reduce the rate of acute complications, pruritus, spread of infection, and duration of absence from school or work with no significant adverse effects if given within 24 hours of illness
    1. Acyclovir is recommended, if it can be initiated within the first 24 hours after the onset or rash, in the following groups:
        a. Otherwise, healthy, nonpregnant individuals 13 years of age or older
        b. Some experts also suggest oral acyclovir for secondary household cases who typically have most severe infection
    2. If therapy can be initiated within the first 24 hours of rash onset, prescribe oral acyclovir 20 mg/kg/dose in 4 divided doses for 5 days; maximum dose is 800 mg per dose QID. Patient should be maintained in a well-hydrated state
    3. Intravenously administered acyclovir is recommended for treatment of immunocompromised patients
    4. In the pregnant woman with uncomplicated varicella, oral acyclovir therapy is not advised, because of unknown risks to fetus. Intravenous therapy should be considered for pregnant women with serious viral mediated complications of varicella

B. Measures to control pruritus:
    1. Can apply calamine or cetaphil lotion to lesions
    2. Prescribe hydroxyzine (Atarax). Adult dosage is 25 mg TID/QID
    3. Alternatively, can prescribe diphenhydramine HCl (Benadryl). Adult dosage is 25-50 mg TID/QID
    4. Daily baths with baking soda or Aveeno may relieve pruritus and prevent bacterial superinfection
    5. Cut patient's nails

C. Symptomatic treatment to reduce fever and discomfort: Use acetaminophen (Tylenol) (see section on FEVER for dosage); NEVER USE ASPIRIN IN YOUNG ADULTS

D. Control Measures: Patients may return to school/work on the sixth day after the onset of the rash or in mild cases, after all the lesions are crusted

E. Care of Exposed Persons: Administration of varicella-zoster immune globulin (VZIG) within 72-96 hours after exposure to varicella; may prevent or modify the disease (obtain VZIG from American Red Cross Blood Services)
    1. VZIG should be given to the following persons if they have had signficant exposure such as residing in same household, indoor face-to-face contact, hospital contact:
        a. Immunocompromised persons known to be susceptible
        b. Susceptible, pregnant women
        c. Newborns whose mothers have had onset of varicella within 5 days before or within 2 days after delivery
        d. Hospitalized premature infant
            (1) ≥28 weeks gestation whose mother has no history of varicella or seronegativity
            (2) <28 weeks of gestation or ≤1000 g regardless of maternal history
        e. Dosage: One vial VZIG containing 125 units is given for each 10 kg of body weight. The maximum dose is 625 units or 5 vials
        f. Because of the availability of acyclovir, it is no longer recommended that normal adults who have close contact with infected patient use VZIG

2. Postexposure prophylactic administration of varicella vaccine is not FDA-approved but it may be effective in preventing or reducing clinical symptoms of the contact and carries little risk

F. Active or primary immunization is recommended for the following patients:
   1. Healthy adolescents and adults: prescribe two doses of vaccine 4 to 8 weeks apart
   2. Adults: vaccination of susceptible adults is encouraged (two doses 4-8 weeks apart); priority given to persons at high risk for complications such as health care personnel and family contacts of immunocompromised individuals, those at high risk for exposure, and non-pregnant women of child-bearing age
   3. Vaccination is contraindicated in individuals with moderate to serious illness, immunocompromised persons, patients receiving corticosteroids, persons with acute lymphocytic leukemia, and persons with allergies to vaccine component
      a. Salicylates should not be administered for 6 weeks and VZIG should not be given for 3 weeks after vaccine
      b. Vaccine should not be given for at least 5 months after patient has taken VZIG

G. Follow Up
   1. Teach patients to identify potential complications such as secondary skin infections, central nervous system problems, and pneumonia
   2. In uncomplicated cases, no follow up is needed

REFERENCES

American Academy of Pediatrics. (1997). Summaries of infectious diseases. In Peter, G. (Ed.). 1997 Red Book: Report of the committee on infectious diseases (24th ed.). Elk Grove Village, IL: Author.

American College of Physicians. (1997). Clinical guideline, part 1: Guideline for laboratory evaluation in the diagnosis of Lyme disease. Annals of Internal Medicine, 127, 1106-1108.

American College of Rheumatology and the Council of the Infectious Diseases Society of America (1993). Appropriateness of parenteral antibiotic treatment for patients with presumed Lyme disease. Annals of Internal Medicine, 119, 518.

Centers for Disease Control and Prevention. (1996). Prevention of varicella: Recommendations of the Advisory Committee on Immunization Practices. MMWR,45(No. RR-11), 1-27.

Centers for Disease Control and Prevention. (1997). Prevention and control of influenza: Recommendations of the Advisory Committee on Immunization Practices. MMWR, 46(No. RR-9), 1-25.

Committee on Infectious Diseases. American Academy of Pediatrics. (1993). Vitamin A treatment of measles. Pediatrics, 91(5), 1014-1015.

Cozad, J. (1996). Infectious mononucleosis. Nurse Practitioner, 21 (3), 14-28.

Dajani, A.S., Ayoub, E., Bierman, F.Z., Bisno, A.L., Denny, F.W., Durack, D.T., Ferrieri, P., Freed, M., Gerber, M., Kaplan, E.L., Karchmer, A.W., Markowitz, M., Rahimtoola, S.H., Shulman, S.T., Stollerman, G., Takahashi, M., Taranto, A., Taubert, K.A., & Wilson, W. (1993). Guidelines for the diagnosis of rheumatic fever: Jones criteria, updated 1992. Circulation, 87, 302-307.

Dajani, A., Taubert, K., Ferrieri, P., Peter, G., Shulman, S. and other committee members. (1995). Treatment of acute streptococcal pharyngitis and prevention of rheumatic fever: A statement for health professionals. Pediatrics, 96, 758-764.

Dajani, A.S.,Taubert, K.A., Wilson, W., Bolger, A.F., Bayer, A., Ferrieri, P., Gewitz, M., Shulman, S.T., Nouri, S., Newburger, J.W., Hutto, C. Pallasch, T.J., Gage, T.W. Levison, M.E., Peter, G., & Zuccaro, G. Jr. (1997). Prevention of bacterial endocarditis: Recommendations by the American Heart Association. JAMA, 277, 1794-1801.

Dattwyler, R.J., Luft, B.J., Kunkel, M.J., et al. (1997). Ceftriaxone compared with doxycycline for the treatment of acute disseminated Lyme disease. New England Journal of Medicine, 337, 289-294.

Habif, T.P. (1996). Clinical dermatology: A color guide to diagnosis and therapy (3rd ed.). St. Louis: Mosby.

Nightingale, S.L. (1997). Public health advisory: Limitations, use, and interpretation of assays for supporting clinical diagnosis of Lyme disease. JAMA, 278, 805.

Smith, D.L. (1997). Cat scratch disease and related clinical syndromes. <u>American Family Physician, 55,</u> 1783-1789.

Spach, D.H., Liles, W.C., Campbell, G.L., Quick, R.E., Anderson, D.E. & Fritsche, T.R. (1993). Tick-borne diseases in the United States. <u>The New England Journal of Medicine, 329</u>(13), 936-945.

Still, M.M., & Ryan, M.E. (1997). Pitfalls in diagnosis of Lyme disease. <u>Postgraduate Medicine, 102,</u> 65-72.

Straus, S.E., Cohen, J.E., Tosato, G., & Meier, J. (1993). Epstein-Barr virus infections: Biology, pathogenesis, and management. <u>Annals of Internal Medicine, 118,</u> 45-55.

Tugwell, P., Dennis, D.T., Weinstein, A., Wells, G., Shea, B., Nichol, G., Hayward, R., Lightfoot, R., Baker, P., & Steere, A.C. (1997). Clinical guideline, part 2: Laboratory evaluation in the diagnosis of Lyme disease. <u>Annals of Internal Medicine, 127,</u> 1109-1121.

Vernon, M.E., & Igal, L.H. (1997). Recognition and management of Lyme disease. <u>American Family Physician, 56,</u> 427-436.

Zangwill, K.M., Hamilton, D.H., Perkins, B.A. (1993). Cat scratch disease in Connecticut: Epidemiology, risk factors, and evaluation of a new diagnostic test. <u>New England Journal of Medicine, 329,</u> 8-13.

CHAPTER 7

Skin Problems in Adults

CARE OF DRY AND OILY SKIN

I.   Definition: Care aimed at preserving or restoring the normal physiologic state of the skin

II.   Pathogenesis

    A.   Dry skin results from reduced water content of the stratum corneum and may result from exposure to irritating substances (household/industrial chemicals), decreased humidity, and frequent or prolonged exposure to water

    B.   Oily skin is a result of excess sebum production by sebaceous glands which are largest and most numerous on face, chest, and upper back

III.   Clinical Presentation

    A.   Dry skin presents as scaly, dry appearing skin which feels dry to touch, and is most often located on extensor surfaces of legs and arms

    B.   Dry skin may appear at any age, but is more common among the elderly with the legs being the most commonly affected

    C.   Dry skin is sensitive (that is, easily irritated) and usually pruritic

    D.   Oily skin presents as moist appearing, shiny skin which feels oily to touch and is most often located on face, chest, and upper back

    E.   Oily skin may occur at any age, but is most common among young adults

IV.   Diagnosis/Evaluation

    A.   History
        1.   Inquire about distribution, onset, duration
        2.   Ask about skin cleansing practices, occupational, and household exposures
        3.   Ask about treatments tried and results

    B.   Physical Examination
        1.   Examine entire skin surface
        2.   For patients complaining of dry skin, focus on legs, extensor surfaces, and hands, where drying is likely to be worse
        3.   For oily skin, focus on face, upper back, and chest

    C.   Differential Diagnosis
        1.   Atopic dermatitis
        2.   Contact dermatitis
        3.   Ichthyosis
        4.   Dyshidrotic eczema

    D.   Diagnostic Tests: None indicated

V.   Plan/Management

    A.   For dry skin, the following recommendations should be provided to patients

---

ADVICE FOR PATIENTS WITH DRY SKIN

➡ Soak, rather than shower, immersed in water no warmer than 90° for 10 minutes (**Note:** Experts in previous years discouraged frequent bathing–daily soaking is now recommended for dry skin)

➡ Use a mild, non-drying synthetic detergent (syndet) bar such as Dove, Caress or Eucerin and rinse well

➡ A waterless liquid cleanser such as Cetaphil or Aquanil may also be used, especially for washing face

➡ Omit use of bubble baths and bath oils which pose hazard (falls)

➡ Pat skin dry–brush away excess water with hands, then pat or blot skin with towel

➡ Apply moisturizers from the following list after bathing and while skin is somewhat moist to seal moisture into skin

➡ **Note:** Lotions are the least moisturizing but the most acceptable to patients; ointments are the most moisturizing but patients dislike the greasy feel of ointments

Moisturizing Lotions	**Moisturizing Creams**	**Moisturizing Ointments**
Petrolatum-based	Petrolatum-based	Petrolatum-based
Dermasil	Purpose Dry Skin Cream	Vaseline Pure Petroleum Jelly
SML Lotion	Cetaphil Cream	(Fragrance, preservative, and
Moisturel Lotion	Keri Cream	lanolin free)
Replenaderm		
Mixtures of lanolin and petrolatum	Mixtures of lanolin and petrolatum	Mixtures of lanolin and petrolatum
Eucerin Lotion	Eucerin Creme	Aquaphor Natural Healing
Lubriderm Lotion		Ointment
Nivea Moisturizing		(Fragrance and preservative free)
Without lanolin or petrolatum	Without lanolin or petrolatum	
Corn Huskers Lotion	Neutrogena Norwegian	
Cetaphil Lotion	Formula Hand Cream	

    B.   For patients with extremely dry skin, products containing urea or lactic acid may be helpful (**Note:** Urea and lactic acid remove excess adherent scales and make skin more pliable but use cautiously, as erythema and peeling may occur)

UREA CREAMS AND LOTIONS

Cream 10% (Aquacare, Nutraplus)
Cream 20% (Carmol 20)
Lotion 10% (Aquacare, Carmol 10)

LACTIC ACID-CONTAINING LOTIONS

5% (LactiCare)
12% (Lac-Hydrin) [a Rx product]

Caution: Lactic acid-containing preparations may cause burning or stinging

---

    C.   For oily skin, the following recommendations should be provided to patients

---

ADVICE FOR PATIENTS WITH OILY SKIN

➡ Use a deodorant soap such as Dial or Safeguard containing an antibacterial or a mildly drying soap (Ivory)
➡ Avoid using preparations containing oils
➡ Use an astringent or toner on face
➡ For women, use cosmetics such as those listed here

COSMETICS FOR WOMEN WITH OILY SKIN			
Allercreme	Matte-Finish Makeup (Waterbase, oil free)	Lancome	Maquicontrol, Oil-Free Liquid Makeup
Charles of the Ritz	T-Zone Controller	Mary Kay cosmetics	Oil-Free Foundation (Fragrance and oil-free)
Clinique	Pore Minimizer Makeup (Fragrance and oil free) Stay True Oil-Free (For sensitive skin, SPF 15)	Max Factor	Shine-Free Makeup
		Revlon	Spring Water Matte Makeup
		Shisheido	Pureness Oil-Control Makeup
Covergirl	Fresh Complexion, 100% Oil-Free		
Estee Lauder	Tender Matte Makeup (Fragrance and oil free) Simply Sheer Fresh Air Makeup Base, Oil-free		

D.   Follow up: None indicated

BENIGN SKIN LESIONS OF ADULTS

I.   Definition: Cutaneous growths with no malignant potential

II.   Pathogenesis: Variable depending on lesion

III.   Clinical Presentation

BENIGN SKIN LESIONS IN ADULTS: CLINICAL PRESENTATION	

Seborrheic keratosis	Common benign skin tumors of varying coloration, generally seen beginning in middle age
	    May occur in sun-exposed areas; vary in size from 0.2-3.0 cm
	    Sharply circumscribed, waxy, stuck-on appearing papules, fairly symmetrical in shape that know no racial predilection
	    More common on trunk, but also occur on face, scalp, extremities

Stucco keratosis	A variant of seborrheic keratosis; small hypopigmented to white papules found commonly on legs and forearms
	    A marker of aging
	    Usually 1.0-10.0 mm in size; may rub off but often recur

Dermatosis papulosa nigra	Hyperpigmented pedunculated papules common on face and neck of African-Americans and Asians
	    Appear somewhat earlier than seborrheic keratosis, but still considered marker of aging
	    Thought to be a variant of seborrheic keratosis
	    Usually 1-3 mm in size; may be called "moles" by patients who have them

Cherry angiomas	Punctate, mature, vascular papules also called senile hemangiomas
	    A marker of aging but occasionally seen in early adulthood
	    Red to purple non-blanching papules most commonly seen on trunk
	    Overlying surface of these 1-3 mm papules is smooth

Senile sebaceous hyperplasia	Small tumors composed of enlarged sebaceous glands which appear as soft, yellow papules
	    Occurs on face (usually forehead) of older persons
	    Characterized by central umbilication
	    A marker of aging and associated with sun exposure
	    May be confused with basal cell carcinoma

Solar lentigo	Appear as lightly pigmented tan macules with irregular borders in sun-exposed areas
	    Seen in majority of whites over age 60; caused by sun exposure
	    Commonly called liver spots
	    Occur most often on the face and backs of hands

IV.   Diagnosis/Evaluation

    A.   History
        1.   Inquire about onset, and growth rate of lesions
        2.   Ask about new or recently changing lesions
        3.   Inquire about family history of skin tumors

    B.   Physical Examination
        1.   Examine entire skin surface noting hallmark characteristics of lesions
        2.   Use exam to teach patient skin self-exam for malignant lesions

    C.   Differential Diagnosis
        1.   Senile sebaceous hyperplasia: Basal cell carcinoma (has pearly surface rather than dull yellow surface of senile sebaceous hyperplasia)
        2.   Seborrheic keratosis, solar lentigines: Benign intradermal nevus (mole), basal cell carcinoma, malignant melanoma, squamous cell carcinoma

    D.   Diagnostic Tests
        1.   None indicated when lesions are characteristic
        2.   Questionable lesions should be biopsied

V.   Plan/Management

    A.   Provide reassurance that lesions are benign

    B.   Explain that no treatment is required for these very common lesions

    C.   Counsel about sun exposure and need for skin self-exam on regular basis
        1.   Discuss sun protection including use of protective clothing (hat, long-sleeved shirt and pants) use of sun screen with a SPF ≥ 15, avoidance of sun exposure between 10 AM and 4 PM
        2.   Teach patients how to carefully examine skin each month with the help of spouse/friend or mirror, noting any suspect moles; moles that change in size, shape, color, or become symptomatic should be reported to health care provider

    D.   Refer for removal for cosmetic purposes if patient desires

    E.   Treatment of solar lentigo can usually be done without referral using **one** of the following

TREATMENT OF SOLAR LENTIGO
Use of liquid nitrogen on lesions for 10 seconds or less is usually effective Melanocytes are very sensitive to liquid nitrogen Easily destroyed with very small amounts and short exposure times Lesions may heal with hypopigmentation
Tretinoin (Retin A) 0.025%, 0.05%, 0.1% cream, supplied in 20, 45 g tubes or (Renova), available as .05% cream, supplied in 40, 60 g tubes May be prescribed QD for at least 4-6 months to lighten lesions and prevent new lesions from appearing (**Note**: Warn patient about photosensitivity with this product)

    F.   Patients can be referred to The Skin Cancer Foundation Web site for patient education handouts including color pictures

Skin Cancer Foundation Web site: http://www.derm-infonet.com/Moles.html

    G.   Follow Up: None required unless changes in lesions occur

CANCERS OF THE SKIN (SQUAMOUS CELL, BASAL CELL, & MALIGNANT MELANOMA)

I. Definition: Malignant cutaneous neoplasms found in humans

II. Pathogenesis

    A. Squamous cell carcinoma (SCC)
        1. Atypical squamous cells originate in epidermis and proliferate
        2. Cells then penetrate the epidermal basement membrane and proliferate into the dermis producing SCC

    B. Basal cell carcinoma (BCC)
        1. Cells of BCC resemble those of basal layer of epidermis
        2. BCC grows by direct extension and requires surrounding stroma to support growth
        3. Major etiologic factor is solar radiation

    C. Malignant melanoma
        1. Arises from cells of the melanocyte system; begins either de novo or develops from a preexisting lesion
        2. Initially grows superficially and laterally, confining itself to epidermis and papillary dermis
        3. Vertical growth then occurs with penetration of reticular dermis and subcutaneous fat

    D. Malignant tumors are a result of cumulative cellular effects of ultraviolet radiation and inability of skin to mount a defense to ultraviolet light

    E. Fair skin and sun exposure are important predisposing factors

III. Clinical Presentation

CANCERS OF THE SKIN: CLINICAL PRESENTATION	
Squamous cell carcinoma	➡ Accounts for about 20% of all skin cancers ➡ Occurs most often in middle-aged and elderly population ➡ Most common in sun-exposed areas; also arises in skin damaged by thermal burns or chronic inflammation ➡ The lower lip is a frequent location, particularly in smokers ➡ May metastasize, especially tumors arising from trauma sites ➡ Usual appearance is a firm irregular papule with a scaly, keratotic, bleeding, and friable surface
Basal cell carcinoma	➡ The most common skin cancer with 400,000 new cases occurring each year in the US ➡ Usually develops in 6th or 7th decade of life but is becoming more common in younger individuals ➡ Commonly found on the head and neck ➡ Fair-skinned persons, persons living in sunny climates, and elderly persons are at increased risk ➡ A slow growing tumor that occurs in both men and women and rarely metastasizes ➡ Tumor takes many forms. Most common is the nodular form -- a pearly colored nodule with fine telangiectasia over the surface and a depressed center or rolled edge
Malignant melanoma	➡ Accounts for less than 5% of all skin cancers but responsible for over 60% of deaths due to skin cancer ➡ Incidence and mortality rates have risen rapidly in past few decades ➡ Frequently affects young people; median age is early 40s ➡ Risk factors include fair skin and hair and intermittent heavy sun exposure; acute episodic exposure appears to be more of a risk factor than constant mild exposure ➡ Has ability to metastasize to any organ, including brain ➡ Melanomas tend to have Asymmetry, Border irregularity, Color variegation, and Diameter greater than 6mm

IV. Diagnosis/Evaluation

   A. History
      1. Question regarding any skin changes/new growths
      2. Determine family and personal history of malignant melanoma
      3. Ask about history of acute blistering sunburns and chronic sun exposure
      4. Inquire about prior radiation, thermal injury, cigarette smoking

   B. Physical Examination
      1. Examine entire surface of skin for suspicious lesions
      2. Use magnifying glass to assist in visualization of surface characteristics
      3. All pigmented lesions should be carefully evaluated
      4. Count and measure lesions mapping size and location in chart
      5. For accurate measurement, use a lesion measurement tool
      6. A hair dryer is helpful in examining the scalp; can also use cotton-tipped applicator to examine scalp

> **Lesion Measurement Tool**
> To order MediRules, which are disposable plastic sheets
> for measuring the size of lesions or wounds:
> Briggs Corp.
> 7887 University Bend
> DesMoines, IA 50306
> 1-800-247-2343

   C. Differential Diagnosis
      1. Actinic keratosis
      2. Leukoplakia
      3. Common nevus
      4. Seborrheic keratosis
      5. Solar lentigo

   D. Diagnostic Tests: Arrange for biopsy of lesions suggestive of malignancy

V. Plan/Management

   A. Patients suspected of having skin cancer should be referred to a dermatologist or surgeon for biopsy

   B. Early diagnosis and intervention are crucial (see BENIGN SKIN LESIONS OF ADULTS for recommendations about patient teaching); refer patients to the following web site for good information about skin cancer and prevention

> American Academy of Dermatology web site:
> http://www.AAD.org

   C. Educate patients about importance of sun exposure protection (wearing hat/long-sleeves, avoiding mid-day sun, using sun screen with an SPF of ≥15)

   D. Follow Up: By dermatologist

ACNE ROSACEA

I. Definition: Chronic, acneiform disorder of middle-aged and older adults characterized by vascular dilation of the central face

II. Pathogenesis

   A. Causes of rosacea are unknown

   B. Most experts believe that it is primarily a vascular disorder

   C. *Helicobacter pylori* may also play a role in the disorder

III. Clinical Presentation

   A. A common dermatosis, occurring in about 5% of persons in the US

   B. Onset is typically between ages 30 and 50 years of age, and occurs most often in fair-skinned persons of northern and eastern European descent

   C. Characteristically, affected individuals have facial flushing, especially with increases in skin temperature, ingestion of hot or spicy food, and alcohol consumption

   D. Over time, the flushing frequently develops into persistent erythema of the face and fine telangiectases develop as a result of the continual vascular engorgement
      1. Edema, papules, and pustules appear, most often on the central portion of the face
      2. Skin of upper and lower eyelids, skin below the eyes, and above the nasolabial folds becomes edematous, giving the areas a "baggy" look

   E. In the final stages of the disease, erythema of the face is deep and persistent, there are numerous telangiectatic blood vessels, particularly in the paranasal area, and pustules, papules, and nodules are prominent; in addition, edema and enlarged pores, especially of the nose are evident
      1. Rhinophyma, the red, bulbous nose of rosacea, occurs almost exclusively in men
      2. It is the end result of increase in connective tissue of the nose due to chronic inflammation, vascular dilation, and sebaceous gland hyperplasia

   F. Almost 60% of patients with rosacea have some eye involvement including blepharitis and conjunctival injection; the **most common** problem, however, is dry eye syndrome

IV. Diagnosis/Evaluation

   A. History
      1. Inquire about onset, initial symptoms, progression of symptoms over time
      2. Ask about associated symptoms such as dry eyes, red eyes, lid involvement
      3. Ask what makes the condition worse; specifically, ask about the effects of hot ambient temperatures, effects of eating hot or spicy foods, or ingesting alcohol
      4. Ask about treatments tried and results

   B. Physical Exam
      1. Examine facial skin for characteristic distribution (central facial area) and for characteristic erythema, papules, pustules, and telangiectasia
      2. Examine eyelids for scaling, erythema, and sclera and conjunctiva for hyperemia

C. Diagnostic Tests: None indicated

D. Differential Diagnosis
    1. Acne vulgaris
    2. Seborrheic dermatitis
    3. Contact dermatitis
    4. Photosensitivity reaction

V. Plan/Management

A. Provide patient with information about the disorder and emphasize that control rather than cure is the goal of treatment

B. Counsel patient to cleanse the face twice daily with a soapless cleanser such as Aquanil or Cetaphil
    1. Patient should avoid use of soaps, scrubs, astringents, and toners which often cause burning and stinging
    2. Women should use makeup which is hypoallergenic and should avoid products which may cause irritation (see NONACNEGENIC COSMETICS FOR WOMEN table in section on ACNE VULGARIS)

C. Treatment of choice is **combination** therapy with a systemic antibiotic and a topical antibiotic
    1. Systemic antibiotics are effective for treating inflammatory lesions, papules, pustules, as well as flushing, erythema, and telangiectases
    2. Topical antibiotics are effective for reducing erythema, resolving inflammatory papules and pustules and allow for long-term control without subjecting the patient to systemic effects caused by oral antibiotics
    3. Topical agents and systemic antibiotics should be started at the same time with the aim of tapering off the systemic antibiotic over a period of 5-8 months and continuing to use the topical antibiotic for maintenance

D. Choose one of the oral antibiotics from the following table

SYSTEMIC ANTIBIOTICS USEFUL IN TREATMENT OF ROSACEA		
Generic (Trade) Name	**Dosing**	**Comment**
Tetracycline (Sumycin)	500 mg BID x 4-6 weeks (Available as 250, 500 mg caps)	- Reduce dose to 500 mg QD (AM or PM) as soon as significant improvement occurs - Then, continue treatment for next 4-6 weeks - If remission continues, decrease the dose to 250 mg QD for an additional 4-6 weeks - If skin is clear after treatment, discontinue systemic treatment at this point - If flares occur, return to lowest dose (250 mg) QD
Erythromycin (E-Mycin)	500 mg BID x 4-6 weeks (Available as 250 mg tabs)	- Follow the same pattern as Tetracycline (above) [decreasing dose every 4-6 weeks]
Doxycycline (Vibramycin)	100 mg QD tapering to every other or every 3rd day (Available as 50, 100 mg caps)	- Follow the same pattern as with Tetracycline (above) [decreasing dose every 4-6 weeks]

E.   Choose one of the topical antibiotics from the following table

TOPICAL AGENTS USEFUL IN THE TREATMENT OF ROSACEA	
Metronidazole, 0.75% gel or cream (Metrogel and Metrocream)	❖ Apply BID ❖ Use gel in patients with oily skin and cream in patients with dry skin. **(Note:** Recently became available in 1% concentration which can be dosed QD) ❖ Women may apply makeup over the medication ❖ Supplied as gel--30, 45 g; cream--45 g OR
Sulfacet--R lotion	❖ Apply BID ❖ Supplied as 25 g

F.   Provide counseling to patient in terms of what to expect and the need for continuing therapy in most cases; provide patient with resources such as those contained in the following table

> **The National Rosacea Society**
> 800 S. Northwest Highway, Suite 200
> Barrington, IL 60010
> 1-888-NO BLUSH (662-5874)
>
> Materials provided include educational information for health care providers and patients
> Newsletter called "Rosacea Review" is also published by the society
> Call the toll free number for more information
> or visit the web site at www.rosacea.org

G.   Environmental and lifestyle factors may trigger flares
1.   Identification of the factors is an individual process
2.   Factors that cause problems in one patient may not in another
3.   Among common triggers are sun, stress, heat, alcohol, spicy foods, exercise
4.   Provide patient with counseling regarding how to deal with common triggers identified above (e.g., sun screen, use of hats in sun, stress management techniques, etc.)
5.   Men should consider use of electric shaver which is less irritating than safety razor

H.   Patients with dry eye syndrome can relieve symptoms with use of artificial tears
1.   Advise patient to use drops as soon as eyes begin feeling dry or before engaging in activities that are drying to eyes such as looking at computer screen or jogging
2.   Product examples, all OTC, are Hypotears and Hypotears PF (preservative-free)

I.   Patients with blepharitis can be treated as described in section on BLEPHARITIS

J.   Patients with moderate to severe telangiectasia and rhinophyma may require surgical intervention and should be referred for treatment

K.   Follow up: Every 4-6 weeks when initiating therapy, then less frequently when the condition begins to become controlled

ACNE VULGARIS

I. Definition: A disease of the pilosebaceous unit that is most intense in areas where sebaceous glands are numerous

II. Pathogenesis

    A. A number of factors and events work in concert to make the pathogenesis of acne multifactorial in nature

    B. Excessive sebum produced by the androgen-dependent sebaceous glands, combined with excessive numbers of desquamated cells from the walls of the sebaceous follicles cause obstruction of the follicles (which are located primarily on the face and upper trunk)

    C. As a consequence of this obstruction, a microcomedo is formed that may eventually evolve into either a comedo or an inflammatory lesion

    D. A resident anaerobic organism, *Propionibacterium acnes* (found in very low numbers on normal skin) finds the environment created by the excessive sebum and desquamated follicular cells very conducive to growth and produces chemotactic factors and proinflammatory mediators that may lead to inflammation

III. Clinical Presentation

    A. Acne is the most common skin disorder, affecting almost 80% of persons at some point in their lives, most often between the ages of 11 and 30
        1. Acne begins in the pre-pubertal period when the adrenal glands begin secreting increased amounts of adrenal androgens which leads to increased production of sebum
        2. Androgen production and sebaceous gland activity are further stimulated with gonad development during puberty

    B. Most patients with acne are probably hyperresponsive to androgens rather than overproducers of androgens; androgen excess, however, has been implicated in the development of acne

    C. **Comedonal acne** represents the **earliest** clinical expression of acne, occurring in the pre-teen and early teenage years
        1. Characteristic lesions are noninflammatory comedones located on central forehead, chin, nose, paranasal area
        2. Comedones are open (blackheads) or closed (whiteheads)
        3. Colonization with *P. acnes* has not yet occurred; thus, no inflammatory lesions are present

    D. **Mild inflammatory acne** usually develops in teenagers **after the first phase** of non-inflammatory comedonal acne; also occurs in adult women in their 20s
        1. Characterized by scattered small papules or pustules with a minimum of comedones
        2. Arises from microcomedones in which two factors are present
            a. Abnormal desquamation of epithelial cells in the follicles
            b. Proliferation of *P. acnes*

    E. **Inflammatory acne** represents the **final** phase in the evolution of acne from noninflammatory comedonal acne, to small numbers of inflammatory lesions on the face, to a more generalized eruption, first on the face, and then on the upper trunk
        1. Most patients with acne have inflammatory acne, with comedones, papules, and pustules on the face and trunk

2. In a minority of patients, large, deep inflammatory nodules (called cysts) develop reflecting the presence of a very destructive type of inflammation
3. Cystic acne requires prompt attention since ruptured cysts may result in scar formation

IV. Evaluation/Diagnosis

    A. History
        1. Question regarding onset, type of lesions, distribution
        2. In females, question about history of cyclic menstrual flares, use of oral contraceptives
        3. Inquire about types of cleansers and lubricants used on face
        4. Document previous treatments and results

    B. Physical Examination
        1. Examine skin to determine form of acne:
            a. Comedonal acne--noninflammatory comedones
            b. Mild inflammatory acne--scattered small papules or pustules with a minimum of comedones
            c. Inflammatory acne -- comedones, papules, and pustules on the face and trunk
            d. Inflammatory acne with large, deep inflammatory nodules
        2. Determine areas of involvement
        3. Use chart such as the one below to document location, type, and number of lesions during initial and follow up visits:

CHART OF ACNE LESIONS BY TYPE, NUMBER, AND VISIT			
Location		Date of Visit	
	1:_____ 2:_____	3:_____	4:_____
R Cheek			
L Cheek			
Forehead			
Nose			
Chin			
Other (Back/Chest)			

    C. Differential Diagnosis
        1. Rosacea
        2. Steroid Rosacea
        3. Molluscum contagiosum
        4. Folliculitis

    D. Diagnostic Tests: None indicated

V. Plan/Management

    A. Explain the mechanism of acne and treatment plan to the patient
        1. Emphasize that little improvement may be evident for 2-3 months
        2. Use written patient education materials to reinforce teaching

    B. Counsel patient regarding the following general measures:
        1. Wash affected area gently with mild soap (Purpose, Basis) no more than 2-3 x day (emphasize that use of topical agents such as soaps and astringents have no effect on sebum production but only remove sebum from the surface of the skin which has little value therapeutically)
        2. Avoid picking at lesions to prevent scarring
        3. Avoid oil-based cosmetics, hair styling mousse, and face creams which have no effect on sebum production but do increase the amount of oil on the face

4. Use cleansers such as Cetaphil lotion, nonacnegenic moisturizers such as Moisturel, and cosmetics from the table that follows

NONACNEGENIC COSMETICS FOR WOMEN			
Allercreme	Matte-Finish Makeup (Waterbase, oil free)	Lancome	Maquicontrol, Oil-Free Liquid Makeup
Charles of the Ritz	T-Zone Controller	Mary Kay cosmetics	Oil-Free Foundation (Fragrance and oil-free)
Clinique	Pore Minimizer Makeup (Fragrance and oil free) Stay True Oil-Free (For sensitive skin, SPF 15)	Max Factor	Shine-Free Makeup
		Revlon	Spring Water Matte Makeup
		Shisheido	Pureness Oil-Control Makeup
Covergirl	Fresh Complexion, 100% Oil-Free		
Estee Lauder	Tender Matte Makeup (Fragrance and oil free) Simply Sheer Fresh Air Makeup Base, Oil-free		

5. Dietary factors have no effect on sebum production; thus patient should be counseled to eat a normal, well-balanced diet

C. Treatment of acne is outlined in the following table

Comedonal Acne

Treatment Aims	Treatment	Comments

Reduce or counteract abnormal desquamation of follicular epithelium	Topical comedolytic agents are the treatment of choice
	Select a comedolytic agent from the following list
	
	Comedolytic agents
	Topical tretinoin (Retin-A) available as cream, gel, or liquid
	  Cream: 0.025, 0.05, and 0.1% concentrations, supplied as 20 g, 45 g
	  Gel: 0.01, 0.025% concentrations, supplied as 15 g, 45 g
	  Liquid: 0.05% concentration, supplied as 28 mL
	Apply QD, at bedtime, beginning with a lower concentration of the cream, gel, or liquid and increasing if local irritation does not occur
	(**Note**: Considered the standard against which all other comedolytics are judged)
	
	Adapalene (Differin), [a naphthoic derivative with retinoid activity] available as gel or solution
	  Gel: 0.1%, supplied as 15 g, 45 g
	  Solution: 0.1%, supplied as 30 mL
	Apply QD at bedtime, beginning with a lower concentration of the solution or gel, and increasing if local irritation does not occur
	(**Note**: Causes less irritation than topical tretinoin and is often effective in patients who cannot tolerate topical tretinoin)
	
	Azelaic acid (Azelex) [has both comedolytic and antibacterial effects], available as cream (one concentration only): supplied as 30 g
	Apply BID, in the morning and evening to clean dry skin
	(**Note**: Also causes less irritation than tretinoin; may cause hypopigmentation which may be desirable for some patients)
		Advise patient to apply thin layer of the topical agent to the entire face, not just the individual lesions
		Warn about increased photosensitivity--patient must apply sunscreen daily for **any** sun exposure
		Gels are usually preferred in hot/humid climates and creams in cold/dry climates
		Several months may be necessary to achieve good results
		Treatment should be continued until no new lesions are developing

(continued)

193

TREATMENT OF ACNE (CONTINUED)

Treatment Aims	Treatment	Comments
Reduce or counteract abnormal desquamation of follicular epithelium Prevent proliferation of *P. acnes*	**Mild Inflammatory Acne** Topical therapy with a combination of a comedolytic **and** an antibiotic is the treatment of choice Select a comedolytic agent from the list on the previous page Select an antibiotic agent from the list below (**Note**: When used in combination, **once** daily dosing for the comedolytic and the antibiotic is acceptable; each product should be used at separate time of day: Use comedolytic in AM and antibiotic in the PM. **The BID dosing schedule for both comedolytic and antibiotic agents in the lists given here are the dosing recommendations when the agents are used alone!**) **Topical antibiotics** Benzoyl peroxide, (Benzac) available as a gel with alcohol-base in 5, 10% concentrations; also available as aqueous-base gel (Benzac-W) in 2.5, 5, 10% concentrations Both products supplied as 60 g Apply QD to clean, dry skin (**Note**: Very effective anti-*P. acnes* agent; major disadvantage is irritation which can be minimized by using lower concentrations and water-base form) Erythromycin, 2% solution (A/T/S) and gel (A/T/S GEL) [alcohol base] Supplied as solution--60 mL and gel--30 g Apply BID to clean, dry skin Clindamycin, 1% (Cleocin-T) available as solution, pads, lotion, and alcohol-base gel Supplied as solution--30, 60 mL; pads--boxes of 60; lotion--60 mL; gel--30 g, 60 g Apply BID to clean, dry skin Benzoyl peroxide **plus** erythromycin (Benzamycin), contains 3% erythromycin and 5% benzoyl peroxide in gel form (alcohol base) Supplied as gel--23.3 g, 46.6 g Apply BID to clean, dry skin (**Note**: Considered by experts to be the **most effective** topical antibiotic therapy against *P. acnes*)	Most patients respond to treatment after 2-4 weeks Treatment should be continued until no new lesions develop, then slowly discontinued

(continued)

194

Treatment Aims	Treatment	Comments
	Inflammatory Acne	
Reduce or counteract abnormal desquamation of follicular epithelium	Topical therapy with comedolytic **and** systemic antibiotic therapy Select a comedolytic agent from list on the previous page Select an antibiotic from the following list	Deciding between topical and systemic antibiotics should be guided by two factors: Extent of skin involvement and severity of inflammation
Prevent proliferation of *P. acnes* and the resultant inflammation produced by the organism	**Oral antibiotics**	**Do not use tetracycline derivatives** in pregnant or nursing mothers
	Doxycycline (Vibramycin), available as 50, 100 mg caps 100 mg BID x 1 day, then 50 mg BID; dose can be reduced to 50 mg QD after improvement	Patients treated with oral antibiotics may also be given topical antibiotics once the oral dose is reduced to a maintenance level
	Minocycline (Minocin), available as 50, 100 mg caps 50 mg BID; dose can be reduced to 50 mg QD after improvement	
	(**Note**: Above two agents are more lipid-soluble than tetracycline and erythromycin and are generally considered to be more effective than tetracycline and erythromycin)	
	Tetracycline (Achromycin V), available as 250, 500 mg caps 1 gram/day in 2 divided doses, then 125-500 mg/day with further reduction after improvement	
	Erythromycin (E-Mycin), available as 250, 333 mg tabs 500 mg BID or 333 mg BID, with reduction after improvement	

195

D. Refer patients with widespread, nodular cystic lesions to a dermatologist for treatment aimed at therapy to suppress sebum production

E. Follow Up: Three follow up visits (over 8-10 weeks) are generally needed to establish a successful treatment program.
   1. For patients with comedonal and mild inflammatory acne on topical agents:
      a. Use chart to document location, type, and number of lesions to determine treatment response on each visit
      b. Adjust strength and frequency of topical agents depending on irritation and effectiveness
      c. If skin dryness is a problem that interferes with compliance, suggest use of a nonacnegenic moisturizer such as Moisturel, Purpose lotion, or Neutrogena Moisture after application of gel, or switch to a cream preparation
   2. For patients with inflammatory acne using **topical** comedolytics as well as **oral** antibiotics:
      a. Do a., b., and c. in E.1. above.
      b. Begin tapering oral antibiotic dose by 4-6 weeks into treatment (depending upon when development of new inflammatory lesions ceases); once the oral dose is reduced to a maintenance level, can add topical antibiotics to provide control
      c. Most patients require prolonged courses (months) or frequent, intermittent courses before complete and final remission occurs. **Consult PDR regarding need to monitor blood, renal, and hepatic function in patients on long-term antibiotic use!**
   3. For patients who are not on a successful treatment program after a total of 10-12 weeks of therapy, referral to a dermatologist is indicated

ATOPIC DERMATITIS

I. Definition: Extremely pruritic skin disorder involving cutaneous hypersensitivity

II. Pathogenesis

   A. Exact pathogenesis is unknown, but abnormalities of the immune system have been documented

   B. Epidermal barrier dysfunction and increased genetic susceptibility are also believed to be causative factors

III. Clinical Presentation

   A. Generally, begins in infancy/childhood, has periods of remission, exacerbation, and resolves by age 30. Highest incidence is among children

   B. Abnormally dry skin and lowered threshold for itching are significant factors

   C. Itching occurs in paroxysms and may be severe, especially in evenings

   D. Once itch-scratch cycle is established, characteristic lesions are created

   E. Patterns of inflammation begin with severe pruritus and erythema. As skin changes are produced by scratching, skin becomes dry and scaly (xerosis)

   F. Several patterns of lesions may be produced: erythematous papular lesions that become confluent; diffuse erythema and scaling; lichenification (thickening of dermis with accentuation of skin lines)

G.   Atopic dermatitis is divided into 3 phases which are outlined in the following table

ATOPIC DERMATITIS	

Infant phase (birth to 2 years)	Usually appears at about 3 months of age especially during cold, dry weather
	    Erythema and scaling of cheeks, chin with sparing of perioral and paranasal areas is frequently seen and there is sparing of the diaper area as well. May have generalized eruption of papules that are erythematous and scaly
	    Exudative lesions (oozing, weeping) are typical in infancy

Childhood phase (2-12 years)	Characteristic appearance at this age is flexural area involvement; perspiration produced by act of flexing and extending stimulates itching and itch-scratch cycle
	    Erythematous papules coalesce into plaques and scratching produces lichenification
	    Exudative lesions are seen less frequently

Adult phase (12 years to adult)	New onset as adult is rare
	    Onset of puberty may be associated with exacerbation
	    Localized inflammation of flexural areas with lichenification is most common pattern
	    Hand dermatitis occurs much more frequently in the adult phase

IV.   Diagnosis/Evaluation

    A.   History
        1.   Inquire about personal or family history of atopy -- allergic rhinitis, asthma, atopic dermatitis -- and age of onset
        2.   Question about itching, appearance and distribution of lesions, if dermatitis is chronic or chronically relapsing
        3.   Question regarding hand dermatitis
        4.   Ask about routine skin care at home including frequency of bathing and products used

    B.   Physical Examination
        1.   Have patient disrobe completely
        2.   Examine the skin methodically and determine the extent of the eruption and its distribution
        3.   Determine the primary lesion and the nature of the secondary lesions
        4.   Examine flexural areas for erythema and scaling but also look for lichenification in these areas
            a.   Examine the hands. Look for erythema and scaling on dorsal aspects of hands
            b.   Look for dry, fissured fingertip pads

    C.   Differential Diagnosis
        1.   Contact dermatitis, irritant or allergic
        2.   Seborrheic dermatitis
        3.   Nummular dermatitis
        4.   Scabies
        5.   Tinea

    D.   Diagnostic Tests: None indicated

V.   Plan/Management

    A.   Emphasize to patient that this is a chronic condition and exacerbating factors must be controlled for successful management

B. Counsel patient how to control exacerbating factors using guidelines in the following table

---

KEYS TO REDUCING OR ELIMINATING FACTORS THAT PROMOTE DRYNESS AND INCREASE DESIRE TO SCRATCH

- Keep environment slightly cool and well humidified (home or office humidifiers)
- Avoid frequent hand washing
- Daily soaks in tepid water using syndet bars such as Dove or soap substitutes such as Cetaphil or Aquanil is acceptable
- Wear 100% cotton clothing; avoid wool and synthetics
- Use fragrance-free laundry products such as Ivory Snow Flakes, Cheer-Free
- Recognize that emotional stress can worsen but not cause the disorder

---

C. Systematic lubrication of the skin must be done daily
  1. Bathing should always be followed by immediate application of emollients applied after patting the skin dry
  2. Remind patient to lubricate skin more frequently during winter months
  3. Recommend moisturizers from the table below
  4. Lotions are the least moisturizing but the most acceptable to patients; ointments are the most moisturizing but patients dislike the greasy feel of ointments

---

RECOMMENDED MOISTURIZERS

Moisturizing Lotions
  Petrolatum-based
    Dermasil
    Moisturel Lotion
    Replenaderm Lotion

  Mixtures of lanolin and petrolatum
    Eucerin Lotion
    Lubriderm Lotion
    Nivea Moisturizing Lotion

  Without lanolin or petrolatum
    Corn Huskers Lotion
    Cetaphil Lotion

Moisturizing Creams
  Petrolatum-based
    Purpose Dry Skin Cream
    Cetaphil Cream
    Keri Cream

  Mixtures of lanolin and petrolatum
    Eucerin Creme

  Without lanolin or petrolatum
    Neutrogena Norwegian Formula Hand Cream

Moisturizing Ointments
  Petrolatum-based
    Vaseline Pure Petroleum Jelly
    (Frangrance, preservative, and lanolin free)

  Mixtures of lanolin and petrolatum
    Aquaphor Natural Healing Ointment
    (Fragrance and preservative free)

D. To reduce inflammation, may use topical corticosteroids applied thinly 2x/day until controlled (up to 14 days)
  1. Triamcinolone acetonide ointment 0.1% (Aristocort ointment 0.1%, supplied as 15, 60 g) [use lower potency such as hydrocortisone cream, 2.5% on face and intertriginous areas]
  2. Apply lubricant to inflamed area 3-4x/day also
  3. Once inflammation is controlled, continue frequent daily use of emollients only
  4. Use the topical corticosteroid of the lowest potency that will control the condition

E. Pruritus control is important for all patients (see following table)

PRURITUS CONTROL USING PHARMACOLOGIC INTERVENTIONS

Oral Antihistamines

Hydroxyzine (Atarax), supplied as 10, 25, 50, 100 mg tablets

25-50 mg/dose TID PRN

A single dose at bedtime is frequently all that is necessary

Oral Antihistamines for Use in the Daytime (Nonsedating)

Loratadine (Claritin) 10 mg tabs QD or fexofenadine (Allegra) 60 mg caps BID

Begin with 10 mg every other day; then 10 mg/day

Supplied as Claritin Reditabs, 10 mg, which are dissolved on tongue and swallowed with or without water

Supplied also as Claritin syrup, 1 mg/1 mL (alcohol free, dye free)

Important to prescribe nonsedating antihistamines for patients who must work or attend school or who have other daytime responsibilities that require alertness

Topical Antipruritic Agents

Sarna lotion, Prax lotion and Itch-X gel are all OTC products

Cetaphil with menthol 0.25% and phenol 0.25% is an Rx product

Topical agents may be used in addition to or instead of oral antihistamines

Topical Antihistamines

Doxepin HCL cream 5% (Zonalon) may be used for short-term **(<8 days)**

FDA approved for use in atopic dermatitis and lichen planus

Supplied as 30, 45 g

Apply QID PRN in addition to topical steroids

May cause drowsiness and contact dermatitis

F.   Counsel patient to avoid exposure to chemicals, and to use gloves for protection when engaging in "wet work"

G.   Consider referral to a specialist for patients who have severe skin eruptions or for those who do not respond to conservative treatment after a 2 week trial

H.   Follow up visit should be monthly, then every 3 months until using lubricants only, then every 6 months
1.   Patient should understand that this is a chronic, recurrent disorder and should be offered practical counseling on each visit regarding ways to deal with the disorder
2.   Reliable patients should be given ample refills of topical corticosteroids so that they can control the condition themselves (if there is not a concern about overuse/inappropriate use)

DYSHIDROSIS (POMPHOLYX)

I.   Definition: A disease of unknown etiology that disrupts the skin of the palms and soles

II.   Pathogenesis

A.   The name dyshidrosis implies, incorrectly, an abnormality of sweating

B.   The cause of dyshidrosis is unknown, but there may be some relationship to stress

III. Clinical Presentation

A.   Condition is characterized by itchy vesicles on the palms, side of fingers, and soles (acute phase)

B.   After 3-4 weeks vesicles slowly resolve, and are replaced by scaling, redness, and lichenification (chronic phase)

C.   Waves of vesiculation may occur

D.   Moderate to severe itching usually precedes the emergence of the vesicles

IV.   Diagnosis/Evaluation

    A.   History
        1.   Question about location of lesions, onset, duration, and changes in lesions over time
        2.   Ask about associated symptoms
        3.   Inquire about skin allergies
        4.   Ask about treatments tried and results

    B.   Physical Examination
        1.   Examine lesions looking for vesicles, or if the acute process has ended, exfoliation of skin revealing a red, cracked base
        2.   Examine all skin areas to determine if vesicles are located in areas other than palms and soles

    C.   Differential Diagnosis
        1.   Contact dermatitis
        2.   Tinea
        3.   Atopic dermatitis
        4.   Pustular psoriasis of palms and soles (with this disease, vesicles are cloudy with purulent fluid and pain is the chief complaint); referral is needed

    D.   Diagnostic Tests: Skin patch testing for cell mediated allergy may be arranged if problem perseveres or if allergy is suspected

V.   Plan/Management

    A.   Topical corticosteroids: Triamcinolone acetonide cream, 0.025% (Aristocort cream, 0.025%) TID x 14 days **AND**

    B.   Oral antibiotics: Erythromycin (as base) [E-Mycin] 250 mg QID x 10 days **AND**

    C.   Cold wet compresses: Apply cold, sopping wet compresses (consisting of 4-8 layers) to affected area; leave in place at least 30 minutes; repeat 3-4 x day

    D.   Follow up: None indicated

CONTACT DERMATITIS

I.   Definition: Skin inflammation due to irritants (irritant contact dermatitis) or allergens (allergic contact dermatitis)

II.   Pathogenesis

    A.   Irritant contact dermatitis
        1.   Damage to one of the components of the water-protein-lipid matrix of the outer layer of the epidermis of the skin caused by irritants including chemicals, dry, cold air, and friction
        2.   An eczematous response in the skin is produced that is nonallergic in origin

B. Allergic contact dermatitis
1. A form of cell mediated immunity that occurs in 2 phases
2. The sensitization phase which occurs when allergens penetrate the epidermis and produce proliferation of T lymphocytes (sensitization phase; can take days or months)
3. In the elicitation phase, the antigen-specific T lymphocytes present in the skin combine with the subsequent exposures to the allergen to produce inflammation

III. Clinical Presentation

A. Irritant contact dermatitis
1. Intensity of inflammation is related to the concentration of the irritant and the exposure time
2. Everyone is at risk for the dermatitis, but people vary in their response to the irritant
3. Frequent hand washing with harsh detergents is a very common cause
4. Mild irritants cause erythema, dryness, and fissuring
5. Chronic exposure can cause oozing, weeping lesions

B. Allergic contact dermatitis
1. A genetically predisposed hypersensitivity reaction
2. May correspond exactly to contactant (e.g., fabric treatments, clothing, nickel in jewelry)
3. Poison ivy, oak, and sumac produce more cases of allergic contact dermatitis than all other contactants combined
   a. Observe for highly characteristic sharply demarcated linear lesions caused from leaves brushing skin or from streaking oleoresin when scratching
   b. Classic lesions are vesicles and blisters on erythematous base
   c. Diffuse patterns may occur when oleoresin is contacted from contaminated pets or smoke from burning plants

C. Distribution often provides clues to diagnosis
1. Scalp and ears: Hair care products, jewelry
2. Eyelids: Cosmetics, contact lens solution
3. Face/neck: Cosmetics, cleansers, medications, jewelry
4. Trunk/axilla: Clothing, deodorants
5. Arms/hands: Poison oak, ivy, sumac, soaps, detergents, frequent hand washing chemicals, jewelry, rubber gloves
6. Legs/feet: Clothing, shoes
7. Preservatives in OTC and prescriptive topical products may produce dermatitis at area of application

D. Older persons usually have relatively little vesiculation or inflammation and instead have scaling as a prominent feature of the eruption

E. The most common causes of allergic contact dermatitis in the elderly are topical medications, including neomycin, furacin, vitamin E, lanolin, and adhesives in transdermal medications

IV. Diagnosis/Evaluation

A. History
1. Question regarding location of eruption, time and rate of onset (abrupt or insidious), and associated symptoms such as pruritus
2. Ask about occupation and recreational pursuits
3. Question regarding exposures to such substances as chemicals, detergents, medications, poison plants, lubricants, cleansers, and rubber gloves, both at home and at work or in recreational pursuits
4. Obtain family history, personal history of allergies, treatments tried and results

B. Physical Examination
1. Examine skin to determine the location of the inflammation
2. Determine the primary lesion
3. Determine the distribution of the eruption as a clue to diagnosis

C.   Differential Diagnosis
    1.   Atopic dermatitis (usually more chronic, occurs in flexural distribution, onset in childhood)
    2.   Scabies (usually begins in fingerwebs, wrists, spreading to groin, axilla; other household contacts are symptomatic)
    3.   Nummular dermatitis (discrete, coin-shaped, erythematous, scaling plaques)
    4.   Dermatitis herpetiformis (usually localized to elbows, knees, buttocks, posterior scalp)

D.   Diagnostic Tests: None indicated

V.   Plan/Management

A.   For both types of contact dermatitis, the first step in management is to identify the offending agent and limit or eliminate further exposure

B.   Pruritus control is important for all patients

PRURITUS CONTROL USING PHARMACOLOGIC AND NONPHARMACOLOGIC INTERVENTIONS

Oral Antihistamines

Hydroxyzine (Atarax), supplied as 10 mg/5mL syrup and 10, 25, 50, 100 mg tablets
Dosing: 25-50 mg TID PRN
A single dose at bedtime is frequently all that is necessary

Oral Antihistamines for Use in the Daytime (Nonsedating)

Loratadine (Claritin) 10 mg tabs QD or fexofenadine (Allegra) 60 mg caps BID
Begin with 10 mg every other day; then 10 mg/day
Supplied as Claritin Reditabs, 10 mg, which are dissolved on tongue and swallowed with or without water
Supplied also as Claritin syrup, 1 mg/1mL (alcohol free, dye free)

Important to prescribe nonsedating antihistamines for patients who must work or attend school, or who have other daytime responsibilities that require alertness

Topical Antipruritic Agents

Sarna lotion, Prax lotion and Itch-X gel are all OTC products
Cetaphil with menthol 0.25% and phenol 0.25% is an Rx product
Topical agents may be used in addition to or instead of oral antihistamines

Nonpharmacologic Treatment Modalities to Soothe Itchy Skin

Cool tub baths with or without colloidal oatmeal can provide relief
Topical compresses (washcloths wet with plain water and kept in freezer) can be applied to affected skin for 15-20 minutes, 3-4 x day

---

C.   When skin involvement is limited but the dermatitis is moderate, not mild, treatment with topical corticosteriods is indicated
    1.   Prescribe intermediate potency preparation such as Diflorasone diacetate 0.05% cream, or high potency preparation such as betamethasone dipropionate 0.05% cream or lotion
        a.   Apply thin layer 1-2 x daily; do not occlude
        b.   Maximum 14 days of treatment
        c.   Do not use on face, groin, or axillary area; use hydrocortisone 2.5% cream on these areas
        d.   Always exclude viral disease before use of a topical steroid
    2.   When skin involvement is generalized, the face and groin areas are involved, and pruritus is poorly controlled with topical therapies, use of an oral corticosteroid may be indicated
        a.   Prednisone: 50 mg/day x 2 days, 45 mg/day x 2 days, 40 mg/day x 2 days, 30 mg/day x 2 days, 20 mg/day x 2 days, 10 mg/day for 2 days, and 5 mg/day x 2 days (for a total of 14 days of treatment)
        b.   Avoid dose packs as dosage is usually inadequate
    3.   Oral steroids are not appropriate for use in irritant contact dermatitis and for use as chronic therapy

D.   Follow Up
        1.   None indicated if dermatitis is mild
        2.   Follow up in 2-3 days for moderate dermatitis requiring topical or oral corticosteroid
              treatment

KERATOSIS PILARIS

I.   Definition: An eruption consisting of sterile pustules on the posterolateral aspects of the upper arms, anterior thighs, and the buttocks that is common in person with atopic dermatitis

II.   Pathogenesis

        A.   Unknown

        B.   One theory is that the condition is caused by a disorder in keratinization so that follicular plugging with keratin debris occurs

        C.   A second theory is that it represents a response to drying of the skin surface; the scaling produced is trapped in follicular opening

III.   Clinical Presentation

        A.   Commonly occurs in individuals with atopic dermatitis with children, adolescents, and young adults most often affected

        B.   Appears as small, pinpoint, follicular papules and pustules on the extensor aspects of the extremities, and the buttocks–a "gooseflesh" appearance

        C.   The affected skin surface feels rough and dry; hair in the center of the papule/pustule confirms a follicular location

        D.   Condition is aggravated by cold, dry climates, and is usually associated with extremely dry skin

IV.   Diagnosis/Evaluation

        A.   History
              1.   Ask about location of eruption, onset, duration, and appearance of lesions
              2.   Determine if there is a history of atopic dermatitis
              3.   Ask if condition gets better or worse at any time of the year
              4.   Question about associated symptoms (there should be none)

        B.   Physical Examination
              1.   Examine skin, focusing on areas typically affected -- extensor aspects of arms, legs, and the buttocks
              2.   Feel affected areas for rough skin; examine all skin surfaces for signs of dryness

        C.   Differential Diagnosis
              1.   Microcomedones of acne (distribution of acne is face, chest, upper back)
              2.   Molluscum contagiosum (lesions are waxy-appearing with central umbilication)
              3.   Drug eruption (drug eruption usually has acute onset and keratosis pilaris is chronic)

        D.   Diagnostic Tests: None indicated

V. Plan/Management

    A. Mild forms: Lubricants applied to moist skin immediately after bathing are usually effective (see CARE OF DRY AND OILY SKIN for table of moisturizers)

    B. Moderate to severe forms
        1. Lubricants and keratolytics (to remove keratin debris from the follicles) are effective
        2. Lactic acid 12% cream (Lac-Hydrin) or a urea lotion 10% (Carmol 10), applied BID usually control the condition

    C. Advise patient to soak daily for 10 minutes in tepid water, to use bars such as Dove, Purpose, or Basis, and to apply moisturizers after bathing while skin is still damp after having been patted dry (**Note:** Persons who shower typically use hotter water than those who take tub baths–experts now recommend daily soaks in tepid water to keep skin hydrated)

    D. Follow up: None indicated

SEBORRHEIC DERMATITIS

I. Definition: A common, chronic, inflammatory disease with a characteristic pattern for different age groups

II. Pathogenesis

    A. The yeast *Pityrosporum ovale* is believed to play a role in the etiology

    B. Both genetic and environmental factors seem to influence onset and course of disease

III. Clinical Presentation

    A. Affects all age groups, but is most common in adults age 20-50 or older

    B. An extremely common condition which waxes and wanes and may be aggravated by stress

    C. Mild seborrheic dermatitis presents as fine, dry, white or yellow scale, on an inflamed base

    D. More severe eruptions appear as dull, red plaques with thick, white or yellow scale in a diffuse distribution

    E. Occurs in seborrheic areas--scalp, eyebrows, paranasal, nasolabial fold, external ear canals, posterior auricular fold, and presternal areas

    F. Seborrheic dermatitis is one of the most common early cutaneous manifestations of HIV infection

IV. Diagnosis/Evaluation

    A. History
        1. Question regarding onset, duration, and location of lesions
        2. Inquire about personal or family history of seborrheic dermatitis
        3. Question regarding immunosuppressed status
        4. Ask about treatments tried and results

    B. Physical Examination
        1. Examine skin for characteristic lesions: fine, dry, white or yellow scale on inflamed base or dull, red plaques with thick white or yellow greasy appearing scale
        2. Determine distribution

C. Differential Diagnosis
1. Psoriasis (lesions are usually on elbows/knees and consist of thick, silvery scales; facial involvement is less common; psoriasis of scalp may be difficult to differentiate from seborrheic dermatitis)
2. Tinea capitis/faciale (fungal culture/KOH prep can help differentiate; tinea faciale is usually unilateral)
3. Acne rosacea (central facial erythema and a significant flushing component are present with this condition; also telangiectasia and inflammatory papules may be present)

D. Diagnostic Tests: None indicated if typical lesions, distribution

V. Plan/Management

A. Adults with seborrheic dermatitis should be treated as follows

---

TREATMENT OF SEBORRHEIC DERMATITIS

For scalp involvement, medicated shampoos may be prescribed
◆ Selenium sulfide: Exsel, Selsun blue (OTC)
◆ Coal tar: Denorex, T/Gel, Tegrin (OTC)
◆ Above shampoos must be left on a minimum of 5-10 minutes before rinsing
◆ Ketoconazole: Nizoral (Rx): Use 2-3x/week x 1 month; may need to use once a week for maintenance

For scalp involvement, topical corticosteroid lotions/solutions may also be used on the scalp if shampoo fails to control the condition after 2-3 weeks, or for initial treatment of moderate to severe scalp involvement
◆ Intermediate potency drug such as betamethasone valerate 0.1% lotion, available in 20, 60 mL bottles may be used BID for 2 weeks; after 2 weeks, use hydrocortisone lotion, 1% or 2.5% QD for control, tapering to every other day and then discontinuing over the next 2 weeks
◆ Should be used only on scalp and not on face and should not be used for maintenance therapy

For face/groin involvement, low-potency agents such as hydrocortisone 1% cream or lotion, QD or BID to control erythema and scale; lotion works best in eyebrows

For facial involvement that is unresponsive to topical steroids, may use Ketoconazole 2% cream QD to address a possible yeast component (**Note**: May be used as a combination treatment with topical steroids, applied at different times during the day)

For chest involvement, medicated shampoos may be used on chest skin; may also use triamcinolone 0.1% lotion BID OR ketoconazole (Nizoral) 2% cream BID until clear; then use once or twice weekly

---

B. Recalcitrant cases should be referred to a specialist for management

C. Follow up: Not indicated except in treatment failures

IMPETIGO AND ECTHYMA

I. Definition: Bacterial skin infection caused by invasion of the epidermis by pathogenic *Staphylococcus aureus* or *Streptococcus pyogenes,* or a combination of these organisms

II. Pathogenesis

A. Microscopic breaks in the epidermal barrier allows penetration by two major pathogens *S. aureus* and/or *S. pyogenes*

B. The depth of invasion in impetigo is superficial; the entire epidermis is involved in ecthyma

C. Poststreptococcal glomerulonephritis may follow skin infections involving strains of nephritogenic streptococci; rheumatic heart disease is not a sequelae of this infection

III.   Clinical Presentation

   A.   Impetigo begins as small (1-2 mm) superficial vesicles with fragile roofs that are quickly lost; vesicles rupture leaving erosions covered by moist, honey-colored crusts

   B.   Multiple lesions are usually present, and face and extremities are the **most common** sites of involvement

   C.   The terms bullous and nonbullous impetigo have been used to describe two patterns of infection with bullous impetigo suggesting staphylococcal origin and nonbullous, streptococcal origin. The preferred term presently is simply, "impetigo," since differentiation is difficult based on appearance, and many infections are caused by both organisms

   D.   In ecthyma, ulcers form with a dry, dark crust, and surrounding erythema; lesions are usually found on legs

   E.   Both ecthyma and impetigo may occur simultaneously

   F.   Both infections occur most frequently in children but also occur in adults

   G.   Enhanced by poor hygiene and warm, moist climates; disease is self-limiting

IV.   Diagnosis/Evaluation

   A.   History
      1.   Question about location of lesions, onset, duration, and any associated symptoms
      2.   Ask if other family members are affected; treatments tried and results

   B.   Physical Examination
      1.   Examine skin (focus on areas of typical involvement--face, arms, legs) looking for erosions covered by moist, honey-colored crusts that characterize impetigo, and firm, dry, dark crusts with surrounding erythema that characterize ecthyma
      2.   Check for regional lymphadenopathy

   C.   Differential Diagnosis
      1.   Tinea (with tinea, there is central clearing, and KOH test is positive)
      2.   Herpes simplex infections (HSV is characterized by clusters of lesions, and prodromal illness)
      3.   Second-degree burn may be confused with ecthyma (careful history is important; Gram's stain for bacteria should be negative unless burn site contaminated with bacteria)
      4.   Allergic contact dermatitis (itching is prominent symptom in allergic contact dermatitis)

   D.   Diagnostic Tests: None required as clinical features are so characteristic; if uncertain about diagnosis, perform Gram's stain of fluid from intact vesicle/pustule looking for gram-positive cocci in clusters (*S. aureus*) or chains (*S. pyogenes*)

V.   Plan/Management

   A.   For multiple lesions, oral antibiotics are the preferred therapy

   B.   Treatment of choice is dicloxacillin 250 mg QID x 10 days (supplied as caps, 250, 500 mg)

   C.   Erythromycin (E-Mycin) 250 mg QID x 10 days (supplied as 250 mg, 500 mg)

   D.   Cephalexin (Keflex) 500 mg BID x 10 days (supplied as caps 250 mg, 500 mg; tabs, 250, 500 mg). **Note:** Better compliance with this drug than with either dicloxacillin or erythromycin

E. Please note that strains of staphylococci resistant to erythromycin have been encountered in US; thus dicloxacillin is the drug of choice

F. If only a few lesions are present, consider use of topical mupirocin ointment (Bactroban) applied TID x 7-10 days or until all lesions have cleared (**Note:** Reevaluate if no response in 3-5 days)

G. Gentle washing of lesions to remove loose crusts may be helpful and must be done if mupirocin is used; scrubbing of lesions with antibacterial soaps has not been shown to be effective and is not routinely recommended

H. Good hand washing and personal hygiene are recommended to reduce likelihood of spread; use of a mild antibacterial soap such as Lever 2000 for bathing may be helpful

I. Follow up is not routinely recommended but is indicated for resistant or recurrent cases

CELLULITIS

I. Definition: An acute, diffuse, inflammation of the skin and subcutaneous structures characterized by hyperemia, edema, and leukocytic infiltration

II. Pathogenesis

A. Invasion of bacteria (usually pathogenic streptococci) into the dermis and subcutaneous fat with subsequent spread through the lymphatics

B. *Haemophilus influenzae* and *Staphylococcus aureus* are also frequent causative organisms

C. May develop in apparently normal skin, but more often trauma to the skin provides a portal of entry for invading organisms

III. Clinical Presentation

A. Erythema, warmth, edema, and pain are usual clinical features

B. Fever, chills, malaise, and lymphadenopathy are also frequently present

C. Typically, there is a preceding wound or trauma to the skin which compromises lymphatic drainage

D. Findings that signal an emergent condition are listed in the following table

INDICES OF AN EMERGENT CONDITION
-Extensive cellulitis -Fever, or other signs and symptoms of septicemia -Diminished arterial pulse in a cool, swollen, infected extremity -Presence of cutaneous necrosis -Closed space infections of the hand -Periorbital cellulitis because of proximity to brain -Immunosuppressed or diabetic host

E. Erysipelas, a distinctive type of superficial cellulitis is virtually always caused by group A streptococci

F. In erysipelas, infection is more superficial, with margins that are more clearly demarcated from normal skin than in cellulitis

G. Lower legs, face, and ears are most frequently involved in erysipelas

H. Lymphatic involvement ("streaking") is prominent in erysipelas which also differentiates it from other types of cellulitis

IV. Diagnosis/Evaluation

A. History
1. Question about location, onset, duration, degree of spread, and presence of pain
2. Ask if there was a preexisting wound or trauma to involved area
3. Determine if systemic symptoms are present (fever, chills, malaise)

B. Physical Examination
1. Vital signs and BP to determine if febrile, and to evaluate cardiovascular status
2. Examine involved area of skin to determine how extensive infection is, degree of erythema, presence of purulent discharge, presence of necrotic tissue
3. Examine adjacent skin/lymph nodes to determine presence of "streaking," degree of lymphadenopathy

C. Differential Diagnosis
1. Pressure erythema
2. Contact dermatitis
3. Swelling over septic joint

D. Diagnostic Tests
1. Obtain Gram's stain and culture and sensitivity of wound before treatment is instituted
2. Obtain CBC and blood cultures if cellulitis is extensive or associated with marked systemic toxicity

V. Plan/Treatment

A. Treatment of erysipelas and cellulitis depends on the patient's condition and underlying risk factors

B. Refer for hospitalization any patient with emergent conditions described in section III.D. (above)

C. Most patients with erysipelas and localized cellulitis can be treated with oral antibiotics

D. For uncomplicated cases, choose ONE of the following antibiotics, and **treat for 10-14 days** (except for Zithromax):
1. Oxacillin: Adults: 500 mg QID, OR
2. Cephalexin (Keflex) 500 mg BID (supplied as caps, 250, 500 mg; tabs, 250, 500 mg) OR
3. Erythromycin (E-Mycin) 250 mg QID(supplied as tabs, 250 mg, 500 mg) OR
4. Azithromycin (Zithromax) supplied as Z-Pak (6 tabs): 500 mg on day 1, then 250 mg/day on days 2-5

E. In all cases, antibiotic therapy may require changing based on culture results and clinical response

F. Local measures such as immobilization, elevation, application of moist heat (3-4 x day for 15-20 minutes) should be used with all patients to provide symptomatic relief and speed resolution of the infection

G. Follow up in 48 hours to determine response to therapy

FOLLICULITIS, FURUNCULOSIS, AND CARBUNCULOSIS

I. Definition: Bacterial invasion of the follicular wall

II. Pathogenesis

   A. Most commonly due to *Staphylococcus aureus*

   B. Other organisms may be involved, and, in general, the microbiology of cutaneous infection reflects the microflora of the part of body involved

III. Clinical Presentation

   A. Folliculitis is inflammation of the hair follicle caused by infection, chemical irritation, or injury

   B. Furuncle (abscess or boil) is a deep folliculitis, consisting of a walled-off, pus filled mass that is painful, firm, or fluctuant

   C. Furuncle may appear at any site, but most often occurs in areas of friction (waistline, groin, buttocks, axilla)

   D. Carbuncles are aggregates of infected follicles located deep in dermis; it points and drains through multiple openings

   E. Carbuncles are painful and systemic signs such as chills, fever may be present. Occur in areas with thick dermis (back of neck, lateral aspect of thigh)

IV. Diagnosis/Evaluation

   A. History
      1. Ask about location, appearance of lesion, onset, duration, and if purulent drainage is exuding from surface
      2. Inquire about associated symptoms of pain and systemic symptoms of fever and chills
      3. Inquire about frequency of occurrence

   B. Physical Examination
      1. Take temperature to determine if systemic involvement
      2. Inspect lesion(s) for signs of local inflammation (erythema, swelling, and pustular surface)
      3. Palpate surface of lesion for fluctuance, indicating accumulation of purulent matter; palpate adjacent lymph nodes

   C. Differential Diagnosis
      1. Acne pustules
      2. Keratosis pilaris
      3. Epidermal cyst
      4. Hidradenitis suppurativa

   D. Diagnostic Tests: Wound culture should be done to verify antibiotic choice

V. Plan/Management

A. For folliculitis, application of 5% benzoyl peroxide gel (Desquam-X) BID x 10 days is usually sufficient
1. Alternative: Erythromycin 2% solution (A/T/S) BID x 10 days
2. Clindamycin solution (Cleocin T) BID x 10 days may also be used

B. For carbuncles and furuncles, frequent warm, moist compresses provide relief and promote localization and spontaneous draining

C. Incision and drainage is commonly required for carbuncles and furuncles

D. Systemic antistaphylococcal antibiotics should be used to treat furuncles and carbuncles
1. Treatment of choice is dicloxacillin 250 mg QID x 10 days (supplied as caps, 250, 500 mg)
2. Alternative treatment is cephalexin (Keflex) 500 mg BID (supplied as caps, 250, 500 mg; tabs, 250, 500 mg)

E. Refer patients with cutaneous abscesses located on face, scalp, and neck

F. Culture recurrent abscesses and refer patients for evaluation for diseases that may underlie recurrent furunculosis: Immunodeficiency, diabetes mellitus, alcoholism, malnutrition, and severe anemia

G. To prevent recurrence, stress role of good hygiene to patient and family. Most useful: frequent hand washing and daily skin cleansing with an antibacterial soap such as Dial or Hibiclens antimicrobial skin cleanser

H. Follow Up: None indicated

CANDIDIASIS

I. Definition: Skin and mucous membrane infections caused by the yeast-like fungus, *Candida albicans*

II. Pathogenesis: *C. albicans* is part of the normal flora of skin and mucous membranes; invasion of the epidermis occurs when moisture, warmth, and breaks in epidermal barrier allows overgrowth

III. Clinical Presentation

A. **Oral** cavity: In immunocompromised patients, acute process presents as white plaque on erythematous base (thrush). Tongue is almost always involved; may spread into trachea, esophagus, and angles of mouth, and become a chronic process

B. **Intertriginous** areas: Occurs most often in obese individuals (inframammary, axillary, neck, and inguinal body folds). Presents as red, moist, glistening plaque or moist red papules and pustules

C. **Vagina**: Appears as a cheesy discharge with white plaques on erythematous base. External genitalia becomes red, swollen, with some skin erosions (see GYNECOLOGY section for discussion of vulvovaginal candidiasis)

D. **Male genitalia**: Occurs mainly in uncircumcised but also occurs in circumcised. Multiple, round red erosions on glans and shaft (candida balanitis); usually painful. Often involves scrotum whereas tinea spares scrotum

E.   **Nails**: A common result of thumb/finger sucking. Non-tender erythema and swelling at nail margin

F.   Pain, discomfort usually symptoms regardless of site. Itching usually occurs with vulvovaginitis

IV.   Diagnosis/Evaluation

    A.   History
        1.   Inquire about location of lesions, medications used (e.g., inhaled steroids or oral corticosteroids) and underlying chronic conditions (diabetes, HIV+)
        2.   If vagina, penis involved, ask about associated symptoms of discharge, itching, and pain

    B.   Physical Examination
        1.   Examine skin, mucous membranes, and nails for characteristic lesions
            a.   White plaques on erythematous base (oral); red moist plaques with satellite lesions (intertriginous)
            b.   Red erosions on glans, shaft (penis); non-tender erythema of nail margins (nail)
            c.   For vulvovaginal candidiasis, see under GYNECOLOGY
        2.   Palpate adjacent lymph nodes

    C.   Differential Diagnosis
        1.   Oral
            a.   Geographic tongue
            b.   Aphthous stomatitis
            c.   Leukoplakia
        2.   Intertriginous areas
            a.   Miliaria
            b.   Bacterial
        3.   Vaginal: See GYNECOLOGY section
        4.   Male genitalia
            a.   Bacterial
            b.   Psoriasis
            c.   Tinea
        5.   Nails
            a.   Bacterial
            b.   Tinea

    D.   Diagnostic Tests
        1.   None indicated when typical lesions present
        2.   Potassium hydroxide (KOH) wet mount that is positive for pseudohyphae and budding spores confirms the diagnosis

V.   Plan/Management

    A.   Oral candidiasis: For the majority of patients, topical treatments are effective

---

TREATMENT FOR ORAL CANDIDIASIS

Topical treatment is preferred for limited disease in normal hosts
- ➡ Nystatin (Mycostatin) oral suspension (100,000 U/mL) QID x 10 days
  - 4-6 mL (1/2 dose in each side of mouth)
  - Medication should be retained in mouth as long as possible before swallowing
- ➡ Clotrimazole (Lotrimin) 10 mg troches: Dissolve 1 PO 5x day for 2 weeks

Systemic therapy is necessary for moderate to severe disease that occurs in immunocompromised persons (see HIV/AIDS section for treatment recommendations)

    B.   For candidal vaginitis, see GYNECOLOGY section

    C.   Candida balanitis: For limited disease, select one of the topical agents from the following table

TREATMENT FOR CANDIDA BALANTITIS
➡ Nystatin cream, 2-3x day for 10 days
➡ Miconozole (Monistat-Derm) or clotrimazole (Lotrimin) cream 2x day for 10 days
➡ Econazole (Spectazole) cream, BID x 10 days
➡ Relief occurs quickly once treatment begins; remind patient to use for 10 days even though pain is gone

D.   Candida intertrigo: Select one of the topical agents from the table

TREATMENT FOR CANDIDA INTERTRIGO
➡ Nystatin cream applied 2-3x day after thorough drying of the skin x 10 days
➡ Econazole (Spectazole) cream; apply BID x 10 days
➡ Clotrimazole (Lotrimin) cream, solution, lotion; apply BID x 10 days
➡ Ketoconazole (Nizoral) cream; apply QD x 10 days
➡ Counsel regarding weight reduction and elimination of conditions leading to maceration of skin
➡ If there is maceration, use wet Burrow's compress 3-4x day for 15-20 minutes to promote drying
➡ Advise patient to expose areas to light and air several times a day to promote drying

E.   Candida paronychia (chronic): The following treatment is recommended

TREATMENT FOR CANDIDA PARONYCHIA
➡ 3% thymol in 95% ethanol (must be compounded by pharmacist) TID
➡ **In adddition,select one** of the following to be used BID 2-4 weeks
• Clotrimazole (Lotrimin) solution
• Ciclopirox (Loprox) lotion
• Ketoconazole (Nizoral) cream
➡ Advise patient to avoid excess exposure to water
➡ For refractory cases, refer to specialist

F.   Treat predisposing factors. Rule out HIV+ and diabetes mellitus in patients with recurring infection

G.   Follow up is not indicated; patient should return if no improvement after 2 weeks and drug from another class should be prescribed

TINEA VERSICOLOR

I.   Definition: Common non-inflammatory fungal infection of the skin caused by lipophilic yeast

II.   Pathogenesis

A.   Fungal infection of skin caused by *Pityrosporum orbiculare*

B.   *P. orbiculare* is part of normal flora; overgrowth occurs for unknown reasons

III.   Clinical Presentation

A.   Occurs at any age, but most likely to occur in adolescence and young adulthood

B.   Presents as multiple small, circular macules of various colors -- white, pink, or brown -- thus the name "versicolor"

C. Infection is limited to the outermost layers of the skin; lesions enlarge rapidly and have mild scaling

D. Upper trunk most commonly affected, rarely located on face; may itch, but usually asymptomatic; not contagious

E. Proliferation exacerbated by heat, humidity, pregnancy, corticosteroid therapy, oral contraceptives, and immunosuppression

F. Infection is most evident in summer because the organism produces azelaic acid, a substance that inhibits pigment transfer to keratinocytes

IV. Diagnosis/Evaluation

A. History
1. Ask about location, onset, duration, and appearance of lesions
2. Inquire if associated symptoms present
3. Ask if any medications, including oral contraceptives are being taken
4. Determine if patient is immunocompromised

B. Physical Examination
1. Examine skin for characteristic lesions
2. Use Wood's light to look at skin. While not useful as a diagnostic aid (because fluorescence is not predictably present) can demonstrate extent of the infection better than ordinary light

C. Differential Diagnosis
1. Vitiligo
2. Tinea corporis
3. Seborrheic dermatitis
4. Pityriasis alba

D. Diagnostic Tests
1. Microscopy of KOH-cleared scrapings
2. Short, curved hyphae and clusters of round yeast cells "spaghetti and meatballs" are diagnostic

V. Plan/Management

A. For limited disease, **topical** therapies are usually effective. Select **one** from the following from the table below

TREATMENT FOR TINEA VERSICOLOR USING TOPICAL THERAPIES
Selenium sulfide 2.5% lotion (Selsun), supplied as 4 oz ❖ Applied and then washed off **after** 24 hours; repeat once each week for a total of 4 weeks **OR** ❖ Applied daily x 7 days, rinsing off after 10 minutes ❖ Advise patient to apply Selsun from neck down ❖ Allow skin to repigment for one month; if not cleared in one month, have patient repeat above treatment ❖ Repeat the treatment monthly until satisfactory result obtained; treatment is cheap and usually effective Sulconazole (Exelderm) supplied as cream, 15, 30 g and solution, 30 mL ❖ Apply once or twice daily for 3 weeks Ketoconzaole (Nizoral) supplied as shampoo, 4 oz ❖ Apply to damp skin in affected area with wide margins ❖ Lather, and leave in place for 5 minutes ❖ One application should be sufficient (No need to repeat) ❖ Repeat treatment if necessary Ketoconazole (Nizoral) cream, supplied as 25, 30 g ❖ Apply QD x 2 weeks

B. Use **oral therapies** for extensive or recalcitrant infection
  1. Ketoconazole (Nizoral) 400 mg PO x 1 dose. Small risk of liver toxicity with this drug **OR**
  2. Fluconazole (Diflucan) 200 mg PO QD x 5 days

C. Tell patients that clearing may be temporary; since infection is caused by an inhabitant of normal skin, it often recurs

D. Recommend prophylactic monthly use of selenium sulfide lotion (especially during summer) to prevent recurrences

E. Advise that treatment does not repigment the skin; once the infection is cleared up, the skin with normally repigment itself, but it will take 2 months or longer

F. Follow Up: None indicated

DERMATOPHYTE INFECTIONS

I. Definition: Infections by a group of fungi that have the ability to infect and survive only on keratin

II. Pathogenesis

  A. Causative organisms belong to 3 genera:
   1. Microsporum
   2. Trichophyton
   3. Epidermophyton

  B. Predisposing factors include debilitating diseases, poor nutrition, poor hygiene, tropical climates, and contact with infected persons or animals

III. Clinical Presentation

  A. Tinea capitis, or ringworm of the scalp
   1. Rarely occurs in adults
   2. Erythema and scaling of the scalp with patchy hair loss are characteristic
   3. Usually asymptomatic unless kerion, a tender, boggy, lesion representing a hypersensitivity reaction to the fungal infection is present

  B. Tinea corporis, or ringworm of the body and face (excluding beard area in men)
   1. Occurs in all age groups; more common in warm climates
   2. Lesion is generally circular, erythematous, well-demarcated with a raised, scaly, vesicular border
   3. The central area becomes hypopigmented, and less scaly as the active border progresses outward
   4. Pruritus is common

  C. Tinea cruris, or ringworm of the groin and upper thighs
   1. Frequent in males, usually obese ones; rare in females
   2. Eruption is sharply demarcated, scaling patches; usually extremely pruritic
   3. Involvement of the scrotum is uncommon (unlike candidal infections in which scrotal involvement is common)

  D. Tinea pedis, or ringworm of the foot
   1. Common infection in adolescents and adults (uncommon in prepubertal children)
   2. Lesions are fine, vesiculopustular or scaly and usually itch

3. Any area of the foot may be involved, but likely to occur on the instep or between the toes

E. Tinea unguium, or ringworm of the nails (onychomycosis)
1. Occurs in adolescents and adults; rare in children
2. May occur simultaneously with hand or foot tinea or present independently
3. Usually involves only 1 or 2 nails; toenails more often than fingernails
4. Distal thickening and yellowing of the nail plate are characteristic features

IV. Evaluation/Diagnosis

A. History
1. Question regarding onset, duration, distribution, morphology of lesions, and presence of symptoms
2. Question regarding contact with others (or infected dogs, cats) with similar lesions, symptoms
3. Ask about predisposing conditions -- sweaty feet, occlusive footwear
4. Inquire about treatments used and outcomes

B. Physical Examination
1. Examine skin to determine type, distribution of lesions
2. Use of Wood's light may aid in exam as some species cause tinea to fluoresce (pale or brilliant green). The most common fungus infecting the scalp, *T. tonsurans* does not fluoresce. Also, lint, scales, serum exudate, and hair preparations containing petrolatum fluoresce a bluish or purplish color which may be misleading

C. Differential Diagnosis
1. Seborrheic dermatitis
2. Psoriasis
3. Alopecia areata
4. Atopic dermatitis
5. Contact dermatitis

D. Diagnostic Tests

DIAGNOSTIC TESTS FOR DERMATOPHYE INFECTIONS

Microscopic examination for fungus
❖ Scrape the border of lesion with a sterile scalpel blade (No. 15) moistened with tap water to contain scales; can also "pluck" 2 or 3 hairs using a hemostat. Transfer specimen to slide with a small droplet of plain water
❖ Add 1 or 2 drops of KOH solution, put on coverslip and warm the slide carefully for 15-30 seconds with a flame
❖ Examine the specimen under low power with minimal illumination
❖ Identify hyphae -- thin, often branching strands of uniform diameter; switch to high dry (43X) objective to confirm finding
❖ While a positive exam establishes the diagnosis, a negative test does not rule out the disease
Dermatophyte test medium (DTM)
❖ Using a hemostat, remove 5-10 hairs from a scaling area or rub a moistened 2 x 2 gauze vigorously over an area of scaling and alopecia
❖ Inoculate the plucked hair/scrapings from the gauze directly onto the culture medium and incubate at room temperature (with cap on loosely)
❖ After 1-2 weeks, phenol red indicator in agar will turn from yellow to red in area surrounding dermatophte colony

---

V. Plan/Management

A. Treatment for tinea capitis is contained in the table below

TREATMENT FOR TINEA CAPITIS
Tinea capitis requires systemic antifungal therapy Griseofulvin microsize (Grifulvin V), supplied as 250, 500 mg tabs; 125 mg/5 mL suspension ❖ 500 mg/day in a single dose x 4-8 weeks ❖ Take with high fat food such as whole milk, peanut butter, ice cream to enhance absorption ❖ 4-6 weeks of therapy are needed; some patients require longer ❖ Continue medication for 2 weeks after clinical resolution Selenium sulfide, 2.5% shampoo, used 2x week for 2 weeks may reduce fungal shedding ❖ If kerion present, a short course of oral steroid therapy to reduce inflammation and prevent scarring of scalp may be needed ❖ Prednisone 25-50 mg for 7-10 days is recommended ❖ Taper dose over last half of therapy ❖ Cutting hair, shaving head, wearing cap unnecessary ❖ Advise patient that hair regrowth is slow

B. Treatment for tinea corporis, pedis, and cruris is outlined in the table below

TREATMENT FOR TINEA CORPORIS, PEDIS, AND CRURIS			
Topical Antifungal Agents	Supplied As	Dosing	Duration of Treatment
Miconazole (Monistat-Derm)	Cream, 15 g, 1 oz, 3 oz	BID	Tinea corporis, cruris--2 wks Tinea pedis--1 month
Terbinafine (Lamisil)	Cream, 15, 30 g	QD or BID for tinea corporis, cruris; BID for tinea pedis	Tinea Corporis, cruris--2 wks Tinea pedis--1 month
Econazole (Spectazole)	Cream, 15, 30 g	QD	Tinea corporis, cruris--2 weeks Tinea pedis--1 month
Ciclopirox (Loprox)	Cream, 15, 30 g Lotion, 30, 60 mL	BID	Up to 4 weeks
Ketoconazole (Nizoral)	Cream, 15, 30, 60 g	QD	Tinea corporis, cruris--2 wks Tinea pedis--6 wks
Oxiconazole (Oxistat)	Cream, 15, 30 g Lotion, 30 mL	QD or BID	Tinea corporis, cruris--2 wks Tinea pedis--4 wks
Sulconazole (Exelderm)	Cream, 15, 30, 40 g Solution, 30 mL	BID in tinea pedis (use cream only) QD or BID for tinea corporis, cruris	Tinea corporis, cruris--3 wks Tinea pedis--4 wks

ORAL THERAPIES FOR RECALCITRANT OR RECURRENT INFECTIONS	
Type	Treatment
Tinea corporis	Terbinafine (Lamisil), 250 mg, QD x 2-4 weeks, OR Fluconazole (Diflucan), 150 mg/week for up to 4 weeks
Tinea pedis	Terbinafine, 250 mg, QD x 2-6 weeks Fluconazole, 150 mg/week for up to 4 weeks
Tinea cruris	No oral therapies approved by FDA

C. Treatment for onychomycosis is outlined in the table below; select **one** of the following

TREATMENT FOR ONYCHOMYCOSIS
Medication: Terbinafine (Lamisil) **Dosing**: 250 mg QD x 6 weeks for fingernails 250 mg QD x 12 weeks for toenails
Medication: Itraconazole (Sporanox) **Dosing**: 200 mg BID x 1 week each month for 2-3 months for fingernails 200 mg BID x 1 week each month for 3-4 months for toenails
Laboratory monitoring for abnormal liver function and signs of hematologic abnormalities are required when these medications are prescribed Consult PDR for details relating to drug interactions and adverse events
Topical agents from the list above TREATMENT FOR TINEA CORPORIS, CRURIS AND PEDIS may also be used BID **when treatment with oral therapy has been completed**; these agents may be used 2-3x week for several months

D. Follow Up: Every 2-4 weeks for patients receiving long-term (more than 2 week) oral antifungal treatment to monitor LFTs and CBC

SCABIES

I. Definition: Skin infestation of the mite, *Sarcoptes scabiei*

II. Pathogenesis

   A. A fertilized female mite excavates a burrow in the stratum corneum and deposits eggs and fecal pellets

   B. The larvae hatch and reach maturity in about 14 days, mate, and repeat the cycle

   C. Humans are the source of infection with transmission occurring most often by close personal contact

   D. A hypersensitivity reaction rather than a foreign-body response is responsible for the intense pruritus

   E. Incubation period in persons without previous exposure is 4-6 weeks

III. Clinical Presentation

   A. Occurs mainly in children, young adults; also among institutionalized persons of all ages (e.g., elderly in nursing homes)

   B. Primary lesions are burrows, vesicles, and papules
      1. Burrows appear as gray or skin-colored ridges up to a few centimeters in length; scratching destroys burrows, so they may be difficult to find
      2. Vesicles are isolated, pinpoint and filled with serous fluid; may contain mites
      3. Papules are small, isolated, represent a hypersensitivity reaction and rarely contain mites

   C. Secondary lesions with erythema and scaling caused by scratching are present in more chronic cases

D.   A generalized urticarial rash may occur, especially in infants and the elderly. This condition, called Norwegian scabies, is the result of penetration of the underlying epidermis by hundreds of mites

E.   Common sites of involvement are hands (90%), especially fingerwebs, flexor aspects of the wrists, belt line, thighs, navel, intergluteal cleft, penis, areola, and axillae

F.   Main symptom is intense itching which is usually more intense at night and the diagnosis should be considered with widespread pruritus presenting primarily with skin excoriation

IV.   Diagnosis/Evaluation

A.   History
1.   Question regarding onset, duration, morphology and location of lesions
2.   Ask if itching is present, and if it is worse at night
3.   Ask about exposures to friends or family members with similar symptoms
4.   Inquire what treatments have been tried and their effectiveness

B.   Physical Examination
1.   Examine the skin for typical burrows
2.   Pay particular attention to the hands, especially the fingerwebs and wrists (flexor aspect), axillary folds, belt line, navel, penis, areas surrounding the areolae
3.   A magnifying glass and good lighting are essential

C.   Differential Diagnosis
1.   Atopic dermatitis
2.   Allergic and irritant contact dermatitis
3.   Papular urticaria
4.   Pediculosis

D.   Diagnostic Tests
1.   Microscopic identification of mite, ova, or feces proves the diagnosis. Two ways to do this:
       a.   Locate tiny black dot at end of burrow; insert a 25 gauge hypodermic needle at dot. Mite, ova, or feces (dot) will stick to it and can be transferred to immersion oil on slide; cover with slip and examine under low power
       b.   Slice off whole burrow with sterile scalpel blade (No. 15) held parallel to skin; put slice on slide, add immersion oil, cover with slip and examine under low power
2.   If no burrows are found, no diagnostic test indicated

V.   Plan/Management

A.   Use a scabicide from the following table

TREATMENT OF SCABIES
Drug of choice is 5% permethrin (Elimite) cream → Apply cream over the entire body below the head → Remove by bathing in 8-14 hours → Of drugs available to treat scabies, this drug is safest for use in pregnant and lactating women Alternatives: Lindane (Kwell, Scabine) and crotamiton (Eurax) cream or lotion → Apply as for permethrin cream above → Lindane, remove in 8-12 hours → Crotamiton, remove in 48 hours; repeat application for 2 to 5 days → *Caution: Lindane should not be used in pregnant women*

B. Control Measures/Patient Education
    1. Prophylactic therapy recommended for household members; therefore all household members should be treated simultaneously to prevent reinfection **(Note:** Lindane should not be used in children <2 years of age)
    2. Launder all clothing and bedding in hot water and hot drying cycle
    3. Clothing that cannot be laundered should be placed in plastic storage bags for at least a week. (Parasites cannot survive off the skin for longer than 3-4 days)
    4. Advise patient that pruritus may continue a week after cure due to local irritation (see CONTROL OF PRURITUS table below)
    5. Follow up: None indicated unless patient fails to respond to treatment

---

PRURITUS CONTROL USING PHARMACOLOGIC AND NONPHARMACOLOGIC INTERVENTIONS

Oral Antihistamines
Hydroxyzine (Atarax), supplied as 10 mg/5 mL syrup and 10, 25, 50, 100 mg tablets
Dosing: 25-50 mg TID PRN
A single dose at bedtime is frequently all that is necessary

Oral Antihistamines for Use in the Daytime (Nonsedating)
Loratadine (Claritin) 10 mg tabs QD or fexofenadine (Allegra) 60 mg caps BID
Begin with 10 mg every other day; then 10 mg/day
Supplied as Claritin Reditabs, 10 mg, which are dissolved on tongue and swallowed with or without water
Supplied also as Claritin syrup, 1 mg/1 mL (alcohol free, dye free)

Important to prescribe nonsedating antihistamines for patients who must work or attend school, or who have other daytime responsibilities that require alertness

Topical Antipruritic Agents
Sarna lotion, Prax lotion and Itch-X gel are all OTC products
Cetaphil with menthol 0.25% and phenol 0.25% is an Rx product
Topical agents may be used in addition to or instead of oral antihistamines

Nonpharmacologic Treatment Modalities to Soothe Itchy Skin
Cool tub baths with or without colloidal oatmeal can provide relief
Topical compresses (washcloths wet with plain water and kept in freezer) can be applied to affected skin for 15-20 minutes, 3-4 x day

---

PEDICULOSIS (LICE)

I. Definition: Infestation with one of the three species of lice that infest humans

    A. *Pediculus humanus* var. *capitis* (head louse)

    B. *Pediculus humanus* var. *corporis* (body louse)

    C. *Pthirus pubis* (pubic or crab louse)

II. Pathogenesis

    A. Transmission of head lice occurs by direct contact with infested persons or through hats, brushes, and combs

    B. Fomites play a major role in transmission of body lice, but almost no role in transmission of pubic lice, which are transmitted through sexual contact

    C. Ova hatch in a week; lice feed on human blood

    D. Incubation period from laying of eggs to hatching of first nymph is 6-10 days; mature lice (capable of reproducing) do not appear until 2-3 weeks later

III. Clinical Presentation

CLINICAL PRESENTATION OF LICE

Pediculosis capitis (head lice)
- Most common in children but adults are also affected; African Americans are less likely than other races to become infested
- Head lice are not responsible for the spread of any disease
- Most commonly seen in hair on back of the head near nape of neck
- Nits (ova) are cemented to hair shaft and may be seen; few adult lice are seen
- Head lice can survive only 1-2 days away from the scalp
- Excoriation from scratching, secondary bacterial infections, and cervical adenopathy are common

Pediculosis corporis (body lice)
- Generally found on persons with poor hygiene; lice cannot survive away from blood source for longer than 10 days
- Body lice are vectors of disease including typhus, trench fever, and relapsing fever
- Excoriation and secondary bacterial infection are common
- Body lice and nits may be found in seams of clothing

Pediculosis pubis (pubic lice)
- Highly contagious; chance of acquiring from one exposure is about 90%
- Common in adolescents and young adults; African-Americans and other racial groups are affected with same frequency
- Pubic hair is most common site of infestation, but can also infest hair on chest, abdomen, and thighs
- Infested adults may spread pubic lice to eyelashes of children
- Frequently coexists with other sexually transmitted diseases

IV. Diagnosis/Evaluation

    A. History
        1. Determine if nits, lice have been visualized and when they were first noticed
        2. Ask if itching present, especially nocturnal; determine if itching is generalized or localized
        3. Question if nits, lice present in close contacts

    B. Physical Examination
        1. Examine appropriate body part for lice, nits; a magnifying glass is helpful
        2. Examine skin of infested site for excoriation secondary to scratching
        3. If body lice suspected, examine seams of clothing for lice

    C. Differential Diagnosis
        1. Scabies
        2. Neurotic excoriation

    D. Diagnostic Tests
        1. Identification of eggs, nymphs, and lice with naked eye or magnifying glass
        2. Microscopic exam usually unnecessary

V. Plan/Management

    A. The following products are recommended for the treatment of head lice

TREATMENT OF HEAD LICE

Permethrin 1% cream rinse (Nix) OTC
- Apply cream rinse to shampooed, rinsed, and towel dried hair (and scalp)
- Leave on for 10 minute; rinse
- A single treatment is usually adequate, but some experts recommend retreatment 7-10 days after the initial treatment

Lindane 1% shampoo (Kwell shampoo)
- Do not use in pregnant women
- Apply to dry hair until thoroughly wet.; allow to remain for 4 minutes
- Add water to lather, rinse thoroughly
- Repeat application in 7-10 days is often recommended

Pyrethrins 0.33% shampoo, gel (A-200) (RID) OTC
- Apply to area until thoroughly wet, massage in, wait 10 minutes, rinse
- Use gel for body lice, shampoo for head or pubic lice

B. To remove nits for aesthetic reasons (not necessary to prevent spread)
   1. Soak hair with white vinegar for 30-60 minutes, or use a commercial formic acid rinse (Step 2) made for this purpose
   2. Use fine-tooth comb to mechanically remove nits
   3. With heavy involvement, a haircut may be preferable to tedious nit removal (child should not be forced to have hair cut, however, if he/she would find it humiliating)

C. Combs and brushes should be soaked in hot water with pediculicide shampoo for 15 minutes

D. Treatment of pubic lice is described below

TREATMENT OF PUBIC LICE

For the treatment of pubic lice, any of the pediculocides listed above for treatment of head lice are effective
➡ Retreatment is recommended in 7-10 days following initial treatment
➡ All sexual contacts of persons with pubic lice should be treated

---

E. Treatment of body lice is described below

TREATMENT OF BODY LICE

For the treatment of body lice, pediculocides are not necessary
➡ Treatment consists of improving hygiene and laundering clothing
➡ Infested clothing should be washed and dried at very hot temperatures to kill lice

---

F. Household and other close contacts should be examined and treated if they have head or body lice; bed mates should be treated prophylactically (**Note:** Lindane should not be used in children <2 years of age)

G. Clothing, bedding should be laundered in hot soapy water and dried on hot cycle or dry cleaned

H. Follow Up: Unnecessary

CUTANEOUS LARVAE MIGRANS

I. Definition: A skin disease caused by infected larvae of cat and dog hookworms with *Ancylostoma braziliense* and *Ancylostoma caninum* the usual causes; often referred to as creeping eruption

II. Pathogenesis

   A. Ova of *A. braziliense* or *A. caninum* are deposited in cat or dog feces

   B. Larvae in soil or sand penetrate human skin that contacts soil

III. Clinical Presentation

   A. A disease of persons likely to come into contact with sandy soil contaminated with cat/dog feces (i.e., gardeners, sunbathers, outdoor workers)

   B. Disease is most prevalent in the southeastern part of the US

   C. Classically presents as pruritic, erythematous, thread-like (or serpiginous) lesions that advance about 1 cm/day

   D. Lesions are usually located on feet, hands, buttocks, or upper thighs; excoriation may obscure the otherwise typical serpiginous lesion

221

IV. Diagnosis/Evaluation

    A. History
        1. Inquire about location, onset, duration, and if pruritus is present
        2. Ask if sitting or playing in soil/sand has occurred recently

    B. Physical Examination: Examine skin for typical serpiginous, thread-like lesions; look for signs of scratching

    C. Differential Diagnosis
        1. Tinea
        2. Urticaria
        3. Erythema chronicum migrans
        4. Scabies

    D. Diagnostic Tests: None indicated

V. Plan/Treatment

    A. Treatment of choice is topical application of oral thiabendazole suspension (Mintezol); apply suspension to affected areas QID x 7-10 days

    B. Alternative: Albendazole (Albenza) 200 mg tabs; 400 mg PO x 3 days (nonpregnant adults only)

    C. Patient Education: Should be advised not to sit, lie, or walk barefoot on wet soil or sand in areas where cats or dogs are likely to deposit feces

    D. Follow Up: None indicated

PSORIASIS

I. Definition: A chronic, relapsing hyperproliferative inflammatory disorder of the skin of unknown cause

II. Pathogenesis

    A. Believed to be a T-lymphocyte-mediated disease with secondary keratinocyte hyperproliferation

    B. The antigen-activating signals responsible for the T-lymphocyte infiltration into the psoriatic lesions are unknown

    C. Numerous initiating factors are postulated including local trauma, infection, stress, use of certain medications

    D. In sum, inappropriate stimulation of immune-mediated inflammation appears to be a major factor in the pathogenesis

III. Clinical Presentation

    A. Affects about 2% of the population in North America with the mean age of onset between 20-30 years
        1. Fewer than 10% of patients have onset during childhood
        2. About 60% of patients develop lesions before age 35

B. Males and females are equally affected and about 30% of patients have a family history of the disorder
   1. Patients are likely to have history of chronic dandruff, and chronic scaling of ears
   2. Past medical history of many patients is positive for other autoimmune diseases

C. Several distinct clinical variants of psoriasis exist, but the most common forms are the plaque-type and the guttate form

D. Plaque-type lesions are distinctive; begin as purplish, red, scaling papules that coalesce to form plaques with adherent silvery-white scale that are easily distinguishable from normal skin
   1. Scale reveals bleeding points when removed (called Auspitz sign)
   2. Most common sites are extensor surfaces of the elbows and knees
   3. Scalp, umbilicus, intergluteal cleft are also common sites
   4. Bilateral symmetrical involvement of the extremities is a consistent feature (**Note**: Scalp psoriasis is typically asymmetrical, probably due to habitual scratching or picking at one area rather than another)

E. Guttate form is characterized by multiple, scattered papules and plaques, 1-2 cm in diameter, with an acute eruptive onset
   1. Trunk is the predominant site of involvement
   2. In children and young adults, frequently occurs after a streptococcal infection

F. May also affect the palms, soles, or fingernails
   1. Nail pitting (small pits or yellow-brown spots--called oil spots in the nail bed) is the best known nail abnormality
   2. Distal separation of the nail plate from the bed is also a sign of the disorder producing a whitish to yellowish discoloration of the nail plate

G. Pruritus is not a common symptom, but appearance of the lesions may be altered by patients scratching or picking at the lesions

H. About 5% of patients will develop psoriatic arthritis, a distinct form of arthritis in which rheumatoid factor is negative; distal interphalangeal (DIP) joint disease is the most common expression

I. May be the first sign of HIV+; usually has explosive onset in this group of patients and facial involvement is often significant

IV. Diagnosis/Evaluation

   A. History
      1. Inquire about location and appearance of lesions, onset, and duration; if there are bleeding points when thick scale is removed
      2. Ask if nail pitting, arthritis, particularly in DIP joints of fingers or toes
      3. Ask about past history of chronic dandruff, scaling of external ear and canal
      4. In young adults with abrupt onset of symptoms, ask about recent streptococcal infection (pharyngitis)
      5. Also ask about HIV+ status in cases where onset is abrupt
      6. Ask about treatments tried and results
      7. Review past medical history, particularly presence of other autoimmune disorders
      8. Assess the impact of the disease on the patient's quality of life
      9. Ask about family history of psoriasis in first-degree relatives

   B. Physical Examination
      1. Examine entire body surface beginning with scalp and including soles of feet
      2. Look for characteristic lesions, particularly on extensor surfaces, keeping in mind that symmetry of distribution and classic silvery scale are the hallmarks of the plaque-form of the disease (which is by far the most common)
      3. Use tongue blade to scrape over a lesion surface to elicit the fine pinpoint bleeding referred to as Auspitz sign

4.   Quantify the extent of the disease by using the guidelines below (see ESTIMATING BODY SURFACE AREA)

5.   Examine nails for pitting and joints in fingers and toes for inflammatory changes

C.   Differential Diagnosis
1.   Seborrheic dermatitis
2.   Nummular dermatitis
3.   Atopic dermatitis
4.   Pityriasis rosea

D.   Diagnostic Tests
1.   None indicated for cutaneous manifestations only; shave biopsy may be necessary to differentiate this disorder from other papulosquamous diseases
2.   If joint inflammation present, order rheumatoid factor levels, erythrocyte sedimentation rate, and uric acid levels

V.   Plan/Management

A.   Education of the patient and the family is the first step in management
1.   Emphasize that the disorder is not contagious (patients are often treated as though it were by others, even family members and friends)
2.   Most patients believe that psoriasis adversely affects their lives; provide patient with opportunities to discuss feelings in this area
3.   Counsel patient regarding elements of a healthy lifestyle, including well-balanced diet, frequent exercise, moderate alcohol intake, and avoidance of all tobacco products
4.   Discuss the role of stress (from acute illnesses such as respiratory tract infections and from psychosocial sources such as family difficulties, work related problems)
5.   Shaving (face in men, armpits and legs in women) should be done very cautiously to avoid trauma to the skin; moisturizers should be applied afterwards
6.   Provide patient with information about the National Psoriasis Foundation (NPF), a nonprofit organization that can be a major resource for patient education

---

National Psoriasis Foundtion
6600 SW 92nd Avenue, Suite 300
Portland, Oregon 97223-7195
(800) 723-9166
http://www.psoriasis.org

B.   Treatment for psoriasis is divided into three major categories: topical, ultraviolet light, and systemic therapy

C.   All patients with psoriatic involvement of greater than 10% of body surface area (BSA) or with moderate to severe disease should be referred to a dermatologist for management; many of these patients are candidates for phototherapy and/or systemic therapy

D.   Most patients whose involvement is less that 10% of total BSA can be treated with topical therapy alone (**Note**: This generalization does not apply to forms of psoriasis such as hand and foot psoriasis which may have less than 5% of BSA involvement but which can be very disabling)

ESTIMATING BODY SURFACE AREA (BSA) IN ORDER TO QUANTIFY THE DISEASE

✦   The palm of the patient's hand represents approximately 1% BSA
✦   Using that diameter as a guide, estimate the degree of involvement
✦   Involvement of less than 10% (see V. D. above for exceptions) indicates that this patient is a candidate for topical therapy alone (at least initially) and management in a primary care setting is probably appropriate

E. Recommendations below are for mild to moderate disease in which less than 10% of body surface is affected
    1. Aim of treatment is to bring the psoriasis into remission or an inactive state
    2. Selected residual lesions on some parts of the body may need to be left rather than treated aggressively

F. A basic principle in the management of psoriasis is daily lubrication and moisturization of the skin (see section on CARE OF DRY AND OILY SKIN for recommendations regarding moisturizers)

G. Topical corticosteroid preparations are the most frequently used topical agents for treatment of psoriasis and are considered first-line therapy by most experts

---

TOPICAL STEROID THERAPY FOR BODY AND EXTREMITIES

➡ **Initiate therapy** with a preparation from the high potency classification (**Note**: This is different from recommendations in previous years in which the least potent agents were tried first, and then more potent agents were used when treatment failures occurred)

➡ **Choose one** of the following:
  • Betamethasone dipropionate 0.05% (Diprolene AF) cream **OR**
  • Triamcinolone acetonide 0.5% cream or ointment (Aristocort)

➡ **Instruct patient** on appropriate use of topical steroid
  • Apply BID and apply no more often than this
  • Use only the amount that will easily rub into skin in a minute or two
  • Apply gently
  • Always wash hands after application so that medication is not inadvertently applied to other areas such as face, groin
  • Use for two weeks only

➡ After 2 weeks of topical therapy with a high potency agent, choose **one** of the following (**either 1 OR 2**) for the next phase of therapy (**Note:** Institute either 1 or 2, not both!)
  ✦ Provide a 1 week break from topical steroid therapy, and then institute a second 2-week course using the same medication (assuming, of course, that patient had a good response with first course and had no adverse reactions)
    • Provide a 1 week break, and then institute a third 2-week course using the same medication
    • Many patients have a remission lasting 8 weeks or longer after three 2-week treatment cycles
    • After this response (complete or almost complete remission), once or twice weekly application of the same potency topical steroid often maintains clearing **OR**
  ✦ Taper the high potency topical steroid to once or twice a week and use the nonsteroidal calcipotriene as maintenance therapy
    • Calcipotriene (Dovonex) is a synthetic Vitamin B_3 derivative that is believed to reduce epidermal differentiation and T-lymphocyte proliferation
    • Dovonex is available as a cream or ointment and should be applied BID
    • Patients may prefer to use the cream during the day since it is more cosmetically acceptable and the ointment at bedtime
    ★ Thus, calcipotriene is used as combination therapy with the high potency topical steroid
    ★ A recommended approach is to use the high potency topical steroid BID on weekends and calcipotriene BID during the week

---

H. Topical therapy for scalp depends on the degree of scalp involvement as well as the degree of patch thickening; treatment of the scalp is outlined below

---

TREATMENT OF THE SCALP

The scalp is often one of the most difficult areas to treat
  ➡ For very dense lesions on the scalp prescribe clobetasol propionate 0.05% scalp application (Cormax) 3-4 times weekly for one week only (**Note:** This is a super high potency topical steroid; should be used a total of 3-4 times during a one week period, applied at bedtime)
  ➡ For less dense lesions, a medium-potency topical steroid oil (Derma-Smooth/PS Topical Oil under occlusion with a shower cap at bedtime may be used 3-4 x week for a total of two weeks)
  ➡ For minimal scalp involvement, recommend a medicated shampoo that contains a keratolytic agents such as salicylic acid (T/Sal), tar (T/Gel) or a combination of these ingredients (Ionil T Plus)
  ➡ Minimal scalp involvement may also be treated with a low potency topical steroid solution such as fluocinolone acetonide 0.01% (Synalar), supplied in 20, 60 mL bottles, and for use after shampooing

---

I.   Topical therapy for face, flexural folds, and genitalia is described in table below

---

TOPICAL THERAPY FOR FACE, FLEXURAL FOLDS, AND GENITALIA

➡ Should be with low potency agents such as hydrocortisone 1% cream or an intermediate agent such as desonide 0.05% cream or lotion
  ✦ Treatment should be BID
  ✦ Treat for no longer than 2 weeks
  ✦ Explain to patient that pulse therapy (once or twice a week) should be used for maintenance

---

J.   Daily and regular sunlight exposure is beneficial to 4 out of 5 psoriasis patients; advise patients to avoid sunburn (short time in sun with no sun exposure during 4 hour period around noon)

K.   Follow Up: In 2-3 weeks in all patients in whom therapy has been initiated; then, monitor for side effects every 2 to 3 months

PITYRIASIS ROSEA

I.   Definition: A common, benign, often asymptomatic, self-limiting skin eruption of unknown etiology

II. Pathogenesis: Unknown, but some evidence suggests it is viral in origin

III. Clinical Presentation

   A.   More than 75% of cases are in persons 10-35 years of age

   B.   Incidence is higher during cold months

   C.   In its typical form, a 2-10 cm round-to-oval lesion (the herald patch) appears on the trunk
       1.   Precedes the appearance of the generalized eruption by 7-14 days
       2.   Herald patch usually has central clearing

   D.   The herald patch is followed by a generalized eruption consisting of multiple, erythematous (appears as hyperpigmentation in dark-skinned patients) macules progressing to papules which enlarge and become oval; a fine scale is present

   E.   Long axes of oval lesions tend to run parallel to each other, creating a "Christmas tree" distribution on trunk

   F.   Lesions usually last 4-8 weeks and mild itching is common

IV. Diagnosis/Evaluation

   A.   History
       1.   Question regarding recent occurrence of herald patch and location and presence of other lesions
       2.   Question regarding medications currently taking
       3.   Question if symptoms such as pruritus are present

   B.   Physical Examination
       1.   Examine skin for characteristic lesions; look specifically for herald patch which is usually on trunk
       2.   Determine distribution of lesions, looking to see if long axes of oval-shaped lesions are parallel to each other
       3.   Check the mucous surfaces, palms, and soles which are spared by pityriasis rosea

C. Differential Diagnosis
1. Tinea corporis
2. Tinea versicolor
3. Viral exanthems
4. Drug eruptions
5. Syphilis

D. Diagnostic Tests: **Always** order VDRL or RPR as syphilis can mimic this disorder

V. Plan/Management

A. No therapy is required, but symptomatic management of pruritus may be indicated

---

PRURITUS CONTROL USING PHARMACOLOGIC AND NONPHARMACOLOGIC INTERVENTIONS

Oral Antihistamines
Hydroxyzine (Atarax), supplied as 10 mg/5mL syrup and 10, 25, 50, 100 mg tablets
Dosing: 25-50 mg TID PRN
A single dose at bedtime is frequently all that is necessary

Oral Antihistamines for Use in the Daytime (Nonsedating)
Loratadine (Claritin) 10 mg tabs QD or fexofenadine (Allegra) 60 mg caps BID
Begin with 10 mg every other day; then 10 mg/day
Supplied as Claritin Reditabs, 10 mg, which are dissolved on tongue and swallowed with or without water
Supplied also as Claritin syrup, 1 mg/1 mL (alcohol free, dye free)

Important to prescribe nonsedating antihistamines for patients who must work or attend school, or who have other daytime responsibilities that require alertness

Topical Antipruritic Agents
Sarna lotion, Prax lotion and Itch-X gel are all OTC products
Cetaphil with menthol 0.25% and phenol 0.25% is an Rx product
Topical agents may be used in addition to or instead of oral antihistamines

Nonpharmacologic Treatment Modalities to Soothe Itchy Skin
Cool tub baths with or without colloidal oatmeal can provide relief
Topical compresses (washcloths wet with plain water and kept in freezer) can be applied to affected skin for 15-20 minutes, 3-4 x day

---

B. Sunlight exposure to the point of minimal erythema will hasten disappearance of lesions and decrease itching; caution against sunburn

C. Follow Up: None required

LICHEN PLANUS

I. Definition: A chronic, inflammatory, cutaneous and mucous membrane reaction pattern of unknown etiology usually affecting middle-aged adults

II. Pathogenesis

A. Cause is unknown

B. Possibly due to cell-mediated immune response to epidermal cell antigens

C. Genetic factors may play a role in etiology; familial cases are more severe

III.   Clinical Presentation

    A.   Age of onset is usually between 30-70 years

    B.   Clinical features of lichen planus (5 Ps): pruritic, planar (flat-topped), polyangular, purple, papules, or plaques

    C.   Number of lesions varies from a few chronic lesions to a generalized eruption

    D.   Close inspection of the surface of lesion reveals a lacy, reticulated pattern of whitish lines (called Wickham's striae)

    E.   Oral mucous membrane lichen planus can occur without cutaneous disease
        1.   Lesions may be on tongue, lips, but most common site is buccal mucosa
        2.   Mucous membrane involvement may consist only of the lace-like lesions

    F.   Five to ten percent of patients have nail changes ranging from minor dystrophy to total nail loss

IV.   Diagnosis/Evaluation

    A.   History
        1.   Question about appearance and location of lesions, onset, duration (whether a chronic or acute process)
        2.   Ask if lesions are pruritic
        3.   Question about presence of lesions in mouth
        4.   Ask if any first-degree relatives have a similar eruption

    B.   Physical Examination
        1.   Examine the involved skin looking for flat-topped, polyangular, purple papules
        2.   Use a magnifying glass to inspect the surface of lesions for reticulated pattern of whitish lines
        3.   Examine oral cavity, particularly the buccal mucosa, the most common site; look for Wickham's striae on the buccal mucosa

    C.   Differential Diagnosis
        1.   Drug eruption
        2.   Psoriasis
        3.   Aphthous stomatitis
        4.   Leukoplakia
        5.   Thrush

    D.   Diagnostic Tests: None indicated

V.   Plan/Management

    A.   Mouth lesions: Triamcinolone acetonide 0.025% cream in an adhesive base (Orabase) BID for 1-2 weeks; medication should be carefully placed on oral lesions, and not rubbed in as rubbing in disrupts adhesive properties of Orabase

    B.   Body lesion (not mucous membrane): Triamcinolone acetonide 0.1% cream (Aristocort, supplied as 15, 60 g) applied 2-3 x day for 1-2 weeks (Caution patient about steroid atrophy)

    C.   Treatment for pruritus is outlined in the section on PITYRIASIS ROSEA

    D.   Follow up: Not indicated

HERPES SIMPLEX

I. Definition: Cutaneous infections with herpes simplex viruses which are large, enveloped DNA viruses of two types that have major genomic and antigenic differences

    A.   HSV-1 is usually associated with oral/labial infections

    B.   HSV-2 is usually associated with genital infections (Genital herpes is considered under SEXUALLY TRANSMITTED DISEASES)

II. Pathogenesis

    A.   HSV-1 and HSV-2 are epidermotropic viruses with infection occurring within keratinocytes

    B.   Transmission is only by direct contact with active lesions, or by virus-containing fluid such as saliva or cervical secretions in persons with no evidence of active disease

    C.   Inoculation of the virus into skin or mucosal surfaces produces infection, with an incubation period of 2-12 days

    D.   About 48 hours after entering the host, the virus transverses afferent nerves to find host ganglion
        1.   The trigeminal ganglia are the target of the oral virus -- primarily HSV-1
        2.   The sacral ganglia are the target of the genital virus -- most often HSV-2

    E.   Upon reactivation, the virus retraces its route, causing recurrence in the cutaneous area affected by the same nerve root, but not necessarily in the original site

    F.   Generally HSV-1 is associated with infection of the lips, face, buccal mucosae, and throat; HSV-2, with the genitalia (see SEXUALLY TRANSMITTED DISEASES section for a full discussion of this topic)

    G.   An increasing number of genital herpes cases are attributable to HSV-1

III. Clinical Presentation

    A.   Three clinical stages define the course of herpes viruses: primary infection, latency, and recurrent infection

    B.   During primary infection with HSV-1 virus, the following usually occurs:
        1.   Lesions may appear 2-14 days following inoculation; lesions are typically grouped vesicles on an erythematous base, usually located on the lips, facial area, buccal mucosa, and throat
        2.   Vesicles rupture, leaving erosions that slowly form crusts; crusting signals the end of viral shedding; lesions are intraepidermal and usually heal without leaving a scar
        3.   There may be tenderness, pain, mild paresthesia, or burning prior to eruption of lesions; some persons have no prodrome
        4.   Persons may be asymptomatic during the primary infection stage, or may have fever, myalgia, malaise, or cervical lymphadenopathy

    C.   During the second clinical stage called latency, the virus remains dormant in the ganglia

    D.   During the recurrent or third clinical stage, the virus is reactivated and travels down the peripheral nerves to the site of the initial infection, causing the characteristic focal infection; recurrent infection is not inevitable and may be triggered by one or more of the following:
        1.   Local skin trauma
        2.   Sunlight exposure
        3.   Systemic changes such as menses, fatigue, or fever

    E.   The severity of the disease increases with age

IV.   Diagnosis/Evaluation

    A.   History
        1.   Question regarding location, onset, duration, and appearance of lesions; ask if pain, burning, or paresthesia present prior to eruption
        2.   Ask about associated symptoms of fever, myalgia, malaise
        3.   Ask regarding previous occurrence of similar lesions, symptoms
        4.   Inquire about exposures to infected persons

    B.   Physical Examination
        1.   Examine lesions for characteristic location, distribution, and appearance
        2.   Check for cervical lymphadenopathy

    C.   Differential Diagnosis
        1.   Erythema multiforme
        2.   Pemphigus

    D.   Diagnostic Tests
        1.   Tzanck preparation
        2.   Use of a commercially available rapid office test such as Kodak SureCell Herpes (uses enzyme immunoassay for HSV)
        3.   Most definitive test: Viral culture
            a.   Unroof vesicle and scrape the material with Dacron-tipped swab
            b.   Place swab in viral transport media
            c.   Viral detection usually requires 1-3 days after inoculation

V.   Plan/Management

    A.   Treatment of primary episode of mild to moderate HSV that is localized
        1.   For symptomatic management of lesions of the mouth
            a.   Apply viscous xylocaine (Lidocaine) 2% directly to lesion, or use 5 mL as an oral rinse before meals to facilitate eating
            b.   Apply Orabase, a dental protective paste QID to prevent irritation of lesion by teeth
            c.   Diphenhydramine (Benadryl) elixir mixed 1:1 with aluminum hydroxide/magnesium hydroxide (Maalox) may also be used QID as an oral rinse in both children and adults
            d.   Sucking on frozen juice bars, drinking ice water can also be helpful
        2.   For symptomatic management of lesions of the lip
            a.   Apply ice to reduce swelling
            b.   Use Blistex to prevent drying and reduce pain
            c.   Use sun-screen containing lip protectants prior to sun exposure
        3.   Use acetaminophen (Tylenol) PO for pain relief

    B.   Treatment of recurrent herpes simplex infections involving lips/face
        1.   Recommend symptomatic treatment as above
        2.   Topical antiviral agents may help speed healing and reduce pain
            a.   Penciclovir (Denavir) 1% cream; apply Q 2 hours while awake for 4 days
            b.   Begin treatment at earliest sign of symptoms (supplied as 2 g)

    C.   Immunocompromised patients with persistent intraoral or extralabial lesions
        1.   Acyclovir, 200 mg PO 5 x/day x 7 days OR
        2.   Valacyclovir, 500 mg PO BID x 5 days
        3.   Famciclovir, 500 mg PO BID x 7 days
        4.   **If suppressive** therapy is indicated, prescribe Acyclovir, 200-400 mg PO BID

    D.   Follow Up: None indicated

HERPES ZOSTER (SHINGLES)

I. Definition: A cutaneous viral infection, usually involving skin of a single dermatome but may involve one or two adjacent dermatomes

II. Pathogenesis: Caused by a reactivation of the varicella virus that remained in latent form in the basal ganglia after primary infection

III. Clinical Presentation

   A. Persons of all ages are affected but incidence increases with age with 75% of cases occurring in persons over age 50

   B. Dermatomal pain, itching, or burning may be severe and often begins 4-5 days before the eruption appears (see Figure 7.1)

   C. Preeruptive hyperesthia along the dermatome is a predictive sign

   D. Fever, headache, and malaise may precede the eruption

   E. Eruption begins with erythematous plaques and the distribution is dermatomal and unilateral
      1. Vesicles arise in clusters from the erythematous base, become cloudy with purulent fluid in 3-4 days, then form crust which falls off in 2-3 weeks
      2. Successive crops continue for about a week

   F. The trunk is affected in the majority of herpes zoster cases and fewer than 1% of cases are bilateral

   G. Usually resolves over 2 weeks, but elderly or debilitated persons may have a prolonged and difficult course

   H. Postherpetic neuralgia (pain lasting longer than 6 weeks after infection) occurs frequently in the elderly and can be debilitating

   I. Herpes zoster may be an early clinical sign of HIV infection and should be suspected when the disease occurs in young adults, or when a case is protracted, recurrent, or involves more than one dermatome

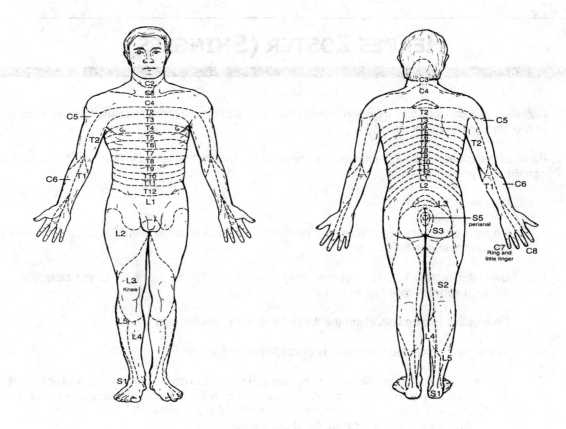

Figure 7.1. Dermatomes.

IV. Diagnosis/Evaluation

    A. History
        1. Inquire when the eruption began and ask about appearance and distribution of the lesions
        2. Question if there was preeruptive pain, itching, or burning in the affected dermatome several days before the eruption
        3. Ask about history of prior varicella infection
        4. Question regarding immunosuppressed status

    B. Physical Examination
        1. Examine skin for characteristic lesions and distribution (grouped vesicles on an erythematous base in a dermatomal distribution with unilateral involvement)
        2. Determine if there is ophthalmic involvement

    C. Differential Diagnosis
        1. Varicella
        2. Herpes simplex
        3. Poison ivy
        4. Cellulitis

    D. Diagnostic Tests
        1. If lesions and course are atypical, consider viral antigen smear or viral cultures
        2. If patient is young adult, or if this is a recurrent, protracted case, consider HIV testing

V.   Plan/Management

   A.   Suppression of pain, inflammation, and infection is goal of therapy

   B.   Use NSAIDs for pain, fever

   C.   Wet compresses using Burrow's solution or cool tap water can be applied for 30 minutes several times a day

   D.   The following groups of patients are candidates for systemic therapy
         1.   Patients with outbreak that is <72 hours in duration
         2.   Patients with outbreak that is >72 hours in duration but in whom new lesions are still developing
         3.   All patients >50 years of age
         4.   Immunosuppressed patients

   E.   Recommendations for oral systemic therapy for immunocompetent **adults** with outbreak limited to one dermatome are as follows:
         1.   Valacyclovir (Valtrex), 1 g TID x 7 days (supplied as 500 mg tabs), OR
         2.   Famciclovir (Famvir), 500 mg TID x 7 days (supplied as 500 mg tabs)
         3.   Each dose should be taken with at least 8 oz water

   F.   Adults who are HIV+ with outbreak limited to one dermatome should be treated with acyclovir 800 mg PO 5 x/day OR famciclovir 500 mg PO TID x 7 days

   G.   Treatment with intravenous drugs may be necessary in the following situations: More than one dermatome involved, involvement of the trigeminal nerve, dissemination or if is a concern

   H.   Management of patients with postherpetic neuralgia
         1.   Patients who continue to have pain that persists more than 1 month after lesions have healed require close follow up for pain control and support
               a.   NSAIDs dosed properly are the first-line therapy
               b.   Narcotics such as Tylenol #3 may be needed short term to get pain under control
               c.   Capsaicin cream (Zostrix) [OTC] may be applied topically 3-4x/day for up to 4 weeks; should not be used on open, weeping lesions
                     (1)   Most useful for localized involvement
                     (2)   Advise patient to avoid eyes and wash hands thoroughly after application
               d.   Lidocaine-prilocaine cream (EMLA) may also be used
                     (1)   Apply generously to affected area
                     (2)   May use occlusion with plastic wrap
         2.   Amitriptyline dosed at 10-25 mg at HS and increasing up to 75mg/day may be helpful in some patients
               a.   Anticholinergic side effects may limit acceptability
               b.   Warn patient about sedation
               c.   Use cautiously in elderly
         3.   Patients with pain that is refractory should be referred to a pain clinic for management

   I.   For secondarily infected lesions, apply mupirocin (Bactroban) cream TID for 10 days (**Note:** Cream formulation is recommended for secondary infections)

   J.   Isolate patient from neonates, pregnant women, and immunosuppressed persons since the active lesions are potentially infectious, though this is rare

   K.   Follow up in 1-3 days after diagnosis; then again in 7-10 days

MOLLUSCUM CONTAGIOSUM

I. Definition: A benign, viral disease of the skin characterized by discrete, white to flesh-colored, dome-shaped papules

II. Pathogenesis

    A. Caused by a poxvirus that induces epidermal cell proliferation

    B. Humans are the only known source of the virus and infectivity is relatively low

    C. Spreads by direct contact, including sexual contact, or by fomites

    D. Incubation period varies between 2-7 weeks and may be as long a 6 months

III. Clinical Presentation

    A. More common in children and adolescents, but may also occur in adults

    B. Tiny (2-5 mm), early lesions are shiny, white to flesh-colored, dome-shaped discrete papules with a firm, waxy appearance
        1. As lesions mature, the center becomes soft and umbilicated
        2. Usually number of lesions ranges from 2-20

    C. Lesions occur in groups; usually on genital area in adults

    D. Erythema may surround the lesions as a result of inflammation from scratching or may be a hypersensitivity reaction

    E. Self-limiting; usually spontaneously clears in 6-9 months

    F. A common, cutaneous manifestation of HIV+ infection

IV. Diagnosis/Evaluation

    A. History
        1. Inquire about location, appearance of lesions, onset and duration
        2. Ask about past medical history, HIV+ infection

    B. Physical Examination
        1. Examine skin looking for lesions in groups, 3-5 mm in size, with a waxy appearance
        2. Magnification may assist in seeing central umbilication in more mature lesions
        3. Palpate the lesions to reveal their solid versus fluid-filled nature (wear gloves)

    C. Differential Diagnosis
        1. Basal cell carcinoma
        2. Epidermal cyst
        3. Wart
        4. Herpes simplex

    D. Diagnostic Tests: None indicated

V. Diagnosis/Treatment

    A. For small number of asymptomatic lesions that are stable (not spreading), observe for spontaneous resolution over next few months

    B. If patient prefers, removal via curettage of the central core or via liquid nitrogen therapy is also an option

C. Another option is to use one of the following topical agents for removal
1. Duofilm (available as 15 mL) OR
2. Viranol solution (available as 10 mL) OR
3. Duoplant (available as 7.5 mL gel), OR
4. Tretinoin 0.01% or 0.025% gel (available as 15 g)
   a. Products should be used sparingly at bedtime
   b. Dead skin should be removed nightly with washcloth before reapplying preparation
   c. Use petroleum jelly to protect the surrounding skin

D. Follow Up: None required

WARTS

I. Definition: Virus-induced epidermal tumors

II. Pathogenesis

   A. Wart virus is located within epidermal cell nucleus

   B. Cells proliferate to form a mass which remains confined to the epidermis

III. Clinical Presentation

   A. May appear at any age but commonly occur in younger age groups

   B. Warts are transmitted by touch and commonly appear at sites of trauma on the hands, periungual regions from biting, and on plantar surfaces from weight bearing

   C. Most warts resolve in 12-24 months without treatment

   D. Generally, warts are asymptomatic except for plantar warts which may be painful

   E. Presentation is variable depending on type:
     1. Common warts (*verruca vulgaris*) may arise anywhere on body and appear as solitary flesh-colored papule with a scaly, irregular surface
     2. Filiform warts are usually seen on face (lips, nose, eyelids) and appear as thin projections on a narrow stalk
     3. Flat warts (*verruca plana*) are usually located on face and extremities and appear in groups as flat-topped, skin-colored papules
     4. Plantar warts occur on weight-bearing areas of the feet; papule is pushed into skin and verrucous surface appears level with skin surface
     5. Venereal warts are considered under SEXUALLY TRANSMITTED DISEASES section

IV. Diagnosis/Evaluation

   A. History
     1. Question about location, onset, duration, and if any symptoms are present
     2. Ask about treatments tried and results

   B. Physical Examination
     1. Examine lesion looking for characteristic appearance
     2. Use hand lens to aid in visualizing surface characteristics

C. Differential Diagnosis
    1. Calluses (have smooth rather than rough irregular surface)
    2. Lichen planus (look for Wickham's striae)
    3. Seborrheic keratosis (have stuck on appearance with horn cysts visible on close inspection)

D. Diagnostic Tests: None indicated

V. Plan/Management

A. Common wart: Topical salicylic acid preparations applied at bedtime for 6-8 weeks; may use liquid nitrogen in cooperative patients
    1. Examples of 17% concentrations are Occlusal HP, Duoplant, Compound W, Duofilm, Wart-Off; all are OTC and in liquid form
    2. An example of a 15% solution in karaya gum base patches for use on isolated thicker lesions is Trans Ver Sal (40 patches of varying size with securing tapes and emery file)

B. Filiform wart: Refer for removal by snip excision

C. Flat wart: Refer for removal; these warts are resistant to treatment and are usually located in cosmetically important areas

D. Plantar wart: Use 40% salicylic acid plasters; examples are Mediplast and Duofilm Patch
    1. Plaster is cut to size of wart and applied over wart
    2. Plaster is removed in 24-48 hours and pliable dead white keratin is removed with pumice stone
    3. Process is repeated every 24-48 hours until wart is removed (usually 6-8 weeks)
    4. Pain relief occurs early because a large part of wart is removed in first few days of treatment

E. Follow Up: None indicated

REFERENCES

Abramowicz, M. (1998). Drugs for parasitic infections. The Medical Letter, 40(1017), 1-11.

American Academy of Pediatrics, Committee on Infectious Diseases. (1997). Red book: Report of the committee on infectious diseases (24th ed.). Elk Grove Village, IL: Author.

Bernhard, J.D. (1994). Itch: Mechanisms and management of puritus. New York: McGraw-Hill.

Bikowski, J. (1997). Rosacea: The great imitator. Family Practice Recertification, 19(10), 61-75.

Bisno, A.L., & Stevens, D.L. (1996). Streptococcal infections of skin and soft tissues. New England Journal of Medicine, 334, 240-245.

Choo, P.W., LaRussa, P., Seward. J., & Weber, D. (1997, Dec). Management and prevention of varicella-zoster. Patient Care, 31-48.

Fisher, G.J., Wang, Z., Datta, S.C., Varani, J., Kang, S., & Voorhes, J.J. (1997). Pathophysiology of premature skin aging induced by ultraviolet light. New England Journal of Medicine, 337, 1419-1428.

Gilchrest, B.A. (1997). Treatment of photodamage with topical tretinoin: An overview. Journal of the American Academy of Dermatology, 36(3), S-27-35.

Goldstein, B.G., & Goldstein, A.O. (1997). Practical dermatology. St. Louis: Mosby.

Habif, T.P. (1996). Clinical dermatology. St. Louis: Mosby.

Kligman, A.M. (1997). The treatment of acne with topical retinoids: One man's opinions. <u>Journal of the American Academy of Dermatology, 36</u>, S-92-95.

Leyden, J.J. (1997). Therapy for acne vulgaris. <u>New England Journal of Medicine, 336</u>, 1156-1162.

Leyden, J.J. (1998). Emerging topical retinoid therapies. <u>Journal of the American Academy of Dermatology, 38</u>, S1-4.

Lowe, N.J. (1997, May). Managing acne in adult women. <u>Patient Care</u>, 30-43.

Menter, A. (1997). Psoriasis in primary care: Diagnosis and management. <u>Family Practice Recertification, 19</u>(Suppl. 5), 1-33.

Reifsnider, E. (1997). Common adult infectious skin conditions. <u>Nurse Practitioner, 22</u>(11), 17-33.

Rosen, T., & Ablon, G. (1997, Sept). Cutaneous herpes virus infection update. <u>Consultant</u>, 2443-2455.

Sadick, N.S. (1997). Current aspects of bacterial infections of the skin. <u>Dermatologic Clinics of North America, 15</u>(2), 341-346.

Wilkin, J.K. (1994). Rosacea: Pathophysiology and treatment. <u>Archives of Dermatology, 130</u>, 359-362.

Problems of the Eyes

BLEPHARITIS

I. Definition: Inflammation of the eyelid margins

II. Pathogenesis:

A. Often due to infection (usually Staphylococcal)

B. May also be caused by hypersecretory or inflammation of sebaceous glands (often associated with seborrhea of face/scalp)

C. May be associated with conjunctivitis

III. Clinical Presentation

A. A common, chronic problem which usually begins in early childhood and continues throughout adulthood

B. Characterized by hypertrophy and desquamation of the epidermis near the lid margin which results in erythema and scaling of the lid border

C. Main complaint is redness of the eyelid margin but burning and discomfort of the eyes may be additional symptoms

D. Severe cases may produce purulent discharge and over time permanent changes in the eyelid structure can occur (lost lashes and distortion of lid contour)

E. Patient usually has a history of recurrent chalazia and hordeola

IV. Diagnosis/Evaluation

A. History
    1. Determine onset and duration of symptoms
    2. Ask about presence of flaking, crusting at lid margins
    3. Inquire about eye pain, visual disturbances, dry eyes and tearing
    4. Ask about past episodes and previous treatments
    5. Inquire about previous and present skin problems, particularly of the face and scalp
    6. Ask about chronic exposure to irritants such as smoke, cosmetics, and chemicals
    7. Inquire about frequency of eye rubbing

B. Physical Examination
    1. Determine visual acuity
    2. Perform a complete eye examination, paying particular attention to the following components:
        a. Inspect eyelid margins with magnifying glass for crusting, scaling, erythema, and ulcers
        b. Examine sclera and conjunctiva for abnormalities
        c. Palpate lid margins and lid for masses
    3. Palpate for preauricular adenopathy

C. Differential Diagnosis
    1. Chalazion, stye, conjunctivitis, and keratitis may result from blepharitis
    2. Sebaceous cell carcinoma is a rare condition, but should be suspected if blepharitis persists despite extensive treatment

D. Diagnostic Tests: None are usually indicated

V.   Plan/Management:

   A.   If an underlying source of the lid irritation can be identified, it is important to treat the source as the first step in management
      1.   If seborrheic dermatitis of the scalp and face is present, institute appropriate treatment (see section on SEBORRHEIC DERMATITIS for treatment recommendations)
      2.   If rosacea is present, institute treatment (see section on ROSACEA for treatment recommendations)
      3.   If dry eyes are present, advise patient to use agents such as Cellufresh or Lacrisert

   B.   For patients with **acute** phase of blepharitis, the following treatment should be instituted
      1.   Instruct patient in eye hygiene
         a.   Patient should be directed to scrub eyelids with wet washcloth (or cotton-tipped applicator) and baby shampoo (or commercial cleansing pads such as Eye Scrub or Lid Wipes SPF) in order to remove crusts and scale
         b.   Scrubs should be repeated up to four times a day depending on symptoms
         c.   May also apply warm, moist compresses for 15 minutes throughout the day
      2.   If condition is moderate to severe, prescribe erythromycin, 5 mg/g (Ilotycin)   ophthalmic ointment BID x 7 days OR sulfacetamide sodium 10% (Bleph-10) available as ophthalmic solution or ointment (solution: 1-2 drops Q3H during day; ointment: QID and at HS) x 7 days

   C.   For patients with chronic blepharitis, the following treatment is recommended
      1.   Instruct patient to continue daily eye hygiene of the lid margins
      2.   For flares, also use warm moist compresses throughout day and apply ophthalmic antibiotics intermittently when needed

   D.   For severe blepharitis, referral to an ophthalmologist is indicated

   E.   Follow Up
      1.   None needed for mild cases
      2.   Reevaluate moderate cases in 10-14 days

CATARACT

I.   Definition: A decrease in the transparency of the crystalline lens to the degree that vision is disturbed

II.   Pathogenesis

   A.   Protein coagulations form opaque areas in the crystalline lens of the eye for unknown reasons

   B.   Occurs most often as a natural process of aging

   C.   Other causes are metabolic, congenital, drug-induced, ocular trauma, and ocular conditions such as chronic anterior uveitis

III.   Clinical Presentation

   A.   Cataract is the most common cause of decreased visual acuity in adults; ninety-five percent of persons >65 years of age have some degree of lens opacity

   B.   Approximately 1 million cataract extractions are done each year in the US; worldwide, cataract accounts for 1.7 million cases of treatable blindness

   C.   A gradual, painless, progressive loss of vision occurs over time, and many patients are unaware of vision problems

D. Complaints of cloudy, foggy, or blurred vision are common

E. Glare is one of the symptomatic manifestations of light scattering and is experienced when person looks at a point source of light and sees a diffusion of bright white and colored light which reduces visual acuity; glare interferes with night driving

F. Distortion occurs making straight edges appear wavy or curved; patient may complain of double vision (double vision caused by cataract is usually monocular versus binocular)

G. Often, color perception is altered so that colors are seen differently (loss of contrast sensitivity)

H. Cataract may occur in only one eye (monocular) or may mature more rapidly in one eye than in the other

I. Factors that influence the risk of adult-onset cataract include excessive ultraviolet B radiation exposure, diabetes mellitus, corticosteroid therapy, tobacco and alcohol use, and low antioxidant vitamin use

IV. Diagnosis/Evaluation

A. History
1. Inquire regarding onset of decreased vision, and if one or both eyes are involved
2. Ask about increased problems with glare and if changes in ways colors are seen has occurred in recent months
3. Inquire about presence of risk factors (see III., I., above)
4. Ask if any recent injury to eye has occurred
5. Obtain medication and past medical history

B. Physical Examination
1. Measure visual acuity at both near and far distances (**Note**: Most common objective finding associated with cataracts is decreased visual acuity)
2. Check pupillary reaction to light (**Note**: Pupillary reaction is unaffected by a cataract)
3. Observe for leukokoria (white pupil) seen in mature cataracts
4. Assess visual fields by confrontation (**Note**: Visual fields should be full or only mildly limited)
5. Examine the red reflex with the ophthalmoscope set on +4 (black) diopters at about 20 cm from patient (**Note**: Examination will reveal a black lens opacity against the red-orange pupillary light reflex)

C. Differential Diagnosis
1. Macular degeneration
2. Diabetic retinopathy

D. Diagnostic Tests: Additional testing should be done by the ophthalmologist (**Note**: Cataracts are best evaluated by slit-lamp examination)

V. Plan/Management

A. Ophthalmology referral for evaluation
1. Decision to obtain cataract surgery is based on degree of functional impairment
2. Patient should weigh the risk and benefits associated with surgery

B. Nonsurgical management by the ophthalmologist includes changing lens prescription, use of strong bifocals or magnification, and appropriate illumination

C. Patient should be informed that cataract does not need to be removed unless there is impairment of normal activities

D.   Progression of cataract formation may be slowed by decreasing amount of sun exposure (wearing of hat and dark glasses when outdoors), smoking cessation, and increasing antioxidant vitamin ingestion

E.   Follow Up: By ophthalmologist

CHALAZION

I.   Definition: Focal chronic inflammation of a meibomian gland

II.   Pathogenesis

   A.   Chronic granuloma from obstructed meibomian gland

   B.   May occur as a result of a chronic hordeolum

   C.   Secondary infection of the surrounding tissues may develop

III.   Clinical Presentation

   A.   Usually hard, non-tender nodule is found on midportion of the tarsus, away from the lid border; may develop on lid margin if the opening of the duct is involved and can present with lid tenderness, pain, and swelling

   B.   Chalazia which become infected result in painful swelling of the entire lid

   C.   Small chalazia may resolve spontaneously without treatment

   D.   History of chronic blepharitis and prior excision of chalazia is often present

IV.   Diagnosis/Evaluation

   A.   History
      1.   Determine onset and duration of symptoms
      2.   Inquire about pain or tenderness of the lid
      3.   Inquire about any changes in visual acuity level
      4.   Ask about past episodes and previous treatments

   B.   Physical Examination
      1.   Assess visual acuity
      2.   Perform a complete eye examination, paying particular attention to the following components
         a.   Inspect eyelids for inflammation and masses
         b.   Palpate eyelids for masses and tenderness
         c.   Evert the eyelid and examine inner surface for pointing
         d.   Inspect sclera and conjunctiva for abnormalities
      3.   Palpate for preauricular adenopathy

   C.   Differential Diagnosis
      1.   May be associated with a hordeolum and blepharitis
      2.   Sebaceous cell carcinoma is a rare condition which should be considered

   D.   Diagnostic Tests: None indicated

V. Plan/Management

    A. Small, asymptomatic chronic chalazia do not require treatment and usually disappear spontaneously within a few months

    B. If chalazia are large or if there is secondary infection, treatment is needed
        1. Apply warm, moist compresses for 15 minutes throughout the day
        2. Prescribe erythromycin, 5 mg/g (Ilotycin) ophthalmic ointment BID x 7 days OR polymyxin B-trimethoprim drops (Polytrim) BID x 7 days

    C. If the chalazion does not respond to conservative therapy, patient should be referred to an expert for injection of the lesion or incision and curettage

    D. Follow Up
        1. Small chalazia do not require follow up
        2. Follow up for chalazia that do not respond to conservative therapy should be with ophthalmologist

CONJUNCTIVITIS

I. Definition: Inflammation of the conjunctiva characterized by vascular dilation, cellular infiltration, and exudation

II. Pathogenesis

    A. Conjunctivitis can be caused by bacterial or viral agents, by allergic reaction, or by toxic factors

    B. Acute bacterial conjunctivitis
        1. *Staphylococcus aureus* (probably the most common cause of bacterial conjunctivitis and the most common causative organism in adults)
        2. *Streptococcus pneumoniae* (more commonly a causative organism in children rather than adults)
        3. *Haemophilus influenzae* (more commonly a causative organism in children rather than adults)

    C. Hyperacute bacterial conjunctivitis
        1. Most commonly caused by *Neisseria gonorrhoeae* and less often by *Neisseria meningitidis*
        2. Occurs in adults via autoinoculation from infected genitalia

    D. Ocular chlamydial infections are of two types
        1. Trachoma is associated with serotypes A through C and causes a chronic keratoconjunctivitis which frequently results in blindness; this condition is rare in the US but occurs in rural areas of developing countries, particularly Africa, Asia, and the Middle East
        2. Inclusion conjunctivitis is associated with serotypes D through K and is a common, primarily sexually transmitted disease that occurs in the US

    E. Viral conjunctivitis
        1. Usually caused by adenovirus
        2. *Herpes simplex* virus is a less common cause

    F. Noninfectious conjunctivitis
        1. Allergic conjunctivitis (hay fever conjunctivitis)
        2. Contact lens associated
        3. Toxic (often occurs as a chemical reaction in patients using ocular medications)

III.   Clinical presentation

A.   Acute bacterial conjunctivitis
1.   Characterized by acute onset of mucopurulent or purulent discharge with burning, irritation, and tearing
2.   Eyelids are often edematous with matting of the eyelashes upon awakening
3.   Inflammation is more prominent in the palpebral conjunctiva than in the bulbar conjunctiva with mild injection of the conjunctival vessels
4.   Typically, the infection begins in one eye and then becomes bilateral in 2 to 5 days
5.   Usually the condition is self-limited but antibiotics can shorten the time course of infection

B.   Hyperacute bacterial conjunctivitis
1.   A severe, sight-threatening ocular infection most often affecting sexually active young adults; organism is transmitted from genitalia to hands, and then to eyes
2.   Characterized by marked yellow-green purulent discharge that is bilateral, lid edema, erythema, and chemosis
3.   Preauricular lymphadenopathy often present

C.   Chlamydial conjunctivitis in adolescents and adults
1.   Usually presents in young sexually active persons between the ages of 18 and 30
2.   Transmission occurs most often via autoinoculation from infected genital secretions
3.   Typically, an indolent infection which is characterized by a thin, mucoid discharge
4.   Patient may have photophobia and enlarged, tender preauricular nodes
5.   Subacute or chronic in nature, with patients presenting with symptoms that have been present for as long as 6 months

D.   Viral conjunctivitis due to adenoviruses
1.   Often occurs in community epidemics and is highly contagious
2.   Usual modes of transmission are contaminated fingers and swimming pool water
3.   Onset is usually acute and discharge is usually watery
4.   A mild injection of the conjunctiva lasting 3-4 days is often present
5.   Always self-limited and rarely results in sequelae

E.   Viral conjunctivitis due to herpes simplex
1.   Type 1 herpes simplex virus is the type that is usually involved in ocular disease
2.   Occurs very infrequently especially in view of the fact that by age 60, approximately 97% of all persons have been infected with type 1 HSV, and less than 1% of these infections present as ocular disease
3.   May be accompanied by fever blister on lip or face
4.   Preauricular nodes are usually enlarged
5.   Occurs most frequently in immunosuppressed persons

F.   Noninfectious conjunctivitis
1.   **Allergic**: Itching is the hallmark of this condition; systemic manifestations of hay fever such as rhinorrhea and sneezing which is usually seasonal may also be present
       a.   Characterized by itchy, red eyes, with discharge that is watery and bilateral
       b.   Eyelids may be edematous and have a cobblestone appearance
       c.   **Note**: Vernal catarrh is a serious form of allergic conjunctivitis and is seen most often in children and adolescents (more common in male African Americans); may result in severe corneal ulceration and loss of vision
2.   **Contact lens associated**: Soft contact lenses are most often involved
       a.   Ocular irritation with erythema, pruritus, and mucoid discharge is common
       b.   Characteristic papillae are present on the upper tarsal conjunctiva
3.   **Toxic**: Presents most commonly in patients using ocular medication
       a.   Discharge is usually watery or mucoid
       b.   Chemosis may be present but no preauricular nodes are palpable
       c.   Examination will reveal a follicular and papillary response

IV.   Diagnosis/Evaluation

    A.   History
        1.   Inquire regarding onset and duration of symptoms (Is the condition acute, subacute, chronic, or recurrent?)
        2.   Determine if condition is unilateral or bilateral; ask about the type and amount of discharge
        3.   Determine if ocular pain, photophobia, or blurred vision (that fails to clear with a blink) are present
        4.   Ask if itching and other symptoms of seasonal allergic rhinitis are present
        5.   Ask about contact with a person with "pink-eye"
        6.   Inquire about personal and family history of hay fever, allergic rhinitis
        7.   Obtain past medical and medication history, specifically asking about use of any ocular medications (including OTCs)

    B.   Physical Examination
        1.   Determine visual acuity, visual fields, pupillary function and extraocular movements
        2.   Examine eyelids for inflammation or tenderness
        3.   Examine sclera and conjunctiva for hyperemia and edema; check cornea for clarity
        4.   Determine type of discharge
        5.   Examine face for presence of herpes labialis or a dermatomal vesicular eruption suggesting shingles
        6.   Palpate for regional lymphadenopathy

    C.   Differential Diagnosis: Patients typically present with the main complaint of red eye; there is need to distinguish conjunctivitis from other conditions causing red eye
        1.   In conjunctivitis, redness of the conjunctiva is diffuse, pain is minimal, and vision, pupil size, and reactivity are normal
        2.   Acute angle-closure glaucoma presents with severe ocular pain, headache, and blurred vision
        3.   Iritis presents with pain, moderately decreased vision, dull and swollen iris, and sluggishly reacting pupil; injection is usually bulbar near limbus
        4.   Blepharitis may have similar presentation as conjunctivitis with burning and itching of the conjunctiva, but with blepharitis there also is inflammation of lid margins
        5.   Corneal abrasions usually have a history of trauma with mild to moderate bulbar injection and a foreign-body sensation

    D.   Diagnostic Tests
        1.   Culture and smears of discharge are usually not recommended for mild conjunctivitis with a suspected viral, bacterial, allergic, or toxic origin
        2.   If there is severe inflammation as occurs with hyperacute conjunctivitis, or if the condition is chronic or recurrent, a culture is indicated
        3.   If testing for chlamydia is indicated based on history, enzyme immunoassays for Chlamydia organisms or DNA assays may be used

V.   Plan/Management

    A.   Acute bacterial conjunctivitis: If treatment is based on clinical diagnosis alone, select a broad spectrum topical antibiotics such as ONE of the following
        1.   Erythromycin ointment (Ilotycin): Apply small amount 2-3x/day for 7-10 days
        2.   Polymyxin B-trimethoprim solution (Polytrim): 1 gtt Q 3-4 hours (maximum 6 doses/day) x 7-10 days
        3.   Sodium sulfacetamide 10% solution (Bleph-10): 1-2 gtts Q 2-3 hours during day for 7-10 days (**Note**: About 50% of staphylococci are now resistant to the sulfonamides)

    B.   Hyperacute bacterial conjunctivitis: Systemic antibiotics are required and most patients with this condition should be admitted to the hospital for IV therapy

C. Chlamydial conjunctivitis: Prescribe systemic antibiotics Doxycycline (Vibramycin) 100 mg BID for 7 days
1. Once a diagnosis has been established, a genital work-up of the patient and sexual partner is indicated
2. Pregnant and lactating women: Use erythromycin, 250 mg QID x 21 days
3. Diagnosis of chlamydial disease should prompt investigation for other sexually diseases, including syphilis, gonorrhea, hepatitis B and HIV infection

D. Viral infections primarily due to adenoviruses
1. Usually self-limiting and treatment is supportive (application of cold compresses and use of topical vasoconstrictor)
2. Antiviral agents have not proven to be effective
3. Topical antibiotics are not necessary as secondary bacterial infection is uncommon

E. Viral infection due to herpes simplex
1. Refer to ophthalmologist
2. Never prescribe steroid medication if herpes simplex virus is a possibility as steroid preparations can enhance proliferation of virus and result in permanent eye damage

F. Allergic conjunctivitis
1. Prescribe cromolyn sodium (Crolom) ophthalmic solution: 1-2 gtts 4 times a day OR
2. Patanol solution, an antihistamine/mast cell stabilizer: 1-2 gtts BID at 6-8 hour intervals
3. Systemic antihistamines are also often recommended: Loratadine (Claritin), supplied as 10 mg tabs and Reditabs, dosing 10 mg QD

G. Toxic conjunctivitis
1. Eliminate the suspected medication
2. Prescribe mild ocular lubricants such as Tears Naturale or Naturale Free to promote comfort
3. Suggest frequent cold compresses

H. Contact lens associated conjunctivitis
1. Discontinuation of contact lens use is curative, but is not often acceptable to patient
2. Trials of stopping the use of various agents and substituting others (example, change the contact lens solution) or changing the type of contact lens may be helpful

I. Refer the patient for expert management if any of the following occur
1. There is no improvement in 24-48 hours
2. Patient has moderate to severe ocular pain, decreased visual acuity, abnormal eye exam
3. Infection from herpes simplex virus

J. Patient Education
1. Instruct patients to instill medication in the inner aspect of the lower eyelid
2. Teach patients that infection is easily spread to unaffected eye and to other household members
3. The role of frequent handwashing in limiting the spread of ocular infections cannot be overemphasized
4. Discuss with patient that eye secretions are contagious for 24 to 48 hours after therapy begins
5. Patients with viral infections should be instructed that the ocular infection is contagious for at least seven days after the onset

K. Follow Up
1. If no improvement in 24-48, or if condition worsens, patient should return for referral for expert care
2. No follow up is indicated for mild cases which resolve without problems

GLAUCOMA

I. Definition: A group of ocular disorders characterized by elevation of intraocular pressure (IOP) accompanied by characteristic optic nerve damage and/or visual field loss via capillary microinfarction causing optic nerve ischemia

II. Pathogenesis

    A. Glaucoma can be generally classified into three categories: developmental, open-angle, and angle-closure glaucoma (**Note**: The two primary types of glaucoma--open-angle and angle-closure glaucoma are classified according to the anatomy of the anterior chamber angle)

    B. Developmental: Characterized by an anterior chamber angle defect caused by abnormal differentiation of embryonic tissue

    C. Primary Open-Angle Glaucoma (POAG)
        1. An abnormality in the trabecular angle tissue causing resistance to fluid flow
        2. Condition is not secondary to another condition

    D. Primary Angle-Closure Glaucoma
        1. Relative pupillary block is the mechanism of angle closure
        2. Resistance to fluid flow of aqueous humor between posterior iris surface and lens related to their close approximation at the pupil

III. Clinical Presentation

    A. Glaucoma is the second leading cause of blindness is the US, and is prevalent in nearly 3-4% of the population over age 70

    B. Risk factors include high intraocular pressure (IOP), older age, African-American race, and family history of glaucoma; evidence supporting a link between myopia, diabetes, high blood pressure, and glaucoma is very weak

    C. In developmental glaucoma, affected infants tend to be irritable, photophobic, and have some degree of tearing
        1. Infants keep their eyes closed most of the time and, after eye-hand coordination has developed, constantly rub at their eyes
        2. Penlight exam reveals diffuse haziness with a bluish appearance of the cornea

    D. Primary open-angle glaucoma (POAG) is by far the most prevalent form of the disorder
        1. Onset of the disorder is slow and insidious, with central visual acuity affected late in course; usually bilateral
        2. Signs include elevated IOP and increased cup-to-disc ratio as well as other signs that are detectable through slit-lamp examination
        3. A significant number of patients with open-angle glaucoma have intraocular pressure below 21 mm Hg (as measured by tonometry), a condition which is referred to as normal tension glaucoma
        4. Intraocular pressure **alone** is not the primary determinant for diagnosis

    E. In primary angle-closure glaucoma (a relatively rare condition), manifestations of angle closure depend on the extent and reversibility of the pupillary block
        1. Angle-closure glaucoma is most likely to occur in persons of Asian descent
        2. Patients may complain of unilateral headache (same side as affected eye), visual blurring, nausea, and photophobia
        3. Angle-closure glaucoma is an ophthalmologic emergency as irreversible eye damage can occur if left untreated

F.   Present standard for determining visual loss in glaucoma is the visual-field test, an automated examination that is reserved for the ophthalmologist's office

IV.   Diagnosis/Evaluation

    A.   History
        1.   Inquire about onset and duration of symptoms, and if one or both eyes are affected
        2.   In adults, ask about difficulties with peripheral vision, and if symptoms of headache, photophobia, visual blurring are present
        3.   In infants, ask parents if child is resistant to opening eyes, if tearing is present, and if infant rubs eyes
        4.   Inquire about family history of eye disease

    B.   Physical Examination
        1.   Quickly examine external eye for swelling, ptosis, injection of conjunctiva, tearing, and corneal clarity
        2.   If emergent condition not suspected, visual acuity testing should be performed (may be normal in persons with glaucoma)
        3.   Measurement of intraocular pressure using a hand-held device such as the Shiötz tonometer is a useful screening approach (provides gross measurement only)
            a.   Normal intraocular pressure is 10-20 mm Hg
            b.   Women have slightly higher pressures than men
            c.   Asians may have higher intraocular pressures than African Americans and Caucasions
        4.   Measure peripheral vision using direct confrontation (provides gross measurement of visual fields)
        5.   Fundoscopic exam may reveal notching of the cup and a difference in cup-to-disc ratio between the two eyes

    C.   Differential Diagnosis
        1.   Conjunctivitis
        2.   Acute uveitis
        3.   Macular degeneration

    D.   Diagnostic Test: None except those described under Physical Examination (Further evaluation should be performed by the ophthalmologist who bases diagnosis on the appearance of the optic nerve [i.e., color and contour] and findings on visual field examination, testing which requires highly specialized equipment)

V.   Plan/Management

    A.   Angle-closure glaucoma is an ocular emergency; if this condition is suspected, immediate referral to an ophthalmologist is indicated

    B.   All patients who present with complaints of ocular pain, photophobia, visual blurring, or sudden loss of vision should be immediately referred for emergency care by an ophthalmologist

    C.   Infants with tearing, rubbing eyes, and resistance to opening eyes should be referred to a pediatric ophthalmologist for immediate care

    D.   If primary open-angle glaucoma suspected based on physical examination, refer to ophthalmologist for evaluation

    E.   Follow Up: By ophthalmologist

HORDEOLUM (STYE)

I.   Definition: Acute inflammation of the follicle of an eyelash or the associated gland of Zeis (sebaceous) or Moll (apocrine sweat gland)

II.   Pathogenesis: An acute infectious process involving the sebaceous, sweat or meibomian glands of the eyelid usually caused by *Staphylococcus aureus*

III. Clinical Presentation

    A.   More common in children and adolescents than adults

    B.   Patient often presents with sudden onset of localized tenderness, redness, and swelling of the eyelid

    C.   May occur in crops because the infecting pathogen may spread from one hair follicle to another

    D.   May point to the conjunctival side of the lid (internal hordeolum involving the meibomian glands) or may involve the lid margin (external hordeolum involving the sebaceous or sweat glands)

IV.   Diagnosis/Evaluation

    A.   History
        1.   Determine onset and duration of symptoms
        2.   Inquire about pain and visual disturbances
        3.   Ask about past episodes and previous treatments

    B.   Physical Examination
        1.   Assess visual acuity
        2.   Inspect eyelids for inflammation, swelling, and discharge
        3.   Palpate eyelids for induration and masses
        4.   Evert the eyelid and examine inner surface for pointing
        5.   Examine sclera and conjunctiva for abnormalities
        6.   Palpate for preauricular adenopathy

    C.   Differential Diagnosis: The main differential diagnosis is chalazia; chalazia point on the conjunctival side of the eyelid and do not usually affect the margin of the eyelid

    D.   Diagnostic Tests: None indicated

V.   Plan/Management

    A.   Apply warm, moist compresses for 15 minutes throughout the day

    B.   Prescribe erythromycin, 5 mg/g (Ilotycin) ophthalmic ointment BID x 7 days OR polymyxin B-trimethoprim drops (Polytrim) BID x 7 days

    C.   Cleanse eyelids daily with a neutral soap (e.g., Ivory or Neutrogena)

    D.   If not responsive to medical therapy, refer to expert for incision and drainage

    E.   If crops of styes occur, diabetes mellitus must be excluded and patient should be told not to rub eyes; some authorities recommend a course of tetracycline to stop recurrences

F. Patient Education
    1. Advise patient that good periorbital hygiene will help prevent recurrence
    2. Advise against wearing eye makeup until clear and disposing of all old make up as it may be contaminated.

G. Follow Up: None indicated

UVEITIS

I. Definition

    A. A general term, referring to inflammation of the uveal tract

    B. Uveitis is often divided into the following:
        1. Anterior uveitis or iritis
        2. Intermediate uveitis or cyclitis (inflammation of the ciliary body)
        3. Posterior uveitis or choroiditis or retinitis

II. Pathogenesis

    A. Etiology of anterior uveitis
        1. Juvenile rheumatoid arthritis (most common)
        2. Fuch's heterochromic iridocyclitis
        3. Sarcoid
        4. Syphilis
        5. Ankylosing spondylitis
        6. Tuberculosis
        7. Trauma
        8. Herpes Simplex
        9. Kawasaki disease

    B. Etiology of intermediate uveitis is unknown

    C. Etiology of posterior uveitis
        1. Toxoplasmosis (most common)
        2. Cytomegalovirus
        3. Tuberculosis
        4. AIDS

III. Clinical Presentation

    A. In clinical practice, anterior, intermediate and posterior uveitis overlap in their clinical presentation

    B. Uveitis occurs most frequently in adults with those in the 20-50 year age group affected most often; there is a marked decrease in incidence in persons over age 70

    C. Males are affected twice as often as females (for most, but not all forms of uveitis)

    D. Signs and symptoms of uveitis may be unilateral or bilateral, with isolated or repeated episodes

    E. Patients may be asymptomatic or present with acute onset of deep aching pain, photophobia, and blurred vision

    F. Particularly if the patient has posterior uveitis, there may be a complaint of vision with numerous floaters

G.   Pupil constriction is common and the pupil may be irregular in shape

H.   Ciliary flush or injection of the bulbar conjunctiva around the limbus is often present

I.   The vitreous may be cloudy and retinal patches (yellow-white) may be noted on funduscopy

J.   Complications of uveitis include band keratopathy, glaucoma, and cataracts

K.   If patients are seen early in the course of their condition and treated, prevention of permanent eye damage is possible

IV.   Diagnosis/Evaluation

A.   History
1.   Determine onset, duration, and course of symptoms
2.   Ask about accompanying symptoms such as tearing, photophobia, decreased visual acuity
3.   Ask about previous eye problems and treatments
4.   Obtain past medical history; particularly the following:
   a.   Sarcoid, tuberculosis, rheumatoid arthritis, ankylosing spondylitis
   b.   Histoplasmosis, toxoplasmosis, syphilis
   c.   Intestinal disease (Whipple's disease, ulcerative colitis), regional enteritis
   d.   Multiple sclerosis, collagen vascular disease
   e.   Immunosuppressive disease (endogenous opportunistic infection)
   f.   Urethritis (rule out retinal vasculitis)
5.   Obtain a sexual history
6.   Inquire about exposure to cats
7.   Because uveitis is associated with many different systemic diseases, it often is necessary to do a complete review of systems

B.   Physical Examination
1.   Observe sclera for circumcorneal flush; observe pupil for size and shape
2.   Check pupillary response to light
3.   Perform funduscopy to ascertain clarity of lens and vitreous; inspect for abnormalities of the retina
4.   Determine visual acuity
5.   Examine for cross photophobia, cover the affected eye and dilate the unaffected eye with a bright light; if pain occurs in the covered eye in response, this is considered abnormally positive
6.   May need to perform complete physical exam if systemic disease is present

C.   Differential Diagnosis (see differential diagnosis under the section CONJUNCTIVITIS for further discussion of "red eye")
1.   Conjunctivitis
2.   Acute angle glaucoma
3.   Cataract
4.   Foreign body

D.   Diagnostic Tests: Numerous diagnostic tests are available and should be performed based on suspected etiology

V.   Plan/Management

A.   Treatment: The damage and secondary complications are severe and may develop rapidly; therefore, in any suspected case of uveitis, an ophthalmology referral is indicated immediately

B.   Follow up by ophthalmologist

VISUAL IMPAIRMENT IN ADULTS

I.   Definition: A decline in vision in one or both eyes

II.   Pathogenesis

   A.   Etiology of impaired vision can be divided into two general categories
      1.   Refractive errors or those problems that can be improved by glasses (common causes: myopia, hyperopia, presbyopia, anisometropia, and astigmatism)
      2.   Non-refractive errors (retinal abnormalities, glaucoma, cataract, retinoblastoma, eye muscle imbalance, and systemic disease with ocular manifestations) that cannot be corrected by glasses alone

   B.   For clear vision, light must focus precisely on the retina
      1.   In nearsightedness, or myopia, light is focused in front of the retina and the person sees near objects best
      2.   In farsightedness, or hyperopia, light is focused behind the retina and the person sees far objects best

   C.   Myopia is a condition in which objects can be seen clearly if held close enough to the eye (the person is "nearsighted"); person typically has no problem with reading or close work

   D.   Hyperopia is called farsightedness, and means that the individual cannot see near objects

   E.   Presbyopia develops as part of the aging process; the lens becomes less resilient, does not thicken as readily, and poor near vision (presbyopia) occurs
      1.   In an attempt to compensate for this decrease in vision, the person holds reading material farther away to aid in accommodation
      2.   Eventually, reading glasses become necessary

   F.   Anisometropia is a state in which there is a difference in the refractive error of the two eyes; condition may be congenital or acquired (due to asymmetric age changes or disease)

   G.   Astigmatism is a condition in which curvature variations of the optical system result in unequal light refraction and impaired vision

   H.   Pathophysiology of conditions causing non-refractive errors is dependent on the condition

III. Clinical Presentation

   A.   Refractive errors remain the most common cause of decreased visual acuity in adults

   B.   Adults with refractive errors most often complain about difficulty with near vision (hyperopia)
      1.   They may also complain of headache, fatigue, and blurred vision when doing tasks requiring extended use of eyes for near vision
      2.   Onset is usually slow with a gradual decline in ability to see near objects well
      3.   Almost 100% of adults require glasses by age 60 in order to see well for both far and near circumstances

   C.   Presbyopia usually begins in middle-age (45-55); symptoms of presbyopia include the following
      1.   Longer reading distance required (objects less than 20 cm away cannot be brought into focus)
      2.   Inability to focus on close work and excessive illumination required
      3.   Greater difficulty with close work occurs as day progresses

   D.   Astigmatism can begin in either childhood or adulthood and can be easily corrected if it causes blurred vision or eye discomfort

E. Adults with non-refractive errors have impaired vision at both near and far distances
   1. Patients with open-angle glaucoma are usually asymptomatic until neural damage has occurred; visual dysfunction in glaucoma is first expressed in the mid-peripheral field of vision (central vision functions such as acuity remain relatively intact until late in the disease process)
   2. Patients with cataract complain of poor visual acuity and problems with glare; children with cataract may be observed to have nystagmus of the wandering or searching type (nystagmus of the blind)
   3. Patients with retinal detachment may complain of lightning flashes and abrupt vision loss
   4. Patients with uveitis may complain of pain of the globe and photophobia
   5. Patients with age-related macular degeneration may complain of gradual loss of vision

F. Visual acuity correctable by glasses or contact lenses to 20/200 or worse in both eyes, or visual fields <10° centrally, constitutes legal blindness in the US

IV. Diagnosis/Evaluation

A. History
   1. Determine if vision in one or both eyes is impaired and if both near and far vision are affected
   2. Ask if there are associated symptoms of eye discomfort, increased tearing, cloudy vision, or flashing lights
   3. Ask about chronic or past eye problems, previous treatments and response
   4. Ask if there is a family history of eye disease

B. Physical Examination
   1. Examine external eye for swelling, ptosis, injection of the conjunctiva, and corneal clarity
   2. Determine extraocular movement
   3. Measure peripheral vision by direct confrontation (recognizing that this is only a very gross assessment of visual fields)
   4. Elicit red reflex and perform fundoscopic exam
   5. Determine visual acuity

KEY POINTS TO KEEP IN MIND IN THE ASSESSMENT OF VISUAL ACUITY IN ADULTS

General Principles for Testing
❖ It is essential to test each eye independently, with the other eye occluded
❖ Use of a hand held occluder is usually satisfactory
❖ Subjects who wear corrective glasses should be tested with and without glasses

❖ Measure far vision using Snellen chart (read at 20 feet away) and near vision using hand-held Rosenbaum Pocket Vision Screening Card [Use the Tumbling E chart for adults who cannot read--patient identifies the direction that E is open by pointing in that direction]

❖ Pinhole vision is tested if the patient is unable to read the 20/30 line
❖ Place a pinhole aperture in front of the eye to ascertain any improvement in acuity (the pinhole will correct for any uncorrected refractive error due to nearsightedness, farsightedness, and astigmatism)
❖ Through the pinhole, a patient with refractive error should read close to 20/20
❖ If the pinhole fails to improve the patient's visual acuity, another cause for reduced vision such as opacities in the ocular media, or macular or optic nerve disease should be suspected

---

C. Differential Diagnosis
   1. Refractive errors
   2. Non-refractive errors (common causes: glaucoma, cataract, retinal detachment, uveitis, macular degeneration, strabismus, and amblyopia)

D. Diagnostic Tests: None indicated

V.   Plan/Management

A.   Indicators requiring further evaluation are outlined in the table below

PATIENTS REQUIRING FURTHER EVALUATION
• Visual acuity of 20/30 or worse
• More than a **one-line** difference between eyes

B.   If the cause of the impaired vision is not believed to be a refractive error, refer to ophthalmologist for further evaluation

C.   Patients with acute onset of impaired vision need immediate referral for emergency care

D.   Patients requiring visual acuity determination for purposes of legal blindness or disability determination or for any medicolegal cases should be referred to an ophthalmologist

E.   Follow Up: By ophthalmologist or optometrist

REFERENCES

American Academy of Pediatrics, Committee on Practice and Ambulatory Medicine. (1996). Eye examination and vision screening in infants, children, and young adults. Pediatrics, 98(1), 153-1577.

Bedrossian, E.H. (1997, March). Treatment of hordeolums: Styes and chalazia. Hospital Medicine, 59-64.

Carter, S.R. (1998). Eyelid disorders: Diagnosis and management. American Family Physician, 57, 2695-2702.

Cataract Management Guideline Panel. (1993). Cataract in adults: Management of functional impairment. Clinical Practice Guideline, Number 4. Rockville, MD: US Department of Health & Human Services, Public Health Service. Agency for Health Care Policy and Research (AHCPR) (Publication No. 93-0542).

Centers for Disease Control and Prevention. (1998). 1998 Sexually transmitted diseases treatment guidelines. MMWR, 47, (No. RR-1).

Danyluk, A.W., & Paton, D. (1991). Diagnosis and management of glaucoma. Clinical Symposia, 43(4), 2-29.

Faye, E.F. (1998). Living with low vision. Postgraduate Medicine, 103(5), 167-178.

Garcia, G.E., & Pavan-Langston, D. (1996). Refractive errors and clinical optics. In D. Pavan-Langston (Ed.), Manual of ocular diagnosis and therapy. Boston: Little-Brown.

Grove, A.S. (1996). Eyelids and lacrimal system. In D. Pavan-Langston (Ed.), Manual of ocular diagnosis and therapy. Boston: Little-Brown.

Klein, T.B., & Koller, W.C. (1998). Glaucoma. In R.E. Rakel (Ed.), Conn's current therapy. Philadelphia: Saunders.

Morrow, G.L., & Abbott, R.L. (1998). Conjunctivitis. American Family Physician, 57, 735-745.

Neher, J.O. (1997). Eye problems of aging: Cataracts, glaucoma, and macular degeneration. In R.B. Taylor, D. Haxby, & C. Blem (Eds.), Manual of family practice. Boston: Little, Brown.

Pavan-Langston, D. (1996). Ocular examination: Techniques and diagnostic tests. In D. Pavan-Langston (Ed.), Manual of ocular diagnosis and therapy. Boston: Little-Brown.

Podolsky, M.M. (1998). Exposing glaucoma. Postgraduate Medicine, 103(5), 131-151.

Quigley, H.A. (1993). Open-angle glaucoma. The New England Journal of Medicine, 328(15), 1097-1104.

Ragge, N.K. & Easty, D.L. (1990). Immediate Eye care. St. Louis: Mosby.

Schachat, A.P. (1995). The red eye. In L.R. Barker, J.R. Burton, & P.D. Zieve (Eds.), Principles of ambulatory medicine. Baltimore: Williams & Wilkins.

Schachat, A.P. (1995). Common problems associated with impaired vision: Cataracts and age-related macular degeneration. In L.R. Barker, J.R. Burton, & P.D. Zieve (Eds.), Principles of ambulatory medicine. Baltimore: Williams & Wilkins.

Schachat, A.P. (1995). Glaucoma. In L.R. Barker, J.R. Burton, & P.D. Zieve (Eds.), Principles of ambulatory medicine. Baltimore: Williams & Wilkins.

Sutherland, J.E., & Mauer, R.C. (1997). Conjunctivitis and other causes or red eye. In R.B. Taylor, D. Haxby, & C. Blem (Eds.), Manual of family practice. Boston: Little, Brown.

Trudo, E.W., & Stark, W.J. (1998). Cataracts. Postgraduate Medicine, 103(5), 114-126.

US Department of Health and Human Services, Office of Disease Prevention and Health Promotion. (1994). Put prevention into practice. Washington, DC: Author.

Varma, R. (1997). Essentials of eye care. Philadelphia: Lippincott-Raven.

Weber, C.M., & Eichenbaum, J.W. (1997). Acute red eye. Postgraduate Medicine, 101(5), 185-196.

Zwaan, J. (1993). Styes and chalazia. In R.A. Dershewitz (Ed.), Ambulatory pediatric care. Philadelphia: Lippincott.

CHAPTER 9

Problems of the Ears, Nose, Sinuses, Throat, Mouth and Neck

HEARING LOSS

I.   Definitions: Reduction in a person's ability to perceive sound

    A.   Hearing loss is measured according to hearing thresholds (the softest tone heard by patient at a given frequency) during pure tone audiometric testing
1. Normal hearing: 0 to 25 decibels (dB)
2. Mild impairment: 26 to 40 dB
3. Moderate impairment: 41 to 55 dB
4. Moderately severe: 56 to 70 dB
5. Severe: 71 to 90 dB
6. Profound: 91 dB and above

    B.   Conductive hearing loss occurs when sound is inadequately conducted through the external or middle ear to the sensorineural apparatus of the inner ear

    C.   Sensorineural hearing loss occurs when sound is normally carried through the external and middle ear but there is a defect within the inner ear which results in sound distortion

II. Pathogenesis

    A.   Common causes of conductive hearing loss
1. Impacted cerumen
2. Foreign bodies
3. Otitis externa
4. Benign tumors of middle ear
5. Carcinoma of external auditory canal and/or middle ear
6. Eustachian tube dysfunction
7. Otitis media
8. Serous otitis media with effusion
9. Cholesteatoma
10. Otosclerosis
11. Tuberculosis of the temporal bone

    B.   Common causes of sensorineural hearing loss
1. Congenital and neonatal hearing loss may be hereditary (albinism, Alport's syndrome, User's syndrome, or Waardenburg's syndrome) or caused by maternal rubella, prematurity, traumatic delivery, or other infections during the perinatal period
2. Presbycusis which occurs because of atrophy of the basal end of the organ of Corti, a loss in number of auditory receptors, vascular changes, and stiffening of the basilar membranes
3. Noise exposure
4. Meniere's disease (see VERTIGO section)
5. Acoustic tumors (see VERTIGO section)
6. Trauma
7. Other diseases
    a. Syphilis
    b. Paget disease
    c. Collagen diseases
    d. Endocrine disease such as diabetes mellitus or hypothyroidism
    e. Bacterial meningitis
    f. Tuberculosis of the temporal bone
    g. Basilar migraines
    h. Viral illnesses such as mumps, cytomegalovirus, and herpes zoster
    i. Demyelinating processes such as multiple sclerosis

8. Drug ototoxicities
   a. Antibiotics such as streptomycin, neomycin, gentamicin, and vancomycin
   b. Diuretics such as ethacrynic acid and furosemide
   c. Salicylates
   d. Antineoplastic agents such as cisplatin

III. Clinical presentation of common causes of hearing loss

   A. About 4% of persons under 45 years and 29% of those over 65 years have handicapping hearing loss

   B. In conductive hearing loss (most common), sensitivity to sound is diminished, but clarity is unchanged; if volume is increased to compensate for loss, the hearing is normal
      1. Serous otitis media
         a. Most frequent cause of hearing loss in children and an important factor of hearing loss in adults
         b. Patient usually has fullness and decreased hearing in one or both ears
      2. Otosclerosis is associated with slow, progressive hearing loss (usually bilateral) beginning in second or third decade of life
         a. Most common cause of progressive conductive hearing loss in young adults
         b. Hereditary condition of unknown etiology in which there is an irregular ossification in the bony labyrinth of the inner ear, particularly of the stapes
         c. Patients have tinnitus and hearing loss which may progress to deafness
         d. On physical examination, the tympanic membrane (TM) is normal

   C. Sensorineural hearing loss is most commonly seen in elderly persons who have sound distortion
      1. Presbycusis is a slowly progressive problem in persons over age 65 years
         a. Frequently, patients are unaware of their hearing problems
         b. Results in a decrease in speech discrimination (cannot understand speech even when spoken loudly)
         c. Patients often have tinnitus and hypersensitivity to noise
      2. Noise-induced hearing loss
         a. Early in condition there is isolated pure tone loss at 4000 Hertz (Hz) unilaterally or bilaterally
         b. Pure tone loss progresses to other frequencies with increased exposure
      3. Acoustic neuroma presents with tinnitus and unilateral, unexplained hearing loss
      4. Meniere's disease is characterized by episodic vertigo, fluctuating sensorineural hearing loss, and roaring tinnitus (see VERTIGO section)

   D. Hearing loss may be erroneously diagnosed as dementia or behavioral problems in the elderly

IV. Diagnosis/Evaluation

   A. History
      1. Question about nature of onset of hearing loss (unilateral, bilateral, progressive, acute versus chronic, fluctuating)
      2. Inquire about associated symptoms such as fever, ear pain, discharge from ear, vertigo, tinnitus, and neurologic disturbances
      3. Explore predisposing factors such as exposure to noise, trauma, barotrauma (air plane travel or diving), antecedent viral infection, and medication use
      4. Obtain a thorough past medical history
      5. Ask about family history of hearing loss and neoplastic diseases
      6. Question patient about the impact of the hearing loss on activities of daily living

B. Physical Examination
1. Perform visual examination of TM and external auditory canal
2. Perform pneumatic otoscopy to determine mobility of TM
3. Perform clinical hearing test: whispered voice should be done with the patient using a finger to occlude the opposite ear to prevent crossover
4. Perform Weber and Rinne tests (see table that follows)

TUNING FORK TESTS		
	Weber Test	Rinne Test
Procedure	Strike fork and hold in middle of forehead or apex of skull and ask patient to localize sound	Strike fork, then place firmly on mastoid tip [(measure of bone conduction (BC)], and ask patient to raise hand when sound is no longer present; then move fork so that it resonates beside ear [measure of air conduction (AC)]
Conductive Loss	Sound louder in ear in which patient perceives the hearing loss	In affected ear, sound is louder when on mastoid tip than beside ear (BC>AC)
Sensorineural Loss	Sound louder in unaffected ear	In normal ear or ear with sensorineural hearing loss, the sound is louder beside the ear than on the mastoid tip (AC>BC)

5. Complete head, neck and cranial nerve examination are often indicated; craniofacial and ophthalmic abnormalities are often present in persons with congenital or hereditary hearing loss disorders

C. Differential Diagnosis: See common causes of hearing loss under pathogenesis; important to determine the following:
1. Is hearing loss acute versus chronic? (acute hearing loss almost always requires immediate intervention such as removal or cerumen or treatment with antibiotics with otitis media)
2. Is hearing loss conductive versus sensorineural?

D. Diagnostic Tests
1. Puretone audiometry characterizes the extent of impairment; air-conduction and bone-conduction measurements are made for sounds of varying intensity (decibels) and frequency (Hertz or cps): Indicated for all cases of chronic hearing loss and in cases of acute hearing loss when the etiology is uncertain
    a. Presbycusis: higher frequency loss at 8000 than at 4000 cycles (smooth, ski slope curve)
    b. Noise-induced hearing loss: high frequency loss, greatest at 4000 cycles and improvement at 8000 cycles
    c. Conductive hearing loss: Low frequency hearing loss (125-500 cycles)
2. Vestibular testing should be considered if there are tinnitus and vertigo: electronystagmometry, rotational tests, and posturography are useful adjuncts
3. Computerized tomography should be considered if tumors and bony lesions are suspected
4. Magnetic resonance imaging should be considered if acoustic neuromas are diagnostic possibilities
5. Fluorescent treponemal-antibody-absorption test should be ordered if there is a possibility of late latent syphilis
6. Tympanometry should be considered to assess TM stiffness
7. Impedance audiometry evaluates middle ear function by testing tympanic membrane compliance and acoustic reflex thresholds

V. Plan/Management

A. Referral to otolaryngologist is needed for patients with acute hearing loss who do not have an apparent diagnosis or for patients with apparent treatable acute or chronic causes for hearing loss who do not improve with appropriate treatments

B. Referral to audiologist is needed for patients with chronic deficits who may benefit from a hearing device

C. Most patients with otosclerosis and congenital or acquired causes of conductive hearing loss can be helped by surgical procedures

D. Aural rehabilitation is often beneficial for patients with sensorineural hearing loss
   1. Hearing aids are the mainstay of therapy
   2. Inexpensive auditory amplifiers are available and include telephone receiver amplifiers and radio and television earphones
   3. Cochlear implants stimulate the eighth cranial nerve directly and can provide sound awareness for patients with severe hearing loss
   4. Lip reading and sign language may be helpful

E. Patient Education
   1. Discuss ways to enhance communication with the patient's family such as facing patient, obtaining their attention before speaking, speaking slowly, using gestures, and only speaking louder or moving closer if the patient states that it is helpful; in the older patient there is often some difficulty in discriminating consonants (take time to carefully enunciate all words to patient)
   2. Because many patients are embarrassed about wearing a hearing aid, emphasize that today's hearing aids are small and less noticeable; inform patient that due to advanced technology, today's hearing aids are more efficient
   3. Discuss prices of hearing aids: older analog models range from $500 to $2000 whereas digital hearing aids with better sound quality may cost $3000; medicare does not cover cost
   4. Discuss prevention of hearing loss
      a. Ear plugs or ear muffs with tight seal may reduce noise by 10-30 dB
      b. People vary in their susceptibility to noise-induced trauma, but typically if sound causes pain, tinnitus, or temporary blocking of ear, extended exposure to this noise will cause permanent hearing loss
      c. Limit exposure to loud noise; prolonged or repeated exposure to any noise above 85 dB can cause hearing loss; most lawn mowers, motorcycles, chainsaws, and powerboats produce noise > 85 dB; personal stereos, rock concerts, and firecrackers may produce noise at 140 dB or more

F. Follow up is dependent on the type and cause of the hearing loss

IMPACTED CERUMEN

I. Definition: Obstruction of the ear canal by cerumen (earwax)

II. Pathogenesis

   A. Cerumen is produced by the ceruminous glands in the outer portion of the canal and is a naturally occurring lubricant and protectant of the external ear canal

   B. While cerumen is normally cleared from the ears through the body's natural mechanisms, excessive accumulation may occur and partially or totally occlude the canal

III. Clinical Presentation

   A. Commonly occurs in the elderly and industrial workers

   B. Ear pain may be present if cerumen hardens and touches the tympanic membrane, or if the external canal is irritated by build up of hardened cerumen

C.   Symptoms may include pain, itching, and sensation of fullness on the affected side; conductive hearing loss may also be present with total occlusion of the canal

D.   Removal of cerumen may be necessary in the following situations
1.   Accumulation is causing the patient to have a problem with decreased hearing, tinnitus, feeling of fullness, vertigo, or ear discomfort
2.   Accumulation is causing the patient no problem, but is obstructing the examiner's view of the tympanic membrane

IV.   Diagnosis/Evaluation

A.   History
1.   Ask about onset, and if ear discomfort or a feeling of fullness is present
2.   Ask how ears are usually cleaned (Are cotton-tipped swabs used?)
3.   Ask if wax removal has been required in the past
4.   Determine if patient has history of previous ear surgery with resultant scarring and increased risk of perforation (cerumen removal procedure is **contraindicated** if patient responds positively)

B.   Physical Examination
1.   Examine both ear canals
2.   Attempt to visualize the tympanic membranes around the wax to ascertain intactness
3.   Test hearing to determine if the affected ear is the only hearing ear (if so, referral to a specialist is indicated)

C.   Differential Diagnosis
1.   Foreign body
2.   Otitis media
3.   Otitis externa

D.   Diagnostic Tests: None indicated

V.   Plan/Management

A.   Removal of cerumen using either the curette or irrigation technique is usually successful and both techniques are described in tables that follow

B.   The irrigation technique takes longer than the curette technique and is usually implemented when the curette technique fails or is poorly tolerated by patient; irrigation technique rarely fails

C.   Cerumen solvents that are commercially available are not recommended because they frequently make the condition worse

D.   To prevent recurrences, direct patient to apply 1 or 2 drops of baby oil in each ear once or twice weekly to help soften wax; patient may also use a squeeze bulb syringe filled with lukewarm water to gently irrigate canals every month or so (best to do about 10 minutes after oil has been instilled into canals)

E.   Follow Up: None indicated unless cerumen removal fails

REMOVAL USING CURETTE TECHNIQUE	
Equipment needed/types of curette	Metal and plastic Metal curettes are either rigid or flexible Plastic are the flex-loop ear curette
Positioning patient	Seat comfortably on exam table and explain procedure and the importance of remaining still
Visualize cerumen	Using otoscope, look into the canal using posterior traction on helix
Select the appropriate curette	Gently remove the impacted cerumen, working through the otoscope or by direct vision (after having identified where the impaction is and keeping in mind the anatomy of the external auditory canal)
If hard wax is encountered	Stop the procedure and instill a few drops of mineral oil into the canal to soften for 10 minutes and then resume removal
If wax appears to be adherent to the tympanic membrane itself	Removal must be via gentle irrigation (see technique in the table that follows)
Immobilization	Absolutely necessary to avoid risk of perforation and trauma to the ear canal!
If removal is via direct vision	Use the otoscope to assess progress during procedure

REMOVAL USING IRRIGATION TECHNIQUE	
Equipment needed	Use a soft-tipped syringe such as a 22-gauge butterfly intravenous catheter tubing with needle and butterfly removed and a 20 to 50 cc syringe, or A bulb syringe, or A water jet device such as Water-Pik
Irrigate with lukewarm water	**Caution**: Use of cold or hot water may lead to dizziness and nausea! Squirt water on your wrist to verify that temperature is correct
Positioning patient	Place in supine postion, or seat comfortably on exam table Cover the patient's shoulder with towel Instruct the patient to tilt head toward side being irrigated and place a small kidney-shaped basin under the ear to catch water (patient can hold basin)
Visualize cerumen	Use otoscope to determine location
Place the tip of the tubing or syringe just inside the canal	Infuse the water with a moderately strong and steady force If the water jet irrigator is used, set at **lowest** setting to reduce risk of perforation
Direct the jet of water superiorly toward the occiput	Allow for space in the canal for the return of water and cerumen **Do not** direct the stream of water onto the tympanic membrane Try to direct the stream of water past the plug of cerumen so as to create outward pressure on it
Evaluate the effluent	Sometimes an intact plug of cerumen is expelled and at other times the effluent will be tinted yellow but no obvious plug will be seen
Reassess progress using the otoscope	It will be necessary to dry the external canal with gauze for good visualization
If pain or bleeding occur	STOP!
If the irrigation is not successful after a few minutes	Terminate the procedure
Instruct the patient to	Instill 1-2 drops of baby oil in the affected ear twice a week to soften wax, or Use 3 drops of hydrogen peroxide and water solution (1:1 solution) in affected ear 2-3 times a week
Ask the patient to return	In one week for evaluation and removal of cerumen

263

OTITIS EXTERNA

I. Definition: Inflammation of the external auditory canal

II. Pathogenesis

    A. Predisposing factors
        1. Frequent exposure to moisture (e.g., swimming; humid, warm climates), aggressive cleaning of the canal, or trauma
        2. Allergies or skin conditions such as psoriasis or seborrhea

    B. Pathogens
        1. Bacteria: *Pseudomonas* species, staphylococci coliform, *Proteus* species and anaerobes
        2. Fungi (account for 9% of cases): *Candida* and *Aspergillus*

III. Clinical Presentation

    A. Ear pain (occurs approximately 85% of cases) may begin gradually or suddenly; increases when pressure is placed on the tragus or when the pinna is moved; pain may increase with movement of jaw

    B. Sensation of fullness or obstruction of the ear occurs early in the process

    C. Itching may occur and it may be the predominant symptom with fungal infections

    D. Purulent discharge and conductive hearing loss may occur

    E. Systemic symptomatology such as fever or chills is uncommon

    F. An uncommon, serious complication is malignant or necrotizing external otitis which can lead to cranial neuropathies and infection of the temporal bone
        1. Characterized by deep-seated nocturnal pain and granulation tissue at the bony-cartilaginous junction
        2. Foul-smelling, purulent drainage and facial nerve paralysis and cranial neuropathies may be present
        3. Most common in elderly male diabetics and immunocompromised persons

IV. Diagnosis/Evaluation

    A. History
        1. Ask about the location of pain/discomfort and time of onset
        2. Ask about the occurrence of itching, and bleeding/purulent exudate
        3. Question about hearing loss
        4. Ask about frequency of swimming
        5. Obtain history of recent ear trauma; ask type of ear cleaning method
        6. Ask if there is a history of previous episodes and risk factors such as diabetes and immunosuppression

    B. Physical Examination
        1. Determine if febrile
        2. Assuming the ear is extremely tender, carefully examine the external canal with the otoscope; the following are signs of otitis externa:
            a. Erythema and edema of the canal
            b. Weeping secretions, purulent otorrhea, and exudate or crusting of the skin
        3. Apply pressure to the tragus and move the pinna, noting degree of tenderness

       4.   If possible, observe the tympanic membrane which is usually normal; edema may impede observation

       5.   Palpate the infra-auricular cervical lymph nodes for signs of lymphadenitis

  C.   Differential Diagnosis
       1.   Cyst, furuncle or abscess
       2.   Carcinoma
       3.   Herpes zoster oticus (characterized by tiny vesicles which may be difficult to visualize; pain usually precedes eruption of vesicles)
       4.   Otitis media
       5.   Mastoiditis
       6.   Foreign body

  D.   Diagnostic Tests: Culture should be performed if resistance to initial management occurs

V.   Plan/Management: Objectives are to decrease edema and pain and restore the acidic pH, flora, cerumen and canal epithelium to normal

  A.   Referral is recommended whenever malignant otitis externa cannot be ruled-out or for severe, recalcitrant infections and recurrent otitis externa

  B.   Before treatment, remove all exudative and epidermal debris
       1.   Best approach is to use a Frazier suction tip (5F or 7F) or a cotton-tipped metal applicator
       2.   Otherwise, use gentle irrigation with isotonic saline; irrigation of the canal should be done cautiously until perforation is ruled out

  C.   If swelling prevents the passage of topical medications, insert cotton wick
       1.   Insert by gently twisting the wick into the canal
       2.   Patient should place drops on wick for first two days, then remove wick and place drops directly in canal

  D.   Ear drops containing combinations of antibiotics, hydrocortisone, and propylene glycol are effective in treating bacterial infections: Use polymyxin B sulfate, neomycin, hydrocortisone (Cortisporin Otic suspension): Dose: 4 drops in canal, QID x 7 days

  E.   If cortisporin suspension causes localized reaction due to neomycin, switch to tobramycin, dexamethasone (TobraDex) 4 gtts. TID or QID x 7 days; Ciprofloxacin hydrochloride and hydrocortisone otic suspension (Cipro HC Otic) and ofloxacin otic solution 0.3% (Fioxin Otic), both 3 drops BID for 7 days are other effective topical agents

  F.   For fungal infections prescribe one of the following for 7 days:
       1.   Acetic acid, aluminum acetate solution (Otic Domeboro) 5 drops QID
       2.   Propylene glycol solution of acetic acid (Vosol) 5 drops QID
       3.   Clotrimazole (Lotrimin) solution 3 gtts. BID for 5-7 days

  G.   Severe cases require systemic antibiotics
       1.   Prescribe Ciprofloxacin (Cipro) 500 mg BID
       2.   Consider consultation with ENT specialist

  H.   Advise patient to keep moisture out of ear for 4-6 weeks. May bathe or shower but plug ear with cotton impregnated with petroleum jelly. Swimming is not permitted

  I.   Teach patients to prevent recurrence
       1.   Discuss importance of keeping ear canals as dry as possible and not inserting any objects into ears to clean them
       2.   Advise to instill 2-3 drops of 1:1:1 solution of vinegar/isopropyl alcohol/water after each contact with water
       3.   Use ear plugs while swimming, showering or shampooing

4. Remind of importance of avoiding strong jets of water from shower heads or dental water jet systems
5. Instruct in proper way to clean ears (see section on IMPACTED CERUMEN)

J. Follow Up
1. If properly treated, otitis externa should resolve in 7 days; mild cases do not require follow-up
2. Moderate and severe case should return to office in 3 days and 24 hours, respectively

ACUTE OTITIS MEDIA

I. Definition: Presence of fluid in the middle ear in association with signs and symptoms of acute local or systemic illness; other terms synonymous with acute otitis media (OM) include suppurative otitis media, acute bacterial otitis media, and purulent otitis media

II. Pathogenesis

A. Single most important factor is eustachian tube dysfunction which prevents effective drainage of middle ear fluid
1. Typically, patient has an antecedent event such as an infection or allergy which results in edema and congestion of the mucosa of the nasopharynx, eustachian tube, and middle ear
2. The congestion of the eustachian tube impedes the flow of middle ear secretions
3. Negative pressure often increases which further pulls fluid into the middle ear
4. As middle ear secretions increase microbial pathogens grow resulting in otitis media; common pathogens are as follows:
   a. *Streptococcus pneumoniae*
   b. *Haemophilus influenzae*
   c. *Moraxella catarrhalis*
   d. Viruses
   e. Other bacteria such as *Streptococcus pyogenes* and *Staphylococcus aureus*
5. Recently, there has been an increase in infections due to beta-lactamase producing organisms *(M. catarrhalis* and *H. influenzae)* and drug-resistant *S. pneumoniae*

B. Recurrent episodes of otitis media may be related to anatomical or physiological eustachian tube abnormality

C. Predisposing factors to developing otitis media include the following:
1. Active or passive smoking
2. Caucasian or Native American race
3. Male gender
4. Congenital disorders such as cleft palate and trisomy 21
5. Family history of otitis media

III. Clinical Presentation

A. Commonly seen following a viral upper respiratory infection

B. Symptoms include the following:
1. Patients may be asymptomatic or have ear pain, otorrhea, hearing loss and/or vertigo
2. Fever is a common but not a universal symptom
3. Other less common symptoms include nausea, vomiting, and diarrhea

C. Complications include hearing loss, perforation of eardrum, cholesteatoma, acute mastoiditis, meningitis, and epidural abscess

D. Diagnosis is based on the appearance of the tympanic membrane (TM), the following are characteristic:
1. Full or bulging TM
2. Absent or obscured bony landmarks
3. Distorted light reflex
4. Decreased of absent mobility of TM by pneumatic otoscopy
5. Erythema of TM is an inconsistent finding; TM may be red due to crying or vascular engorgement due to fever rather than infection
6. Bullae may form between layers of TM; often associated with *Mycoplasma pneumoniae*

IV. Diagnosis/Evaluation

A. History
1. Determine onset and duration of symptoms
2. Ask about ear pain, fever, irritability
3. Inquire about hearing loss, tinnitus and dizziness
4. Ask about drainage from ear
5. Inquire about associated symptoms such as nasal congestion, headache, sore throat, mouth pain, cough, hearing loss
6. Carefully document the number and if possible dates of previous occurrences; ask about successes and failures of previous treatments
7. Determine whether an upper respiratory infection preceded the fever or ear pain
8. Inquire about history of allergies and other risk factors such as active or passive smoking and congenital disorders such as cleft palate

B. Physical Examination
1. Measure vital signs
2. Inspect conjunctivae, pharynx, and nasal mucosa
3. Palpate sinuses
4. Palpate for auricular and cervical adenopathy
5. Examine auricle and external auditory canal
6. Carefully examine tympanic membranes bilaterally for position, color, degree of translucency and mobility (may require removal of cerumen)
   a. Position: Process of the malleus should be visible but not prominent through the membrane; retraction and bulging indicate effusion
   b. Color: Normal TM is gray; an amber color often indicates an effusion; erythema may indicate infection but also may be due to crying, severe coughing, or vascular engorgement
   c. Translucency: Middle ear landmarks should be visible through the TM; air fluid level, bubbles, and inability to visualize middle ear landmarks suggest effusion
   d. Mobility: Normal ear will move with pneumatic otoscopy; **to be diagnosed with acute otitis media there must be presence of fluid in middle ear; this can only be detected with pneumatic otoscopy**
7. Perform a lung examination
8. When a healthy adult has ear pain and the examination of the ear is completely normal, a more thorough evaluation of the head and neck is essential
   a. Examine mouth and teeth for dental disorders
   b. Assess functioning of temporomandibular joint
   c. Assess nose and pharynx for nasopharyngeal carcinoma
   d. Assess cranial nerves to detect neurological problems which could be associated with intracranial neoplasms

C. Differential Diagnosis [Health care providers can generally detect OM 90% of time when it is present, but over diagnosis frequently occurs (as high as 40%)]
1. External otitis media
2. Transient middle ear effusion may result with flying or traveling in high altitudes (barotrauma)
3. Mastoiditis
4. Furuncle

<ol start="5">
<li>Temporomandibular joint dysfunction</li>
<li>Mumps</li>
<li>Dental abscess</li>
<li>Tonsillitis</li>
<li>Foreign body</li>
<li>Trauma</li>
</ol>

D. Diagnostic Tests
1. Usually no diagnostic tests are ordered
2. Rarely, may perform tympanocentesis for culture and sensitivity of middle ear effusion in toxic patients, patients with complications such as mastoiditis, immuno-compromised patients, patients in whom treatment is unsatisfactory or who have recurrent infections
3. Tympanometry may be indicated in recurrent cases and when there is suspicion of fluid behind the TM without clinical signs
4. Acoustic reflectometry helps diagnose OM by analyzing sound pressure and reflected sound in the eardrum
5. Consider ordering sinus films in patients with recurrent otitis media or otitis media with effusion
6. Consider audiometry post treatment

V. Plan/Management

A. General management concepts (see following table)

GENERAL CONCEPTS OF MANAGEMENT	
1. Be cautious	Remember favorable natural history of OM (80% of cases resolve spontaneously)
2. Prescribe antibiotics sparingly	-Antibiotics improve resolution by only about 15% -Antibiotics increase risk of bacterial resistance

3. Modify risk factors	Improve odds of resolution:
	  -Avoid passive smoking
	  -Control food and inhalant allergies
	  -Treat sinusitis

4. Avoid unproven therapies	-Antihistamines/decongestants -Homeopathy and naturopathy -Folk remedies such as "sweet oil"

B. Some experts only recommend antibiotics for patients with pus drainage, recurrent infections, and history of serous otitis media or ear tubes; most experts, however, recommend antibiotics to reduce the development of delayed suppurative complications such as mastoiditis
1. Use first-line antibiotics for initial empiric treatment (see following table)

RECOMMENDED FIRST-LINE ANTIBIOTICS FOR MEDICAL MANAGEMENT		
Generic (Trade) Name *Duration of treatment*	Dosing	Comment
Amoxicillin (Amoxil) *10 day treatment**	250-500 mg tabs TID	-Inexpensive, few adverse effects -In 1998 still recommended as **drug of choice** for initial therapy -Disadvantage: Not effective against beta-lactamase producing organisms
Trimethoprim-sulfamethoxazole (Bactrim, Septra) *10 day treatment**	One DS tab BID	-Effective against beta-lactamase producing organisms -**Drug of choice** - pts. allergic to penicillin -Disadvantage:Less effective than amoxil against common pathogen, *S. pneumonia*

* Duration of treatment may be 5-7 days for persons who have mild, uncomplicated AOM, and no underlying medical condition and no history of chronic or recurrent otitis media

2. Use second-line antibiotics for following cases (see following table)
   a. Initial treatment failures
   b. Complicated infections
   c. Patients with ipsilateral conjunctivitis suggesting *H. Influenzae* infection

RECOMMENDED SECOND-LINE ANTIBIOTICS FOR MEDICAL MANAGEMENT

Generic (Trade) Name *Duration of treatment*	Dosing	Comment
Amoxicillin-clavulanate (Augmentin) *10 day treatment**	250-500 mg tabs TID or 875 mg tab BID	-Broad spectrum -15-20% patients have gastrointestinal upset
Azithromycin (Zithromax) *5 day treatment*	500 mg tab QD Day 1; 250 mg Days 2-5	-Broad spectrum
Cefprozil (Cefzil) *10 day treatment**	500 mg tab BID	-Broad spectrum
Cefpodoxime (Vantin) *10 day treatment**	200 mg tab BID	-Broad spectrum -Convenient dosing -Take tabs with food
Cefibuten (Cedax) *10 day treatment**	400 mg cap QD	-Broad spectrum -Convenient dosing -Take suspension on empty stomach; caps may be taken without regard for meals
Cefuroxime (Ceftin) *10 day treatment**	250-500 mg cap BID	-Broad spectrum -Bitter taste -Take with food
Clarithromycin (Biaxin) *10 day treatment**	250-500 mg cap BID	-Broad spectrum -Well tolerated
Loracarbef (Lorabid) *10 day treatment**	200-400 mg caps BID	-Broad spectrum -Must take on an empty stomach

* Duration of treatment may be 5-7 days for patients who have mild, uncomplicated AOM, and no underlying medical condition and no history of chronic or recurrent otitis media

3. Use third-line antibiotics for special cases; for example, infections with resistant *S. pneumoniae* or patients who have difficulty taking a course of oral medications

RECOMMENDED THIRD-LINE ANTIBIOTICS FOR MEDICAL MANAGEMENT

Generic (Trade) Name *Duration of treatment*	Dosing	Comment
Clindamycin (Cleocin) *10 day treatment*	150-300 mg caps QID	-Excellent choice for resistant S. pneumoniae -Take with full glass of water
Ceftriaxone (Rocephin) *1-5 day treatment*	50-75mg/kg/day IM injection - QD	-Useful for refractory cases -Inconsistent findings of efficacy of drug -Reserve as third-line drug and for cases with intra-cranial complications

C. Cases involving penicillin-resistant *S. pneumoniae* (suspect when patient has persistent AOM)
   1. Drug of choice: clindamycin (see previous table)
   2. Alternatives:
      a. High dose amoxicillin (60-80 mg/kg/day)
      b. Ceftriaxone IM (5 day treatment)

D. Management of pain
    1. Usually, an analgesic such as acetaminophen (adults 300-600 mg every 4 hours) is all that is needed; codeine may be prescribed
    2. Topical pain relievers such as Americaine Otic solution, 4 to 5 gtts q 1-2 hours or Auralgan Otic solution every 1-2 hours may be prescribed

E. Nasal and oral decongestants are usually not effective in preventing otitis media, but may provide symptomatic relief of associated symptoms which often accompany otitis media

F. Antihistamines are not recommended unless the predisposing factor for developing otitis media is an allergy; antihistamines may thicken the secretions and aggravate the problem

G. Treatment of persistent, recalcitrant, or subacute otitis media
    1. If no response in 2-3 days and patient is not toxic switch to a second-line antibiotic (see previous table); consider the possibility of infection with penicillin-resistant *S. pneumoniae* (see V.C. for treatment)
    2. Consider consultation with specialist if 2-3 courses of recommended treatments fail

H. Treatment of recurrent infections is controversial; recurrent infections are those in which the middle ear effusion clears between episodes.
    1. Always try preventive measures such as limiting passive smoking, administering vaccines, etc. before prescribing prophylactic antibiotics (see table - General Concepts)
    2. Consult an otolaryngologist for a healthy adult who has recurrent infections because of the remote possibility of nasopharyngeal cancer

I. Treatment of tympanic membrane perforation involves prescription of oral antibiotic supplemented with topical antibiotic such as a combination of neomycin sulfate, polymyxin-ß and hydrocortisone (Cortisporin otic suspension) 4 drops in each ear, 3-4 times a day for maximum of 10 days

J. Consult specialist and consider surgery for following:
    1. Hearing loss bilaterally of 20 dB or more
    2. Chronic or persistent infection with evidence of mastoid involvement
    3. Cholesteatoma formation or chronic perforation
    4. Recurrent infections in healthy adults

K. Follow Up
    1. Return to clinic in 2-3 days if condition is not significantly improved.
    2. Typically, return visits are scheduled several days after completion of drug therapy or recheck in 2-3 weeks from initial visit
    3. For patients treated with prophylactic antibiotics, evaluate every 4 weeks

OTITIS MEDIA WITH EFFUSION

I. Definition: Accumulation of serous fluid in the middle ear longer than 2 or 3 months without signs and symptoms of acute infection (sometimes referred to as serous otitis media)

II. Pathogenesis

A. Loss of patency of the eustachian tube with subsequent negative pressure and effusion behind the tympanic membrane

B. Common causative factors:
    1. Adenoidal hypertrophy
    2. Recent upper respiratory infection
    3. Allergies

4. Deviated nasal septum
5. Post purulent otitis media
6. Rarely due to nasopharyngeal neoplasm

III. Clinical Presentation

A. Effusion may occur in adults but is less common than in children

B. Often asymptomatic or may have mild pain

C. Common symptoms include sensation of stuffiness or fullness in ear or popping and crackling sounds in ear with chewing, yawning or blowing nose

D. A small number of patients may experience vertigo or ataxia

E. Tympanic membrane is often retracted with diffuse light reflex
   1. Bubbles or a fluid level may be present behind the tympanic membrane
   2. Decreased tympanic membrane movement with insufflation (pneumatic otoscopy)

F. Chronic effusion may result in the following:
   1. Hearing loss which, in children, may lead to a delay in language development
   2. Delay of gross motor skills in children

G. Complications are rare, but may include chronic drainage and perforation, cholesteatoma, and facial nerve paralysis

IV. Diagnosis/Evaluation

A. History
   1. Determine onset, duration, character of symptoms
   2. Inquire about rhinitis, cough, and fever
   3. Question about pain and decreased hearing acuity level
   4. Inquire about recent upper respiratory infection and allergies
   5. Inquire about past episodes of otitis media and treatments received
   6. Ask about family history of allergies

B. Physical Examination
   1. Measure vital signs
   2. Examine nasal passages and pharynx
   3. Examine tympanic membranes for fluid level, retraction, diffuse light reflex and/or bubbles
   4. Assess TM mobility with pneumatic otoscopy
      a. Recommended for primary diagnosis
      b. Accuracy of diagnosis with pneumatic otoscopy is 70-79%
   5. Perform Rinne and Weber tests
   6. Palpate neck and jaw for adenopathy
   7. Examine neck and head for anatomical abnormalities

C. Differential Diagnosis
   1. Nasopharyngeal carcinoma
   2. Anatomic abnormalities

D. Diagnostic Tests
   1. Tympanometry (Indirect measure of tympanic membrane compliance and estimate of middle ear pressure)
      a. Often falsely positive due to impacted cerumen, foreign body, TM perforation, or improper placement of instrument tip on the ear canal wall
      b. Pneumatic otoscopy recommended for primary diagnosis, followed by tympanometry as confirmatory test
      c. Tympanogram is flat with an effusion

2. Audiometry
    a. Patients with fluid in both ears for three months should undergo hearing evaluation; prior to three months, audiometry is an option
    b. Hearing impairment is defined as equal to or worse than 20 decibels (dB) hearing threshold level in the better-hearing ear
3. Acoustic reflectometry; experts disagree about the value of this test

V. Plan/Management

A. Nasopharyngeal cancer is a remote possibility in a healthy adult and consultation with an otolaryngologist is necessary if there is suspicion of this condition

B. For asymptomatic patients choose either watchful waiting with vigilant monitoring **OR** antibiotic therapy (consult with specialist)
1. Watchful waiting is sometimes used because of accumulating evidence that antibiotic use increases the risk for both colonization and invasive disease with penicillin-resistant *Streptococcus pneumoniae*; additional rationale for this recommendation:
    a. Most cases spontaneously resolve without antibiotic treatment (about 90%)
    b. Effect of antibiotics is marginal and often short-lived; antibiotics increase short-term resolution by approximately 15%
    c. Incidence of delayed suppurative complications from effusion is small
2. If antibiotic therapy is chosen, prescribe a beta-lactamase stable antibiotic such as the following:
    a. Amoxicillin-clavulanate (Augmentin) 500 mg tabs TID or 875 mg tabs BID
    b. Clarithromycin (Biaxin) 250-500 mg cap BID

C. Assess hearing status and structural integrity of TM with audiometry and pneumatic otoscopy every 3-4 months

D. Consider autoinflation of eustachian tube with plastic nasal cannula attached to balloon

E. Patient education, modification of risk factors, and controlling concurrent illness are important
1. Limit active and passive smoking
2. Treat concurrent illnesses such as sinusitis and allergic rhinitis
3. Emphasize importance of follow up

F. Most studies indicate that decongestants and antihistamines are ineffective; the role of allergies in patients with effusions is still uncertain

G. Adenoidectomy combined with tympanostomy tubes may be beneficial

H. Follow Up
1. Assess every 4-6 weeks or sooner if ear pain or other bothersome symptoms occur
2. If effusion still persists at 6-week follow-up visit, watchful waiting or antibiotic therapy are acceptable approaches
3. If effusion persists at 3-month follow-up visit, hearing evaluation is indicated

CARE OF PATIENT WITH TYMPANOSTOMY TUBES

I.   Definition: Middle ear ventilation tubes placed in tympanic membrane (TM) after myringotomy

II.   Procedure

    A.   Tubes restore hearing to pre-effusion threshold, permit normal vibration of TM and middle ear bones, permit ventilation of middle ear tissues, equalize middle ear and atmospheric pressures, and prevent accumulation of fluid or mucus in middle ear

    B.   Tubes are placed in pars tensa of the tympanic membrane, in any location except the posterosuperior quadrant, overlying the incus and stapes

    C.   Generally, tubes are made of plastic, metal or Teflon and are designed for short-term placement (8-15 months) or long-term placement (>15 months)

    D.   Possible candidates for tube placement:
        1.   Patients with bilateral middle ear effusion and hearing deficiency for more than 3 months; recommended if condition existed for 4-6 months
        2.   Patients with middle ear effusion and structural changes of tympanic membrane
        3.   Experts consider earlier tube placement for patients with recurrent painful ear infections, and craniofacial anomalies

III. Clinical Presentation

    A.   Potential benefits include improvements in communication and hearing

    B.   Potential Risks
        1.   Auditory canal wall laceration, persistent otorrhea, granuloma formation, cholesteatoma and permanent TM perforation
        2.   Structural changes in TM such as flaccidity, retraction and/or tympanosclerosis have occurred; long-term effects on hearing are unknown but estimated as small
        3.   Risks associated with general anesthesia
        4.   Intrusion of tube into middle ear cleft rather than normal extrusion through external ear canal

IV.   Diagnosis/Evaluation

    A.   History
        1.   Question about pain and ear discharge
        2.   Inquire about noticeable changes in hearing and speech

    B.   Physical Examination
        1.   Inspect ear canal for possible tube extrusion and signs of ear discharge
        2.   Inspect TM for placement of tube and color and degree of translucency (TM should be gray and translucent if tube is properly functioning)
        3.   Assess for mobility with pneumatic otoscopy (TM should be immobile if tube is properly functioning)

    C.   Diagnostic tests
        1.   If tube functioning is questionable, order tympanometry which should be flat if tube is properly functioning
        2.   Audiometry helps to confirm status of tube functioning

V.   Plan/Management

A.   In past, an otolaryngologist was responsible for complete care and follow-up of patients with tympanostomy tubes; today, experienced, health care providers in primary care are caring for minor problems with tubes in collaboration with an otolaryngologist

B.   For tubes clogged with dried middle ear effusion, consider consultation with specialist and prescribe topical antibiotic such as Cortisporin otic suspension for 5-7 days; hydrogen peroxide and cerumolytics are **contraindicated**

C.   Posttube otorrhea occurs in 10-30% of patients
1.   Prescribe amoxicillin (Amoxil) 500 mg TID or a beta-lactamase stable antibiotic in areas with prevalence of resistant organisms (see second-line antibiotics under OTITIS MEDIA)
2.   If unresponsive to first course of antibiotics, consider the possibility of water contamination with *Pseudomonas aeruginosa* and *Staphylococcus aureus* and prescribe Cortisporin otic suspension for 5-7 days

D.   Refer the following cases to an otolaryngologist
1.   Recurrent or chronic tube otorrhea
2.   Recurrent episodes of acute otitis media
3.   Occluded tube with middle ear effusion which does not readily clear
4.   Bloody otorrhea
5.   Decreased hearing acuity
6.   Suspicion of cholesteatoma
7.   TM perforation surrounding tube
8.   Retention of tube for more than 2 years

E.   Patient Education
1.   Teach patient to watch for tube extrusion and possible complications such as discharge from ear and fever
2.   Emphasize importance of follow-up visits with otolaryngologist
3.   Wear fitted ear plugs when swimming or bathing especially during diving and head dunking in lakes, ponds, rivers and bath water which may have higher bacterial counts

F.   Follow Up
1.   Typically patients have routine postoperative visits with otolaryngologist at the following times: 2-4 weeks after tube placement; 4-6 months after tube placement; 6-12 months after tube extrusion
2.   Patients should return to primary care provider after treatment for clogged tube or posttube otorrhea

ALLERGIC AND NONALLERGIC RHINITIS

I.   Definition of rhinitis: Inflammation of mucous membranes of the nose, usually accompanied by edema of mucosa and a nasal discharge. Rhinitis may be allergic or nonallergic

II.   Pathogenesis

A.   Allergic rhinitis: An IgE-mediated inflammatory disease involving the nasal mucosa membranes
1.   When a person with a genetic predisposition to allergy is exposed to a strong allergic stimulus, antigen IgE-antibody molecules are produced and bind to mast cells in the respiratory epithelium
2.   Reexposure to offending allergen causes a hypersensitivity to offending allergen and triggers the release of histamines and other mediators
3.   Histamine release results in immediate local vasodilation, mucosal edema, and increased mucous production

4. A late-phase reaction sometimes occurs 4-8 hours after the original reaction in persons with severe disease; results in hyperresponsiveness to antigenic and nonantigenic stimuli and is linked to development of chronic disease
5. Most common form is the seasonal pattern due to inhalant pollen allergens
6. Year-round perennial type which is difficult to diagnose and treat is usually related to house dust mites, mold, cockroaches, and animal dander; in adults, food allergies are a rare cause of rhinitis

B. Nonallergic Rhinitis
1. Vasomotor rhinitis: Perennial nonallergic rhinitis which represents a hyperreactive state of the nasal mucosa
2. Atrophic or geriatric rhinitis: Perennial nonallergic rhinitis resulting from progressive degeneration and atrophy of nasal mucous membranes and bones of nose
3. Rhinitis medicamentosis or rebound rhinitis is due to overuse of topical decongestant
4. Rhinitis of pregnancy is due to hormonal increase (will not be discussed further)

III. Clinical Presentation

A. Allergic rhinitis
1. Onset of symptoms is most common between ages 10-20; rarely begins before age 4 or after age 40
2. Usually involves the triad of nasal congestion, sneezing and clear rhinorrhea
3. Coughing, sore throat, and itching and puffiness of eyes may occur
4. Signs include the following:
   a. Pale, boggy nasal mucosa with clear thin secretions
   b. Enlarged nasal turbinates which may obstruct airway flow
   c. "Allergic shiners" or a dark discoloration beneath both eyes
   d. Cobblestone appearance of the conjunctiva
   e. "Dennie's lines" or extra wrinkles below the lower eyelids
   f. Transverse nasal crease due to chronic upward wiping of the nose
   g. Nasal salute
   h. Mouth-breathing
   i. Short, upper lip
   j. Enlarged tonsils and adenoids
5. Predisposing factors include serous otitis media, chronic sinusitis, asthma, nasal polyposis, respiratory infections, nasal speech, and abnormal facial development

B. Vasomotor rhinitis
1. May be due to abnormal autonomic responsiveness and vascular dilatation of submucosal vessels
2. Vasomotor rhinitis or persistent nasal congestion does not have a correlation to specific allergen exposures
3. Onset is usually in adult life
4. Patients have a rapid onset of nasal congestion and a pronounced and noticeable postnasal drip
5. Triggers of attacks are the following: abrupt changes in temperature and barometric pressure, odors, and emotional stress
6. Negative family history of allergy
7. Nasal smear and skin tests are negative
8. Patients are usually unresponsive to environmental controls and medications

C. Atrophic rhinitis
1. Occurs in older patients who complain of nasal congestion, thick postnasal drip, frequent clearing of throat, and a constant bad smell in nose
2. On physical examination, the nasal airways are patent and the mucosa is dry

D. Rhinitis medicamentosa
    1. When the beneficial effects of topical nasal decongestants subside, a secondary vasodilation occurs, resulting in increased nasal congestion
    2. Addiction may develop as the patient's relief becomes shorter and the rebound more severe within a short time

IV. Diagnosis/Evaluation

A. History
    1. Question about onset, duration, and progression of symptoms
    2. Explore relationship of symptoms to season, place, time of day, and activity
    3. Question about contact with offending allergens and other triggers such as exposure to cold air, ingestion of spicy foods, odors, and changes in temperature and barometric pressure
    4. Question about nasal stuffiness or obstruction, sensation of pressure over and under the eyes, itching of the eyes, nose and pharynx, sneezing, color, consistency, and amount of nasal and postnasal discharges, and sensation of needing to constantly clear throat
    5. Ask about mouth breathing, changes in hearing and smell acuity, snoring during sleep, and fatigue
    6. Inquire about self-treatment, particularly duration and use of nasal sprays
    7. Inquire about family history and past history of allergies

B. Physical Examination
    1. Check pulse and blood pressure as sympathomimetic decongestants may increase both
    2. Measure temperature which should be normal
    3. Inspect eyes for allergic "shiners," tearing, conjunctival injection, lid swelling, and periorbital edema
    4. Palpate for sinus tenderness.
    5. Examine ears to rule out otitis media and to check for serous otitis media
    6. Assess for nasal obstruction and polyps
    7. Inspect nasal mucosa noting color, edema, and type and color of nasal discharge
    8. Assess pharynx for tonsillar enlargement and inflammation
    9. Palpate lymph nodes
    10. Always check breath sounds to rule out concurrent asthma

C. Differential Diagnosis
    1. Upper respiratory infections typically have a history of contagion, presence of fever, purulent nasal discharge, inflamed nasal mucosa, and absence of eosinophils on nasal smear
    2. Sinusitis
    3. Otitis media
    4. Foreign body, if blockage is unilateral
    5. Deviated septum, if blockage is unilateral
    6. Nasal polyps
    7. Endocrine conditions such as hypothyroidism
    8. Pregnancy and oral contraceptives

D. Diagnostic tests (most of the time the diagnosis is made from the history and physical and no tests are required)
    1. Skin testing for allergies is often recommended and the results must be compared with the clinical history; gold standard test
    2. Nasal smear for eosinophils is often helpful and eosinophils are elevated with allergic rhinitis; peripheral eosinophil count is not useful
    3. Serum IgE levels are elevated in 30-40% of patients with allergic rhinitis and increased levels occur in nonallergies. Thus, the test has limited value
    4. In vitro serum allergy tests (radioallergosorbent tests: RAST, FAST, MAST) are expensive and not as specific nor sensitive as skin testing
    5. If there is any question of an infectious process obtain a CBC

V.   Plan/Management
    A.   Allergic rhinitis
        1.   Patient Education: Allergen avoidance is the most effective form of treatment.
            a.   The bedroom is considered the room that must be the most allergen-free
            b.   Try to eliminate dust and allergen exposure in the household (see table that follows)

MEASURES OF ENVIRONMENTAL CONTROL IN THE HOME
➡ Vacuum weekly (some vacuums spread dust and mites, so the vacuum should be cleaned regularly) or perform damp mopping
➡ Dust furniture and all horizontal surfaces weekly with a damp cloth
➡ Encase mattress and pillow in allergen-impermeable cover; wash sheets and blankets in hot water weekly
➡ Remove carpets from bedroom; avoid lying on upholstered furniture; remove carpets laid on concrete
➡ Avoid rubber mattress
➡ Recommend keeping windows and doors closed to decrease influx of mold and pollen; may necessitate air conditioning in the summer (have AC unit professionally cleaned to clear mold/mildew off coils)
➡ Reduce indoor humidity to less than 50%
➡ Eliminate or restrict exposure to pets
➡ To control cockroaches, use poison traps or bait; do not leave food or garbage exposed
➡ Use clothes dryer rather than hanging clothes outside to air dry
➡ Wear high-efficiency mask and long-sleeved shirt when gardening; bathe and change clothes immediately after coming inside

        2.   Drug therapy is indicated when allergen avoidance is ineffective or impractical
        3.   There is no recommended first-line drug of choice; Choice of medication depends on symptoms patient is experiencing as well as adverse reactions of drugs, adherence factors, risk of drug interactions, and cost (See table on the EFFICACY OF PHARMACOTHERAPEUTIC AGENTS)

EFFICACY OF PHARMACOTHERAPEUTIC AGENTS				
Therapeutic Agents	Itching/ Sneezing	Runny Nose	Nasal Blockage	Eye Symptoms
Oral Antihistamines	+++	++	---	+++
Intranasal corticosteroids	+++	+++	+++	+
Oral decongestants	---	+	+++	---
Antihistamine/decongestant combinations	+++	++	++	+++
Nasal decongestants	---	+	+++	---
Cromolyn sodium	++	++	---	---
Intranasal ipratropium	---	+++	---	---

Adapted from Kaiser, H.B., Kay, G.G., & Palakanis, K. (1998). Contemporary issues in the management of allergic disorders: A focus on respiratory and dermatologic manifestations. Clinical Courier, 16 (46), 1-7.

        4.   First generation antihistamines (see table that follows)
            a.   Advantage: Inexpensive; anticholinergic properties may be beneficial for patient who is bothered by rhinorrhea; early onset of action which is useful for intermittent symptoms

    b.   Disadvantage: Numerous adverse effects: drowsiness, impaired performance, anticholinergic effects such as dry mouth, urinary retention and constipation; do not relieve nasal congestion; must be cautious when used in the elderly (particularly persons with benign prostate hypertrophy and narrow angle glaucoma); do not control underlying inflammatory response

    c.   Hydroxyzine is the most potent

    d.   Rule of thumb is to use the smallest dose that is effective

    e.   Slowly titrate drugs beginning with one dose at bedtime for several days, then adding a small morning dose and so on (base titration on symptom control and adverse effects); tolerance to sedative effects usually occurs after 1-2 weeks of continued dosing

    f.   May be necessary to try several antihistamines from different classes before effective one is found; administer 2-3 weeks before switching to an agent of another class; may need to switch occasionally to prevent increased tolerance

5.   Azelastine HCl 0.1% nasal spray (Astelin) is the first topical antihistamine

    a.   Advantage: Effective in reducing allergic symptoms, has good safely profile, and is more beneficial in relieving nasal obstruction than oral antihistamines

    b.   Disadvantage: Few studies to determine long-term effectiveness

    c.   Prescribe 2 sprays per nostril BID

FIRST GENERATION ANTIHISTAMINES	
Ethanolamine	
Diphenhydramine (Benadryl)	25-50 mg TID/QID
Clemastine (Tavist)	1-2 mg BID
Ethylenediamine	
Tripelennamine (Pyribenzamine)	25-50 mg TID/QID
Alkylamine	
Chlorpheniramine (Chlor-Trimeton)	4 mg QID
Brompheniramine (Dimetane)	4 mg QID
Piperazine	
Hydroxyzine (Atarax, Vistaril)	10-25 mg TID/QID
Phenothiazine	
Trimeprazine (Temaril)	2.5 mg QID
Piperidine	
Cyproheptadine (Periactin)	4 mg TID

6.   Second generation antihistamines (see table that follows)

    a.   Advantage: Fewer adverse drug effects and simpler dosing schedule than first-generation antihistamines

    b.   Disadvantage: Expensive; less effective than first-generation antihistamines and other medications in reducing rhinorrhea; no relief for nasal congestion; do not control underlying inflammatory response

COMPARISON OF SECOND GENERATION ANTIHISTAMINES

	Astemizole (Hismanal)	Loratadine (Claritin)	Fexofenadine (Allegra)	Certirizine (Zyrtec)
Dosage Adult	10 mg tab QD (Take on empty stomach)	10 mg tab QD (Initially 10 mg EOD)	60 mg cap BID (Initially 60 mg QD)	10 mg tab QD
Risk of Torsades de Pointes (Cardiotoxicity)	Yes	No	No	No
Sedation	No	No	No	Yes
Dry mouth & urinary retention	No	No	No	Yes
Weight gain	Yes	<astemizole	Not reported	Yes
Interactions	Avoid erythromycin, clarithromycin, keto-conazole, itracon-azole, quinine	None known	None known	Potentiates CNS depression with alcohol & other CNS depressants

7. Oral decongestants are often combined with antihistamines to enhance effectiveness and counterbalance sedative side effects (see table that follows)

COMMON COMBINATION ANTIHISTAMINE/DECONGESTANT PRODUCTS

Antihistamine/-Decongestant	Brand Name	Adult Dose (mg)
Brompheniramine/-phenylpropanolamine	Dimetapp	1 tab q 4 hours
Chlorpheniramine/-pseudoephedrine	Deconamine	1 tab TID/QID
Chlorpheniramine/-pyrilamine/phenylephrine	Rynatan	1-2 tabs BID
Chlorpheniramine/-phenylpropanolamine	Triaminic-12	1 tab q 12 hours
Fexofenadine/pseudoephedrine	Allegra-D	1 tab BID
Loratadine/pseudoephedrine	Claritin-D 12 hr Claritin-D 24 hr	1 tab BID/QD 1 tab QD

8. For patients with significant congestion of mucous membranes, a topical decongestant may be needed first. Topical pharmacotherapy provides direct delivery of drug to nasal mucosa and has minimal side effects but will be ineffective for pulmonary and ocular allergic symptoms. Prescribe phenylephrine HCl (Neo-Synephrine spray or drops) 1-2 sprays or 2-3 drops of 0.25% or 0.5% in each nostril every 3-4 hours; use no longer than 3-4 days

9. Steroid sprays are often drug of choice, particularly for patients who have moderate or severe symptoms (see table that follows for dosing and prescribing information)

   a. Advantages: Control nasal congestion as well as rhinorrhea; few adverse effects; most effective and potent agents available for treatment; controls underlying anti-inflammatory response

   b. Disadvantages: Expensive; slow onset of activity; do not relieve ocular symptoms

INTRANASAL CORTICOSTEROID SPRAYS

Medications	Dose per Actuation	Formulation (Aq/MDI)	Adult Dosage
Beclomethasone dipropionate (Vancenase, Beconase)	42 mcg 84 mcg	+/+ +/0	1-2 sprays each nostril BID-QID 2 sprays each nostril QD
Budesonide (Rhinocort)	32 mcg	0/+	2 sprays each nostril BID or 4 sprays each nostril QD
Dexamethasone (Dexacort)	100 mcg	0/+	2 sprays each nostril BID-TID
Flunisolide (Nasarel)	25 mcg	+/0	2 sprays each nostril BID-TID
Fluticasone propionate (Flonase)	50 mcg	+/0	2 sprays each nostril QD
Mometasone furoate (Nasonex)	50 mcg	+/0	2 sprays each nostril QD
Triamcinolone acetonide (Nasacort)	55 mcg	+/+	2-4 sprays each nostril QD

Aq = Aqueous, MDI = Metered-dose inhaler, + = Available, 0 = Not available

Adapted from Kaiser, H.B., Kay, G.G., & Palakanis, K. (1998). Contemporary issues in the management of allergic disorders: A focus on respiratory and dermatologic manifestations. Clinical Courier, 16 (46), 1-7.

  c. May be combined with antihistamines for enhanced effectiveness

  d. Steroid sprays have a slow onset of activity; warn patients they might <u>not</u> see effects for 2 weeks after initiating therapy

  e. Medication must be used on a regular basis to be effective

10. Oral corticosteroids are reserved for short-term therapy for patients with severe, debilitating disease

11. Mast cell stabilizers are usually reserved for patients with chronic or severe symptoms

  a. Advantages: Good safety profile, control underlying inflammatory response

  b. Disadvantages: Less effective than other therapies in relieving nasal obstruction; frequent dosing makes it difficult for patients to adhere; more expensive than other therapies

  c. These medications prevent symptoms from starting and are generally not beneficial once an attack has started; relief of symptoms may be delayed 3-4 weeks after initiation of therapy

   (1) Recommend over-the-counter, intranasal cromolyn sodium (Nasalcrom) 1-2 sprays in each nostril 3-6x daily at regular intervals; use prophylactically before known or suspected allergen contact

   (2) Nedocromil is considered ten times more potent than cromolyn

   (3) Concomitant use of decongestants may be useful to relieve congestion

12. Application of saline to nasal mucosa acts as a mild decongestant and can liquify mucus and prevent crusting; administer 2-4 times a day

13. Intranasal ipratropium may be used for relief of rhinorrhea with allergic and nonallergic rhinitis

  a. Advantage: excellent safety profile and few adverse reactions

  b. Disadvantage: effective for only rhinorrhea; minimal effect on other symptoms

  c. Prescribe ipratropium bromide 0.03% aqueous solution (Atrovent nasal spray) 2 sprays in each nostril 2-3 times daily

14. Allergic conjunctivitis which often accompanies allergic rhinitis may require flushing eyes with artificial liquid tears; may use naphazoline HCl 0.025% and pheniramine maleate (0.3%) (Naphcon A) ophthalmic solution 1-2 drops every 3-4 hours prn. May also use cromolyn sodium 4% ophthalmic solution (Crolom) 1-2 drops 4-6 times daily

15. For patients with nasal polyps, refer to specialist

16. Patient education

  a. Remind patients with perennial allergic rhinitis to take medications regularly rather than sporadically when symptoms occur

  b. Teach patients to read drug labels before taking over-the-counter medication as many cold products and sleep aids contain antihistamines

  c. Teach patient proper administration of intranasal medications (see following table)

INSTRUCTIONS FOR USE OF INTRANASAL MEDICATION

➡ Clear nasal passages or blow nose before administering medication

➡ Keep head upright and spray medication quickly and firmly into each nostril

➡ Spray medication away from nasal septum

➡ Spray each nostril separately and wait at least 1 minute before second spray

➡ If possible, avoid sneezing or blowing nose for 5-10 minutes after spraying

➡ Cleanse medicine canister device after each use

    17.   Referral to a specialist for allergen immunotherapy is recommended when patients cannot eliminate environmental allergens or have severe symptoms, poor response to medications, long-term need for medications, or presence of secondary complications

B.   Vasomotor rhinitis
1.   Difficult to relieve symptoms; best medication is a nasal spray of physiological saline solution
2.   More thorough cleansing of nose may be accomplished by powered irrigators such as the Grossan irrigator
3.   Topical ipratropium often relieves symptoms
4.   Oral anti-histamines/decongestants and steroid sprays are usually less efficacious than the above recommendations, but for some patients are helpful

C.   Atrophic rhinitis
1.   Recommend mucus-stimulating medication such as guaifenesin 200 mg/5mL (Naldecon Senior EX syrup) 10 mL every 4 hours
2.   If above medication is ineffective, use nasal spray of physiological saline solution; powered irrigators such as the Grossan irrigator may be helpful

D.   Follow up of all types of rhinitis
1.   Schedule follow up visit in 2-3 weeks to review patient education topics and check results of therapies
2.   Schedule quarterly or biannual rechecks depending on patient's level of comfort and health

EPISTAXIS

I.   Definition: Nasal bleeding from any cause

II.   Pathogenesis

A.   The nose acts as a conduit to allow air into the lungs and has a very well vascularized mucosa with a complex interior surface composed of folds and irregularities

B.   The blood supply of the nose comes from both the internal and external carotid systems

C.   The anterior portion of the septum contains a plexus of vessels known as Kisselbach's plexus which is particularly vulnerable to digital as well as direct blunt trauma

D.   Bleeding occurs as a result of disruption of the nasal mucosa, whether due to trauma, inflammation, or neoplasm

E.   More than 90% of bleeds are related to local irritation and most occur in the absence of a specific underlying anatomic lesion

F.   Epistaxis is rarely associated with systemic diseases such as liver disease, hypertension (hypertension does not cause nasal bleeding but may exacerbate the problem), clotting abnormalities, thrombocytopenia, or platelet dysfunction

III.   Clinical Presentation

A.   Approximately 10% of the population experiences at least one significant nosebleed

B.   More common in children than adults and episodes are typically infrequent, mild, and self-limiting

C.   Over 90% of nosebleeds are anterior, and usually involve the Kisselbach's triangle of the anterior portion of the septum

D.   Anterior nosebleeds are generally less severe and easier to control than nosebleeds originating in posterior area of nose

E.   Epistaxis can be severe and difficult to treat in the elderly because bleeding occurs more commonly in the posterior portion of the nose

F.   Epistaxis is rare in hemophiliacs without trauma, but is characteristic of von Willebrand's disease (a heritable coagulation disorder)

IV.   Diagnosis/Evaluation

A.   History
1.   Question about onset and duration of nasal bleeding; ask how frequently does it occur and how much bleeding is there (quantity)
2.   Ask if there has been an increase in nasal mucus production; if yes, determine color, character, and quantity
3.   Ask if nasal obstruction is present, and if so, is it an acute or chronic occurrence
4.   Ask about occupational exposure to irritating chemicals or dust; ask about cocaine use if appropriate
5.   Inquire about the use of oral anticoagulants or drugs with antiplatelet effects (such as aspirin)
6.   Inquire about previous episodes and treatments
7.   Determine if patient has any clotting abnormalities, thrombocytopenia, or platelet dysfunction; is the patient hypertensive? (A **rare** hypertensive patient with severe pressure elevation may experience epistaxis)

B.   Physical Examination
1.   Assess blood pressure and pulse
2.   Use gentle suction with a bulb syringe to remove blood and secretions and make visualization of the involved vessels possible
3.   Locate bleeding site if possible; 90% are in the anterior septum (Kisselbach's plexus). Posterior site is indicated by persistent drainage of blood down the pharynx

C.   Differential Diagnosis
1.   Coagulation disorders
2.   Intranasal foreign bodies
3.   Familial hereditary telangiectasia

D.   Diagnostic Tests
1.   Extensive evaluation should be reserved for those cases that are recurrent or particularly severe
2.   Hemoglobin or hematocrit if significant blood loss suspected
3.   CBC with differential, platelets, PT and PTT if bleeding disorders suspected

V.   Plan/Management

   A.   Use the approaches outlined in the table below

MANAGEMENT OF NOSE BLEEDS
✓ First, apply pressure to anterior nasal septum while head tilted forward; continue pressure for 10-15 minutes
✓ Then, if clot formation and bleeding cessation do not occur, do the following
✱ Place a small piece of cotton soaked in 1:1000 epinephrine or a vasoconstricting nosedrop such as phenylephrine (Neo-Synephrine) into the vestibule of the nose
✱ Press against the bleeding site for 5 to 10 minutes to promote vasoconstriction
✱ Remove to observe for bleeding (almost all venous types of anterior nosebleeds are stopped with this treatment)
✓ If bleeding continues, but has slowed considerably,
✱ Repeat treatment
✱ Apply ice pack over the nose as an additional therapy
✓ Finally, if these remedies fail,
✱ Anesthetize the mucous membrane with 4% lidocaine (apply to cotton ball and hold in place for several minutes)
✱ Apply a silver nitrate stick to the bleeding site

   B.   If still not responsive, refer to local emergency department

   C.   Instruct patient regarding management of simple nose bleeds at home

   D.   Advise increasing humidity in home through use of humidifier, especially during winter months

   E.   Advise liberal use of lubricant such a petrolatum in nares to promote hydration

   F.   All cases that are recurrent or are particularly severe should be referred to a specialist

   G.   Follow Up: None indicated for cases due to local trauma or inflammation

FOREIGN BODY IN THE NOSE

I.   Definition: Presence of object(s) in the nasal cavity

II.   Pathogenesis: Intentional placement of an object in nose, or occasionally accidental placement of a foreign body while person is attempting to sniff or smell the object

III. Clinical Presentation

   A.   Boredom or curiosity may lead a mentally-impaired adult to place an object in his/her nose

   B.   Typically, these objects are soft materials such as tissues, erasers, or clay

   C.   Symptoms include unilateral obstruction, mild discomfort, sneezing; unilateral purulent nasal discharge can also occur over time

   D.   A key feature is that it is unilateral

IV.   Diagnosis/Evaluation

   A.   History
         1.   Inquire about onset and duration of symptoms
         2.   Ask patient/caregiver if this has occurred in the past

   B.   Physical Examination
         1.   Test both nares for patency
         2.   Examine both nares with nasal speculum to visualize the object

   C.   Differential Diagnosis
         1.   Rhinitis
         2.   Sinusitis

   D.   Diagnostic Tests: None indicated

V.   Plan/Management

   A.   Remove secretions with a small suction tip and use topical decongestant such as Neosynephrine to reduce mucosal edema

   B.   Occlude the uninvolved nostril and have the patient blow forcefully out

   C.   If the above intervention is not successful, use alligator forceps if patient is cooperative; instruments introduced into the nasal passage require a steady hand resting on the patient's head

   D.   For uncooperative patient, or when the nasal passage is completely occluded by an expanding foreign object such as plant materials, beans, or other seeds, or when there is marked edema and inflammation, referral to a specialist is indicated

   E.   Follow Up: Instruct patient/caregiver to use saline irrigation 2-3 times/day for 2-3 days, and follow up in 2 days to evaluate healing of mucosa

SINUSITIS

I.   Definition: Acute, subacute, or chronic inflammation of the mucous membranes that line the paranasal sinuses

   A.   Acute sinusitis is the abrupt onset of infection of one or more of paranasal sinuses with resolution of symptoms with therapy

   B.   Subacute sinusitis is the persistent occurrence of purulent nasal discharge despite therapy; epithelial damage is usually reversible, symptoms last <3 months

   C.   Chronic sinusitis occurs with episodes of prolonged inflammation and/or repeated or inadequately treated acute infection; irreversible damage to the mucosa is present, symptoms last >3 months

II.   Pathogenesis

   A.   Etiological factors
         1.   Main factor is obstruction of ostiomeatal unit which leads to lower levels of oxygen within sinuses, decreased clearance of foreign material, and mucus stasis which creates a good environment for pathogens to grow; any factor or condition which blocks flow of secretions can lead to sinusitis:

a. Recent upper respiratory infection
b. Allergic response to airborne allergens (considered an uncommon predisposing factor in adults)
c. Anatomical abnormalities such as deviated septum
d. Adenoidal hypertrophy
e. Diving and swimming
f. Extension of dental abscess
g. Neoplasms
h. Trauma
i. Foreign body

    2. Other patients have problems with mucus stasis due to immune deficiency, immotile cilia syndrome, or cystic fibrosis

B. Pathogens in acute sinusitis
    1. Common
        a. *Streptococcus pneumoniae*
        b. *Haemophilus influenzae* (may be ß-lactamase producing)
        c. *Moraxella catarrhalis* [(may be ß-lactamase producing); prevalence greater among children than adults]
    2. Less common
        a. *Chlamydia pneumoniae*
        b. *Streptococcus pyogenes*
        c. Viruses
        d. Fungi (e.g., *Aspergillus fumigatus*) (more common in patients who are immunosuppressed or have diabetes mellitus)
    3. Penicillin-resistant *Streptococcus pneumoniae* is becoming more common

C. Pathogens in chronic or subacute sinusitis are usually polymicrobial
    1. Anaerobic bacteria
    2. *Staphylococcus aureus*

D. Anaerobes are common in sinusitis resulting from dental infections

III. Clinical Presentation

A. Most sinus disease in adults and children involves the maxillary and anterior ethmoidal sinuses

B. Acute sinusitis is considered a common problem, complicating 5-10% of upper respiratory infections

C. Acute sinusitis has the following characteristics:
    1. Yellow or green nasal discharge with fever
    2. Nasal congestion with an intermittent sore or raw sensation in throat
    3. Complaint of facial pain, toothache, or headache over the affected sinus.
    4. Increased pain with coughing, bending over or sudden head movement
    5. Cough which may worsen with lying down
    6. Early morning periorbital swelling
    7. Fever and malaise are common systemic symptoms
    8. Classic study by Williams & Simel (1993) found that three symptoms (maxillary toothache, poor response to nasal decongestants, and history of colored nasal discharge) and two signs (purulent nasal secretion and abnormal transillumination) were the best predictors of acute sinusitis
        a. According to the Canadian Sinusitis Symposium Panel, acute sinusitis can be ruled out when there are fewer than 2 of the preceding signs and symptoms
        b. When 4 or more of the preceding signs and symptoms are present the likelihood of acute sinusitis is very high

9. According to O'Brien et al. (1998) the clinical diagnosis of sinusitis requires one of the following:
   a. Prolonged nonspecific upper respiratory signs and symptoms without improvement for >10-14 days
   b. More severe upper respiratory tract signs and symptoms such as facial swelling, facial pain , and fever≥39.0°C

D. Thick, tenacious, brown secretions are characteristic of fungal sinusitis

E. Subacute or chronic sinusitis has the following characteristics:
   1. Nasal discharge, nasal congestion, or cough lasting >30 days
   2. Hallmark is dull ache or pressure across midface or headache
   3. Other symptoms include thick postnatal drip, "popping" ears, eye pain, halitosis, chronic cough, and fatigue

F. All types of sinusitis may exacerbate asthma

G. Diabetics and immunosuppressed patients often experience severe, invasive sinus disease

H. Complications of sinusitis include contiguous spread or hematogenous dissemination of infection and can result in life-threatening intraorbital or intracranial suppuration; patients with frontal headaches and associated frontal sinusitis are at greatest risk for intracranial complications

IV. Diagnosis/Evaluation

A. History
   1. Question regarding onset, duration, and seasonality of symptoms
   2. Inquire about the laterality and quality (mucoid, purulent, serous) of nasal discharge
   3. Ask about fever and systemic symptoms such as fatigue
   4. Question about character (dry, productive) and timing (day, night, continual) of cough
   5. Ask patient to describe pain and what aggravates it
   6. Ask about timing and quality of headaches and morning puffiness about the eyes
   7. Ask about history of allergies
   8. Ask about past episodes and treatments
   9. Inquire about past medical history such as diabetes mellitus, immunodeficiency, asthma
   10. Question about smoking, recent trauma to the nose, recent upper respiratory infections
   11. Inquire about family history of allergies, immunodeficiency, chronic respiratory complaints

B. Physical Examination
   1. Determine vital signs
   2. Examine eyes, noting peri-orbital swelling and presence of allergic shiners
   3. Examine nasal mucosa for erythema, edema, and discharge
   4. Determine patency of both nasal nares
   5. Inspect nose for septal deviation and polyps
   6. Examine ears, throat, and mouth for signs of inflammation
   7. Transilluminate and percuss frontal and maxillary sinuses
   8. Examine teeth and gingivae for caries and inflammation; tap maxillary teeth with tongue blade because 5% to 10% of maxillary sinusitis is due to dental root infection
   9. Palpate neck and jaw for lymphadenopathy.
   10. Auscultate heart and lungs.
   11. Perform a neurological examination to rule-out complications

C. Differential Diagnosis:
   1. Dental abscess
   2. Cluster and migraine headaches
   3. Allergic rhinitis
   4. Vasomotor rhinitis
   5. Nasal polyp
   6. Tumor
   7. Uncomplicated upper respiratory infection

D. Diagnostic Tests
1. None indicated for typical presentation and for first episode of acute sinusitis
2. Radiologic studies are not routinely ordered and must be intrepreted cautiously
   a. The common cold often includes radiologic evidence of sinus involvement (abnormal images only reflect inflammation, they do not pinpoint whether the inflammation is viral, bacterial or allergic in origin)
   b. Order radiographs to confirm clinical impression and in following: patients with frontal headaches, refractory cases, when complications are suspected, and when diagnosis is unclear.
      (1) Sinus x-rays
         (a) Need antero-posterior, lateral and occipitomental (Waters view) views.
         (b) An air-fluid level or complete opacification of the sinuses and thickening of the mucosal lining are most diagnostic
         (c) Accuracy of diagnosing ethmoid disease is questionable with x-rays
      (2) Computerized tomography (CT scan) is gold standard of radiographic study, but is reserved for recalcitrant cases and patients in need of surgery
3. To confirm diagnosis of maxillary and frontal sinusitis and to identify causative pathogen, obtain sinus aspirates by antral puncture (impractical in most primary care settings)
4. Flexible fiber optic rhinoscopy, after the topical application of a vasoconstrictor and anesthetic may be indicated
5. CBC with differential indicated for severely, ill patients
6. Allergy testing when the history suggests an allergic disease

V. Plan/Management

A. Treatment of acute sinusitis and acute episodes in patients who have subacute and chronic sinusitis includes antibiotics and drugs to reduce obstruction of the ostiomeatal unit
   1. Antibiotics for acute sinusitis are similar to those recommended for otitis media (see tables on pages of recommended antibiotics in OTITIS MEDIA section); duration of antibiotic therapy is 10-14 days or 7 days beyond the point of resolution of signs and symptoms
      a. Amoxicillin (Amoxil) 500 mg TID is the first-line drug
      b. Prescribe trimethoprim sulfamethoxazole (Bactrim) 1 double strength tab q 12 hours for patients allergic to penicillin
   2. Patients with chronic sinusitis are likely to have acute exacerbations; for these acute episodes prescribe a beta-lactamase stable antibiotic and extend therapy for a total of 2-4 weeks; prescribe one of following:
      a. Amoxicillin/clavulanate (Augmentin) 500 mg TID or 875 mg BID
      b. Clarithromycin (Biaxin) 500 mg tab every 12 hours
      c. See table for other recommended second-line antibiotics in OTITIS MEDIA section
   3. Decongestants or saline nasal spray at the time of diagnosis of acute sinusitis and in acute episodes of subacute and chronic sinusitis can improve patency of ostiomeatal unit
      a. Topical decongestants should be used no longer than 3-4 days. Use phenylephrine (Neo-Synephrine spray or drops) 1-2 sprays or 2-3 drops of 0.25% or 0.5% in each nostril every 3-4 hours
      b. Oral decongestants are not as effective as topical agents but can be used for a longer time period
         (1) Use cautiously in patients with hypertension
         (2) Suggest pseudoephedrine hydrochloride (Sudafed) 60 mg, 1 tablet every 4-6 hours or Pseudoephedrine sulfate (Afrin) 120 mg, 1 tablet every 12 hours

B. For recurrent acute infections or for persons with acute sinusitis or acute exacerbations who do not have a clinical response to first antibiotic in 48 to 72 hours, prescribe a beta-lactamase-stable agent or second-line drug (see OTITIS MEDIA section)

C. Acute sinusitis due to dental infection: Prescribe amoxicillin clavulanate (Augmentin)

D. Unresponsive cases may be due to infection with *Chlamydia pneumoniae*; trial with doxycycline (Vibramycin) 100 mg caps every 12 hours for 10-14 days or clarithromycin may be beneficial

E. Treatment of fungal infections involves surgery and broad-spectrum antibiotics for intercurrent bacterial infections

F. Treatment of chronic sinusitis
1. Prescribe: Nasal steroids sprays such as beclomethasone dipropionate (Beconase, Vancenase) 1-2 sprays in each nostril BID; triamcinolone acetonide (Nasacort AQ) or mometasone furoate (Nasonex) both prescribed 2 sprays in each nostril QD and then may decrease as symptoms improve
2. Do not use topical steroids when patient has an acute episode of sinusitis

G. Oral antihistamines should not be used unless patient has allergies. Antihistamines tend to slow the movement of secretions out of the sinuses

H. Referral to a specialist is needed for the following:
1. Exquisite pain with palpation or percussion of the face
2. Possibility of cellulitis
3. Periorbital swelling

I. Functional endoscopic sinus surgery which removes only affected tissue has revolutionized surgical treatment of sinus disease

J. Patient Education
1. Instruct patient to return for further evaluation if symptoms are not improved within 48 hours
2. Teach patient about the complications of sinusitis, particularly the need to return if there is swelling in the periorbital area
3. Humidify the air
4. Increase fluid intake
5. Steam inhalation and warm compresses often help relieve pressure
6. Avoid allergens and excessively dry heat
7. Avoid swimming/diving and air travel during acute period
8. Avoid use of antihistamines unless there is an allergic basis to disease
9. Encourage cessation of smoking
10. Teach proper application of nasal sprays (see table on instructions for use of intranasal medications in ALLERGIC RHINITIS section)
11. Patients who have recurrent sinusitis should be instructed to begin decongestants at the first sign of sinusitis to facilitate sinus drainage and decrease development of infection

K. Follow Up
1. If no decrease in symptoms in 48-72 hours, patient should be reevaluated; refer to specialist if symptoms are actually worsening.
2. Schedule return visit for 10-14 days.
3. Patients with chronic sinusitis who do not have marked improvement in four weeks with continuous medical therapy may be candidates for needle aspiration of a maxillary sinus or sinus surgery

PHARYNGITIS

I. Definition: Inflammation of the pharynx and surrounding lymph tissue (tonsils)

II. Pathogenesis

A. Viruses are the most common pathogens; the following are common viral infections
1. Infections due to rhinovirus, adenovirus, parainfluenza, coronavirus, and echovirus
2. Herpangina due to Coxsackie virus and echovirus
3. Hand-Foot-and-Mouth disease due to Coxsackie virus

4. Infectious mononucleosis caused by Epstein-Barr virus
5. Human Immunodeficiency Virus (HIV)

 B. Bacteria (listed common to rare)
  1. Group A β-hemolytic *streptococcus*
  2. *Neisseria gonorrhoea*
  3. *Corynebacterium diphtheriae*
  4. *Streptococci of Lancefield Groups C and G* (often associated with contaminated food)

 C. Other atypical agents usually in adults include *Mycoplasma pneumoniae* and *Chlamydia trachomatis* (rare)

 D. Fungus: *Candida albicans*

 E. Peritonsillar abscess: Often due to anaerobic bacteria, but can be due to Group A *streptococci*, *Haemophilus influenzae*, or *Staphylococcus aureus*

 F. Noninfectious causes
  1. Allergic rhinitis or post-nasal drip
  2. Mouth breathing
  3. Trauma from heat, alcohol, irritants such as marijuana or sharp objects
  4. Subacute thyroiditis in females

III. Clinical Presentation

 A. Herpangina
  1. Small oral vesicles or ulcers may be on tonsils, pharynx, or posterior buccal mucus
  2. Fever, headache, and malaise often accompany sore throat

 B. Hand-Foot-and-Mouth syndrome: usually oral lesions and sore throat accompanied by lesions on hands and feet; may have lesions on arms, legs, buttocks as well

 C. Infectious mononucleosis: May have exudative tonsillitis with fever, fatigue, lymphadenopathy, and palatal petechiae (see section on INFECTIOUS MONONUCLEOSIS)

 D. Primary HIV infection resembles signs and symptoms of mononucleosis with sorethroat, fever, malaise, myalgia, photophobia, lymphadenopathy, and rash; duration is few days to 2 weeks

 E. Pharyngitis due to *Group A β-hemolytic streptococcus*
  1. Commonly seen in 15-40% of school age children; uncommon occurrence in adults
  2. Symptoms include fever >101°F, headaches and sore throat with dysphagia
  3. Erythema of tonsils and pharynx with white or yellow exudate
  4. Tender and enlarged anterior cervical lymph nodes are often present
  5. Erythematous "sand paper" rash and Pastia's lines (petechiae in flexor skin creases of joints) occur with scarlet fever
  6. Abdominal pain, vomiting, and headache may occur whereas upper respiratory symptoms suggest other causes of pharyngitis
  7. Without proper antimicrobial treatment, streptococcal pharyngitis can lead to serious suppurative (direct extension from pharyngeal infection) and nonsuppurative complications (arise from immune responses to acute infection)
   a. Suppurative adenitis involving tender, enlarged nodes
   b. Scarlet fever (suppurative) (see section on SCARLET FEVER)
   c. Peritonsillar abscess (suppurative) (discussed later)
   d. Glomerulonephritis (nonsuppurative) which appears 1-3 weeks after pharyngeal infection (proper treatment with antimicrobials does not prevent)
   e. Rheumatic fever (nonsuppurative) (see section on RHEUMATIC FEVER)

 F. Pharyngitis due to *Corynebacterium diphtheriae*
  1. Gray adherent membrane on the nasal mucosa, tonsils, uvula or pharynx
  2. Bleeding occurs when membrane is removed

G. Pharyngitis due to *Neisseria gonorrhoea* and *Chlamydia trachomatis*
   1. Seen in those patients who practice orogenital sex and sexually abused individuals
   2. Commonly presents as a chronic sore throat

H. Pharyngitis due to *Mycoplasma pneumoniae*
   1. Uncommon in children <5 years of age, but seen in adolescents and adults
   2. Signs and symptoms indistinguishable from streptococcal disease

I. *Candida albicans*
   1. Thin diffuse or patchy exudate on mucous membranes
   2. Patients have history of antibiotic use or are immunosuppressed

J. Peritonsillar abscess
   1. Most commonly occurs after an episode of tonsillitis
   2. Often presents with gradually increasing unilateral ear and throat pain
   3. Dysphagia, dysphonia, drooling, and trismus are common
   4. The affected tonsil is usually grossly swollen medially and erythematous and may displace uvula and soft palate to contralateral side
   5. Swelling and erythema of the soft palate is noted
   6. Fluctuance may be felt with palpation of affected side
   7. Enlarged and very tender lymph nodes are usually present

IV. Diagnosis/Evaluation

A. History
   1. Determine onset and duration of symptoms
   2. Question about rhinorrhea and coughing (suggestive of viral agent)
   3. Inquire regarding trismus, excessive drooling and dysphagia (suggestive of peritonsillar abscess)
   4. Ask about lesions in the mouth (suggestive of herpangina, hand-foot-mouth syndrome, and thrush)
   5. Inquire about skin changes and exanthems (rash with scarlet fever)
   6. Determine other associated symptoms such as abdominal pain, headache, and fatigue
   7. Ascertain that sore throat is not significantly reducing intake of fluids
   8. Inquire about possible streptococcal exposure
   9. Inquire about immunization status
   10. If applicable, inquire about sexual practices

B. Physical Examination
   1. Do not attempt to examine the pharynx of a patient who has drooling, stridor or trouble breathing (may have epiglottitis)
   2. Measure vital signs
   3. Inspect skin for color and exanthems
   4. Palpate skin for texture and turgor, noting whether the skin has a "sand paper" rash
   5. Inspect mouth for lesions and thrush
   6. Examine ears for concurrent otitis media or effusion
   7. Visualize throat and pharynx for exudate and swelling (unilateral swelling occurs with peritonsillar abscess)
   8. Palpate neck and jaw for adenopathy
   9. Completely examine pharynx
   10. Assess for nuchal rigidity
   11. Auscultate chest
   12. Depending on history of sexual activity, may need to perform genitourinary examination
   13. Palpate abdomen

C. Differential Diagnosis
   1. Stomatitis
   2. Rhinitis or sinusitis with post nasal drip
   3. Epiglottitis
   4. Thyroiditis

D. Diagnostic Tests
1. Perform rapid strep test (sensitivity may be as low as 60%)
2. Perform throat culture: It is advisable to collect the rapid antigen strep and the throat culture at the same time; if rapid test is negative and suspicion is high, send throat culture
3. Consider heterophil agglutination, or mono spot test
4. Consider CBC with differential; expect WBC elevation with bacterial infection and WBC decrease with viral agent
5. Consider culture for gonorrhoea
6. Consider viral cultures of throat and mouth lesions

V. Plan/Management

A. For viral pharyngitis (i.e., herpangina, hand-foot-and-mouth disease, and infectious mononucleosis), treatment is symptomatic

B. Antibiotic treatment for possible and probable strep throat: According to some experts such as Schwartz et al. (1998), never prescribe an antibiotic without a positive throat culture or positive antigen-detection test
1. Therapy is aimed at preventing complications such as rheumatic fever
2. Begin therapy on all patients suspected of strep throat and who have a history of rheumatic fever, appear toxic, have clinical scarlet fever, have symptoms suggesting peritonsillar abscess
3. Treatment of choice is oral or intramuscular penicillin
   a. Adults: Penicillin V (Pen-Vee-K) 500 mg BID or TID for at least 10 days
   b. Benzathine penicillin 1,200,000 units IM
      (1) Be familiar with signs, symptoms and treatment of anaphylaxis and observe patient for 30 minutes after injection.
      (2) Bring medication to room temperature before injecting to reduce discomfort
4. Alternative antibiotics:
   a. Erythromycin: Prescribe erythromycin estolate (E-mycin) 500 mg BID for 10 days
   b. Cefadroxil monohydrate (Duricef): Prescribe 500 mg capsules BID for 10 days; Do not use in patients with allergies to penicillin
5. Treatment of patient who has recurrence of streptococcal pharyngitis shortly after completing recommended antibiotic therapy includes one of following:
   a. Retreat with same antibiotic
   b. Prescribe an alternative oral antibiotic
   c. Administer IM dose of benzathine penicillin G
6. Treatment of streptococcal pharyngeal carriers
   a. Antibiotics are not indicated except for the following:
      (1) During outbreaks of acute rheumatic fever or poststreptococcal glomerulonephritis
      (2) During an outbreak of strep. pharyngitis in a closed or semi-closed community
      (3) Family history of rheumatic fever exists
      (4) Multiple episodes of documented, symptomatic strep. pharyngitis continue to occur within a family over weeks despite appropriate antibiotic therapy
      (5) Family with excessive anxiety of strep. pharyngitis
      (6) When tonsillectomy is considered due to chronic strep carriage
   b. To eliminate carriage, prescribe clindamycin (Cleocin) 20 mg/kg/day (maximum 1.8 g/day) in three divided doses for 10 days

C. Pharyngeal gonorrhea is usually treated with ceftriaxone (Rocephin) 250 mg IM

D. Diphtheria needs immediate specialist consult and is usually treated with equine antitoxin and penicillin or erythromycin; notify public health department

E. For pharyngitis due to mycoplasma pneumoniae and *Chlamydia trachomatis*, treat with erythromycin (E-mycin) 500 mg BID for 10 days

F. *Candida albicans* (see section on CANDIDIASIS)

G. Peritonsillar abscess needs an immediate referral to a specialist
　　1. Initially, in outpatient setting, prescribe drug of choice, penicillin, and a pain medication
　　2. Needle aspiration, incision and drainage, or abscess tonsillectomy are current surgical approaches to management

H. Patient Education
　　1. Teach parents and patients to immediately call office if the pain becomes more severe or if dyspnea, drooling, difficulty swallowing, and inability to fully open mouth develop
　　2. Advise increased fluid intake
　　3. May use hard candy, lozenges or warm saline gargles to soothe throat
　　4. Patients with streptococcal pharyngitis should not return to school or work until they have been on antibiotic therapy for a full 24 hours
　　5. Reinforce that patients will usually feel well in 24-48 hours, but that it is important to take full 10-day course of antibiotic to prevent complications, particularly rheumatic fever

I. Follow Up
　　1. If no significant improvement in 3-4 days patient should return to health care provider
　　2. Patients with streptococcal pharyngitis: Posttreatment throat cultures are indicated only for patients who have high risk for rheumatic fever or who are still symptomatic after treatment

APHTHOUS STOMATITIS

I. Definition: Chronic Inflammation of the oral mucosal tissue with ulcers often called canker sores

II. Pathogenesis: Etiology is uncertain, but the following factors play an important role:

A. Immunopathologic processes
　　1. Common in persons with leukemia, neutropenia, and human immunodeficiency virus infection
　　2. Increased prevalence in patients with autoimmune diseases such as Crohn's disease, Behcet's syndrome, Reiter's syndrome, and ulcerative colitis

B. Allergies; coffee, chocolate, potatoes, cheese, figs, nuts, citrus fruits, and gluten are predisposing factors

C. Stress

D. Viral and bacterial pathogens

E. Trauma

F. Nutritional deficiencies such as vitamin B_{12}, folate, and iron

G. Hormones

H. Medications such as antihypertensives, antineoplastics, gold salts, and nonsteroidal anti-inflammatory drugs

III. Clinical Presentation

A. Peak onset is between 10 and 19 years of age

B. Less prevalent in men and in chronic smokers

C. In approximately 1/3 of patients, reoccurrences continue for numerous years

D. Lesions divided into 3 classifications: minor, clusterform ulcers, and major
    1. Minor: Lesions appear on vestibular and buccal mucosa, tongue, soft palate, fauces, and floor of mouth; rarely do lesions appear on attached gingiva and hard palate as occurs with herpetic ulcers
        a. Most common type
        b. Occasionally, patient may have a burning prodrome
        c. Lesions usually occur singly
        d. Lesions start as indurated papules that progress to ulcers (1 cm) which are covered by a yellow fibrinous membrane and surrounded with an erythematous halo; lesions are never vesicular as occurs in herpetic stomatitis
        e. No fever or lymphadenopathy is noted
        f. Typically lesions heal in 7-14 days and tend to recur
    2. Clusterform:
        a. Typically present as crops of small (1-5 mm) painful ulcers from 3 to over 12
        b. Lesions are intially round or oval and later coalesce to form large ulcers with irregular margins
    3. Major:
        a. This severe form presents with lesions that are large (>0.5 cm), and takes 6 weeks or longer to heal with possible scarring
        b. Severe pain, tender lymphadenopathy and facial edema are sometimes present

IV. Diagnosis/Evaluation

A. History
    1. Ask about onset and duration of symptoms
    2. Inquire about fever and systemic symptoms
    3. Question regarding nutritional deficiencies and stressors
    4. Ask about past episodes and treatments received
    5. Inquire about systemic diseases
    6. Inquire regarding contact with irritants or allergens

B. Physical Examination
    1. Determine vital signs
    2. Assess hydration status; patients may not be drinking fluids due to mouth pain
    3. Perform complete head, ears, eyes, nose, mouth, and throat exam; note location, number and distribution of lesions
    4. Palpate neck and jaw for adenopathy
    5. Auscultate chest

C. Differential Diagnosis
    1. Oral cancer (consider if lesions are present for more than 6 weeks, are unresponsive to therapy, and have unusual presentations such as indurated or rolled borders)
    2. Oral candidiasis (white patches in mouth) (see CANDIDIASIS section)
    3. Hand-foot-and-mouth disease (lesions on hands and feet as well as mouth)
    4. Herpes simplex virus (vesicles form before ulcers develop) (see HERPES SIMPLEX section)
        a. In primary herpes simplex, lesions are confined to pharynx, tonsils and soft palate
        b. In secondary herpex simplex, lesions are at the vermillon border of lips
    5. Vincent's stomatitis (uclers appear on gingivae and are covered by purulent, gray exudate)
    6. Herpangina
        a. More common in children than adults
        b. Distinctive papular, vesicular, and ulcerative, multiple lesions on anterior tonsillar pillars, soft palate, tonsils, pharynx, and posterior buccal mucosa
    7. Acute necrotizing ulcerative gingivitis
    8. Trauma due to dental appliances or rough surfaced teeth
    9. Varicella (chicken pox)
    10. Pemphigus (presence of bullous lesions in mouth and other parts of body)

D. Diagnostic Tests
    1. Usually none indicated
    2. May do Vitamin B_{12}, folate and iron levels if nutritional deficiencies are suspected
    3. CBC with differential to assist in ruling out anemias
    4. Consider Tzanck smear for distinguishing herpetic stomatitis from other causes
    5. Biopsy is needed if cancer is suspected

V. Plan/Management

A. Pharmacologic treatment of minor lesions include one of following:
    1. Liquid antacids or 3% hydrogen peroxide/water solution, 1:1 as a gargle
    2. UlcerEase is a sodium bicarbonate based mouth rinse which acts as a soothing, cleansing, and buffering agent
    3. Xylocaine (Lidocaine 2%) viscous solution. May apply to lesions every 3 hours or use 15 mL as a gargle or mouthwash and swallow every 3 hours (maximum 8 doses/day).
    4. Diphenhydramine (Benadryl) elixir mixed 1:1 with attapulgite (Kaopectate) or aluminum hydroxide, magnesium hydroxide (Maalox). May be used as mouth rinse QID
    5. Amlexanox 5% (Aphthasol) adhesive oral paste. Start at earliest onset of symptoms; apply 1/4 inch to each ulcer QID. Wash hands after application. Continue until ulcer heals.
    6. Corticosteroid creams can provide pain relief and promote healing, but be cautious as they worsen viral infections; apply thin layer of triamcinolone acetonide 0.1% (Kenalog) in paste vehicle, Orabase, after meals and HS (moderate potency)

B. For acute clusterform lesions, treat simultaneously with the following two syrups:
    1. Tetracycline syrup (Sumycin) 250mg/10mL syrup QID for 7-14 days; rinse for 2 minutes and swallow; contraindicated in pregnant women
    2. Dexamthasone elixir (Decadron); rinse for 2 minutes QID and then expectorate
    3. Remind patient not to eat or drink for 20 minutes after this treatment

C. Treat severe recurrent aphthous ulcers with one of following:
    1. May require oral corticosteroids:
        a. Initially, prescribe prednisone 60 mg/day with tetracycline syrup QID
        b. Once lesions begin to heal, decrease prednisone by 5 mg (55mg/day) for 2 weeks, then 50 mg for 2 weeks and so on until 20 mg/day is reached; then give 20 mg every other day, tapering to 15 mg every other day, etc.
    2. Ask pharmacist to mix clobetasol propionate 0.05% (Temovate) ointment with an equal amount of Orabase; dry ulcer site lightly and apply sufficient paste to cover lesion three to six times daily

D. Patient Education
    1. Stress the importance of good oral hygiene
    2. Encourage good nutrition and increased fluid intake
    3. Avoid spicy, salty, and acidic foods and drinks
    4. Use soft-bristled toothbrush and avoid foods with sharp surfaces and talking while chewing
    5. Aphthous ulcers are not contagious, so no danger in spreading

E. Follow Up
    1. In severe cases, reschedule in 2-3 days
    2. Consult specialist if not healed in 2-3 weeks

TOOTHACHE (PULPITIS)

I.   Definition: A suppurative process that usually results from pulpal infection

II. Pathogenesis

   A.   Inflammation involving pulp tissue, the central portion of the tooth containing vital soft tissue, occurs due to injury of some type

   B.   Dental caries, a disease of the calcified tissues of the teeth, is the most frequent type of injury that causes pulpitis

   C.   Diverse flora, including gram-positive anaerobes and Bacteroides are the organisms most often involved in the infectious process

III. Clinical Presentation

   A.   Constant, throbbing pain is the most frequent presenting complaint

   B.   Affected tooth is extremely sensitive to touch and pain is intensified with the application of heat or cold (thermal sensitivity)

   C.   Tooth may be slightly extruded so that occlusal contact gives rise to exquisite pain

   D.   The affected area of the jaw is tender to palpation

   E.   Systemic manifestations may or may not be present and are usually limited to regional lymphadenopathy, malaise, and fever

IV. Diagnosis/Evaluation

   A.   History
        1.   Inquire about recent toothache
        2.   Inquire about occurrence of fever and chills
        3.   Inquire about heart murmur or defect
        4.   Determine type of medication taken for pain relief and when it was last taken

   B.   Physical Examination
        1.   Determine if febrile
        2.   Inspect and gently percuss teeth to determine location of affected tooth
        3.   Examine adjacent tissue for signs of inflammation
        4.   Observe for facial symmetry and examine jaw in area for signs of cellulitis
        5.   Auscultate heart (risk of sepsis and complications increase with valvular disease)
        6.   Examine for regional lymphadenopathy

   C.   Differential Diagnosis
        1.   Mumps
        2.   Cellulitis
        3.   Pericoronitis (painful wisdom teeth)

   D.   Diagnostic Tests: Should be done by dentist who will see patient

V.   Plan/Management

   A.   Patients with toothaches generally fall into one of three categories ranging from least to most serious and should be managed as follows

Category 1: Patients who are afebrile, with no extraoral swelling (no facial asymmetry present) or intraoral swelling
- ✓ Prescribe analgesics: Acetaminophen (300 mg) with codeine (30 mg) (Tylenol #3), 1-2 tabs, every 4 hours.
- ✓ Recommend warm salt water rinses (swish and spit) every 3-4 hours
- ✓ Refer to dentist within 24 hours

Category 2: Patients who have either slight extraoral or intraoral swelling, or who have a low-grade fever
- ✓ Prescribe analgesics (as above) and
- ✓ Prescribe antibiotics: Treatment of choice is Penicillin V (Pen-Vee-K): 250-500 mg Q 6 hours x 5-7 days.
- ✓ Patients allergic to penicillin should be treated with erythromycin; consult PDR for dosing recommendations
- ✓ Recommend warm salt water rinses (swish and spit) every 3-4 hours
- ✓ Refer to dentist within 12-24 hours

Category 3: Patients who have fever ≥101F (38.5°) with intraoral and/or extraoral swelling (causing facial asymmetry)
- ✓ Emergency consultation and treatment by dentist is needed
- ✓ Management must be immediate because the consequences of delayed treatment can be serious and occasionally life threatening!

B.   Treatment by the dentist for these three categories of toothache varies from extraction to root canal to incision and drainage, and to hospitalization for IV antibiotic therapy for patients with cellulitis

C.   Follow up should be done by dentist

PERIODONTAL DISEASE

I.   Definition: General term used to describe diseases that destroy the gingival and bony structures that support the teeth

A.   Usually divided into two types, gingivitis and periodontitis

B.   Major difference in the two types is that in periodontitis there is loss of supporting bony structure of the teeth

II.   Pathogenesis

A.   Poor dental hygiene which allows plaque to accumulate on the teeth is the major causative factor

B.   Initiating factors in the development of periodontal disease include bacterial plaque and calculus
1.   The initial changes in healthy gingiva after only a few days of plaque accumulation include an acute inflammation of the junctional epithelium (attachment of the gingiva to the enamel surface of the tooth)
2.   Within 2-4 weeks after the beginning of plaque formation, the gingivitis becomes established
3.   At some point, chronic gingivitis may progress to periodontitis, which is characterized by suppuration, bone loss, loss of attachment, pocket formation, tooth mobility, and loss of teeth

C.   Systemic factors that alter inflammatory and immune responses so that the host's defenses against bacteria or their metabolites are compromised include the following:
1.   Hormonal--pregnancy gingivitis is an exaggerated inflammatory response that may be caused by hormonal changes, especially in the third trimester
2.   Nutritional--Vitamin C deficiency in the development of periodontal disease is well established
3.   Drug Therapy--hyperplasia is associated with the use of phenytoin (Dilantin), cyclosporine, and calcium channel blockers

D. Local factors that modify the immunoinflammatory response and contribute of the progress of plaque-induced periodontal disease include the following:
1. Trauma from occlusion (bruxism) which tends to accelerate pocket formation and bone loss
2. Food impaction which occurs most frequently due to an impinging overbite
3. Mouth breathing and continued exposure and drying of the facial gingiva of the maxillary anterior teeth

III. Clinical Presentation

A. Approximately two-thirds of young adults and 80% of middle-aged and older adults suffer from periodontal disease

B. Most common cause of tooth loss in adults; occurs at all ages, but increases in prevalence and severity with age

C. Whereas dental caries damages the tooth itself, the supporting structures for the tooth, the gingiva, cementum, alveolar bone, and periodontal membrane are damaged by periodontal disease

D. Gingivitis presents in one of four forms: acute, subacute, recurrent, and chronic
1. Acute form, is characterized by rapid onset, short duration, and pain
2. Subacute form is less severe than acute
3. Recurrent form reappears after treatment or spontaneous remission
4. Chronic (most common form) is characterized by slow onset, long duration, and most often painless

E. Early signs of gingivitis include the following:
1. Inflammation of the gingiva (the normally coral-pink gingiva becomes bright red due to increased vascularity and decrease in keratinization)
2. Increased gingival fluid secretion
3. Bleeding from the gingival sulcus (usually with brushing)

F. Both acute and chronic forms produce changes in the gingiva which normally has a firm, resilient consistency
1. In acute forms (acute, subacute), gingiva appears diffusely edematous
2. In chronic forms (recurrent, chronic), gingiva has a fibrous appearance that pits with pressure

G. Major complication of untreated gingivitis is periodontitis
1. Patients with periodontitis present with red, bleeding gums, unpleasant taste in mouth, but usually has no pain (unless acute infection superimposed on chronic process)
2. Signs of gingivitis as described above are present and there is also periodontal pockets around the teeth containing purulent matter
3. As periodontitis progresses, teeth loosen, spread apart, causing difficulty chewing and pain
4. Eventually, destruction of the alveolar bone occurs and teeth are deprived of support and lost

IV. Diagnosis/Evaluation

A. History
1. Ask about onset and duration of symptoms
2. Ask about bleeding from gums after brushing
3. Inquire regarding dental hygiene habits
4. Question about bruxism, mouth breathing, and problems with occlusion
5. Obtain medication history

B. Physical Examination
    1. Examine teeth and gingiva for presence of plaque, and for hyperplasia or recession of gums
    2. Examine gums for areas of erosion
    3. Determine if gingival hyperplasia is generalized or localized

C. Differential Diagnosis
    1. Dental abscess
    2. Stomatitis

D. Diagnostic Tests: None indicated.

V. Plan/Management

A. Treatment of the four forms of gingivitis described above usually requires 1-3 dental visits and is aimed at elimination of local etiologic factors (plaque and calculus) which will result in a reversal of the gingival inflammation
    1. Plaque and calculus are removed using appropriate instruments
    2. Patients are instructed in proper plaque control measures (use of soft-bristled toothbrush that facilitates cleaning of teeth and gingiva; use of dental floss)
    3. Patients are scheduled for return visits for professional cleaning every 6 months
    4. Mouthwashes such as Peridex are helpful in the treatment of gingivitis
    5. Colgate Total is the first toothpaste FDA approved to prevent gingivitis (as well as cavities; it reduces plaque up to 50% and contains the antibacterial triclosan)

B. Patients with phenytoin-induced gingival hyperplasia usually require periodontal surgery

C. Mouth-breathing associated gingivitis usually is difficult to correct, but good plaque control can control the process in most cases

D. Most patients with periodontitis can be effectively treated although early diagnosis and referral are important
    1. The first phase of treatment is similar to that for gingivitis described above
    2. Phase 2 of treatment involves surgery to improve the gingival architecture that remains

E. Follow up should be by the dentist to whom patient was referred

CERVICAL ADENITIS

I. Definition: Acute pyogenic infection of a cervical lymph node

II. Pathogenesis

A. Usually reactive or secondary to an upper respiratory tract infection or dental infection; less frequently due to trauma

B. Pathogens:
    1. *Staphylococcus aureus* and *Streptococcus pyogenes* account for 80% of unilateral cervical adenitis
    2. Increasingly, anaerobic pathogens are being identified
    3. Less common pathogens: viruses and group B streptococci

III.   Clinical Presentation

A.   Less common in adults than children

B.   Typically, patient has a low-grade or no fever, malaise, and an upper respiratory infection or dental infection

C.   Usually presents as tender, soft, warm, rapidly enlarging lymph node with erythema of the overlying skin; node ranges from 2-6 cm.

D.   Most common site is the submandibular and anterior cervical areas

IV.   Diagnosis/Evaluation

A.   History
   1.   Ascertain duration and onset of node enlargement
   2.   Ask if node is increasing in size and whether overlying skin has changed in color
   3.   Ask about pain during eating which suggests parotid gland involvement
   4.   Question about dysphagia, odynophagia, strider, speech disorders, or a sensation of a lump in the throat
   5.   Inquire about associated constitutional symptoms
   6.   Question about recent infections, trauma, insect bites, pet scratches, TB contact, drug usage, and foreign travel

B.   Physical Examination
   1.   Measure vital signs
   2.   Observe for general state of health
   3.   Carefully examine scalp and face for skin lesions
   4.   Assess for facial-nerve weakness which can be caused by a parotid gland tumor
   5.   Thoroughly examine head, ears, eyes, nose, throat and mouth
   6.   Carefully examine neck for other masses and nuchal rigidity
   7.   Carefully palpate cervical mass to determine exact anatomic location, presence of tenderness, mobility, and consistency; examine skin overlying node for color
   8.   Thoroughly examine areas of lymph nodes
   9.   Inspect skin for lesions and rashes
   10.   Assess respiratory status
   11.   Palpate abdomen for organomegaly

C.   Differential Diagnosis (see Figure 9.1 for common location of masses of the neck)
   1.   Congenital cysts (these conditions need referral and usually surgery) (seen primarily in children)
        a.   Thyroglossal duct cyst (located at midline and typically moves with swallowing or tongue protrusion)
        b.   Branchial cleft cysts (small dimple or opening anterior to middle portion of the sternocleidomastoid muscle)
        c.   Cystic hygromas (fluid-filled, compressible mass in the posterior triangle just behind the sternocleidomastoid muscle and the supraclavicular fossa)
   2.   Salivary gland disorders; salivary glands are located in area of lymph nodes and enlarged glands may be confused as cervical adenitis; care must be taken to distinguish glands from nodes; for example, enlargement of the parotid gland obliterates the angle of the mandible

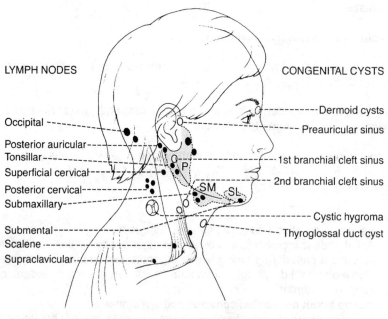

LYMPH NODES   CONGENITAL CYSTS

Occipital

Posterior auricular
Tonsillar
Superficial cervical
Posterior cervical
Submaxillary

Submental
Scalene
Supraclavicular

Dermoid cysts
Preauricular sinus

1st branchial cleft sinus
2nd branchial cleft sinus

Cystic hygroma
Thyroglossal duct cyst

P = Parotid gland, S = Submandibular gland, SL = Sublingual gland

Figure 9.1. Common Location of Masses of the Face and Neck.

3. Cervical lymphadenopathy (see section on LYMPHADENOPATHY); in children most single neck masses are due to cervical lymphadenopathy but in adults >40 years, 80% of isolated solitary neck masses are due to malignant neoplasm
    a. Viral infections (most common)
        (1) Often due to herpesviruses, adenoviruses, enteroviruses, and Ebstein-Barr virus
        (2) Nodes are typically bilateral, discrete, oval, soft, and minimally tender
    b. Bacterial infections of the upper respiratory tract and mouth
    c. Cat Scratch Disease (see CAT SCRATCH DISEASE section)
    d. Atypical mycobacterium
    e. Toxoplasmosis
    f. Systemic disorders such as lupus, rheumatoid arthritis, sarcoidosis, histoplasmosis
4. Malignancy
    a. Neck mass is usually persistent and enlarging
    b. 80% of tumors in adults are associated with tobacco and alcohol use
    c. Node is often supraclavicular, firm and fixated to skin and underlying tissue
    d. Patient often has persistent fever, weight loss, voice change, hearing loss, voice change
    e. On physical examination, patient may have lesion in oral cavity or pharynx or unilateral nasal obstruction
5. Generalized lymphadenopathy is usually caused by systemic disease (see LYMPHADENOPATHY section)
6. Thyroid nodules or goiters may be confused with enlarged nodes

D. Diagnostic Tests
1. Ultrasound is helpful in establishing whether mass is solid, cystic, or fluctuant
2. In moderately or severely ill patient, consider CBC, sedimentation rate, throat culture, and blood culture
3. PPD should be considered if tuberculosis is suspected
4. Heterophil tests or titers for Epstein-Barr virus, cytomegalovirus, and *Toxoplasma* may be indicated to rule-out specific viral infections
5. Consider aspiration and culture in patients who have large, fluctuant nodes which do not respond to initial therapy
6. Biopsy of node is needed when malignancy is suspected

V. Plan/Management

    A. For patient who appears well with minimal pain, close observation for 2-3 days and symptomatic treatment may be all that is needed
        1. Prescribe analgesic such as tylenol or nonsteroidal anti-inflammatory agent
        2. Warm compresses every 4 hours

    B. For the patient with moderate to severe adenitis prescribe one of following antibiotics:
        1. Amoxicillin/clavulanic acid (Augmentin) 500 TID or 875 mg BID
        2. Cephalexin (Keflex) 500 mg BID

    C. Adults who fail to improve with antibiotic therapy or who have warning symptoms and signs of malignancy need referral to specialist

    D. Patient Education
        1. Emphasize that patient should immediately return if difficulty of swallowing or breathing occurs
        2. Reinforce that follow-up is important if symptoms persist

    E. Follow Up
        1. Return to clinic if symptoms not resolved in 2-3 days
        2. For the patient who appears well and is treated only symptomatically, reevaluate symptoms at 3-5 day intervals; some nodes take many weeks to regress but other nodes regress spontaneously within 2-3 weeks without pharmacological treatment
        3. Reevaluate patients who are treated with antibiotics after completion of therapy
        4. Individualize follow-up for of patients who are at risk for systemic or serious disorders

REFERENCES

Armstrong, W.B., & Giglio, M.F. (1998). Is this lump in the neck anything to worry about? How to recognize warning signs of an abnormal mass. Postgraduate Medicine, 104, 63-78.

Ash, M.M. (1992). Oral pathology: An introduction to general and oral pathology for hygienists. Philadelphia: Lea & Febiger.

Barnett, E.D. (1997). Comparison of ceftriaxone and trimethoprim-sulfamethoxazole for acute otitis media. Pediatrics, 99, 23-28.

Bisno, A.L. (1996). Acute pharyngitis: Etiology and diagnosis. Pediatrics, 97 (Suppl), 949-954.

Bojrab, D.I., Bruderly, T., & Abdulrazzak, Y. (1996). Otitis externa. Otolaryngologic Clinics of North America, 29(5), 761-782.

Brunton, S. (1997). Allergic rhinitis: Breaking the cycle of disease and treatment. Family Practice Recertification, 19, 14-32

Burgett, F. (1993). Periodontal disease. In J.A. Regezi & J. Sciubba (Eds.), Oral pathology: Clinical-Pathologic correlations. Philadelphia: Saunders.

Consensus Conference Proceedings. (1995). The chronic airway disease connection: Redefining rhinitis. Los Angeles: UCCLA School of Medicine, Office of Continuing Medical Education.

Connolly, A.A.P., & MacKenzie, K. (1997). Paediatric neck masses--a diagnostic dilemma. Journal of Laryngology and Otology, 111, 541-545.

Culpepper, L., & Froom, J. (1997). Routine antimicrobial treatment of acute otitis media: Is it necessary. JAMA, 278, 1643-1645.

Dowell, S.F., Marcy, S.M., Phillips, W.R., Gerber, M.A., & Schwartz, B. (1998). Otitis media--principles of judicious use of antimicrobial agents. Pediatrics, 101, 171-174.

Eden, A.N., Fineman, P., & Stool, S.E. (1996). Managing acute otitis: A fresh look at a familiar problem. Contemporary Pediatrics, 13,(3), 64-65,70,73-85.

Ferguson, B.J. (1997). Allergic rhinitis: Recognizing signs, symptoms, and triggering allergens. Postgraduate Medicine, 101, 110-131.

Forzley, G.J. (1994). Cerumen impaction removal. In J.L. Pfenninger, & G.C. Fowler (Eds.), <u>Procedures for primary care physicians</u>. St. Louis: Mosby.

Goroll, A.H., May, L.A., & Mulley, A.G., Jr. (1995). Management of aphthous stomatitis. In A.H. Goroll, L.A. May, & A.G. Mulley, Jrs. (Eds.), <u>Primary care medicine.</u> Philadelphia: Lippincott.

Gwaltney, J.M., Jones, J.G., & Kennedy, D.W. (1997). Medical management of sinusitis: Educational goals and management guidelines. <u>Annals of Otology, Rhinology, and Laryngology, Suppl. 167,</u> 22-30.

Hathaway, T.J. (1994). Acute otitis media: Who needs posttreatment follow-up? <u>Pediatrics, 94,</u> 143-147.

Haynes, J.H., & Newkirk, G.R. (1994). Removal of foreign bodies from the ear and nose. In J.L. Pfenninger, & G.C. Fowler (Eds.), <u>Procedures for primary care physicians</u>. St. Louis: Mosby.

Hays, G.L. (1997). Diseases of the mouth. In R.E. Rakel (Ed.), <u>1997 Conn's current therapy</u>. Philadelphia: Saunders.

Herendeen, N.E., & Szilagyi, P.G. (1997). Cystic and solid masses of the face and neck. In R.A. Hoekelman et al., (Ed.). <u>Primary Pediatric Care,</u> St. Louis: Mosby.

Herzon, F.S. (1995). Peritonsillar Abscess: Incidence, current management practices, and a proposal for treatment guidelines. <u>Laryngoscope, 105,</u> 1-17.

Isaacson, G., & Rosenfel, R.M. (1996). Care of the child with tympanostomy tubes. <u>Pediatric Clinics of North America, 43,</u> 1183-1193.

Kaiser, H.B., Kay, G.G., & Palakanis, K. (1998). Contemporary issues in the management of allergic disorders: A focus on respiratory and dermatologic manifestations. <u>Clinical Courier, 16</u> (46), 1-7.

La Rosa, S. (1998). Primary care management of otitis externa. <u>Nurse Practitioner, 23</u>(6), 125-133.

Little, D.R., Mann, B.L., & Sherk, D.W. (1998). Factors influencing the clinical diagnosis of sinusitis. <u>The Journal of Family Practice, 46,</u> 147-153.

Low, D.E., Desrosiers, M., McSherry, J., Garber, G., & other Canadian Sinusitis Symposium Panel. (1997). A practical guide for the diagnosis and treatment of acute sinusitis. <u>Canadian Medical Association Journal, 156</u> (6 suppl.), S1-S14.

MacLeod, D.K. (1998). Common problems of the teeth and oral cavity. In L.R. Barker, J.R. Burton, & P.D. Zieve (Eds.), <u>Principles of ambulatory medicine</u>. Baltimore: Williams & Wilkins.

Mirza, N. (1996). Otitis externa: Management in the primary care office. <u>Postgraduate Medicine, 99</u>(5), 153-158.

Noble, S.L., Forbes, R.C., & Woodbridge, H.B. (1995). Allergic rhinitis. <u>American Family Physician, 51,</u>837-846.

O'Brien, K.L., Dowell, S.F., Schwartz, B., Marcy, S.M., Phillips, W.R., & Gerber, M.A. (1998). Acute sinusitis--principles of judicious use of antimicrobial agents. <u>Pediatrics, 101,</u> 174-177.

Otitis Media with Effusion in Young Chidren Guideline Panel. (1994). <u>Otitis Media with Effusion in Young Children: Clinical Practice Guideline, No. 12.</u> (ACHPR Publication No. 94-0622) Rockville, MD.

Parsons, D.S. (1996). Chronic sinusitis: A medical or surgical disease? <u>Otolaryngologic Clinics of North America, 29,</u> 1-9.

Parsons, D.S., & Van Leeuwen, R.N (1997). Otitis externa. In Rakel, R. E. (Ed.), <u>Conn's current therapy</u>. Philadelphia: W.B. Saunders.

Pellett, F.S., Cox, L.C., & MacDonald, C.B. (1997). Use of acoustic reflectometry in the detection of middle ear effusion. <u>Journal of American Academy of Audiology, 8,</u> 181-187.

Perkins, A. (1997). An approach to diagnosing the acute sore throat. <u>American Family Physician, 55,</u> 131-138.

Peterson, M.J., & Baughman, R.A. (1996). Recurrent aphthous stomatitis: Primary care management. <u>Nurse Practitioner, 21,</u> 36-47.

Roark, R., & Berman. S. (1997). Continuous twice daily or once daily amoxicillin prophylaxis compared with placebo for children with recurrent acute otitis media. <u>Pediatric Infectious Disease Journal, 16,</u> 376-381.

Root, P., & Paul, D. (1996). Hearing loss. In M.B. Mengel and L.P. Schwiebert, (Eds.). <u>Ambulatory medicine: The primary care of families</u> (3rd ed.). Stamford, CT: Appleton & Lange.

Rosenfeld, R.M. (1996). An evidence-based approach to treating otitis media. <u>Pediatric Clinics of North America, 43,</u> 1165-1181.

Ruckenstein, M.J. (1995). Hearing loss: A plan for individualized management. <u>Postgraduate Medicine, 98,</u> 197-214.

Schantz, N.V. (1994). Management of epistaxis. In J.L. Pfenninger, & G.C. Fowler (Eds.), <u>Procedures for primary care physicians</u>. St. Louis: Mosby.

Schwartz, B., Marcy, S.M., Phillips, W.R., Gerber, M.A., & Dowell, S.F., (1998). Pharyngitis--principles of judicious use of antimicrobial agents. <u>Pediatrics, 101,</u> 171-174.

Smith, L.J. (1995). Diagnosis and treatment of allergic rhinitis. <u>Nurse Practitioner, 20</u>, 58-66.

Weiss, J.C., Yates, G.R., & Quinn, L.D. (1996). Acute otitis media: making an accurate diagnosis. <u>American Family Physician, 43,</u> 1200-1206.

Williams, J.W., & Simel, D.L. (1993). Does this patient have sinusitis? Diagnosing acute sinusitis by history and physical examination. <u>JAMA, 270,</u> 1242-1246.

CHAPTER 10

Problems of the Upper Airways, Lower Respiratory System

ASTHMA

I.   Definition: Chronic inflammatory disorder of the airways which causes bronchial hyperresponsiveness to stimuli and recurrent episodes of respiratory symptoms which are usually associated with reversible airflow obstruction

II. Pathogenesis

    A.   Inflammation plays a central role
        1.   Results from complex interactions among many cells and cellular elements (mast cells, eosinophils, T lymphocytes, macrophages, neutrophils, and epithelial cells)
        2.   Inflammation is associated with airway obstruction, airway hyperresponsiveness, respiratory symptoms, and disease chronicity

    B.   Airway obstruction leads to airflow limitation and is usually widespread, recurrent, variable and reversible either with treatment or spontaneously; obstruction is due to the following:
        1.   Acute bronchoconstriction results from airway hyperresponsiveness after exposure to a variety of stimuli such as allergens, drugs (aspirin, nonsteroidal anti-inflammatory drugs), stimuli (exercise, cold air, irritants) and possibly stress
        2.   Airway wall edema and mucosal thickening are caused by increased microvascular permeability and leakage
        3.   Chronic mucus plug formation sometimes occurs in severe, intractable cases
        4.   Airway wall remodeling may develop in severe cases, causing persistent abnormalities in lung function which are unresponsive to treatment

    C.   Factors contributing to asthma severity:
        1.   Inhaled allergens such as animal allergens, house-dust mites, outdoor allergens, indoor fungi, and cockroaches
        2.   Occupational exposures
        3.   Irritants such as tobacco smoke and pollution
        4.   Rhinitis/sinusitis
        5.   Gastroesophageal reflux
        6.   Sensitivity to aspirin, other nonsteroidal anti-inflammatory drugs, and sulfites
        7.   Topical and systemic beta-blockers
        8.   Viral respiratory infection

    D.   Adult-onset asthma may be related to allergies, but some adults have coexisting sinusitis, nasal polyps, and sensitivity to aspirin or nonsteroidal antiinflammatory drugs; occupational exposure to workplace materials may also be a factor

III. Clinical Presentation

    A.   Underdiagnosis and inappropriate therapy are major factors in morbidity and mortality

    B.   Typically, symptoms begin in childhood or adolescence, but can develop in adulthood

    C.   Exercise-induced bronchospasm occurs with loss of heat and/or water from lung during exercise; cough, shortness of breath, chest pain or tightness, wheezing or endurance problems may develop during exercise

    D.   Spectrum ranges from few mild episodes in a lifetime to daily debilitating symptoms; classification of asthma severity is based on symptoms and lung function before treatment (see following table)

CLASSIFICATION OF THE SEVERITY OF ASTHMA*

Step/ Category	Symptoms**	Nighttime Symptoms	Lung Functions
STEP 4 Severe Persistent	✦Continual symptoms ✦Limited physical activity ✦Frequent exacerbations	Frequent	✦FEV$_1$ or PEF ≤60%predicted ✦PEF variability >30%
STEP 3 Moderate Persistent	✦Daily symptoms ✦Daily use of inhaled short-acting beta$_2$-agonist ✦Exacerbations affect activity ✦Exacerbations are ≥2 times a week	>1 time a week	✦FEV$_1$ or PEF >60%-<80% predicted ✦PEF variability >30%
STEP 2 Mild Persistent	✦Symptoms >2 times a week but <1 time a day ✦Exacerbations may affect activity	>2 times a month	✦FEV$_1$ or PEF ≥80% predicted ✦PEF variability 20-30%
STEP 1 Mild Intermittent	✦Symptoms ≤2 times/week ✦Asymptomatic & normal PEF between exacerbations ✦Exacerbations brief (from a few hours to few days) intensity may vary	≤2 times a month	✦FEV$_1$ or PEF ≥80% predicted ✦PEF variability <20%

*The presence of one of the features of severity is sufficient to classify patient in that category. A patient should be assigned to the most severe grade in which any feature occurs.
**Patients at any level of severity can have mild, moderate, or severe exacerbations.

Adapted from National Institutes of Health. National Heart, Lung, and Blood Institute. (1997). The Expert Panel Report 2: Guidelines for the Diagnosis and Management of Asthma. National Asthma Education Program. NIH Publ. #97-4051. Bethesda, MD.

IV. Diagnosis/Evaluation

    A.   History
        1.   Identify the symptoms likely to be due to asthma (see table on KEY INDICATORS)

KEY INDICATORS OF ASTHMA

✔ Wheezing

✔ History of any of the following:
    ✦ Cough worse at night or in early morning
    ✦ Recurrent difficulty breathing
    ✦ Recurrent tightness in chest

✔ Reversible airflow limitation and diurinal variation as measured by peak flow meter

✔ Symptoms occur or are worsened by any of the following:
    ✦ Exercise, viral infection, animals, house-dust mites, mold, smoke, pollen, changes in weather, laughing, hard crying, airborne chemicals or dusts, menses

✔ Symptoms occur or worsen at night, awakening the patient

Adapted from National Institutes of Health. National Heart, Lung, and Blood Institute. (1997). The Expert Panel Report 2: Guidelines for the Diagnosis and Management of Asthma. National Asthma Education Program. NIH Publ. #97-4051. Bethesda, MD.

        2.   Assess onset and duration of symptoms (number of days/nights per week/month)
        3.   Determine whether symptoms are seasonal, continuous, episodic, or diurnal
        4.   Determine profile of asthma attacks or exacerbations
        5.   Assess past and present management strategies and responses
        6.   Inquire about factors known to be related to asthma
        7.   Determine family history of asthma, allergy, sinusitis, rhinitis, or nasal polyps
        8.   Assess impact of disease such as effects on family, finances, school, work, activity, sleep, and behavior
        9.   Assess patient's and family's perceptions such as knowledge level, understanding of treatments, sociocultural beliefs
      10.   For persons with occupational asthma, inquire about number of sick days taken from work per month
      11.   At each follow-up visit assess whether the goals of therapy are being met

B.   Physical Examination
1.   Determine pulse rate and respiratory rate
2.   Assess for signs of dehydration such as delayed capillary refill, poor skin turgor, and dry mucous membranes
3.   Observe for use of accessory respiratory muscles, retractions, nasal flaring, diaphoresis, and cyanosis.
4.   Observe for hyperexpansion of thorax (hunched shoulders or chest deformity)
5.   Observe for flexural eczema or other manifestations of allergic skin conditions
6.   Assess for nasal discharge, mucosal swelling, frontal tenderness, postnasal discharge, nasal polyps, and allergic shiners (dark discoloration beneath both eyes)
7.   Auscultate and percuss lungs
     a.   Wheezing during forced exhalation is no longer believed to be a reliable indicator
     b.   In mild, intermittent asthma, wheezing may be absent between attacks; in severe asthma wheezing may be absent due to diminished breath sounds
8.   Perform a complete cardiac examination

C.   Differential Diagnosis
1.   Underdiagnosis of asthma is common
2.   Remember that recurrent episodes of coughing and wheezing are usually due to asthma; the following should be included in the differential diagnosis:
     a.   Vocal cord dysfunction can cause recurrent wheezing
     b.   Enlarged lymph nodes, tumors
     c.   Pulmonary infections such as pneumonia, tuberculosis, mycoplasma and respiratory syncytial virus disorder
     d.   Gastroesophageal reflux
     e.   Chronic obstructive pulmonary disease
     f.   Congestive heart failure
     g.   Pulmonary embolism
     h.   Cough secondary to drugs such as ACE inhibitors

D.   Diagnostic Tests; regular monitoring of pulmonary function is essential, particularly for patients who do not perceive their symptoms until airways are severely obstructed
1.   Spirometry tests
     a.   Recommended at following intervals:
          (1)   Time of diagnosis
          (2)   After treatment when symptoms and peak flow reading are stabilized to document attainment of normal airway function
          (3)   Every 1-2 years to monitor maintenance of airway function
     b.   More frequent testing is needed in the following cases: to check accuracy of peak flow, when precision is needed to determine treatment response, and when peak flow readings may be unreliable such as when patients are elderly or have neuromuscular problems
2.   Order an exercise challenge test to confirm exercised-induced bronchospasm
3.   Other tests to consider: chest x-ray or CBC if infection is suspected; skin testing or in vitro testing for patients with persistent asthma exposed to perennial indoor allergens
4.   Peak expiratory flow (PEF) meters
     a.   **Should be used to monitor lung function not to confirm diagnosis**
     b.   Daily monitoring is not mandatory for all patients, but is important for patients after an exacerbation and for patients with moderate-to-severe, persistent asthma
     c.   Teach patients to determine their best PEF (see table that follows)

PATIENT EDUCATION OF THE PEAK FLOW METER

1. Demonstrate and have return demonstration of use of peak flow meter
    ● Stand, do not sit
    ● Place indicator at bottom of numbered scale
    ● Take deep breath
    ● Close lips around mouthpiece
    ● Blow out as hard and fast as possible in a single blow
2. Teach patient to repeat #1 two more times and record the best of the three blows
3. Instruct patients how to determine their personal best peak flow number
    ● Take readings twice a day for 2-3 weeks: upon awakening or between 12 noon & 2:00 p.m.
    ● Take readings before and after inhaling beta$_2$-agonist
4. Explain that personal best peak flow numbers are categorized into zones to help patients self-manage their illness and to assess progression of disease and need for additional therapy
    ● Green Zone: 80% of patient's personal best and denotes good control
    ● Yellow Zone: 50-<80% of patient's personal best and denotes caution and the need to take a short-acting inhaled beta$_2$-agonist
    ● Red Zone: <50% of patient's personal best and denotes severe asthma exacerbation and the need to take short-acting inhaled beta$_2$agonist and call health care provider or emergency room or go directly to hospital
5. Explain to patient that once their personal best peak flow is documented they may decrease peak flow readings to once a day in the morning. If morning reading is <80% of personal best, instruct patient to monitor more frequently

Adapted from National Institutes of Health. National Heart, Lung, and Blood Institute. (1997). The Expert Panel Report 2: Guidelines for the Diagnosis and Management of Asthma. National Asthma Education Program. NIH Publ. #97-4051. Bethesda, MD.

V.   Plan/Management

A.   Referral to an asthma specialist is recommended in the following situations:
      1.   Life-threatening or severe, persistent asthma (step 4) is present
      2.   Goals of asthma therapy are not fulfilled after 3 to 6 months of treatment
      3.   Signs and symptoms are atypical or diagnosis is uncertain
      4.   Other illness such as sinusitis, gastroesophageal reflux, of chronic obstructive pulmonary disease complicate the airway disease
      5.   Immunotherapy is a treatment consideration
      6.   Continuous oral corticosteroids or high-dose inhaled corticosteroids or two bursts of oral steroids in 1 year are needed

B.   Control of the factors contributing to asthma severity is important
      1.   Instruct patient to avoid the following:
            a.   Allergens (see table: MEASURES OF ENVIRONMENTAL CONTROL in section: ALLERGIC AND NONALLERGIC RHINITIS)
            b.   Environmental tobacco smoke
            c.   Exercise when levels of pollution are high
            d.   Beta-blockers
            e.   Foods containing sulfite and other foods to which they are sensitive
      2.   Caution patients with severe, persistent asthma, nasal polyps, or a history of sensitivity to aspirin or nonsteroidal anti-inflammatory drugs that there is risk of severe and possibly fatal exacerbations when using these drugs
      3.   Treat patients for rhinitis, sinusitis, and gastroesophageal reflux if present
      4.   Recommend annual influenza vaccination

C. General pharmacological principles; a stepwise pharmacological approach is recommended (see Table on Stepwise Approach in Adults)

STEPWISE APPROACH FOR MANAGING ASTHMA IN ADULTS : TREATMENT

Preferred treatments are in bold print.

	Long-Term Control	Quick Relief
STEP 4 Severe Persistent	Daily medications: ■ **Anti-inflammatory: inhaled corticosteroid (high dose)** **AND** ■ Long-acting bronchodilator: either **long-acting inhaled beta$_2$-agonist**, sustained-release theophylline, or long-acting beta$_2$-agonist tablets AND ■ Corticosteroid tablets or syrup long term	■ Short-acting bronchodilator: **inhaled beta$_2$-agonists** as needed for symptoms.
STEP 3 Moderate Persistent	Daily medication: (Initial Plan) ■ Either **Anti-inflammatory: inhaled corticosteroid (medium dose)** OR Inhaled corticosteroid (low-medium dose) and add a long-acting bronchodilator, especially for nighttime symptoms; either **long-acting inhaled beta$_2$-agonist**, sustained-release theophylline, or long-acting beta$_2$-agonist tablets. (Additional Plan) ■ If needed Anti-inflammatory: **inhaled corticosteroids (medium-high dose)** **AND** **Long-acting inhaled beta$_2$-agonist**, sustained-release theophylline, or long-acting beta$_2$-agonist tablets.	■ Short-acting bronchodilator: **inhaled beta$_2$-agonists** as needed for symptoms.
STEP 2 Mild Persistent	One daily medication: ■ **Anti-inflammatory**: either **inhaled corticosteroid** (low doses) or **cromolyn or nedocromil** ■ Sustained-release theophylline to serum concentration as alternative, but not preferred, therapy. Zafirlukast or zileuton may also be considered.	■ Short-acting bronchodilator: **inhaled beta$_2$-agonists** as needed for symptoms.
STEP 1 Mild Intermittent	■ No daily medication needed.	■ Short-acting bronchodilator: **inhaled beta$_2$-agonists** as needed for symptoms.

Step down
↓ Review treatment every 1 to 6 months; a gradual stepwise reduction in treatment may be possible.

Step up
↑ If control is not maintained, consider step up. First, review patient medication technique, adherence, and environmental control (avoidance of allergens or other factors that contribute to asthma severity).

Adapted from National Institutes of Health. National Heart, Lung, and Blood Institute. (1997). The Expert Panel Report 2: Guidelines for the Diagnosis and Management of Asthma. National Asthma Education Program. NIH Publ. #97-4051. Bethesda, MD.

1. The dose and dosing interval are dictated by the asthma severity with the goal of suppressing airway inflammation and preventing exacerbations
2. Begin therapy at a high level (short course of systemic corticosteroids plus inhaled corticosteroids or use of medium-to-high dose of inhaled corticosteroids) to promptly control symptoms and then lower level
3. Cautiously and very gradually step down therapy after control is achieved and sustained for several weeks or months
    a. Generally, the last medication added should be the first medication reduced
    b. Inhaled corticosteroids may be reduced 25% every 2-3 months to the lowest dose possible to maintain control

4. Continual monitoring is imperative; control is indicated by the following:
   a. Peak expiratory flow (PEF) less than 10-20% variability
   b. PEF consistently greater than 80% patient's personal best
   c. Minimal symptoms
   d. Minimal need for short-acting inhaled beta$_2$-agonist
   e. Absence of nighttime awakenings
   f. No activity limitations
5. Other actions needed if control is not achieved and sustained at any step
   a. Assess patient adherence and technique in using medication
   b. Step up to next higher step of care or temporarily increase anti-inflammatory therapy such as with a burst of prednisone
   c. Reassess for factors that diminish control
   d. Consult a specialist
6. Long-term control drugs are used daily to maintain control of persistent asthma; quick-relief drugs treat acute symptoms and exacerbations (see following tables)

LONG-TERM CONTROL MEDICATIONS

1. Corticosteroids are the most potent and effective anti-inflammatory agents
   ✓ Oral/systemic form used for prompt control when initiating long-term therapy
   ✓ Inhaled form is preferred for long-term control
   ✓ Benefits outweigh risk of adverse effects; to reduce adverse effects, the following are recommended:
      * Use with spacers/holding chambers
      * Rinse mouth after use
      * Use lowest possible dose to maintain control
      * Do not give varicella vaccine to patients receiving ≥2 mg/kg or 20 mg/day of oral prednisone
   ✓ In postmenopausal women, consider supplements of calcium and vitamin D or estrogen therapy

2. Cromolyn sodium and nedocromil are mild to moderate anti-inflammatory medications
   ✓ Comparison of nedocromil and cromolyn
      * Nedocromil is more potent in inhibiting bronchospasm due to exercise, cold dry air and bradykinin aerosol; more effective in nonallergic patients using inhaled corticosteroids
      * Nedocromil may help reduce dose requirements of corticosteroids

3. Long-acting beta$_2$-agonists are used with anti-inflammatory medications; helpful for nocturnal symptoms
   ✓ Salmetrol **is not used for treatment of acute symptoms or exacerbations**
   ✓ Daily use of these drugs should not exceed 84 mcg (salmeterol: 4 puffs)
   ✓ Even if symptoms improve, patients should **not** stop anti-inflammatory medication

4. Methylxanthines (mainly sustained-release theophylline) are used as adjuvant to inhaled corticosteroids for prevention of nocturnal symptoms
   ✓ Although not preferred, sustained-release theophylline may be alternative for long-term preventive therapy when cost or adherence in using inhaled medications is problematic
   ✓ Essential to monitor serum concentration levels
   ✓ Smoking increases metabolism of theophylline

5. Leukotriene modifiers are alternatives to low doses of inhaled corticosteroids or cromolyn or nedocromil for persons with mild persistent asthma (need more research & experience)
   ✓ Zafirlukast has an interaction effect with warfarin; essential to closely monitor prothrombin times and adjust appropriately
   ✓ Zileuton
      * May infrequently cause liver toxicity; essential to monitor liver enzymes
      * May inhibit metabolism of terfenadine, warfarin, and theophylline
   ✓ Montelukast sodium (Singular)

QUICK-RELIEF MEDICATIONS

1. Therapy of choice is a short-acting beta$_2$-agonist
   - ✓ Use of >1 canister in 1 month signifies poor control & need to begin or increase anti-inflammatory drug
   - ✓ Regularly scheduled, daily use of these drugs is **not** recommended

2. Anticholinergics (ipratropium bromide) may provide additive benefit to inhaled beta$_2$-agonist or may be alternative quick-relief drug for patients unable to tolerate inhaled beta$_2$-agonist

3. Oral/systemic corticosteroids are used for moderate-to-severe exacerbations and can speed resolution of airflow obstruction and reduce rate of relapse

D. Treatment of **Step 1: Mild intermittent asthma in adults**
  1. Prescribe short-acting inhaled beta$_2$-agonist on an as-needed basis (see table)

DOSAGES FOR INHALED BETA$_2$-AGONISTS			
Medication	Dosage Form	Adult Dose	Comments
Short-Acting Inhaled Beta$_2$-Agonists			
	Metered-Dose Inhaler		
Albuterol (Ventolin)	90 mcg/puff, 200 puffs	■ 2 puffs TID-QID prn	■ Increasing or regular use on a daily basis indicates the need for additional long-term-control therapy.
Pirbuterol (Maxair Autohaler)	200 mcg/puff, 400 puffs		
	Dry Powder Inhaler		
Albuterol Rotacaps (Ventolin)	200 mcg/capsule	1-2 capsules Q 4-6 hours prn	
	Nebulizer solution		
Albuterol (Ventolin)	5 mg/mL (0.5%)	1.25-5 mg (.25-1 cc) in 2-3 cc of saline Q 4-8 hours	May mix with cromolyn or ipratropium nebulizer solutions.
Bitolterol (Tornalate)	2 mg/mL (0.2%)	0.5-3.5 mg (.25-1 cc) in 2-3 cc of saline Q 4-8 hours	May not mix with other nebulizer solutions.

Adapted from National Institutes of Health. National Heart, Lung, and Blood Institute. (1997). The Expert Panel Report 2: Guidelines for the Diagnosis and Management of Asthma. National Asthma Education Program. NIH Publ. #97-4051. Bethesda, MD.

  2. Treatment of **exercise-induced bronchospasm**; use one of following:
    a. Short-acting inhaled beta$_2$-agonist 1-2 puffs 5 minutes prior to exercise
    b. Inhaled cromolyn sodium (Intal) or nedocromil (Tilade) 2 puffs 10 minutes prior to exercise
  3. Treatment of **mild exacerbations** due to viral respiratory infections: prescribe short-acting beta$_2$-agonist every 4-6 hours for approximately 24 hours
  4. **Treatment of moderate-to-severe exacerbations:**
    a. Use both of the following:
      (1) Give short-acting beta$_2$-agonist by nebulizer or MDI (with close supervision can give 3 treatments spaced every 20-30 minutes)
      (2) Also, prescribe systemic corticosteroid; patients with history of severe exacerbations should start corticosteroids at first sign of infection (see Table on SYSTEMIC CORTICOSTEROIDS)
    b. Oxygen is recommended for most patients
    c. Careful, vigilant monitoring of patient's condition is paramount

DOSAGES FOR SYSTEMIC CORTICOSTEROIDS			
Medication	**Dosage Form**	**Adult Dose**	**Comments**
Methylprednisolone (Medrol)

Prednisone (Deltasone) | 2, 4, 8, 16, 24, 32 mg tablets

1, 2.5, 5, 10, 20, 50 mg tabs | ■ Short course "burst": 40-60 mg/day as single or 2 divided doses for 3-10 days | ■ The burst should be continued until patient achieves 80% PEF personal best or symptoms resolve. This usually requires 3-10 days but may require longer.
■ Give first dose in AM and last dose by 6 PM |

Adapted from National Institutes of Health. National Heart, Lung, and Blood Institute. (1997). The Expert Panel Report 2: Guidelines for the Diagnosis and Management of Asthma. National Asthma Education Program. NIH Publ. #97-4051. Bethesda, MD.

E. Treatment of **Step 2: Mild Persistent Asthma in Adults**: Use inhaled short-acting beta$_2$-agonist on an as-needed basis as well as one of the following:

1. Inhaled corticosteroids at a low dose (see Table on DOSAGES OF INHALED CORTICOSTEROIDS); when taking several inhaled medications simultaneously, always use beta$_2$-agonist first to open airway and then use steroid inhaler for greater penetration of medication

2. Cromolyn (Intal) or Nedocromil (Tilade) can be tried; however, these medications are more effective in children than adults
    a. Cromolyn
        (1) Metered-Dose Inhaler (MDI) (1 mg/puff): Use 2-4 puffs TID or QID
        (2) Nebulizer (20mg/ampule); for all ages use 1 ampule TID or QID
    b. Nedocromil (MDI 1.75 mg/puff): 2-4 puff BID-QID

3. Sustained-release theophylline is an alternative, but is not preferred because of modest effectiveness and potential for toxicity; prescribe drug to achieve a serum concentration of between 5 and 15 mcg/mL (periodic monitoring is necessary to maintain a therapeutic level); begin dose at 10 mg/kg/day up to 300 mg maximum; usual maximum is 800 mg/day

4. Zafirlukast, zileuton, and montelukast sodium are alternative drugs; long-term treatment uncertain because of lack of research and clinical experience
    a. Zafirlukast (Accolate): One 20 mg tablet BID (take 1 hour before or 2 hours after meals)
    b. Zileuton (Zyflo): 600 mg QID (Available 300 mg and 600 mg tablets); regularly monitor hepatic enzymes
    c. Montelukast sodium (Singular): 10 mg tab QD in evening for individuals >14 years

5. For exacerbations, see V.D.3.4 and V.J.

DAILY DOSAGES OF INHALED CORTICOSTEROIDS			
Drug	Low Dose	Medium Dose	High Dose
Beclomethasone dipropionate 42 mcg/puff 84 mcg/puff	168-504 mcg (4-12 puffs--42 mcg) (2-6 puffs--84 mcg)	504-840 mcg (12-20 puffs--42 mcg) (6-10 puffs--84 mcg)	>840 mcg (>20 puffs--42 mcg) (>10 puffs--84 mcg)
Budesonide DPI: 200 mcg/dose	200-400 mcg (1-2 inhalations)	400-600 mcg (2-3 inhalations)	>600 mcg (>3 inhalations)
Flunisolide 250 mcg/puff	500-1,000 mcg (2-4 puffs)	1,000-2,000 mcg (4-8 puffs)	>2,000 mcg (>8 puffs)
Fluticasone MDI: 44, 110, 220 mcg/puff	88-264 mcg (2-6 puffs--44 mcg) OR (2 puffs--110 mcg)	264-660 mcg (2-6 puffs--110 mcg)	>660 mcg (>6 puffs--110 mcg) OR (>3 puffs--220 mcg)
Fluticasone DPI: 50, 100, 250 mcg/dose	(2-6 inhalations--50 mcg)	(3-6 inhallations--100 mcg)	(>6 inhalations--100 mcg) OR (>2 inhalations--250 mcg)
Triamcinolone acetonide 100 mcg/puff	400-1,000 mcg (4-10 puffs)	1,000-2,000 mcg (10-20 puffs)	>2,000 mcg (>20 puffs)

Adapted from National Institutes of Health. National Heart, Lung, and Blood Institute. (1997). The Expert Panel Report 2: Guidelines for the Diagnosis and Management of Asthma. National Asthma Education Program. NIH Publ. #97-4051. Bethesda, MD.

F.   Treatment of **Step 3: Moderate Persistent Asthma in Adults:** consultation with an asthma specialist is advised
  1.   Initial plan: Choose one of the following three options for initiating step 3 therapy:
    a.   Option 1: Increase inhaled corticosteroid to medium dose (see table)
    b.   Option 2: Add a long-acting bronchodilator to a low-to-medium dose of inhaled corticosteroid; add one of the following long-acting bronchodilators:
      (1)   Inhaled beta$_2$-agonist, salmeterol (Serevent) MDI 21 mcg/puff: In adults use 2 puffs every 12 hours; sustained-release albuterol tablets may be considered but are not preferred
      (2)   Alternatively, may add sustained-release theophylline (see V.E.3)
    c.   Option 3 is least preferred: Establish control with medium-dose inhaled corticosteroid, then lower the dose (but still within the medium-dose range) and add inhaled nedocromil (Tilade) (MDI 1.75 mg/puff): 2-4 puff BID-QID
  2.   Additional plan: if symptoms are not optimally controlled with initial plan in step 3, the following two strategies are recommended:
    a.   Increase inhaled corticosteroid to a high dose
    b.   Add a long-acting bronchodilator (an evening dose may control nocturnal symptoms)
  3.   For exacerbations, see V.D.3.4 and V.J.

G.   Treatment of **Step 4: Severe Persistent Asthma in Adults:** Prescribe oral systemic corticosteroids (see preceding table) and consult specialist
  1.   Prescribe lowest possible dose (single daily dose on alternate days)
  2.   Carefully monitor for adverse side effects such as secondary infections, electrolyte imbalances, hypertension, peptic ulcers, dermal atrophy, carbohydrate intolerance, osteoporosis, cataracts, glaucoma, and psychological effects such as euphoria and depression
  3.   Conscientiously try to reduce systemic corticosteroids once symptoms are controlled; high doses of inhaled corticosteroids have less adverse effects and are preferable to systemic corticosteroids
  4.   For exacerbations see V.D.3.4 and V.J.

H. Special considerations in older adults
   1. Chronic obstructive pulmonary disease may coexist with asthma; trial of systemic corticosteroids will determine whether the airflow obstruction is reversible; if reversible, long-term asthma medication may be beneficial
   2. Adjustments in medication may be needed due to increased adverse effects in the elderly and the effects of co-morbid conditions (heart disease, COPD, diabetes)

I. Treatment of exercise-induced bronchospasm (EIB) (see V.D.2)

J. Home management exacerbations
   1. Increase inhaled beta$_2$-agonist (up to three treatments of 2-4 puffs by MDI at 20 minute intervals or a single nebulizer treatment)
      a. If good response: continue beta$_2$-agonist every 3-4 hours for 24-48 hours; patients on inhaled corticosteroids should double dose for 7-10 days; contact clinician for followup instructions
      b. If response is incomplete: Add oral corticosteroid and continue beta$_2$-agonist and contact clinician within the day
      c. If poor response: Add oral corticosteroid, repeat beta$_2$-agonist immediately; if distress is severe go to emergency department or call 911
   2. Continue more intensive treatment for several days as recovery from exacerbations are often slow

K. Route of administration: inhaled route more effectively delivers medication to lung, has reduced side effects, and the onset of action is shorter than oral medications (see following tables on descriptions and how to use various delivery devices)

AEROSOL DELIVERY DEVICES	
Device/Drugs*	**Therapeutic Issues**
Metered-dose inhaler (MDI) Beta$_2$-agonists Corticosteroids Cromolyn sodium and nedocromil Anticholinergics	Takes coordination to actuate and inhale. Mouth washing is effective in reducing systemic absorption.
Breath-actuated MDI Beta$_2$-agonists	Best for patients unable to coordinate inhalation and actuation (may be particularly useful in elderly). Cannot be used with currently available spacer/ holding chamber devices.
Dry powder inhaler (DPI) Beta$_2$-agonists Corticosteroids	Delivery may be ≥MDI depending on device and technique. Mouth washing is effective in reducing systemic absorption.
Space/holding chamber	Easier to use than MDI alone. Decrease oropharyngeal deposition. Reduce potential system absorption of inhaled corticosteroid preparations that have higher oral bioavailability; recommended for all patients on medium-to-high doses of inhaled corticosteroids. May be as effective as nebulizer in delivering high doses of beta$_2$-agonists during severe exacerbations.
Nebulizer Beta$_2$-agonists Cromolyn Anticholinergics Corticosteroids	Method of choice for high-dose beta$_2$-agonists and anticholinergics in moderate-to-severe exacerbations in all patients. Less dependent on patient coordination or cooperation.

*See additional tables for directions on how to use metered-dose inhaler, dry powder capsules, and nebulizers

Adapted from National Institutes of Health. National Heart, Lung, and Blood Institute. (1997). The Expert Panel Report 2: Guidelines for the Diagnosis and Management of Asthma. National Asthma Education Program. NIH Publ. #97-4051. Bethesda, MD.

DIRECTIONS ON HOW TO USE AN INHALER*

▲ Remove the cap, hold the inhaler upright and shake it

▲ Tilt your head back slightly and slowly exhale

▲ Put the inhaler 1-2 inches from your mouth (open mouth technique) -- OR -- Enclose mouthpiece with your lips (closed mouth technique); do **not** use closed mouth technique for corticosteroids — OR — Use spacer/holding chamber** (slowly inhale or tidal breathe immediately after actuation; actuate only once into chamber per inhalation or if face mask is used, allow 3-5 inhalations per actuation)

▲ Press down on the plunger and take a full, deep, slow, even breath (breathe in through mouth, not through nose)

▲ Hold your breath for 10 seconds, then exhale slowly through your nose

▲ Wait one minute before taking next puff

▲ Rinse your mouth afterward to prevent possible fungal infection

▲ Keep mouth piece clean

*Counsel regarding danger of overuse of inhaler. Patients should be using <u>no</u> more than 1 canister (200 metered dose inhalations of a β-agonist) in a month
**Spacers/holding chambers are particularly recommended for older adults and for patients using inhaled corticosteroids

Adapted from National Institutes of Health. National Heart, Lung, and Blood Institute. (1997). <u>The Expert Panel Report 2: Guidelines for the Diagnosis and Management of Asthma</u>. National Asthma Education Program. NIH Publ. #97-4051. Bethesda, MD.

DIRECTIONS ON HOW TO USE DRY POWDER CAPSULES

● Close mouth tightly around mouthpiece
● Inhale deeply and rapidly
● Minimally effective inspiratory flow is device dependent

DIRECTIONS ON HOW TO USE A NEBULIZER

✦ Measure correct amount of normal saline solution and place into cup (if medicine is premixed, go to step 3)
✦ Measure correct amount of medicine and put into cup with saline solution
✦ Fasten mouthpiece to the T-shaped part and then fasten this unit to the cup OR fasten mask to cup
✦ Put mouthpiece in mouth and seal lips tightly around
✦ Turn on the air compressor machine
✦ Take slow, deep breaths through mouth
✦ Hold breath 1-2 seconds before exhaling
✦ Continue until medicine is depleted from cup (approximately 10 minutes)
✦ Don't forget to clean nebulizer; cleaning removes germs and prevents infection as well as keeps nebulizer from clogging

Adapted from National Institutes of Health. (1992). <u>Teach Your Patients about Asthma: A Clinician's Guide.</u> National Asthma Education Program, Office of Prevention, Education and Control. Publication #92-2737. Bethesda, MD.

L. Patient Education: Establish a partnership with patient and include patient in developing goals and plan; important components of patient education include the following:
1. Basic facts about asthma
2. Roles of medications
3. Discuss asthma triggers and ways to avoid or control them (see V.B.)
4. Review techniques and ask patient to demonstrate use of inhaler, spacer, or nebulizer (many drug failures are due to improper use of equipment)
5. Counsel regarding overuse of inhalers which could result in tachyarrhythmias and death
6. Teach how to recognize symptom patterns that indicate poor asthma control; may need to keep a daily diary of symptoms, peak flow readings, and medications
7. Develop a written action plan based on peak flow readings (see Expert Panel Report 2, 1997, page 131, 138-143)

8. Extensive teaching on exacerbation management is needed
   a. Discuss indicators of worsening asthma, specific recommendations for using beta$_2$-agonist rescue therapy, early administration of systemic corticosteroids, and directions on seeking medical care
   b. Patients at high risk of asthma-related death include those using >2 canisters per month of beta$_2$-agonists, difficulty perceiving airflow obstruction, co-morbidity, severe psychiatric or psychosocial problems, low socioeconomic status, illicit drug use, and prior history of severe exacerbations, intubation, hospitalizations, frequent ER visits

M. Follow Up
   1. For acute exacerbations with incomplete or poor responses see patient within 24 hours and then reevaluate in 3-5 days
   2. After exacerbation has resolved completely, schedule follow up visits every 1-3 months
   3. For patients on theophylline, check serum drug levels after 2 weeks from initiation of therapy; then every 4 months
   4. Follow up for other patients depends on symptom severity, symptom control, knowledge level, social support and other resources; for new asthmatics, frequent visits are important to monitor disease as well as for patient education

BRONCHITIS, ACUTE

I. Definition: Infection of the tracheobronchial tree that causes reversible bronchial inflammation

II. Pathogenesis

   A. Mucous membrane of tracheobronchial tree becomes hyperemic, edematous, with increased bronchial secretions and destruction of epithelium and impaired mucociliary activity

   B. Pathogens
      1. In approximately 95% of cases, the infection is due to a virus such as common cold virus, influenza, adenovirus
      2. *Bordetella pertussis* is the second leading cause
      3. *Mycoplasma pneumonia, Chlamydia pneumoniae, Moraxella catarrhalis* are other less common pathogens
      4. Secondary bacterial invasion by *Streptococcus pneumoniae* and *Haemophilus influenzae* type b may occur but is uncommon in nonsmokers and patients without chronic obstructive pulmonary disease

III. Clinical Presentation

   A. Cough, particularly at night, is hallmark symptom; sputum may be clear or purulent

   B. Most patients are afebrile with mild symptoms

   C. Severe symptoms such as fever, substernal pain, and possibly mucoid sputum production, dyspnea, or bronchospasm with wheezing occur occasionally

   D. Symptoms typically last 7-14 days but may continue for 3-4 weeks

   E. Smokers have more frequent, longer, and more severe episodes than nonsmokers

   F. Some patients with acute bronchitis have an underlying predisposition to bronchial reactivity which may turn into more chronic bronchial inflammation which characterizes asthma; untreated chlamydial infections may have a role in this transition to asthma

G. Adults with acute bronchitis due to pertussis typically have a chronic cough which is often paroxysmal ("whooping"); adults with unrecognized pertussis may transmit pathogen to nonimmune children

IV. Diagnosis/Evaluation

    A. History
        1. Determine onset, duration and characteristics of cough, particularly ask about night coughing
        2. Inquire about frequency and pattern of previous episodes of coughing
        3. Ask about associated symptoms such as fever, pharyngitis, dyspnea, chest pain
        4. Questions about the appearance of the sputum are not considered helpful as purulent sputum is most often related to viral infections
        5. Inquire about infectious illnesses of other household members
        6. Always ask if patient or household members smoke
        7. Inquire about past medical history, particularly respiratory diseases
        8. Determine immunization history of patient and household members

    B. Physical Examination
        1. Assess eyes, ears, nose and throat for signs of inflammation
        2. Palpate and transilluminate sinuses
        3. Perform a heart examination
        4. Perform a complete lung examination; inspect, palpate, percuss, and auscultate
        5. Palpate for lymph nodes

    C. Differential Diagnosis
        1. Pneumonia and acute bronchitis are extremely difficult to differentiate. The following characteristics are more consistent with pneumonia than bronchitis:
            a. High fever
            b. Increased respiratory rate
            c. Rigors and constitutional symptoms
            d. Pleuritic chest pain
            e. Rusty/bloody sputum
            f. Focal crackles on auscultation
            g. X-ray abnormalities
        2. Upper respiratory infection and sinusitis
        3. Tuberculosis
        4. Asthma should be considered in patients who have repetitive episodes of acute bronchitis
        5. Allergies
        6. Cystic fibrosis
        7. Nonpulmonary causes of cough such a congestive heart failure, reflux esophagitis, and bronchogenic tumors

    D. Diagnostic Tests: Acute bronchitis is a diagnosis of exclusion
        1. Order a chest x-ray if the patient has severe symptoms to confirm or rule out the diagnosis of pneumonia
        2. Consider PPD if patient is at risk for tuberculosis
        3. Consider diagnostic pulmonary function testing or provocative testing with a methacholine challenge test when asthma is suspected; to diagnose asthma, abnormalities in tests must persist after the acute phase
        4. Order culture or antigen detection from nasopharyngeal secretions if diagnosis of pertussis is suspected
        5. CBC and sputum cultures are not necessary unless diagnosis is uncertain

V.   Plan/Management

   A.   Antibiotic treatment is recommended in only a few clinical situations because most cases of acute bronchitis are viral; even patients who have a persistent cough (>10 days) usually do not need antibiotics

      1.   Although there is only preliminary evidence, treatment of persistent wheezing with agents effective against Chlamydia species may prevent development of asthmatic symptoms; prescribe doxycycline (Vibramycin) 100 mg BID for 2 to 3 weeks

      2.   For patients with secondary bacterial infections and adults with chronic obstructive pulmonary disease who have a change in color, consistency, and amount of sputum, prescribe 10-day course of erythromycin (E-Mycin) 500 BID or trimethoprim-sulfamethoxazole 800/160 (Bactrim DS) BID or doxycycline

   B.   Although controversial, bronchodilators may relieve symptoms. Consider a trial of inhaled albuterol (Ventolin) 2 puffs every 6 hours for 7 days, especially for patients who have wheezes or rhonchi

   C.   Only symptomatic treatment is needed in most cases

   D.   Antihistamines should be avoided because they dry out secretions; expectorants have not been found to relieve symptoms

   E.   Cough suppressants should be avoided except if patient is unable to sleep due to irritating cough

   F.   Encourage smoking cessation

   G.   Follow Up

      1.   Return to clinic if symptoms persist longer than 7-14 days or if condition worsens; although previously patients with symptoms lasting over one week were treated with antibiotics for a bacterial etiology; today it is recognized that even viral infections may persist for 3 or 4 weeks

      2.   Patients who do not improve after 4 to 6 weeks need further evaluation (see section on COUGH)

CHRONIC OBSTRUCTIVE PULMONARY DISEASE (COPD)

I.   Definition: A complex syndrome of chronic airway obstruction or airflow limitation which is generally progressive and may be accompanied by airway hyperactivity; patients with nonremitting asthma are classified as suffering from COPD, but most frequently COPD is caused by the following two conditions:

   A.   Emphysema is a pathologic diagnosis based on a permanent abnormal dilation and destruction of the alveolar ducts and air spaces distal to the terminal bronchioles

   B.   Chronic bronchitis is a clinical diagnosis based on the presence of a cough and sputum production occurring on most days for at least a 3-month period during 2 consecutive years without another explanation

II.   Pathogenesis

   A.   Emphysema is characterized by airway obstruction, hyperinflation, loss of lung elastic recoil, and destruction of the alveolar-capillary interface which decreases gas exchange

B. Chronic bronchitis is characterized by thickened bronchial walls, hyperplasia and hypertrophied mucous glands, and mucosal inflammation in the bronchial walls, large central airways, and later, in the small airways

C. Predisposing Factors
   1. Tobacco smoke (primary cause - 80-90% of cases)
   2. Recurrent or chronic respiratory infections and hyperresponsive airways such as from asthma or atopy
   3. Occupational and environmental exposure to atmospheres polluted with dust, chemical fumes and "second hand" tobacco smoke
   4. α_1-protease inhibitor deficiency (suspect this in patients under 35 years who have significant COPD symptoms whether or not they smoke)

III. Clinical Presentation

A. Fourth leading cause of death in U.S.; mortality rate has significantly increased in last 20 years

B. In COPD, both elements of emphysema and chronic bronchitis are present but usually one condition predominates

C. COPD begins early in adult life, but significant symptoms do not become apparent until the middle years; most patients have been smoking at least 20 cigarettes per day for 20 or more years before symptoms develop

D. Most common symptom is gradually progressing exertional dyspnea

E. Other symptoms may include chronic cough, wheezing, recurrent respiratory infections, fatigue, weight loss, and lack of libido

F. Signs may include tachypnea, increased use of accessory muscles, increased anterior-posterior chest diameter, hyper-resonance on percussion, decreased heart and breath sounds, prolonged expiration during quiet breathing, wheezes and rhonchi

G. Once COPD is established, the patient's condition tends to gradually worsen; however, early detection of the disease with treatment and modifications in risk factors can significantly alter the disease's course

H. Infection may cause acute respiratory decompensation and is most common cause of death in these patients

I. Pulmonary hypertension and cor pulmonale are caused by chronic hypoxemia which may result in symptoms and signs of right-sided heart failure:
   1. Dyspnea at rest
   2. Fatigue and possibly syncope and angina during exertion
   3. Impaired cognitive function
   4. Peripheral edema, weight gain
   5. Cyanosis and neck vein distension
   6. Holosystolic murmur and S_3 gallop
   7. Hepatomegaly
   8. Erythrocytosis
   9. Renal function abnormalities

J. Left ventricular heart failure can also develop in patients with severe COPD

IV. Diagnosis/Evaluation

A. History
   1. Ask patient to specifically describe how far he/she can walk before becoming dyspneic; determine number of stairs patient can climb before stopping to rest
   2. Explore symptoms and limitations experienced in daily living both at rest and with exercise

3. If cough is present, ask patient to describe onset, characteristics, and amount and color of sputum production
4. Question about signs and symptoms of infection such as chills and fever
5. Inquire about associated symptoms such as fatigue, angina, insomnia, edema, weight gain, changes in voiding, weight loss
6. Determine number of pillows patient sleeps on at night
7. Essential to explicitly ask about patterns of cigarette smoking (age at initiation, quantity smoked per day, and whether or not still smoking); inquire about passive smoking
8. Inquire about occupational and environmental exposure to irritants
9. Thoroughly explore past medical history
10. Consider questioning patients with severe symptoms about their wishes concerning intubation and resuscitation
11. Consider asking patient to complete a health-related quality of life tool

B. Physical Examination
1. Observe general appearance, noting color, posture, gait, affect, and degree of respiratory distress when walking
2. Closely monitor weight
3. Assess vital signs, being alert for fever, tachycardia, and tachypnea
4. Observe for clubbing
5. Observe chest for increased anterior-posterior diameter, retractions, accessory muscle use, and pursed-lip breathing
6. Percuss, palpate, and auscultate lungs (note wheezes, decreased breath sounds, and prolonged forced expiratory time)
7. Auscultate heart
8. Palpate for organomegaly
9. Palpate extremities, assessing for peripheral edema and presence and quality of pulses

C. Differential Diagnosis
1. Consider asthma in younger persons, particularly smokers
2. Congestive heart failure
3. Acute bronchitis

D. Diagnostic Tests
1. All persons with altered lung function as well as persons at risk for COPD should be evaluated with a spirometry; assess airflow obstruction with FEV_1 (forced expiratory volume in one second), FVC (total volume forcibly exhaled), and FEV_1/FVC ratio; spirometry defines severity, helps in determining prognosis, and measures response to therapy and disease progression
   a. Early screening for at risk individuals is important; patients have a large reserve of pulmonary function and usually do not develop COPD symptoms until quite severe airflow obstruction is present
      (1) When the ratio of FEV_1 to FVC (FEV_1/FVC) is one second lower than normally expected, air flow limitation is present
      (2) A decline in the FEV_1 greater than expected (normally there is less than a 30 mL decrease per year) helps identify patients at risk for COPD
   b. Diagnosis of COPD is established when FEV_1/FVC ratio is $\leq 70\%$
   c. Staging of COPD is based on FEV_1 (see Table on COPD Stages)

COPD STAGES			
Stage	Degree	FEV$_1$	Comments
		(% Predicted Value)	
I	Moderate	≥50%	Minimal impact on quality of life without severe hypoxemia; can be cared for by generalist; therapy is primarily preventive
II	Severe	35% to 49%	Significant impact on quality of life; need initial and possibly ongoing evaluation by specialist; therapy is primarily symptomatic
III	Very Severe	≤34%	Profound impact on quality of life; need care of specialist; aggressive therapy indicated

Adapted from Celli, B.R. (1998). Standards for the optimal management of COPD: A summary. Chest, 113, 283S-287S.

    d.   Spirometry 10 minutes after administration of a short-acting beta$_2$-agonist confirms presence and reversibility of airflow obstruction; an increase of ≥15% in FEV$_1$ indicates the presence of a substantial reversible component

2.   For newly diagnosed patients, obtain chest x-ray which is diagnostic only of severe emphysema but is essential to rule out other abnormalities; lung hyperinflation, flattening of diaphragms, and increased retrosternal airspace occur in severe emphysema

3.   For patients 45 years old or younger who have a familial history of emphysema or roentogenographic evidence of panlobular emphysema consider testing for α$_1$-protease inhibitor deficiency

4.   Arterial blood gases (ABGs) are not necessary in Stage 1 but are important to monitor disease progression in Stages II and III; ABGs determine need for oxygen therapy and facilitate diagnosis of respiratory failure

5.   Other testing is usually not needed except in special situations:

    a.   Consider ordering carbon monoxide diffusing capacity when the patient has dyspnea out of proportion to severity of airflow limitation

    b.   Order CBC with differential, gram stain and culture of sputum, and administer tuberculin skin test (PPD) if infection is suspected

    c.   For patients with severe airflow obstruction, order electrocardiogram to assess for cardiac dysfunction and presence of cor pulmonale

V.   Plan/Management

    A.   Prevention of further damage is essential

    1.   Cessation of smoking is the single most important intervention (See section on TOBACCO USE AND SMOKING CESSATION)

    2.   Prevention of infection is important

    a.   Pneumococcal vaccination is recommended with one revaccination 6 years after the first for persons at risk for marked declines in immune function

    b.   Yearly prophylactic vaccination against influenza

    c.   Consider prescribing amantadine (Symmetrel) following exposure to influenza A virus for unimmunized persons who are at high risk for influenza or persons who have acute influenza infection: Over 65 years of age prescribe 100 mg QD; under 65 years prescribe 100 mg BID for 2-7 days depending on patient characteristics or clinical improvement

    3.   Elimination of environmental irritants may be beneficial

    a.   In areas of high ozone environments (e.g., industrialized cities) counsel patients to limit or avoid outdoor activities when the air quality is poor

    b.   Advise patients that extremes in temperature, humidity, high altitudes and air travel can trigger hyperreactivity in irritated airways

    4.   Avoid potentially harmful drugs such as antihistamines, cough suppressants, sedatives, tranquilizers, beta-blockers, and narcotics

5. Early treatment of recurrent and chronic infections is important
   a. Indicators of infection are change in color, consistency, and amount of sputum
   b. Approximately one half of exacerbations are due to bacterial infections; major pathogen is *Haemophilus influenzae* (20-40% of strains are resistant to beta-lactam antibiotics); other bacterial pathogens include *Streptococcus pneumoniae*, and *Moraxella catarrhalis*
   c. Antibiotic therapy is warranted in some patients but not in younger patients who are in stage 1 with mild symptoms and infrequent exacerbations
      (1) For patients ≤60 years with mild-to-moderate impairment of lung function (FEV_1 ≥50% predicted) and who have < four exacerbations per year prescribe one of the following inexpensive antibiotics:
         (a) Erythromycin (E-Mycin) 500 mg QID for 10 days
         (b) Amoxicillin (Amoxil) 500 mg TID for 10 days
      (2) For older patients with moderate or severe impairments and frequent exacerbations prescribe one of the following:
         (a) Clarithromycin (Biaxin) 250-500 mg BID for 10 days
         (b) Amoxicillin-clauvanate (Augmentin) 250-500 mg TID or 875 mg BID for 10 days

B. Pharmacological therapy: use a stepwise approach based on severity of airway obstruction, patient's symptoms, and patient's tolerance to specific drugs
   1. For patients with mild, intermittent, variable symptoms who may or may not have spirometric changes, prescribe beta$_2$-agonist albuterol (Ventolin) or metaproterenol (Alupent), both metered dose inhalers (MDI) with or without spacers, 1-2 puffs TID or QID as needed (prn or rescue therapy) or as prophylaxis before exercise (not to exceed 8-12 puffs in 24 hours)
      a. There is no evidence that early, regular use of these medications alters progression of COPD
      b. Carefully dose these drugs to patients with cardiac disease because of the potential of arrhythmias
   2. For patients with mild, persistent symptoms, prescribe ipratropium regularly and beta$_2$-agonist prn or as maintenance or rescue therapy:
      a. Anticholinergic agent, ipratropium bromide (Atrovent)
         (1) Advantages: Low incidence of side effects and absence of tachyphylaxis
         (2) Prescribe MDI, 2-6 puffs every 6-8 hours (because of slow onset and long duration of action use on a regular basis, not as needed)
      b. Also, may prescribe albuterol (Ventolin) or metaproterenol (Alupent), (MDI), 1-4 puffs TID or QID for rapid relief as needed (prn) or as maintenance therapy on a regular basis
         (1) Albuterol and ipratropium are now available in the same MDI; Combivent 2 puffs QID with maximum of 12 puffs per day
         (2) Nebulized beta$_2$-agonists are usually no more effective than MDIs, but are helpful in patients who have trouble using inhalers
   3. If response to combined ipratropium and beta$_2$-agonist is unsatisfactory or when there is mild to moderate increase in symptoms add the following:
      a. Sustained release theophylline (Theo-Dur) 200-400 mg BID daily or 400-800 mg at HS for nocturnal bronchospasm; additional benefits of theophylline include increase in cardiac output, improved contraction and delayed fatigue of diaphragm, stimulation of respiratory center, and diuresis
         (1) Theophylline has a narrow therapeutic window; titrate dosage to achieve safe levels in range of 8-12 μg/ml
         (2) In a smoker, theophylline dosage is approximately 50% higher than that required by nonsmoker
         (3) In a patient who are elderly and those with fever, hypoxia, congestive heart failure, or liver disease the dosage is 25%-50% lower than dose required of nonsmoker
         (4) Theophylline interacts with several drugs; prescribe cautiously (see table that follows)

MEDICATIONS THAT CAN AFFECT THEOPHYLLINE PLASMA CONCENTRATIONS

Drug	% Decrease in Plasma Concentration	Drug	% Increase in Plasma Concentration
carbamazepine	30	allopurinol (≥600 mg/day)	25
isoniazid	---	cimetidine	70
moricizine	25	ciprofloxacin	40
phenobarbital	25	clarithromycin	25
phenytoin	40	disulfiram	50
rifampin	20-40	enoxacin	300
		erythromycin	35
		estrogen	30
		fluvoxamine	70
		interferon	100
		methotrexate (low dose)	20
		mexiletine	80
		pentoxifylline	30
		propafenone	40
		propranolol	100
		tacrine	90
		ticlopidine	60
		troleandomycin	33-100
		verapamil	20
		zileutron	---

Adapted from Hendeles, L., Jenkins, J., & Temple, R. (1995). Revised FDA labeling guideline for theophylline oral dosage forms. Pharmacotherapy, 15 (4), 409-427.

    b.   In addition, consider use of salmeterol (Serevent) 2 puffs at 12 hour intervals rather than maintenance therapy with short-acting beta$_2$-agonist; particularly beneficial in patients who have reversible disease with nocturnal attacks of wheezing

4.   If response is still suboptimal consider oral corticosteroids such as prednisone (Deltasone) up to 40 mg per day for 10-14 days (effective in less than 20-30% of patients):

    a.   If improvement occurs, wean to low daily or alternate-day dose such as 7.5 mg

    b.   If no improvement occurs, stop immediately

    c.   If steroid appears beneficial, consider possibility of inhaled corticosteroid by MDI, particularly if patient has evidence of bronchial hyperactivity (efficacy of inhaled corticosteroids is not well established); prescribe one of following:

        (1)   Beclomethasone (Beclovent) MDI 2 puffs BID

        (2)   Triamcinolone (Azmacort) MDI 2 puffs BID

C.   For severe exacerbations, consider referral to specialist and evaluate patient for cause and severity such as airway infection, pneumonia, cardiac failure, pulmonary embolism, or spontaneous pneumothorax and initiate one or both of the following regimes:

1.   Administer beta$_2$-agonist in one of the following ways:

    a.   Increase beta$_2$-agonist MDI to 6-8 puffs every 30 minutes to 2 hours

    b.   Prescribe nebulized solution of beta$_2$-agonist such as Albuterol 0.5 mL of a 0.5% solution in 2.5 mL of saline every 30 minutes to 2 hours

    c.   Although not usually required, may administer epinephrine or terbutaline subcutaneous injection 0.1 to 0.5 mL if patient cannot tolerate inhalations AND/OR....

2.   Increase ipratropium and give theophylline and methylprednisolone intravenously

    a.   Increase ipratropium dosage MDI 6-8 puffs every 3-4 hours or prescribe nebulized solution of ipratropium 0.5 mg every 4-8 hours

    b.   Administer theophylline intravenously with calculated dosage to bring serum level to 10-12 μg/mL

    c.   Immediately administer methylprednisolone (Solu-Medrol) 50-100 mg intravenously, then give every 6-8 hours, taper as soon as possible

3.   Administer oxygen to maintain PaO$_2$ above 55 mm Hg and carefully monitor PaCO$_2$ and acid-base status; progressively rising PaCO$_2$ or persistent hypoxemia indicates a need for mechanical ventilation

4.   Prescribe antibiotic if indicated (see treatment of infections under prevention, V.A.5)

D. Considerations when prescribing medications
  1. Frequent errors in medication management are inadequate teaching about how to use inhalers, suboptimal dosing, inadequate monitoring, and failure to advise patient to take medicine before exercising.
  2. Teach patient correct method of using inhaler (see table on Directions on How to Use an Inhaler in the section on ASTHMA)

E. Formal or individualized patient education and pulmonary rehabilitation programs are beneficial
  1. Components of successful programs include individual and family education: information about disease process, smoking cessation, medication administration, maintenance of home oxygen equipment, strategies to attain and maintain normal weight, avoidance of infection, sexual counseling, discussion of extraordinary life-support measures, and exercise training
  2. Encourage exercise
      a. Exercise training has been shown to increase exercise tolerance whereby the patient is able to perform a given level of exercise at a lower oxygen consumption and a lower minute ventilation
      b. Upper extremity training can help lessen diaphragmatic work and concomitant fatigue
      c. Lower-extremity exercise is sometimes beneficial
      d. Purse-lip breathing and diaphragmatic exercises may be helpful
  3. Nutritional therapy
      a. Small frequent feedings may reduce gastric distention, thereby improving diaphragmatic breathing
      b. High fat, reduced carbohydrate (CHO) diet is suggested; increased CHO intake may lead to dyspnea and increased ventilation as a result of a high CO_2 production

F. Supplemental oxygen therapy has been shown to prolong life and improve quality of life in hypoxemic patients
  1. Indications for supplemental oxygen:
      a. Pa O_2 $\leq$55 mm Hg or SaO_2 $\leq$88% breathing ambient air
      b. Pa O_2 56 to 59 mm Hg or SaO_2 89% with concurrent cor pulmonale or polycythemia
      c. Pa O_2 $\geq$60 mm Hg or SaO_2 $\geq$90% with significant exercise- or sleep-induced hypoxemia which reverses with supplemental oxygen or other compelling medical justification
  2. Prescribe oxygen at a flow rate sufficient to produce a PaO_2 $\geq$65mm or a Sa$O_2$$\geq$90% at rest and with activity
      a. Oxygen prescription should include the oxygen dose (L/min), number of hours per day that oxygen is needed, and the type of delivery device (nasal cannula, demand-flow device, reservoir cannula, or transtracheal oxygen catheter); typically given by nasal cannula at flow rates of 0.5 to 4 liters per minute
          (1) Ambulatory oxygen sources which enable patients to exercise are recommended
          (2) Instillation of oxygen directly into the trachea (transtracheal oxygen) using a catheter has both cosmetic and physiologic advantages; almost any patient with chronic, stable hypoxemia can be considered a candidate for this technology
      b. May need to increase flow rate by 1 L/min at night or during exercise
      c. May need to increase flow rate when patient travels by air
  3. Reevaluate patients 1-3 months after initiation of oxygen therapy, because many patients (30-45%) do not need long-term therapy

G. Therapies that are **NOT** effective:
  1. Increased fluid intake is not helpful unless patient is dehydrated
  2. Oral expectorants and nebulized water and salt are not beneficial

3. Postural drainage and chest percussion are only helpful for patients who have excessive secretions or a nonproductive cough
4. Use of iodinated glycerol (Organidin) has not been shown to be effective in previous research, but some clinicians suggest a short-term-trial period for patients with increased amounts of tenacious sputum; discontinue drug if there is no therapeutic benefit; may affect thyroid function with long-term use

H. Consult specialist concerning patient who has cor pulmonale; recommended treatment is oxygen therapy, diuretics and possibly digoxin (in left-sided congestive heart failure only)

I. α_1-antitrypsin augmentation is expensive but is approved for use in patients with this deficiency

J. Hospitalization is usually required for patients who continue to deteriorate with acute exacerbations despite therapy, patients with serious comorbid conditions, patients without home support, patients with altered mentation, and patients with worsening hypoxemia and/or hypercapnia

K. Surgical options are available
1. Lung volume reduction surgery
2. Lung transplantation; selection criteria include the following: Limited life expectancy (<3 years), age <60 years, failure of maximal medical therapy, and no extra pulmonary organ failure

L. Follow Up
1. After an acute attack, contact patient by phone in 24-48 hours
2. If patient is on theophylline, measure drug levels 2 weeks after initiation of therapy and at regular intervals thereafter
3. Schedule follow up visits every 3-6 months for stable, chronic disease
4. Teach patient to immediately consult health care provider when signs and symptoms of respiratory infection or respiratory distress develop

COMMON COLD

I. Definition: An acute, mild and self-limiting syndrome caused by a viral infection of the upper respiratory tract mucosa

II. Pathogenesis

A. Inflammation of all or part of the mucosal membranes from the nasal mucosa to the bronchi

B. Etiology is usually rhinoviruses, coronaviruses, or other viruses

C. Incubation period averages 48 hours with a range of 12 hours to 5 days; maximum viral shedding occurs in first 2-4 days

D. Transmission occurs through direct contact with infectious secretions on skin and environmental surfaces and air-borne droplets

III. Clinical Presentation

    A. Adults average 2-4 colds per year

    B. Characterized by one or more of the following symptoms:
        1. General malaise with low grade or no fever
        2. Nasal discharge, obstruction or congestion
        3. Sneezing/coughing, sore throat and hoarseness
        4. Conjunctivae may be watery and inflamed

    C. Usually self-limited (lasting approximately 5-7 days), but can predispose patient to bacterial infections such as otitis media, sinusitis, pneumonia and exacerbation of chronic conditions such as asthma

IV. Diagnosis/Evaluation

    A. History: Question about the following:
        1. Respiratory distress (wheezing, dyspnea, stridor), inability to swallow, drooling and severe headaches which indicate the need for immediate evaluation
        2. Fever, chills, anorexia, nausea, vomiting and diarrhea
        3. Duration, character, and timing (day and/or night) of cough
        4. Facial, head, ear, throat, or chest pain
        5. Number and seasonal pattern of previous colds within 1 year
        6. Exposure to others with similar symptoms
        7. Medication use
        8. Past medical and family history; particularly history of allergies, asthma, or other respiratory problems
        9. History of tobaccos use and passive tobacco exposure

    B. Physical Examination
        1. Measure temperature, pulse and blood pressure
        2. Examine conjunctivae, ears, nose and throat
        3. Sinus percussion and transillumination
        4. Palpate cervical lymph nodes for enlargement and tenderness
        5. Perform a complete lung examination

    C. Differential Diagnosis
        1. Allergic rhinitis (nasal mucosa may be pale and boggy rather than erythematous and swollen as in common cold)
        2. Foreign body (especially if nasal discharge is unilateral, purulent and malodorous)
        3. Sinusitis
            a. Thick, opaque, and discolored nasal discharge are typical of the common cold and do not indicate a more severe, sinus infection
            b. Symptoms persisting or worsening for >10-14 days with facial swelling and tenderness and mucopurulent sputum are suggestive of sinusitis
        4. Influenza (arthralgias are usually present)
        5. Streptococcal pharyngitis
        6. Otitis media
        7. Pneumonia

    D. Diagnostic Tests
        1. Usually none are indicated
        2. Throat culture or quick strep test if symptomatic or history of streptococcal exposure

V.   Plan/Management

A.   Decongestants cause vasoconstriction and reduce nasal secretions and congestion; topical decongestants are effective for short-term therapy and provide rapid decrease in airway resistance whereas oral decongestants are best when treatment is needed for more than 3-4 days
    1.   Topical decongestants should be used no longer than 3-4 days because of potential for rebound congestion. Suggest one of the following:
        a.   Oxymetazoline hydrochloride 0.05% (Afrin 12-Hour Nasal Spray) 2-3 sprays each nostril BID
        b.   Phenylephrine hydrochloride 1% (Neo-Synephrine Spray) 1 sprays each nostril every 3-4 hours as needed
    2.   Oral decongestants (not as effective); suggest one of the following:
        a.   Prescribe pseudoephedrine hydrochloride (Sudafed) 60 mg, 1 tablet every 4-6 hours
        b.   Pseudoephedrine sulfate (Afrin 12-Hour Tablets) 120 mg, 1 tablet every 12 hours.

B.   Intranasal ipratropium bromide (Atrovent) 2 puffs per nostril TID or QID reduces nasal discharge, severity of rhinorrhea and sneezing; not recommended as first-line agent for these symptoms but may prove useful in patients with disease-state contraindications to oral decongestants such as severe hypertension or angle-closure glaucoma

C.   Conflicting research is available on the benefits of zinc gluconate lozenges
    1.   Dosage is 1 lozenge (Halls Zinc Defense) every 2 hours for 4 days while awake
    2.   Therapy should be initiated within 24 hours of symptom onset
    3.   Adverse effects of bad taste and nausea limit use of lozenges
    4.   Zinc is not safe in pregnancy

D.   Although controversial, some researchers found a decrease in the duration and severity of cold symptoms with the use of Vitamin C

E.   Cough suppressants such as dextromethorphan or codeine may be beneficial when patient is unable to sleep due to irritating cough; but suppression of cough may lead to complications such as pneumonia because the body is unable to clear lungs and airways of unwanted material; recommend that cough suppressant be given only at bedtime

F.   Acetaminophen or nonsteroidal antiinflammatory agents (NSAIDS) such as ibuprofen and naproxen are effective in reducing cough and relieving fever and headaches

G.   Nonpharmacologic approaches to relieve symptoms
    1.   Saline nose drops or sprays: 2-3 drops in each nostril BID to QID of commercial products (Ocean, SalineX) or homemade solution (1/4 tsp salt in 8 oz boiled water)
    2.   Steamy showers or inhalation of steam
    3.   Fluids or hydration help loosen secretions and prevent upper airway obstruction; warm fluids such as tea and chicken soup can increase the rate of mucous flow
    4.   Salt-water gargle for sore throat
    5.   Hard candy or throat lozenge for sore throat and cough

H.   Treatments that are not recommended
    1.   Antihistamines are ineffective because nasal congestion in colds is not mediated by histamine receptors; antihistamines may increase upper airway obstruction by impairing flow of mucus
    2.   With exception of increased water intake, expectorants such as guaifenesin provide no benefit in cold management

I. Patient Education
   1. Review the etiology, course, and proper treatment of the common cold
      a. Explain that colds are caused by viruses which are not eradicated with antibiotics
      b. Reinforce that the indiscriminate use of antibiotics can cause adverse effects such as diarrhea, yeast infection, and drug resistance
   2. Emphasize that cold remedies are to relieve symptoms and prevent complications rather than cure infection
   3. Advise rest and increased oral fluid intake.
   4. Increase humidity of the air at home
   5. Discuss ways to prevent the spread of colds; all household members should frequently wash hands

J. Follow Up: None indicated unless symptoms worsen after 3-5 days, new symptoms develop, or symptoms do not improve or resolve after 10-14 days

COUGH, PERSISTENT

I. Definition: Host defense mechanism to clear airway of secretions and inhaled particles which lasts at least 3 weeks or longer

II. Pathogenesis

   A. The most common causes are postnasal drip from chronic sinusitis or allergic rhinitis, asthma, gastroesophageal reflux, chronic bronchitis due to cigarette smoking or environmental irritants

   B. Other less common causes are physical irritants, foreign body aspiration, tuberculosis, and psychogenic factors

   C. Worrisome causes of coughing include mediastinal or pulmonary masses such as tumors or nodes

   D. In 25% of patients, multiple disorders contribute to a persistent cough

III. Clinical presentation of important causes of persistent cough

   A. Tuberculosis
      1. Initially cough is minimally productive of yellow or green mucus which is worse upon arising in morning
      2. As disease progresses, cough becomes more productive
      3. Associated symptoms include fatigue, night sweats, dyspnea, and hemoptysis

   B. Gastroesophageal reflux
      1. May have history of heartburn, dysphagia, sour or bitter taste in mouth, and frequent use of antacids
      2. Symptoms are often aggravated by meals and relieved by sitting up

   C. Asthma
      1. Often occurs at night or after exercise, laughing, or exposure to cold air
      2. May be seasonal in occurrence and have a strong family history
      3. Cough may be nonproductive or productive but not purulent nor yellow or green in color
      4. Associated symptoms include wheezing and intercostal retractions

   D. Aspirated foreign body
      1. Cough may persist for weeks or even months
      2. Fixed, localized wheezing audible when chest is auscultated

E. Viral infections infrequently last beyond 2 weeks
    1. Often occur during the winter
    2. Cough is often nonproductive
    3. Usually accompanying symptoms are mild and include rhinitis and nasal congestion

F. Bacterial infections such as pneumonia
    1. Cough may be productive and purulent but this is not always the case
    2. Associated symptoms may include fever and respiratory distress

G. Postnatal drip from chronic sinusitis or allergic rhinitis
    1. Involved in approximately 41% of patients with chronic cough
    2. Patient often complains of clear nasal discharge, nasal congestion, tickle in throat, and frequent throat clearing

H. Chronic bronchitis: Patient often has dry, hacking cough which is worse in the morning

I. Carcinoma of the lung
    1. Cigarette smoking accounts for the majority of cases
    2. Characteristic of the cough depends on location of the primary tumor

J. Cough related to psychogenic factors
    1. Disappears during sleep and is worse when attention is drawn to it and during times of emotional stress
    2. Lacks other associated physical symptoms

IV. Diagnosis/Evaluation

A. History
    1. Determine type of onset and duration of cough
    2. Determine characteristics of cough
        a. Productive (white, purulent, bloody) or nonproductive
            (1) Productive cough usually suggests infection
            (2) Rusty-colored sputum suggests pneumonia
        b. Quality (raspy, barking, harsh, wet); paroxysms of cough occur in pertussis, and foreign body aspiration
        c. Temporal occurrence (night, morning, or seasonal)
            (1) Nighttime cough suggests asthma, sinusitis with postnasal drip
            (2) Cough associated with exercise may indicate asthma, cardiac disease (rare), and bronchiectasis
    3. Ask about associated symptoms such as fatigue, rhinitis, epistaxis, tickle in throat, pharyngitis, night sweats, dyspnea, fever, heartburn, hemoptysis, weight loss
        a. Hemoptysis signals concern for tuberculosis, cancer, or foreign body (see section on HEMOPTYSIS)
        b. Weight loss and fever suggest tuberculosis or HIV infection
    4. Ask if the cough is preceded by feeding or choking episodes suggestive of gastroesophageal reflux
    5. Inquire about precipitating factors such as exercise, cold air, laughing
    6. Explore environmental and occupational exposure
    7. Inquire about infectious illness of other household members
    8. Always ask about smoking or the exposure to passive smoking
    9. Ask about medications, particularly angiotensin-converting enzyme (ACE) inhibitors which may produce a dry cough
    10. Explore family history of malabsorption, asthma, and allergies
    11. Inquire about past medical history such as allergies, frequent infectious diseases, obstructive airway disease, cardiac disease

B.	Physical Examination
	1.	Observe patient for signs of respiratory distress such as cyanosis, shortness of breath on ambulating, intercostal retractions, accessory muscle use
	2.	Observe general appearance, noting whether patients appear robust or fatigued and wasted
	3.	Listen for the quality of spontaneous coughing during the interview
	4.	Assess eyes, ears, nose and throat
		a.	Conjunctivitis, rhinitis and pharyngitis suggest infection
		b.	Cobblestoning in oropharynx suggests allergies or chronic sinusitis
	5.	Check for tenderness of sinuses
	6.	Palpate lymph nodes
	7.	Observe for tracheal deviation which suggests mediastinal mass or foreign body aspiration
	8.	Perform a complete lung exam including inspection, palpation, percussion, and auscultation
	9.	Perform a complete cardiac exam as chronic cardiovascular problems may present with persistent coughs

C.	Differential Diagnosis: See pathogenesis section

D.	Diagnostic Tests
	1.	Order tuberculin skin test (PPD) and chest x-ray for unexplained persistent cough
	2.	If diagnosis is unclear after PPD and chest x-ray, order spirometry to detect airway obstruction as in asthma
	3.	Consider a CBC with differential if infection, anemia, carcinoma are likely possibilities
	4.	Cough that is productive should have Wright and gram stains of sputum as well as cultures
	5.	If asthma is suspected, a methacholine bronchoprovocation challenge should be considered
	6.	To uncover silent, pathologic gastroesophageal reflux, 24-hour pH probe monitoring may be needed
	7.	Oximetry may be helpful to quickly evaluate the patient's respiratory status and later may be used to assess response to treatment
	8.	Other possible tests to order depend on characteristics of patient and include sinus x-rays, immunologic testing, allergy testing, or a barium swallow for detecting structural lesions
	9.	More invasive tests such as bronchoscopy may be needed

V.	Plan/Management

	A.	Treat all known causes such as antibiotic therapy for bacterial infections, bronchodilators for asthma, and antihistamines for allergies

	B.	Discuss need to stop cigarette smoking and avoid environmental irritants

	C.	Air humidification and keeping the throat moist are simple suggestions that may be beneficial

	D.	Cough suppressants such as dextromethorphan or codeine may be beneficial in improving sleep and rest (use only at bedtime)

	E.	Expectorants and mucolytic agents are ineffective

	F.	A stepwise approach may be beneficial by progressing from simple to more aggressive diagnostic tests and treatments in patients with persistent mild-to-moderate coughing of unknown etiology
		1.	Initial screen: Eliminate environment irritants (smoking, cough-producing medications, etc.)
		2.	Step 1: Treat empirically for postnasal drip with first generation antihistamine-decongestant combination; add nasal steroids or order CT of sinuses if symptoms persist
		3.	Step 2: Evaluate and treat possible asthma with inhaled cromolyn, steroids, and bronchodilators

4. Step 3: Order chest radiographs and CT of sinuses if asthma is not confirmed; treat specific, identified disease
5. Step 4:
   a. Treat for gastroesophageal reflux disease (GERD) if no abnormalities found in step 3: Antireflux measures and high-dose proton-pump inhibitor
   b. Order endoscopy or 24-hour esophageal pH monitoring
6. Step 5
   a. Perform bronchoscopic examination if no abnormalities are found and previous treatments are unsuccessful
   b. Repeat course of antihistamine-decongestant combination
   c. Consider less common diagnoses such as cancer, tuberculosis, congestive heart failure, sarcoidosis, bronchiectasis, etc.

G. In undiagnosed patients with risk factors for cancer such as smoking or occupational exposure consider referral to specialist

H. Follow Up
1. Frequency of return visits will depend on patient's condition
2. Patients who have a complete work-up with no abnormalities should be seen at least every 1-3 months if their coughing persists

HEMOPTYSIS

I. Definition: Expectoration of both blood-tinged and grossly bloody sputum

II. Pathogenesis

A. Inflammation of the tracheobronchial mucosa is the causative factor in many cases
   1. Minor mucosal erosions can occur from upper respiratory infections and bronchitis
   2. Bronchiectasis
   3. Tuberculosis (TB)
   4. Endobronchial inflammation due to sarcoidosis

B. Bronchogenic carcinoma may injure the mucosa whereas metastatic lung cancer rarely results in hemoptysis

C. Injury to the pulmonary vasculature is an important cause
   1. Lung abscess
   2. Necrotizing pneumonias such as those caused by *Klebsiella*
   3. Aspergillomas
   4. Pulmonary infarction secondary to embolization

D. Elevations in pulmonary capillary pressure can result in hemoptysis
   1. Pulmonary edema
   2. Mitral stenosis
   3. Wegener's granulomatosis
   4. Goodpasture's syndrome
   5. Arteriovenous malformations

E. Bleeding disorders and excessive anticoagulant therapy are additional causes

F. Chest trauma is a less common cause

G. Cryptogenic hemoptysis is hemoptysis in which the patient has a normal or nonlocalizing chest radiograph and nondiagnostic fiberoptic bronchoscopy; 90% of patients experience resolution of hemoptysis by 6 months

H. Acute and chronic bronchitis followed by bronchogenic carcinoma, TB, pneumonia, and bronchiectasis are the most common causes

III. Clinical presentation of important causes of hemoptysis

A. Blood that is coughed is bright red, frothy, has an alkaline pH, and is mixed with sputum rather than hematemesis that is darker brown, has an acid pH, and may be mixed with food particles

B. Blood-streaked sputum is common, usually occurs with nonthreatening conditions, and often arises from the nasal mucosa and oropharynx rather than the lower respiratory tract

C. Bronchitis and bronchiectasis
1. Occasional, blood-tinged sputum is characteristic
2. Patient usually has chronic cough and dyspnea which may be worse in the morning

D. Lung tumors account for about 20% of the cases of hemoptysis
1. Occur most frequently in persons over age 40 and in smokers
2. Patient often have a change in cough pattern
3. Chest ache may be an accompanying symptom

E. Pneumonia
1. Sputum appears red-brown or red-green and is mixed with pus
2. May have fever, pleuritic chest pain, and malaise

F. Pulmonary infarction secondary to pulmonary emboli
1. Characterized by a sudden onset of pleuritic pain in conjunction with hemoptysis
2. Diaphoresis and syncope often are present
3. Signs include tachypnea, tachycardia, rales, fever, shock, fourth heart sound, pleural rub, or cyanosis
4. Frequently patient has a history of phlebitis, calf pain, or immobilization of the legs

G. Pulmonary edema
1. Characteristically has pink, frothy sputum
2. Diaphoresis, tachypnea, tachycardia are present
3. Jugular venous distention, hepatomegaly, and ankle edema may be present

IV. Diagnosis/Evaluation

A. History
1. Inquire about onset and whether hemoptysis is a recurrent problem
2. Explicitly determine that the bleeding is originating from the lungs rather than from vomiting blood or expectorating blood from nasopharyngeal bleeding
3. Ask patient to describe the color, consistency, and characteristics of sputum
   a. Pink sputum is suggestive of pulmonary edema fluid
   b. Putrid sputum suggests a lung abscess
   c. Currant-jelly-like sputum may indicate necrotizing pneumonia
   d. Copious amounts of purulent sputum mixed with blood points toward bronchiectasis
4. Ask patient to quantify amount of bleeding or if possible collect the sputum
5. Inquire about associated symptoms such as recent weight loss, fatigue, persistent cough, dyspnea, wheezing, fever, night sweats, excessive bruising, hematuria
6. Determine whether patient has had recent respiratory inflammation or infection
7. Inquire about past medical history, particularly ask about previous lung, cardiac, hematological, and immunological problems
8. Inquire about exposure to tuberculosis
9. Ask about patterns of cigarette smoking

10. Inquire about history of chest trauma
11. Ask about use of anticoagulant drugs
12. Explore environmental exposure to such things as asbestos
13. Ask about family history of hemoptysis, respiratory, cardiac, and hematological problems
14. Inquire about date of last chest x-ray and tuberculin skin test

B. Physical Examination
1. Assess vital signs, particularly noting fever and tachypnea
2. Observe skin for ecchymosis, telangiectasis and nails for clubbing; clubbing is consistent with neoplasm, bronchiectasis, lung abscess and other severe respiratory problems
3. Examine nose, sinuses and pharynx for source of bleeding
4. Inspect neck for jugular venous distention which is suggestive of heart failure
5. Palpate for lymph nodes; lymphadenopathy is associated with TB, sarcoidosis, and malignancy
6. Perform a complete lung and cardiovascular exam
7. Check for ankle edema

C. Differential Diagnosis: Hemoptysis is a symptom. See pathogenesis for possible causes.
1. Most cases of blood-tinged sputum are upper-respiratory in nature and do not need extensive workup
2. Differentiate hemoptysis from epistaxis, hematemesis and bleeding from nasopharyngeal sources

D. Diagnostic Tests
1. Order chest x-ray
2. Administer tuberculin skin test (PPD) unless there has been a positive PPD in the past
3. Consider Gram stain of sputum for suspected infections, an acid-fast stain for suspected tuberculosis, and cytologic examination of three sputum samples for malignant cells
4. Consider bronchoscopy for patients who smoke, who are over 40 years of age, and who have normal chest x-rays; also consider for patients with persistent, recurrent hemoptysis or massive bleeding
5. Consider ventilation-perfusion scanning or angiography when pulmonary embolization is suspected
6. PT, PTT, platelet count and bleeding time are necessary when more than one site of bleeding is present

V. Plan/Management

A. Consider consultation with a specialist for patients who are at increased risk for malignancy and those cases in which bronchoscopy is indicated

B. Patients expectorating more than 25-50 mL of blood in 24 hours require hospitalization

C. Treat any underlying illness or infection

D. Because blood is irritating to the tracheobronchial tree and triggers a cough response, consider prescribing a mild cough suppressant. However, instruct patient to continue expectorating as mucus and blood can accumulate and cause additional problems

E. Patient Education
1. Instruct patient to record episodes of hemoptysis and collect all blood that is expectorated
2. Instruct patient to return to clinic or emergency room if bleeding increases, has clots, or if patient has respiratory distress, diaphoresis, chest pain, or tachypnea

F. Follow Up
1. For mild blood-streaking of sputum with respiratory infection, all blood streaking should resolve in 2-3 days. If blood-streaking of sputum persists, patient needs a reevaluation
2. Patients with hemoptysis which involves expectoration of blood, not just minimal amounts of blood-streaked sputum, should have follow up visit within 12-48 hours

PNEUMONIA, COMMUNITY-ACQUIRED

I.   Definition: "Acute infection of the pulmonary parenchyma that is associated with at least some symptoms of acute infection and is accompanied by the presence of an acute infiltrate on a chest radiograph or auscultatory findings consistent with pneumonia (altered breath sounds and/or localized rales) and occurs in a patient who is not hospitalized or residing in a long-term care facility for ≥14 days before onset of symptoms" (Barlett, et al., 1998)

II. Pathogenesis

   A.   Mainly results from aspiration of pathogens into the lower respiratory tract from oropharyngeal contents

   B.   Less commonly, pathogens spread to lungs hematogenously from distant foci such as bacterial endocarditis or from aerosolized particles

   C.   Aspirated pathogens are usually cleared before infection develops unless there are alterations in the normal protective mechanisms such as depressed mucociliary transport by ethanol and narcotics or by obstruction of bronchus by mucus or tumors

   D.   Pathogens
      1.   *Streptococcus pneumoniae* is the most common cause of morbidity and mortality from community-acquired pneumonia (CAP); accounts for 2/3s of bacteremic pneumonia
      2.   *Haemophilus influenzae* is becoming a more common pathogen
      3.   *Legionella* species is an important pathogen in severe pneumonias
      4.   Gram-negative pathogens account for 20-40% of causative agents in the elderly
      5.   Pathogens according to the 1993 American Thoracic Society categories:
         a.   Outpatient pneumonia without co-morbidity and 60 years of age or younger (following does not include patients at risk for HIV): *Streptococcus pneumoniae* (pneumococcus), *Mycoplasma pneumoniae*, respiratory viruses, *Chlamydia pneumoniae*, *Haemophilus influenzae*
         b.   Outpatient pneumonia with co-morbidity and/or 60 years of age or older (following does not include patients at risk for HIV):*Streptococcus pneumoniae*, respiratory viruses, *Haemophilus influenzae,* aerobic gram-negative bacilli (predominantly *Enterobacteriaceae*), *Staphylococcus aureus*
         c.   Hospitalized patients with community-acquired pneumonia (excluding patients at risk for HIV): *Streptococcus pneumoniae, Haemophilus influenzae* , polymicrobial (including anaerobic bacteria), aerobic gram-negative bacilli (predominantly *Enterobacteriaceae*), *Legionella* species, *Staphylococcus aureus, C. pneumoniae*, respiratory viruses
         d.   Hospitalized patients with severe community-acquired pneumonia (excluding patients at risk for HIV): *Streptococcus pneumoniae, Legionella* species, aerobic gram-negative bacilli (predominantly *Enterobacteriaceae*), *Mycoplasma pneumoniae*, respiratory viruses

   E.   Bacterial pneumonia is often associated with concurrent viral infection which may suppress the immune system and disrupt the respiratory tract mucosa

III.   Clinical Presentation

A.   In U.S., pneumonia is the sixth leading cause of death, and the number one cause of death from infectious disease

B.   The epidemiology of pneumonia has undergone changes in recent years; pneumonia is increasingly common among elderly patients and those with coexisting illnesses; in the elderly the clinical expression of various types of pneumonia is atypical, obscured, and may even be absent

C.   Symptoms suggestive of pneumonia include the following:
1.   Fever or hypothermia, chills, sweats
2.   New cough with or without sputum production; or, in patient with chronic cough, change in color of respiratory secretions
3.   Chest discomfort and/or dypsnea
4.   Nonspecific symptoms such as fatigue, myalgias, abdominal pain, headaches, and anorexia

D.   Signs include respiratory rate >20/minute, tachycardia, crackles heard on auscultation and signs of consolidation

E.   Complications of pneumonia include the following:
1.   Metastatic infection (meningitis, arthritis, endocarditis, pericarditis, peritonitis and empyema) occurs in as many as 10% of patients with bacteremic pneumonia
2.   Bacteremia, renal failure, heart failure, pulmonary embolus with infarction and acute myocardial infarction

F.   The following are risk factors for mortality: Increased age, alcoholism, active malignancies, immunosuppression, neurological disease, congestive heart failure and diabetes

G.   Increasingly, research has found considerable overlap in the symptoms, signs, and radiographic findings of the various types of pneumonia; even though it is usually not prudent to base empiric treatment on clinical findings, this section summarizes literature on the clinical presentation of pneumonia due to specific pathogens
1.   Pneumococcal pneumonia (due to *S. pneumoniae*)
a.   May occur in previously healthy adults after an upper respiratory infection; but occurs predominantly in elderly and patients with other co-morbid medical conditions
b.   Often presents with abrupt onset of high fever, shaking chills, productive cough of purulent or rusty sputum, headache, prostration, and pleuritic chest pain
c.   Bacteremia occurs in 15-30% of cases
2.   *Haemophilus influenzae*
a.   Predilection for the elderly, cigarette smokers, and patients with chronic obstructive pulmonary disease or pre-existing illnesses but may affect healthy persons
b.   Symptoms similar to other bacterial pneumonias
c.   Often occurs after an episode of influenza
3.   Pneumonia due to staphylococcus species occurs in patients with specific risk factors such as residence in nursing home, alcohol abuse, chronic disease, or during influenza epidemics
4.   *Moraxella catarrhalis*
a.   Occurs in patients with chronic obstructive pulmonary disease or other underlying chronic illness
b.   Symptoms are usually mild and patients do not usually have myalgias, chills, pleuritic chest pain, or extreme prostration
5.   Pneumonia due to gram-negative bacilli rarely occurs in previously, healthy adults
a.   Risk factors include old age, residence in chronic care facility, alcohol abuse, malnutrition, and chronic illness
b.   High risk for complications and high (20-30%) mortality rate

6. Pneumonia due to *M. pneumoniae*
   a. Only 3-10% of all community-acquired pneumonia in adults between age 35-60 is due to *M. pneumoniae*, but common in adults <35 years
   b. Close contact is necessary for transmission and epidemics have occurred in military housing, schools, etc.
   c. Usually symptoms are mild and course is self-limited
   d. Hacking cough, fever, malaise, and headache are common symptoms
   e. Symptoms may last up to 6 weeks despite treatment
7. Pneumonia due to *Chlamydia pneumoniae* has presentation and course similar to pneumonia due to *M. pneumoniae*
8. Pneumonia due to *Legionella pneumophila*
   a. *Legionella* is an opportunistic pathogen; rarely occurs in healthy young children and young adults
   b. Symptoms are severe with a fatality rate of 10-30% of all cases
   c. Unique characteristics are hyponatremia, neurologic symptoms (confusion, headache), gastrointestinal symptoms (nausea, diarrhea), hematuria, and elevated serum transaminase
9. Viral pneumonia
   a. Uncommon in adults except in the immunosuppressed patient
   b. Influenza viruses are most common cause of viral pneumonia with fever, chills, dry hacking cough, and pharyngitis
   c. Respiratory syncytial virus is increasingly being recognized as cause of pneumonia in adults
   d. Cytomegalovirus and herpes simplex viruses cause treatable pneumonia in immunosuppressed patients
   e. Viral pneumonias have more prolonged prodromal illness, milder symptoms, less elevated white count than bacterial pneumonias
   f. Chest x-rays do not usually reveal lobar distribution of infiltrate and pleural effusions as in bacterial pneumonias
10. *Pneumocystis carinii* presents with insidious onset of fever, cough, and dyspnea in the immunocompromised person
11. Pneumonia due to anaerobes is most common in patients with poor dental hygiene; putrid sputum is associated with anaerobic infections

IV. Diagnosis/Evaluation

A. History
   1. Determine whether onset was gradual, involving mild upper respiratory symptoms or abrupt with rapid onset of fever and cough
   2. Inquire about associated symptoms such as rhinorrhea, fever, chills, myalgias, pharyngitis, chest pain, and neurological symptoms
   3. Ask patient to describe cough and sputum
   4. Inquire about recent infectious illnesses in the patient's household
   5. Inquire about past medical history such as acquired immunodeficiency, asthma, chronic obstructive pulmonary disease, smoking history, tuberculosis, alcohol and drug abuse

B. Physical Examination
   1. Assess vital signs
   2. Observe for respiratory disease such as cyanosis, tachypnea, intercostal retractions, accessory muscle use, nasal flaring, and grunting
   3. Assess for signs of dehydration, particularly in the elderly
   4. Auscultate lungs; typical findings are the following:
      a. Localized diminished breath sounds
      b. Rales and tubular breath sounds
      c. Egophony (changes patient's "ee" to what sounds like "ay")

      d.   Bronchophony (voice sounds are louder and clearer than usual)

      e.   Whispered pectoriloquy (whispered sounds are louder and clearer than normal)

5.   Palpate chest for tactile fremitus (palpate for increased areas of vibration as patient says "ninety-nine")

6.   Percuss chest for dullness which is typical over consolidated lung tissue

7.   Perform a cardiac examination

8.   Assess mental status

C.   Differential Diagnosis: There is no combination of clinical findings that can rule in a diagnosis of pneumonia; however, some researchers found that absence of vital sign abnormalities or any abnormalities on chest auscultation substantially lessened the likelihood of pneumonia

1.   Chronic pulmonary diseases such as asthma, chronic bronchitis or emphysema

2.   Atelectasis

3.   Lung abscess

4.   Pulmonary embolism

5.   Damage from physical agents such as near drowning and smoke inhalation

6.   Congestive heart failure

7.   Neoplasms

D.   Diagnostic Tests

1.   Chest radiograph is recommended as respiratory complaints alone are poorly predictive of finding an acute infiltrate on x-ray; order PA and lateral chest x-ray to aid in the following:

      a.   To differentiate pneumonia from other conditions that mimic it

      b.   To uncover specific etiologies or conditions such as lung abscess or pneumonia caused by *Pneumocystis carinii*

      c.   To identify co-existing conditions such as pleural effusion or bronchial obstruction

      d.   To evaluate the severity of disease by identifying multilobar involvement which indicates a severe illness

      e.   As a baseline, to assess response to treatment

2.   Sputum gram stain is desirable; culture of expectorated sputum is optional (even though both tests lack sensitivity and specificity they are helpful in diagnosing infections, especially those caused by *Mycobacterium* species, endemic fungi, and *Legionella* species)

3.   Routine laboratory tests such as CBC, glucose, serum electrolytes, hepatic enzymes, and tests of renal function are helpful in deciding which patients should be hospitalized (<u>always</u> do these tests in patients who are 60 years or older or who have a coexisting illness)

4.   Consider tuberculin skin test (PPD)

5.   In addition, patients in whom hospitalization is likely should have the following: arterial-blood gas analysis, two sets of blood cultures, serologic test for HIV infection, deep cough sputum for gram-stain and culture, test for *Mycobacterium tuberculosis* with acid-fast stain and culture for selected patients (cough >1 month); direct fluorescent antibody stain of sputum or the urinary antigen assay for *Legionella* in selected patients (seriously ill, immunosuppressed, >40 years, or patients nonresponsive to β-lactam antibiotics)

6.   Patients with pleural effusion should have a diagnostic thoracentesis

7.   All patients over 40 and all smokers should have chest x-ray at 4-8 weeks posttreatment to rule out bronchogenic carcinoma which has a similar presentation as pneumonia

V.   Plan/Management

A.   Consider consultation with a specialist for a patient who appears toxic, has hemoptysis, severe dyspnea, a history of a serious, chronic disease

B.   Whether to hospitalize a patient with pneumonia is a dilemma; a model by Fine et al., (1997) can help clinicians make the correct decision (See table that follows); patients in classes I and II can usually be treated at home, class III patients should be admitted for a short observation period; class IV and V patients need traditional inpatient care

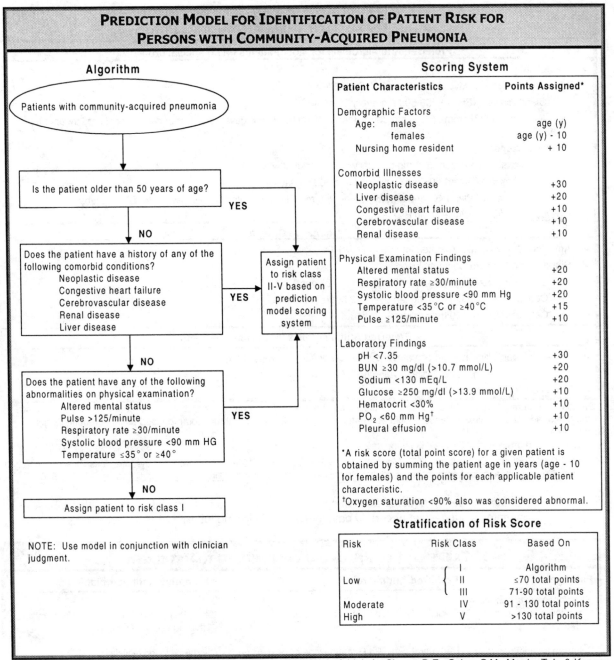

PREDICTION MODEL FOR IDENTIFICATION OF PATIENT RISK FOR PERSONS WITH COMMUNITY-ACQUIRED PNEUMONIA

Algorithm

(Patients with community-acquired pneumonia)

↓

Is the patient older than 50 years of age? — **YES** →

↓ **NO**

Does the patient have a history of any of the following comorbid conditions?
- Neoplastic disease
- Congestive heart failure
- Cerebrovascular disease
- Renal disease
- Liver disease

— **YES** →

↓ **NO**

Does the patient have any of the following abnormalities on physical examination?
- Altered mental status
- Pulse >125/minute
- Respiratory rate ≥30/minute
- Systolic blood pressure <90 mm HG
- Temperature ≤35° or ≥40°

— **YES** →

↓ **NO**

Assign patient to risk class I

Assign patient to risk class II-V based on prediction model scoring system

NOTE: Use model in conjunction with clinician judgment.

Scoring System

Patient Characteristics	Points Assigned*
Demographic Factors	
Age: males	age (y)
females	age (y) - 10
Nursing home resident	+ 10
Comorbid Illnesses	
Neoplastic disease	+30
Liver disease	+20
Congestive heart failure	+10
Cerebrovascular disease	+10
Renal disease	+10
Physical Examination Findings	
Altered mental status	+20
Respiratory rate ≥30/minute	+20
Systolic blood pressure <90 mm Hg	+20
Temperature <35°C or ≥40°C	+15
Pulse ≥125/minute	+10
Laboratory Findings	
pH <7.35	+30
BUN ≥30 mg/dl (>10.7 mmol/L)	+20
Sodium <130 mEq/L	+20
Glucose ≥250 mg/dl (>13.9 mmol/L)	+10
Hematocrit <30%	+10
PO$_2$ <60 mm Hg†	+10
Pleural effusion	+10

*A risk score (total point score) for a given patient is obtained by summing the patient age in years (age - 10 for females) and the points for each applicable patient characteristic.
†Oxygen saturation <90% also was considered abnormal.

Stratification of Risk Score

Risk	Risk Class	Based On
	I	Algorithm
Low	II	≤70 total points
	III	71-90 total points
Moderate	IV	91 - 130 total points
High	V	>130 total points

Adapted from Fine, M.J., Auble, T.E., Yealy, D.M., Hanusa, B.H., Weissfeld, L.A., Singer, D.E., Coley, C.M., Marrie, T.J., & Kapoor, W.N. (1997). A prediction rule to identify low-risk patients with community-acquired pneumonia. New England Journal of Medicine, 336, 243-250.

C. Empiric treatment of pneumonia is often necessary because available diagnostic tests fail to reveal the pathogen in a 40-50% of all cases and most test results (sputum, blood cultures, serologies) are not available at the time of initial presentation
  1. Research has found that patients treated in the early stage of their disease progress better than patients in whom treatment is delayed
  2. Base empiric treatment on the following: presence or absence of coexisting illness, and severity of illness upon clinical presentation (see table that follows)

EMPIRIC OUTPATIENT TREATMENT GUIDELINES*

Preferred Antimicrobials for Most Patients (in no special order)

✓ Macrolides[†]
  + Erythromycin (E-Mycin) 250-500 mg TID or QID
  + Clarithromycin (Biaxin) 250-500 mg every 12 hours
  + Azithromycin (Zithromax) 500 mg day 1, then 250 mg daily for 4 days (take 1 hour before meals or 2 hours after meals)

✓ Fluoroquinolones
  + Levofloxacin (Levaquin) 500 mg tab QD with full glass of water
  + Grepafloxacin (Raxar) 600 mg QD. Available 200 mg tabs
  + Sparfloxacin (Zagam) 400 mg on day 1, then 200 mg QD on remaining days. Available 200 mg tabs

✓ Doxycycline (Vibramycin) 100 mg BID

Alternative Options

✓ Amoxicillin/Clavulanate (Augmentin) 500 mg tab TID

✓ Some second-generation cephalosporins
  + Cefuroxime axetil (Ceftin) 250-500 mg every 12 hours
  + Cepodoxime (Vantin) 200 mg tab every 12 hours with food
  + Cefprozil (Cefzil) 500 mg tab every 12 hours

Preferred Antimicrobials for Selected Patients

✓ Suspected penicillin-resistant *Streptococcus pneumoniae*: Fluoroquinolones

✓ Suspected aspiration: Amoxicillin/clavulanate

✓ Young adult (>17-40 years): Doxycycline

*Duration of treatment varies. Most bacterial infections can be treated until a patient is afebrile for 72 hours. *C. pneumonia, M. pneumonia*, and Legionnaires' disease should be treated for at least 2 weeks. Immunocompromised patients require longer treatments (21 days).
[†]Recommended drugs if *H. influenzae* is suspected

Adapted from Bartlett, J.G., Breiman, R.F., Mandell, L.A., & File, T.M., Jr. (1998). Guidelines from the Infectious Disease Society of America. Community-acquired pneumonia in adults: Guidelines for management. Clinical Infectious Diseases, 26, 811-836.

D.   Treatment can be directed against specific pathogen when it is identified or empirically based on symptoms suggestive of certain pathogens (see following table)

TREATMENT OF PNEUMONIA ACCORDING TO PATHOGEN

Pathogen	Preferred Antimicrobial	Alternative Antimicrobial
Streptococcus pneumoniae Penicillin susceptible (MIC, <0.1 µg/mL)	Penicillin G or penicillin V, amoxicillin	Cephalosporins,* macrolides,[†] clindamycin, fluoroquinolones,[‡] doxycycline
Intermediately penicillin resistant (MIC, 0.1-1 µg/mL)	Parenteral penicillin G, ceftriaxone or cefotaxime, amoxicillin, fluoroquinolones,[‡] other agents based on in vitro susceptibility test results	Clindamycin, doxycycline, oral cephalosporins*
Highly penicillin resistant[§] (MIC, ≥2 µg/mL)	Agents based on in vitro susceptibility results, fluoroquinolones,[‡] vancomycin	
Empirical selection	Fluoroquinolones;[‡] selection based on susceptibility test results in community[¶]	Clindamycin, doxycycline, vancomycin
	Penicillin[#]	Cephalosporins,* macrolides,[†] amoxicillin, clindamycin
Haemophilus influenzae	Second- or third-generation cephalosporins, doxycycline, β-lactam--β-lactamase inhibitor, fluoroquinolines[‡]	Azithromycin, TMP-SMZ
Moraxella catarrhalis	Second- or third-generation cephalosporins, TMP-SMZ, amoxicillin/ clavulanate	Macrolides,[†] fluoroquinolones,[‡] β-lactam--β-lactamase inhibitor
Anaerobes	Clindamycin, penicillin plus metronidazole, β-lactam--β-lactamase inhibitor	Penicillin G or penicillin V, ampicillin/ amoxicillin with or without metronidazole

(continued)

TREATMENT OF PNEUMONIA ACCORDING TO PATHOGEN (CONTINUED)

Pathogen	Preferred Antimicrobial	Alternative Antimicrobial
Staphylococcus aureus[§] Methicillin susceptible	Nafcillin/oxacillin with or without rifampin or gentamicin[§]	Cefazolin or cefuroxime, vancomycin, clindamycin, TMP-SMZ, fluoroquinolones[‡]
Methicillin resistant	Vancomycin with or without rifampin or gentamicin	Requires in vitro testing; TMP-SMZ
Enterobacteriaceae (coliforms: *Escherichia coli, Klebsiella, Proteus, Enterobacter*)[§]	Third-generation cephalosporin with or without an aminoglycoside, carbapenems[**]	Aztreonam, β-lactam---β-lactamase inhibitor, fluoroquinolones[‡]
Pseudomonas aeruginosa[§]	Aminoglycoside plus antipseudomonal β-lactam: ticarcillin, piperacillin, mezlocillin, ceftazidime, cefepime, aztreonam, or carbapenems[**]	Aminoglycoside plus ciprofloxacin, ciprofloxacin plus antipseudomonal β-lactam
Legionella species	Macrolides[†] with or without rifampin, fluoroquinolones[‡]	Doxycycline with or without rifampin
Mycoplasma pneumoniae	Doxycycline, macrolides,[†] fluoroquinolones[‡]	. . .
Chlamydia pneumoniae	Doxycycline, macrolides,[†] fluoroquinolones[‡]	. . .
Influenza A	Amantadine or rimantadine	
Other viruses	None[††]	

Note: TMP-SMZ = trimethoprim-sulfamethoxazole

*Intravenous: cefazolin, cefuroxime, cefotaxime, ceftriaxone; oral: cefpodoxime, cefprozil, cefuroxime

[†]Erythromycin, clarithromycin, or azithromycin

[‡]Levofloxacin, sparfloxacin, grepafloxacin, trovafloxacin, or another fluoroquinolone with enhanced activity against *S. pneumoniae*; ciprofloxacin is appropriate for *Legionella* species, fluoroquinolone-susceptible *S. aureus*, and most gram-negative bacilli

[§]In vitro susceptibility tests are required for optimal treatment; for *Enterobacter* species, the preferred antibiotics are fluoroquinolones and carbapenems

[¶]High rates of high-level penicillin resistance, susceptibility of community strains unknown, and/or patient is seriously ill

[#]Low rates of penicillin resistance in community and patient is at low risk for infection with resistant *S. pneumoniae*

[**]Imipenem and meropenem

[††]Provide supportive care

Adapted from Bartlett, J.G., Breiman, R.F., Mandell, L.A., & File, T.M., Jr. (1998). Guidelines from the Infectious Disease Society of America. Community-acquired pneumonia in adults: Guidelines for management. <u>Clinical Infectious Diseases, 26,</u> 811-836.

    E.   Patient Education
          1.   Increase oral fluids
          2.   Avoid cough suppressants and cigarettes

    F.   Prevention: More emphasis is being placed on the role of vaccination in preventing pneumonia than in the past
          1.   Pneumococcal vaccination is a strategy to control the expansion of drug-resistant pneumococci
               a.   Approximately 90% of penicillin-resistant pneumococci are serotypes covered by the vaccine
               b.   Vaccination is recommended for the following persons: persons ≥65 years, immunocompetent persons ≥2 years who are at increased risk for illness and death because of chronic illness, persons aged ≥2 years with functional or anatomic asplenia, persons aged ≥2 years living in environments in which the risk of disease is high, and immunocompromised persons aged ≥2 years; studies are beginning to find that adults as young as 50 years may also benefit from vaccine
               c.   Revaccination is recommended for all high-risk adults who were initially immunized for at least 5 years or before; revaccinate only once
          2.   Yearly influenza immunization is recommended for at-risk populations and health care workers

G. Follow Up
   1. Contact patient with moderate-to-severe symptoms within 24 hours by phone or see in office
   2. With effective antimicrobial therapy, some improvement in the clinical manifestations of pneumonia should be seen within 48-72 hours; however, antimicrobial therapy should not be changed within first 72 hours unless there is a marked clinical deterioration
      a. Consult specialist if there is little improvement or deterioration after 48-72 hours of therapy
      b. Sampling of lower respiratory tract secretions with bronchoscopy and other diagnostic tests such as computerized tomography are often needed at this point
   3. For patients with moderate and severe symptoms who are improving, schedule return visit in 3-4 days after treatment is initiated to assess response
   4. Then, evaluate patients in 2-3 weeks
   5. For patients >40 years and all smokers, another return visit should be scheduled in 4-8 weeks to obtain second chest x-ray to rule out bronchogenic carcinoma which has a similar presentation as pneumonia

TUBERCULOSIS

I. Definition: Necrotizing bacterial infection most commonly infecting the lungs; other important definitions include the following:

A. Exposure: Applies to a person who has recent contact with an individual with suspected or confirmed, contagious pulmonary tuberculosis (TB) and whose tuberculin skin test is nonreactive and who has a normal physical examination and chest x-ray

B. TB infection: Positive tuberculin skin test in an individual with absent physical findings of disease and a chest x-ray which is either normal or has only granulomas or calcifications in lung and/or regional lymph nodes

C. TB disease: Individual with infection who has signs, symptoms, and x-ray manifestations which are apparently caused by *M. tuberculosis*; disease may be pulmonary or extrapulmonary

II. Pathogenesis

A. Primary or initial infection occurs by inhalation of the etiologic agent, *Mycobacterium tuberculosis*, which is dispersed as droplet nuclei (small airborne particles) from persons with sputum-smear-positive pulmonary tuberculosis (TB) when they cough or sneeze

B. Approximately 90% of primary TB infections remain in a latent or dormant infection stage; persons in this stage are not infectious

C. Active TB disease may develop after periods of stress or at times when the body is undergoing change or fighting an infection

D. The duration of infectivity is variable, but the majority of adult and adolescent patients are noncontagious within a few weeks of starting appropriate therapy; children < 12 years are usually not contagious because their lesions are small and cough is minimal

E. Incubation period from infection to development of a positive reaction to tuberculin skin test is 2-12 weeks

F. Current classification system (see Table that follows) is based on pathogenesis

G. The lungs are the most common sites for clinical TB (85% of cases), but TB is a systemic disease and can result in, disseminated TB (miliary TB), or infections in the bones and joints as well as in the lymphatic, genitourinary, and central nervous systems

	CLASSIFICATION SYSTEM FOR TB	
Class	Type	Description
0	No TB exposure Not infected	No history of exposure Negative reaction to tuberculin skin test
1	TB exposure No evidence of infection	History of exposure Negative reaction to tuberculin skin test
2	TB infection No disease	Positive reaction to tuberculin skin test Negative bacteriologic studies (if done) No clinical or radiographic evidence of TB
3	Current TB Disease	*M. tuberculosis* cultured (if done) or Positive reaction to tuberculin skin test and Clinical or radiographic evidence of current disease
4	Previous TB disease	History of episode(s) of TB or Abnormal but stable radiographic findings Positive reaction to the tuberculin skin test Negative bacteriologic studies (if done) and No clinical or radiologic evidence of current disease
5	TB suspected	Diagnosis pending

Source: US Department of Health and Human Services, Public Health Service, Centers for Disease Control. (1994). Core Curriculum on Tuberculosis.

III. Clinical Presentation

A. From 1985-1993 reported TB cases increased by 14% due to such factors as the HIV epidemic, deterioration in the health-care infrastructure, number of cases among foreign-born individuals, and transmission of TB in congregate shelters

B. Outbreaks of multidrug-resistant TB (MDR-TB) -- resistant to both isoniazid (INH) and rifampin (RIF) -- are a serious concern; these outbreaks have been associated with a high prevalence of HIV infection among the outbreak cases, a high mortality rate, and a high transmission rate of MDR-TB to heath-care and correctional facility workers

C. Presenting symptoms of TB in adults are often vague and may include the following:
   1. Productive, prolonged cough over 3 weeks duration
   2. Chest pain
   3. Hemoptysis
   4. Increased fatigue, malaise, anorexia, weight decrease
   5. Periodic fever, night sweats

D. Symptoms of extrapulmonary TB depend on the site affected: hematuria may occur in TB of the kidney and back pain may occur in TB of the spine

E.   Certain persons are more likely to become infected with *M. tuberculosis* (see table)

INDIVIDUALS AT RISK FOR TB INFECTION

✦ Anyone in close contact with an infectious case

✦ Anyone with associated COPD, diabetes, malignancy, alcoholism, end-stage renal disease, poor nutrition, gastrectomy, stomach bypass surgery for weight loss, chronic malabsorption syndromes, steroid treatment, 10% or more below ideal body weight

✦ Minority groups, homeless, institutionalized groups, persons living in correctional facilities, migrant farm workers, users of intravenous or other street drugs or children who are frequently exposed to adults from the preceding groups

✦ Patients who are HIV positive

Source: U.S. Department of Health & Human Services, Public Health Service, Centers for Disease Control. (1994). Core Curriculum on Tuberculosis.

IV.   Diagnosis/Evaluation

A.   History
1.   Inquire about onset and duration of weight loss, fatigue, fever, night sweats, anorexia, cough, hemoptysis, chest pain as well as localized symptoms in other body organs such as hematuria, enlarged lymph nodes
2.   Ask about history of exposure to TB at home, work, school, or social events
3.   Determine whether patient has had previous TB or active disease; inquire about previous TB treatments
4.   Ask about risk factors
5.   Ask about results and dates of TB skin tests and chest x-rays
6.   Inquire about travel to developing countries where TB is common

B.   Physical Examination
1.   Observe for skin pallor
2.   Palpate for lymphadenopathy
3.   Inspect, palpate, percuss, and auscultate chest (rales in upper posterior chest, bronchovesicular breathing and whispered pectoriloquy are often positive findings in patients with TB)
4.   Complete physical exam is needed if disseminated TB is suspected

C.   Differential Diagnosis
1.   Malignancy
2.   Silicosis
3.   Chronic obstructive pulmonary disease
4.   Asthma
5.   Bronchiectasis
6.   Pneumonia

D.   Diagnostic Tests
1.   Screening is performed to identify infected individuals at high risk for developing TB disease and to identify individuals with TB disease who need treatment; regular tuberculin testing of high risk groups is recommended (no need to repeat PPD on a person with a known positive tuberculin skin test)
a.   Preferred method of screening is the Mantoux tuberculin skin test 5 TU-PPD
(1)   The skin test is the only way to diagnosis TB infection before the infection has progressed to TB disease; generally, takes 2 to 10 weeks after infection for person to react positively to skin test
(2)   Administer intradermal injection of 0.1 mL of purified protein derivative (PPD) tuberculin containing 5 tuberculin units (TU) into volar or dorsal surface of forearm which should produce a discrete pale wheal 6 mm to 10 mm in diameter
(a)   Monitor for reactions 48 hours after application
(b)   Measure only the area of induration and record in millimeters

(3) Interpretation of PPD: PPD is considered positive and indicating primary, latent or active TB in the following cases:

POSITIVE PPDS
✦ ≥5 mm if patient is one of the following: Known or suspected HIV+, had close contact with person with infectious TB, has chest x-ray suggestive of previous TB, injects IV drugs (if HIV status is unknown), and is a child with symptoms suggestive of TB or is immunosuppressed from causes other than HIV infection
✦ ≥10 mm if patient is one of the following: foreign born from area where TB is common, lives in medically underserved area, member of low-income population (including high-risk racial and ethnic groups), lives in long-term care residence, is an IV drug user (if HIV status negative), has medical risk factor, is health care worker in facility where TB patients receive care, is from locally identified high-prevalence group (migrant farm worker or homeless person), is a child <4 years of age
✦ ≥15 mm: all persons with no known risk factor for TB

Adapted from U.S. Department of Health & Human Services, Public Health Service, Centers for Disease Control. (1994). Core Curriculum on Tuberculosis.

(4) Anergy
    (a) Although routine anergy testing is no longer recommended for HIV positive persons, consider anergy on an individual basis in persons with negative skin tests who have the following: HIV infection, severe or febrile illness, overwhelming immunosuppressive therapy, severe or febrile illness or overwhelming TB infection
    (b) Determine anergy by administering two delayed-type hypersensitivity antigens such as mumps, or *Candida* by the Mantoux technique; persons with a reaction ≥3mm are not anergic
    (c) If anergy is present, probability of infection should be evaluated and persons judged at high risk of exposure should be considered for preventive therapy
(5) Two-step testing is used to differentiate boosted reactions from reactions due to new infection and should be performed in adults who will be retested periodically such as health care workers
    (a) Some individuals with TB infection may have a negative skin test when tested several years after an infection; however, the skin test may stimulate their ability to react to tuberculin and cause positive reactions to subsequent tests (boost) which may be misinterpreted as new infections
    (b) To distinguish a boosted reaction from a new infection when the first test is negative, administer a second skin test 1-3 weeks after first test.
        i) If second test is negative: person is uninfected and any subsequent positive test should be classified as a new infection
        ii) If second test is positive: person is infected and should be treated accordingly
b. Chest radiograph or sputum smears may be the recommended first screening test in populations where risk of transmission is high and difficulties in administering and reading tests exist such as jails or homeless shelters
2. Diagnosis of active disease
  a. Order three sputum specimens for **both** smear examination and culture in patients suspected of pulmonary or laryngeal TB
    (1) A presumptive diagnosis of TB can be made with detection of acid-fast bacilli (AFB); results can usually be obtained in 24 hours
    (2) A positive sputum culture for *M. tuberculosis* is essential to confirm diagnosis, but often takes several weeks for results to be obtained
    (3) Drug susceptibility testing should be done on the initial *M. Tuberculosis* isolate; testing should also be performed on additional isolates from patients whose cultures fail to convert to negative within 3 months of beginning therapy, or if there is clinical evidence of failure to respond to therapy

(4) Aerosol induction to stimulate sputum production, bronchoscopy, or gastric aspiration should be done if the patient cannot produce a sputum specimen and there is suspicion of TB

    b. A tuberculin skin test is helpful in making diagnosis and should be applied, but absence of a reaction to the test does not exclude diagnosis

    c. Order posterior-anterior chest x-ray

      (1) Abnormalities are suggestive, but are not diagnostic of TB; x-rays may rule out possibility of pulmonary TB in an asymptomatic person with a positive skin test

      (2) In pulmonary TB, abnormalities are often present in apical or posterior segments of upper lobes or superior segments of lower lobes; in HIV infected persons, other abnormalities are often present

    3. Other tests are ordered after TB is diagnosed. Order baseline measurements of hepatic enzymes, bilirubin, serum creatinine, blood urea nitrogen (BUN), CBC, and platelet count; serum uric acid if pyrazinamide will be prescribed (see V.C. for additional tests needed when drug therapy is used)

V. Plan/Management

    A. Preventive therapy reduces the risk that TB infection will progress to actual disease

      1. Preventive therapy is needed for certain groups of people (see following table)

CANDIDATES FOR PREVENTIVE THERAPY

❖ Skin test positive for persons in the following high-risk groups, regardless of age:
- ✔ Persons with known or suspected HIV infection
- ✔ Close contacts of infectious TB cases
- ✔ Recent tuberculin skin-test converters
- ✔ Previously untreated or inadequately treated persons with abnormal chest radiographs
- ✔ Intravenous drug users
- ✔ Persons with medical conditions which increase the risk of TB

❖ Skin test positive persons in the following high-risk groups who are <35 years of age:
- ✔ Foreign-born persons from high prevalence countries
- ✔ Medically underserved, low income populations, including high-risk minorities
- ✔ Residents of long-term care facilities (including prisons)
- ✔ Locally identified high-prevalence groups (migrant farm workers or homeless persons)
- ✔ Children younger than 4 years of age

❖ Other candidates:
- ✔ Infected persons <35 years of age with no additional risk factors should be evaluated for preventive therapy if reaction to tuberculin test ≥15 mm (priority is lower than groups already listed)
- ✔ Persons who are close contacts with infectious cases should have X-ray regardless of skin test reaction and considered for preventive therapy in following cases: persons in circumstances with high probability of infection, children or adolescents, immunosuppressed persons (close contacts with negative initial reaction should be retested 10 weeks after last exposure to TB)
- ✔ Infants exposed to person with TB should be given a skin test and chest x-ray and started on preventive therapy even if tests are negative because infants <6 months may be anergic; retest again in 3-4 months and at 6 months if initial tests are negative

❖ Consult specialist for pregnant women

Table adapted from U.S. Department of Health & Human Services. (1994). Core Curriculum on Tuberculosis.

      2. Before beginning preventive therapy:

        a. Exclude possibility of current TB which would require multiple drug therapy

        b. Question history of previous preventive therapy

        c. Explore characteristics of person (preventive therapy might **not** be indicated in the following persons: persons at high risk for adverse reactions to isoniazid (INH) such as those with acute or active liver disease, persons who cannot tolerate INH, persons likely to be infected with drug-resistant *M. tuberculosis*, persons who are highly unlikely to complete course of preventive therapy)

3. Drug therapy for prevention of disease is recommended for persons <35 years with positive PPD and no evidence of active disease but is **not** recommended for persons who are ≥35 years unless they are at high risk for developing TB disease because the risk of isoniazid-related hepatitis outweighs the benefits of preventive therapy in this age group (see Table DOSAGES FOR PREVENTIVE THERAPY)
   a. Dispense only a 1-month supply of drug at a time
   b. Monthly question for the following: compliance, symptoms of neurotoxicity (paresthesias of hands and feet), signs of hepatitis

DOSAGES FOR PREVENTIVE DRUG THERAPY	
Type of Patient	**Dosage[†]**
❖ Adults	INH 300 mg QD for 6 months
❖ Adults with HIV infection	INH 300 mg QD for 12 months
❖ Adults with positive skin test and either silicosis or chest x-ray demonstrating old fibrotic lesions	INH 300 mg QD for 12 months or 4 months of INH and rifampin 10 mg/kg/day
❖ Adults with close contacts of infectious patients who have INH-resistant TB	Rifampin 10 mg/kg/day QD for 6 months or Rifampin 300 mg tab BID; 1 hour before meals or 2 hours after meals
❖ Children with close contacts of infectious patients who have INH-resistant TB	Rifampin 10mg/kg/day QD for 9 months

[†] INH can also be given 2x weekly in dose of 15 mg/kg when compliance is doubtful and direct observation is needed

   c. Take special precautions in patients who are at high risk of adverse reactions to INH such as persons ≥35 years, or who have chronic liver disease, peripheral neuropathy (or are predisposed to developing neuropathy such as diabetics), abuse alcohol, are pregnant or inject drugs
      (1) Frequently monitor liver enzymes; if measurements exceed 3-5 times upper limit of normal, discontinue INH
      (2) In patients prone to developing neuropathy, prescribe pyridoxine (10-15mg/day)
   d. New, short-course preventive treatment regimens are currently being investigated

B. Treatment of active disease (uncomplicated, intrathoracic TB): The initial treatment should include four drugs: isoniazid (INH), rifampin (RIF), pyrazinamide (PZA), and either ethambutol (EMB) or streptomycin (SM)
   1. See tables that follow for regimens and dosages of initial drug therapy in adults and in patients with special considerations; when drug susceptibility results are available, the regimen should be altered as appropriate

REGIMEN OPTIONS FOR INITIAL TREATMENT OF PULMONARY AND EXTRAPULMONARY TB

TB without HIV Infection

Option 1	Option 2	Option 3
Administer daily INH, RIF, PZA, and EMB or SM for 8 wks, followed by 16 wks* of INH and RIF daily or 2-3 times/ week** In areas where the INH resistance rate is <4%, EMB or SM may not be necessary for patients with no individual risk factors for drug resistance. Consult a TB medical expert if the patient is symptomatic or smear or culture positive after 3 months.	Administer daily INH, RIF, PZA, and SM or EMB for 2 wks followed by 2 times/week** administration of the same drugs for 6 weeks (by DOT‡), and subsequently, with 2 times/week** administration of INH and RIF for 16 weeks (by DOT).* Consult a TB medical expert if the patient is symptomatic or smear or culture positive after 3 months.	Treat by DOT, 3 times/week** with INH, RIF, PZA, and EMB or SM for 6 months.† Consult a TB medical expert if the patient is symptomatic or smear or culture positive after 3 months.

*For adults with miliary TB, bone and joint TB, or TB meningitis response to therapy should be closely monitored and treatment should be altered accordingly.

**All regimens administered 2 times/week or 3 times/week should be monitored by DOT for the duration of therapy.

†The strongest evidence from clinical trials is the effectiveness of all four drugs administered for the full 6 months. There is weaker evidence that SM can be discontinued after 4 months if the isolate is susceptible to all drugs. The evidence for stopping PZA before the end of 6 months is equivocal for the 3 times/week regimen, and there is no evidence on the effectiveness of this regimen with EMB for less than the full 6 months.

‡DOT = Directly observed therapy.

Table adapted from U.S. Department of Health & Human Services. (1994). Core Curriculum on Tuberculosis.

OPTIONS FOR INITIAL TREATMENT OF PULMONARY AND EXTRAPULMONARY TB IN SPECIAL CIRCUMSTANCES

Smear-and culture negative pulmonary TB	Pulmonary and extrapulmonary TB when PZA is contraindicated
Administer INH, RIF, PZA, and EMB or SM following options 1, 2, or 3 for initial therapy in table above for 8 weeks followed by INH, RIF, PZA, and EMB or SM daily or 2-3 times** per week (DOT) for 8 weeks. If drug resistance is unlikely, EMB or SM may be unnecessary and PZA may be discontinued after 2 months	Administer INH, RIF, and EMB or SM daily for 8 weeks followed by INH and RIF daily or 2 times per week** (DOT) for 24 weeks.* If drug resistance is unlikely, EMB or SM may be unnecessary

*For adults with miliary TB, bone and joint TB, or TB meningitis response to therapy should be closely monitored and treatment should be altered accordingly.

**All regimens administered 2 times/week or 3 times/week should be monitored by DOT for the duration of therapy.

DOSAGE RECOMMENDATION FOR FIRST-LINE DRUGS IN INITIAL TREATMENT OF TB

Drugs	Dosage		
	Daily	2 times/week	3 times/week
Isoniazid	5 mg/kg Max 300 mg	15 mg/kg Max 900 mg	15 mg/kg Max 900 mg
Rifampin	10 mg/kg Max 600 mg	10 mg/kg Max 600 mg	10 mg/kg Max 600 mg
Pyrazinamide	15-30 mg/kg Max 2 gm	50-70 mg/kg Max 4 gm	50-70 mg/kg Max 3 gm
Ethambutol	15-25 mg/kg Max 2.5 gm	50 mg/kg Max 2.5 gm	25-30 mg/kg Max 2.5 gm
Streptomycin	15 mg/kg Max 1 gm	25-30 mg/kg Max 1.5 gm	25-30 mg/kg Max 1 gm

Source: Initial therapy for tuberculosis in the era of multi resistance: Recommendations of the Advisory Council for the Elimination of Tuberculosis. MMWR 42 (No. RR-7) (1993).

2. Rufapentine (Priftin) was FDA approved fall 1998
    a. Administer for 2 months, four 150-mg tablets taken twice weekly with no more than 3 days between doses; use in combination with at least one other antituberculosis drug
    b. Then administer four 150-mg tablets once a week for 4 months with an antituberculosis agent
    c. Do not give Priftin to patients with a history of hypersensitivity to rifamycins
    d. Adverse effects are hyperuricemia, increased liver function tests, neutropenia, pyuria, proteinuria, and lymphopenia
3. Second-line TB drugs may be prescribed after consulting a specialist: capreomycin, kanamycin, ethionamide, para-aminosalicylic acid, cycloserine, ciprofloxacin, ofloxacin, amikacin, clofazimine
4. Treatment of persons with additional medical conditions must be individualized
    a. For patients with impaired renal function avoid streptomycin, kanamycin and capreomycin if possible
    b. In patients with HIV infection duration of treatment is the same as HIV-negative adults; HIV positive adults should be aggressively assessed for response to treatment and treatment should be prolonged if response is slow or suboptimal
5. Treatment of drug-resistant TB
    a. In patients with documented INH resistance during initial four-drug therapy, discontinue INH and continue RIF, PZA, and EMB or SM for entire 6 months -or- treat with RIF and EMB for 12 months
    b. Consult specialist for multidrug-resistant TB
6. Directly observed therapy (DOT) is one method to ensure adherence
    a. DOT requires that a health-care provider or other designated person observe patient while ingesting anti-TB medications
    b. All patients with TB caused by organisms resistant to either INH or RIF and all patients receiving intermittent therapy should receive DOT

C. Monitoring of adults on drug therapy includes the following:
    1. Adults treated for TB should have baseline measurements of hepatic enzymes, bilirubin, serum creatinine or BUN, CBC and platelet count; measure serum uric acid if pyrazinamide is used; test visual acuity if EMB is used; test hearing function if SM is used
    2. At minimum, patients should be seen monthly by provider and assessed for adverse reactions to drugs
    3. Drug interactions: Current literature and package inserts should be consulted
        a. INH and phenytoin interact; monitor serum level of phenytoin
        b. Rifampin may increase the clearance of drugs metabolized by the liver: methadone, coumadin derivatives, glucocorticoids, estrogens, oral hypoglycemic agents, digitalis, anticonvulsants, ketoconazole, fluconazole, cyclosporin; women should use birth control method other than oral contraceptives or Norplant while on rifampin
    4. Specific guidelines for drug monitoring
        a. INH: baseline hepatic enzymes; then, repeat measurements if abnormal or at risk for adverse reactions
        b. Rifampin: baseline CBC, platelets, hepatic enzymes; repeat as needed
        c. PZA: Baseline uric acid and hepatic enzymes; repeat as needed
        d. Ethambutol: baseline and monthly visual acuity and color vision tests
        e. Streptomycin: Baseline hearing test and kidney function; repeat as needed
    5. Monitoring response to therapy includes the following:
        a. Sputum exam at least monthly until conversion to negative; then, at least one sputum at completion of therapy
        b. For patients with multi-drug resistant TB, monthly sputum evaluation should continue for entire course of treatment
        c. Chest radiographs are less important than sputums but chest film at completion of treatment provides a baseline for future comparisons

      d.   Patients with sputum that remains culture positive beyond 3 months should be evaluated for disease due to drug-resistant organisms

      e.   When waiting for drug susceptibility results, continue the original drug regimen or augment regimen with at least three new drugs; **never** add one drug to a failing regimen

D.   BCG vaccination

1.   Vaccination is used in many countries, but is not generally recommended in U.S.

2.   BCG vaccination should be considered on an individual basis among health care workers (HCW) in high-risk settings; HCWs should be informed of variable data about efficacy of BCG vaccination, the interference of BCG vaccination with diagnosing newly acquired TB infection, and possible serious complications of BCG vaccine in immunocompromised persons

3.   BCG vaccination is **not** recommended for HCWs in low-risk settings and is **not** recommended for HIV-infected children or adults

4.   In persons vaccinated with BCG, sensitivity to tuberculin is highly variable; there is no reliable method for distinguishing tuberculin reactions caused by BCG from those caused by natural infections; all BCG-vaccinated persons who have positive skin test should be further evaluated to determine need for preventive therapy

E.   Patient Education: Teach about possible reactions to medicines

1.   INH
    a.   Hepatic toxicity is the most common adverse reaction
    b.   Peripheral neuropathy may be prevented by taking 25 mg of pyridoxine QD

2.   Rifampin
    a.   GI upset, hepatitis, bleeding problems, flu-like symptoms, and rash
    b.   Warn patient that tears, urine, saliva, etc., may turn orange-red; may permanently stain contact lenses

3.   Pyrazinamide: hyperuricemia, gout, hepatitis, joint aches, rash, and GI upset

4.   Ethambutol: Optic neuritis

5.   Streptomycin: Hearing and balance changes and renal toxicity

F.   Patient education also includes discussion of mode of transmission and need to cover nose and mouth when coughing or sneezing; no sharing of eating utensils

G.   Follow Up

1.   Patient must have sputum examination at least monthly until conversion to negative

2.   Patients with multi-drug resistant TB need monthly sputum evaluations for entire course of therapy

3.   Monthly monitoring of adverse reactions to drugs and response to treatment while on drug therapy is essential

4.   Chest films are helpful at completion of therapy

REFERENCES

Advisory Committee on Immunization Practices. (1997). Prevention of pneumococcal disease: Recommendations of the Advisory Committee on Immunization Practices (ACIP). MMWR, 46(RR-8), 1-21.

Advisory Council for the Elimination of Tuberculosis (1993). The initial therapy for tuberculosis in the era of multidrug resistance: Recommendations of the Advisory Council for the Elimination of Tuberculosis. MMWR, 42(RR-7), 1-7

Advisory Council for the Elimination of Tuberculosis and the Advisory Committee on Immunization Practices. (1996). The role of BCG vaccine in the prevention and control of tuberculosis in the United States. MMWR, 42(RR-4), 1-17

American Academy of Pediatrics. 1997. In G. Peter (Ed.). Red Book: Report of the Committee on Infectious Disease. 24th ed. Elk Grove Village, IL: Academy of Pediatrics.

American Thoracic Society (1993). Guidelines for the initial management of adults with community-acquired pneumonia: Diagnosis, assessment of severity, and initial antimicrobial therapy. American Review of Respiratory Disease, 148, 1418-1426.

American Thoracic Society. (1995). Comprehensive outpatient management of COPD. <u>American Journal of Respiratory and Critical Care Medicine, 152,</u>S84-S99.

Bartlett, J.G., Breiman, R.F., Mandell, L.A., & File, T.M., Jr. (1998). Guidelines from the Infectious Disease Society of America. Community-acquired pneumonia in adults: Guidelines for management. <u>Clinical Infectious Diseases, 26,</u> 811-836.

Bartlett, J.G., & Munday, L.M. (1995). Community-acquired pneumonia. <u>New England Journal of Medicine, 333,</u> 1618-1624.

Bergh, K.D. (1998). The patient's differential diagnosis: Unpredictable concerns in visits for acute cough. <u>The Journal of Family Practice, 46,</u> 153-158.

Bertka, K.R. (1997). Managing patients with COPD in the office. <u>Family Practice Recertification, 19</u>(9), 63-86.

Carney, I.K., Gibson, P.G., Murree-Allen, K., Saltos, N., Olson, L.G., & Hensley, M.J. (1997). A systematic evaluation of mechanisms in chronic cough. <u>American Journal of Respiratory Critical Care Medicine, 156,</u> 211-216.

Celi, BR, et al. (1995). Standards for the diagnosis and care of patients with chronic obstructive pulmonary disease. <u>American Journal of Respiratory and Critical Care Medicine, 152,</u> S77-S120.

Celi, BR (1998). Standards for the optimal management of COPD: A summary. <u>Chest, 113,</u> 283S-287S

Ferguson, G.T. (1998). Management of COPD. <u>Postgraduate Medicine, 103,</u> 130-141.

Ferguson, G.T. & Cherniack, R.M. (1993). Management of chronic obstructive pulmonary disease. <u>New England Journal of Medicine, 328,</u> 1017-1022.

Fine, M.J., Auble, T.E., Yealy, D.M., Hanusa, B.H., Weissfeld, L.A., Singer, D.E., Coley, C.M., Marrie, T.J., & Kapoor, W.N. (1997). A prediction rule to identify low-risk patients with community-acquired pneumonia. <u>New England Journal of Medicine, 336,</u> 243-250.

Fine, M.J., Smith, M.A., Carson, C.A., Mutha, S.S., Sankey, S.S., Weissfeld, L.A., & Kapoor, W.N. (1996). Prognosis and outcomes of patients with community-acquired pneumonia: A meta-analysis. <u>JAMA, 275,</u> 134-141.

Glaser V. (Ed.). (September 30, 1997). Bracing for the cold and flu season. <u>Patient Care,</u> 47-62.

Gleason, P.P. & Fine, M.J. (1997). Medical outcomes and antimicrobial costs with the use of the American Thoracic Society Guidelines for outpatients with community-acquired pneumonia. <u>JAMA, 278,</u> 32-39.

Goroll, A.H., May, L.A., & Mulley, A.G., Jr. (1995). Evaluation of hemoptysis. In A.H. Goroll, L.A. May & A.G. Mulley, Jr. (Eds.), <u>Primary care medicine: Office evaluation and management of the adult patient.</u> Philadelphia: J.B. Lippincott.

Grossman, R.F. (1998). The value of antibiotics and the outcomes of antibiotic therapy in exacerbations of COPD. <u>Chest, 113,</u> 249S-255S.

Hayden, F.G., Diamond, L., Wood, P.B., Korts, D.C., & Wecker, M.T. (1996). Effectiveness and safety of intranasal ipratropium bromide in common colds: A randomized, double-blind, placebo-controlled trial. <u>Annals of Internal Medicine, 125,</u> 89-97.

Hemila, H. , & Herman, Z.S. (1995). Vitamin C and the common cold: A retrospective analysis of Chalmers' Review. <u>Journal of American College of Nutrition, 14,</u> 116-123

Hendeles, L., Jenkins, J., & Temple, R. (1995). Revised FDA labeling guideline for theophylline oral dosage forms. <u>Pharmacotherapy, 15</u> (4), 409-427.

Hueston, W.J., & Mainous, A.G. (1998). Acute bronchitis. <u>American Family Physician, 57,</u> 1270-1276.

Institute for Clinical Systems Integration. (1998). Viral upper respiratory tract infection in adults: Differential diagnosis, patient education, and home. <u>Postgraduate Medicine, 103,</u> 71-80.

Iseman, M.D. (1993). Treatment of multidrug-resistant tuberculosis. <u>New England Journal of Medicine, 329</u>(11), 784-790.

Johannsen, J.M. (1994). Chronic obstructive pulmonary disease: Current comprehensive care for emphysema and bronchitis. <u>Nurse Practitioner, 19</u>(1), 59-67.

Latham, B.A. & Morell, V.W. (1996). Viral and atypical pneumonias. <u>Primary Care, 23,</u> 837-849.

Leiner, S. (1997). Acute bronchitis in adults: Commonly diagnosed but poorly defined. <u>Nurse Practitioner, 22</u>(1), 104-117.

Marrie, T.J., Peeling, R.W., Fine, M.J., Singer, D.E., Coley, C.M., & Kapoor, W.N. (1996). Ambulatory patients with community-acquired pneumonia: The frequency of atypical agents and clinical course. <u>American Journal of Medicine, 101,</u> 58-515.

Mello, C.J., Irwin, R.S., & Curley, F.J. (1996). Predictive values of the character, timing, and complications of chronic cough in diagnosing its cause. <u>Archives of Internal Medicine, 156,</u> 997-1003.

Metlay, J.P., Kapoor, W.N., & Fine, M.J. (1997). Does this patient have community-acquired pneumonia? Diagnosing pneumonia by history and physical examination. JAMA, 278, 1440-1445.

Mossard, S.B., Macknin, M.L., Medendorp, S.V., & Mason, P. (1996). Zinc gluconate lozenges for treating the common cold. Annals of Internal Medicine, 125, 81-88.

National Institutes of Health. (1992). Teach your patients about asthma: A clinician's guide. National Asthma Education Program, Office of Prevention, Education and Control. Publication #92-2737. Bethesda, MD.

National Institutes of Health. National Heart, Lung, and Blood Institute. (1997). The Expert Panel Report 2: Guidelines for the Diagnosis and Management of Asthma. National Asthma Education Program, Office of Prevention, Education and Control. NIH Publication #97-4051. Bethesda, MD.

National Lung Health Education Program Executive Committee. (1998). Strategies in preserving lung health and preventing COPD and associated diseases: The National Lung Health Education Program. Chest, 113, 123S-S154S.

Niederman, M.S. (1998). Community-acquired pneumonia: A North American perspective. Chest, 113, 179S-182S.

O'Brien, K.L., Dowell, S.F., Schwartz, B., Marcy, S.M., Phillips, W.R., & Gerber, M.A. (1998). Cough illness/bronchitis--principles of judicious use of antimicrobial agents. Pediatrics, 101, 178-181

Petty, T.L. (1998). Supportive therapy in COPD. Chest, 113, 256S-262S.

Philip, E.B. (1997). Chronic cough. American Family Physician, 56, 1395-1402.

Rosenstein, N., Phillips, W.R., Gerber, M.A., Marcy, M., Schwartz, B., & Dowell, S.F. (1998). The common cold--principles of judicious use of antimicrobial agents. Pediatrics, 101, 181-184.

Senior, R.M., & Anthonisen, N.R. (1998). Chronic obstructive pulmonary disease. American Journal of Respiratory and Critical Care Medicine, 157, S139-S147.

Sullivan, N.C. (1997). Assessment and management of persistent cough in adults. Clinical Excellence for Nurse Practitioners, 1, 417-421.

Turner, R.B. (1997). Epidemiology, pathogenesis, and treatment of the common cold. Annals of Allergy, Asthma, & Immunology, 78, 531-537.

U.S. Department of Health & Human Services, Public Health Service, Centers for Disease Control. (1994). Core Curriculum on Tuberculosis: What the Clinician Should Know (3rd ed.). Publication number 00-5763. Atlanta.

U.S. Department of Health & Human Services, Public Health Service, Centers for Disease Control. (1997). Anergy skin testing and preventive therapy for HIV-infected persons: Revised recommendations. MMWR, 46, (RR-15), 1-10.

Weg, J.G., & Haas, C.F. (1998). Long-term oxygen therapy for COPD: Improving longevity and quality of life in hypoxemic patients. Postgraduate Medicine, 103, 143-155.

Cardiovascular Problems

ATRIAL FIBRILLATION

I. Definition: Disorganized supraventricular tachycardia, ineffective atrial contraction, and irregular, chaotic and often rapid ventricular rate

   A. Acute atrial fibrillation (AF): fibrillation present for less than 3 days

   B. Paroxysmal AF: occurrence of attacks of fibrillation in a patient who typically has normal sinus rhythm; attacks are self-terminating, recurrent, and occur at variable time intervals

   C. Chronic AF: permanent fibrillation rather than brief episodes of symptoms

   D. "Lone" atrial fibrillation: fibrillation without identifiable heart disease or known precipitating factors

II. Pathogenesis

   A. Atrial fibrillation (AF) is frequently triggered by a premature atrial contraction which by re-entry emits multifocal impulses at a rate of 300-700 per minute; these impulses enter the atrioventricular (AV) node randomly and because of the AV node's slower rate of conduction not all of the impulses are conducted resulting in a ventricular rate that is slower than the atrial rate, as well as irregular; less commonly, atrial impulses result in an inadequate or insensitive ventricular response which can lead to severe bradycardia or sudden death

   B. Ineffective emptying of atria due to electrical stimulation from multiple atrial foci leads to hemodynamic instability, ineffective cardiac output, and stasis of blood which may result in thrombus formation and complications such as peripheral embolization and stroke

   C. Factors which predispose patients to develop AF are the following:
       1. Organic heart disease that causes atrial distention such as ischemia or infarction, hypertension, valvular disorders, obstructive cardiomyopathy, rheumatic heart disease, or Wolff-Parkinson-White syndrome
       2. Metabolic diseases such as hyperthyroidism and hypothyroidism
       3. Right atrial stretch due to pulmonary embolus and chronic lung disease
       4. High adrenergic tone secondary to alcohol withdrawal, sepsis, or excessive physical exertion

   D. The most common predisposing factors are coronary artery disease, acute respiratory illness, cardiothoracic surgery, and hyperthyroidism

III. Clinical Presentation

   A. AF is the most common, sustained, cardiac arrhythmia and causes more hospital admissions than any other arrhythmia

   B. Many patients are asymptomatic whereas a few have life-threatening symptoms

   C. Patients with rapid ventricular responses often complain of chest pain, fullness in neck, palpitations, fatigue, dizziness, or syncope secondary to decreased blood pressure

   D. In patients with organic heart disease, AF can lead to hemodynamic decompensation, hypotension, pulmonary edema, cardiac standstill or death

   E. In the past, patients with preexisting left ventricular failure or coronary obstruction had a poor prognosis; today, prognosis is fair if patients are closely followed and participate in cardiac rehabilitation

F. Complications:
1. A major complication is arterial embolization which may lead to stroke
2. AF can cause congestive heart failure (CHF) and severe cardiomyopathy in patients with otherwise normal hearts and restoration of sinus rhythm can reverse both conditions
3. AF increases myocardial vulnerability and decreases the fibrillation threshold which can enhance development of ventricular tachyarrhythmias and sudden death

IV. Diagnosis/Evaluation

A. History
1. Inquire about onset and duration of symptoms
2. Ask patient to describe all symptoms such as palpitations, dizziness, fatigue, calf pain, leg edema, dypsnea
3. Determine whether there is chest pain accompanying the tachycardia which might indicate ischemic heart disease or pulmonary embolism
4. Explore whether there has been a concomitant weight loss or gain, mood change, hair loss, and tremor which are often associated with hyperthyroidism
5. Carefully determine the number of previous episodes of palpitations and what relieved symptoms and what treatment, if any, was initiated
6. Explore precipitating factors such as emotional stress, activity, alcohol or drug use, bath in hot tub
7. Carefully explore previous medical history, focusing on cardiovascular problems, but also addressing pulmonary, endocrine, and neurological systems
8. Ask about family medical history
9. Obtain medication history

B. Physical Examination
1. Observe general appearance and signs of respiratory distress and altered levels of consciousness; note apathetic appearance which may be related to thyroid problems
2. Assess vital signs including postural blood pressure in supine or sitting and standing positions
3. Observe skin for pallor or flushing
4. Perform an eye exam, noting lid lag
5. Assess neck for thyromegaly, jugular venous distention, and carotid artery bruits
6. Perform a complete cardiovascular examination
7. Auscultate lungs
8. Perform a neurological examination, assessing deep tendon reflexes and observing for resting tremors

C. Differential Diagnosis: see factors under pathogenesis

D. Diagnostic Tests
1. Order a 12-lead electrocardiogram (ECG); AF is characterized by absence of P-waves and baseline fibrillatory activity; usually the ventricular rate is irregularly irregular (this finding is very important)
2. Order thyroid function tests
3. Order an echocardiogram
    a. Detects valvular abnormalities, pericardial effusion, enlarged chambers, ventricular contraction abnormalities, or other wall motion abnormalities
    b. Is helpful in predicting the success of cardioversion (a dilated left atrium or severe left ventricular failure has a low success rate)
    c. Transesophageal echocardiograms (TEE) are the most sensitive for identifying left atrial thrombi, but are expensive
4. Consider ordering electrolytes, blood urea nitrogen (BUN), creatinine
5. Ambulatory ECG readings may be necessary (i.e., 24-48 hour Holter monitor)
6. Consider chest x-ray to evaluate cardiomegaly

V.   Plan/Management: Goals of therapy are threefold: control ventricular rate, prevent recurrences (maintain sinus rhythm), and prevent thromboembolism and stroke

A.   Hospitalization is usually required for treatment of acute AF, particularly if ventricular rate is >170 per minute or <50 and patient has underlying cardiac disease (consult cardiologist); patients often revert to sinus rhythm when predisposing factors are removed; otherwise, direct-current-cardioversion (DCC) or intravenous drug therapy is indicated to stabilize patient until oral drug trials are initiated

B.   For patients who have mild stable symptoms with no cardiovascular compromise, oral therapy to control ventricular rate with an AV nodal blocking agent may be the only therapy that is needed; remember, however, these drugs do not convert an acute episode back to sinus rhythm and they do not prevent recurrences of AF; these drugs may also result in an inappropriately low ventricular response (see table that follows)

DRUGS TO CONTROL VENTRICULAR RATE	
Drug	**Dosing**
Digoxin (Lanoxin)	If the heart rate is between 100-120 beats per minute (bpm) begin with a maintenance dose of digoxin 0.25-0.375 mg per day; start with higher doses if rate is >120 bpm (i.e., 1.0-1.25 mg per day)

β-blockers*
  Nadolol (Corgard)
  Atenolol (Tenormin)
	
	40-80 mg daily
	25-100 mg daily

Calcium Channel Blockers*
  Verapamil (Calan)
  Diltiazem (Cardizem)
	
	120-480 mg daily
	90-360 mg daily

*Start at low doses and titrate slowly in elderly patients

1.   Digoxin slows the ventricular rate by blocking conduction through the atrioventricular node
    a.   Digoxin may be used as monotherapy; but recent research suggests that digoxin should usually be given in combination with calcium channel blockers and beta-blockers
    b.   Major disadvantages: Limited effect on exercise heart rate; less effective drug for people who exercise; toxicity can occur relatively rapidly
    c.   Digoxin can play an important role in controlling ventricular response when patient has left ventricular dysfunction
    d.   Reduce dosage of digoxin if patient is also receiving quinidine
2.   Beta-blockers also control ventricular response especially during exercise; these agents may be particularly beneficial when AF is associated with hyperthyroidism or other hyperadrenergic states such as acute myocardial infarction or sepsis
3.   Calcium channel blockers reduce both resting and exercise heart rates
    a.   Best given in a slow release, once daily preparation
    b.   Diltiazem and verapamil are equally effective; the dihydropyridines such as nifedipine are ineffective in AF
    c.   Diltiazem is better than verapamil for patients with poor left ventricular function
4.   Clonidine may also be effective in controlling ventricular response, but further studies are needed

C.   The AV nodal blocking drugs (digoxin, beta-blockers, calcium channel blockers) do not have any specific effect in promoting sinus rhythm; however, they do facilitate hemodynamics which may result in rate control; to restore sinus rhythm direct current cardioversion or pharmacologic cardioversion with an antiarrhythmic drug is often necessary
    1.   Elective direct cardioversion is sometimes the treatment of choice when the duration of the AF is less than 12 months and when the atria are of normal size (not enlarged and boggy)
        a.   Usually, patients are prescribed anticoagulant therapy (i.e., warfarin) for 3-4 weeks prior to cardioversion

  b. Unfortunately, the majority of patients with long-standing AF revert back to AF after cardioversion

  c. Cardioversion is the most effective means of restoring sinus rhythm but can result in embolisms, hypotension, pulmonary edema, and major arrhythmias

 2. Pharmacological conversion involves an antiarrhythmic drug (see table that follows); selection of a drug should be based on potential adverse effects in specific patients; because of dangers of proarrhythmia, drugs are usually initiated in the hospital with continuous cardiac monitoring

ANTIARRHYTHMIC DRUGS*		
Type	**Drug**	**Dose**
IA	Quinidine (Quinaglute) - or - (Quinidex)	324-648 mg q 8 hours (take with fluid and in an upright position) 300-600 mg q 8 hours (take with food in an upright position)
	Procainamide (Procan-SR)	50 mg/kg/day divided in 2 doses q 12 hours
	Disopyramide (Norpace CR)	200-400 mg q 12 hours
IC	Flecainide (Tambocor)	50-150 q 12 hours; Max. 300 mg/day
	Propafenone (Rythmol)	150-300 mg q 8 hours; Max 300mg q 8 hours
III	Sotalol HCl (Betapace)	80-240 mg q 12 hours; Max. 320 mg/day
	Amiodarone (Cordarone)	Initiate in hospital; 800-1200 mg/day in divided doses. After control is achieved, give 400-600 mg/day for one month, then gradually lower to maintenance dose of 200-300 mg/day within 6 months

*Prescribe lower doses in the elderly

  a. Amiodarone affects the repolarization of cardiac cell membranes and research has found it to be one of most effective antiarrhythmic agents

   (1) Also, slows ventricular response which is helpful

   (2) Less risk of proarrhythmia than other agents, but in high doses can cause pulmonary fibrosis, hepatitis and thyroid conditions

   (3) Important to order chest-xray, liver function tests, and thyroid tests every 3 months during first year, then every 6 months

   (4) Monitor drug levels closely for toxicity especially when used in combination with quinidine

  b. Quinidine was the traditional drug of choice, but used less today because of adverse effects

   (1) Causes severe gastric intolerance

   (2) Associated with excessive QT prolongation (torsade de pointes) which is the likely cause of "quinidine syncope", a syndrome precipitated by bradycardia and hypokalemia

  c. Disopyramide has anticholinergic properties and procainamide may cause gastric disturbance and arthralgias, but both drugs are effective

  d. Alternatively, Class IC agents such as flecainide and propafenone which lengthen the PR interval and the width of the QRS interval may be prescribed (may be first-line drugs in patients without coronary artery disease and normal ventricular function)

  e. Class III drugs such as sotalol are newer agents but are probably as effective as other antiarrhythmic drugs (may cause torsades de pointes)

  f. Either avoid Class IA and Class IC drugs in patients who have ischemic heart disease <u>or</u> heart failure or prescribe lower doses of these drugs

 D. Long-term maintenance of sinus rhythm

  1. Approximately 75-85% of patients not maintained on any antiarrhythmic drugs revert to AF in 1-2 years; nonetheless it is reasonable to initially try to maintain sinus rhythm without medications

  2. For patients who have recurrent AF or are likely to have recurrent AF, the following two approaches are acceptable

        a.   Combine antiarrhythmic drugs with AV nodal blocking drugs (digoxin, beta-blockers, calcium channel blockers); continue anticoagulation (this approach is most often recommended)

        b.   Maintain heart rate control with AV nodal blocking drugs and continue anticoagulation

E.   Anticoagulant therapy is recommended for the prevention of stroke and other embolic complications

    1.   Post electrical cardioversion care

        a.   Prescribe warfarin (Coumadin) for 4-6 weeks or indefinitely (see E.2)

        b.   Dose is usually 2.5-5 mg QD

        c.   Titrate dosage to maintain International Normalized Ratio (INR) within 2.0-3.0 range; persons at high risk for embolism (mechanical valves, deep vein thrombosis) should be maintained at INR of 2.5-3.5 range

        d.   Initially, INR should be monitored every 2-3 days until therapeutic level is attained

        e.   After therapeutic level is achieved, monitor INR weekly for several weeks to ensure maintenance of therapeutic level, then every 1-2 months

    2.   Maintenance anticoagulant therapy; monitor INR every 1-2 months (see appropriate dosing and INR ranges in V.E.1)

        a.   All patients over 75 years should be given warfarin

        b.   Prescribe warfarin to patients with chronic AF who are under 75 years of age and who have one of the following 5 features:

            (1)   History of CHF, mitral stenosis, prosthetic heart valves, coronary artery disease

            (2)   Hypertension

            (3)   Diabetes

            (4)   Thyrotoxicosis

            (5)   History of transient ischemic attack or minor nonhemorrhagic cerebrovascular accident

        c.   Patients 65-75 years without any of the five preceding factors should use either warfarin or aspirin

            (1)   If aspirin is used, prescribe buffered aspirin (Ascriptin) 325 mg daily; may be prescribed every other day, particularly in patients predisposed to stroke

            (2)   In elderly, consider children's dose of 80 mg

        d.   Recommend aspirin or nothing in patients under 65 years who have none of the five preceding features

    3.   Patient education in relation to warfarin

        a.   Teach patient to report any signs of bleeding

        b.   Numerous medications such as acetaminophen, some antiarrhythmics, some antibiotics, phenytoin, nonsteroidal antiinflammatory agents, and selective serotonin reuptake inhibitors increase INR: other drugs such a rifampin, carbamazepine, antihistamines, antianxiety agents, and antacids decrease INR

        c.   Foods and beverages such as green tea, alcohol, broccoli, and tomatoes may affect warfarin levels

F.   Patient Education

    1.   Remind patients to quit smoking, avoid sleep deprivation, and limit their use of stimulants (i.e., caffeine, sodas, chocolate) and alcohol

    2.   Teach relaxation techniques to reduce stress

    3.   Teach patients and family members to watch for signs of complications such as extremely rapid heart rate, edema and weight gain, increasing dyspnea on exertion, and chest pain

    4.   Teach signs and symptoms of digitalis toxicity (arrhythmias, anorexia, nausea, vomiting, diarrhea, lethargy, confusion, and visual disturbances such as scotomas and color perception changes) and/or adverse effects of other drugs

    5.   Intensive teaching is needed for patients on warfarin (see V.E.3)

G.   Permanent pacers and/or ablation of atrioventricular junction are alternatives that can be discussed with patients who have disabling symptoms

H. Follow Up: Close follow up is essential
1. Patients who have their first episode of AF should return to clinic within 24-48 hours for reevaluation
2. Patients who were electrically cardioverted should have frequent cardiac monitoring with ECG usually at intervals of less than 1 week, 2 weeks, 1 month, 3 months, and then, every 3 months
3. For patients taking amiodarone order chest x-ray, liver function tests, and thyroid tests every 3 months during first year, then every 6 months
4. Patients on antiarrhythmic agents should have liver enzymes measured the first 4-8 weeks of therapy and patients with risk factors for developing cardiac complications to therapy should have electrocardiograms ordered the first weeks of drug therapy and then in 3-6 months; monitoring of serum levels of drugs every 3-6 months may be helpful to reduce risk of toxicity
5. Patients on digoxin should be carefully monitored for digitalis toxicity (serum drug levels are not routinely ordered); electrolytes, BUN, creatinine and ECG are often ordered 1-2 weeks after therapy is initiated, and then every 1-6 months
6. Monitor INR in patients on warfarin every 2-3 days until therapeutic level is attained; after therapeutic level is achieved, monitor INR weekly for several weeks to ensure maintenance of therapeutic level, then every 1-2 months

CHEST PAIN

I. Definition: Unpleasant sensation in the chest associated with actual or potential tissue damage

II. Pathogenesis

A. Chest pain may emanate from the chest wall and can be associated with musculoskeletal causes such as muscle strain due to exercise and coughing, muscle spasm, costochondritis, and trauma (i.e., rib fractures)

B. Pain originating from the chest wall may also be secondary to neurological disorders such as herpes zoster and nerve root compression

C. Distention of the pleura may produce pain (called pleurisy) and is commonly due to inflammation, infection, and neoplasm

D. Cardiac causes of pain are often due to atherosclerosis; ischemic lactic acidosis and increased prostaglandin at site of coronary artery spasm

E. Gastrointestinal problems due to structural defects such as gastroesophageal reflux (GERD), esophageal spasm, and hiatal hernia or abdominal organ problems resulting from inflammation and infection such as cholecystitis and pancreatitis may produce chest pain

F. Psychogenic disorders due to anxiety, depression, or cardiac neurosis are possible causes

G. Idiopathic causes of chest pain are common, particularly in the pediatric population

III. Clinical Presentation

A. Chest pain due to musculoskeletal factors is variable and may last from a few seconds to several days or even a month or more and may be sharp, dull or aching
1. Pain is aggravated by deep inspiration and cough; the chest is tender on palpation
2. Costochondritis is characterized by sharp, anterior chest pain at the costochondral junction (junction at the anterior ribs and sternum); may have warmth, erythema, and swelling at junction as well

B. Nerve irritation or compression has characteristic types of chest pain (see section on HERPES ZOSTER)
1. Herpes zoster causes pain along dermatomes and typically precedes a persistent, vesicular rash; commonly affects elderly and immunosuppressed patients; patient may have pain along the dermatomes long after the rash has healed
2. Nerve root compression results in pain and motor and sensory deficits (numbness or tingling) in the neck, chest and upper arm

C. Pleural causes of chest pain typically present as pain worsened by deep inspiration and coughing; pleural spasm secondary to cold weather and increased activity may occur
1. Bacterial pneumonia is one of the most common causes of pleuritic pain and is characterized by abrupt onset of fever, chills, leukocytosis, and purulent sputum (see section on PNEUMONIA)
2. Pulmonary embolus (PE) is another common cause of pleuritic pain; patients present with sudden onset of dyspnea, tachypnea, tachycardia, hypotension, and possibly hemoptysis; remember, however, that many patients with PE may be asymptomatic
   a. Rales and a pleural rub may be present; may exhibit decreased or absent breath sounds distal to PE
   b. May progress to acute right failure, pulmonary hypertension, or respiratory arrest
   c. Typically associated with risk factors such as immobility, surgery, pregnancy, oral contraceptives, pelvis or lower extremity trauma
   d. Patents with history of malignancy, deep venous thrombosis, previous pulmonary embolus, congestive heart failure, chronic obstructive pulmonary disease, obesity, and hypercoagulability conditions are more prone to developing a PE
3. Spontaneous pneumothorax or hemothorax secondary to trauma can cause acute, unilateral, stabbing pain with dyspnea
   a. Typically, there is decreased breath and voice sounds over the involved lung or lobe
   b. Incidence is highest in young men or in older patients with chronic obstructive pulmonary disease; other risk factors include cigarette smoking, lung cancer, and Valsalva maneuver
   c. Be on the alert for mediastinal shift and cardiopulmonary compromise in these patients

D. Chest pain due to cardiac diseases may be mild to severe, transient and exertional related or constant
1. Pericarditis may present with pleuritic pain or with steady retrosternal or left precordial pain that resembles angina
   a. Typically, the pain decreases upon sitting and leaning forward
   b. Characterized by a two- or three-component friction rub
   c. Associated signs are fever, tachycardia, pulsus paradoxus, tamponade, elevated sedimentation rate, and leukocytosis
   d. Risk factors include infection, autoimmune disease, recent myocardial infarction, cardiac surgery, malignancy, uremia, drugs such as procainamide, hydralazine, isoniazid
2. Pain with angina pectoris is often shoulder, mid-back, or retrosternal; radiates to the neck, jaw, epigastrium, shoulder, or arm; and is aggravated by exertion or stress; pain typically lasts less than 10 minutes and is relieved with nitroglycerin (see section on ISCHEMIC HEART DISEASE)
3. Patients with myocardial infarction (MI) typically complain of sudden onset of substernal pain which may radiate and is associated with dyspnea, diaphoresis, nausea, vomiting, and anxiety; pain is unrelieved by nitroglycerin and usually lasts 30 minutes or longer (see section on ISCHEMIC HEART DISEASE)
4. Patients with mitral valve prolapse (MVP) are often asymptomatic, but chest pain, fatigue, palpitations (especially when lying supine on left side), lightheadedness, shortness of breath, headaches, and mood swings may be present; only 15% of patients experience moderate to severe symptoms
   a. Pain is usually fleeting and sharp and localized over the central or left chest wall; rarely radiates
   b. Pain is not relieved by nitroglycerin; usually pain is unrelated to exertion

c. Pain may be brief or last for several days

d. In rare cases, MVP can progress to mitral insufficiency with enlargement of left atrium and left ventricle, and congestive heart failure

e. Hallmark diagnostic sign is a mid- to late-systolic click and late systolic murmur

f. Echocardiogram will reveal extent of regurgitation and may reveal an abnormally thickened, redundant mitral valve

5. Dissecting aortic aneurysm often presents with excruciating, tearing, or knifelike pain which is sudden in onset and lasts for hours; less frequently, pain is nagging and constant

a. Usually pain is located in the anterior chest but may be located in the abdomen or back and move as the dissection progresses; often radiates to thoracic area of back

b. Signs include lowered or elevated blood pressure, dissociation of arm blood pressures, absent pulses, paralysis, pulsus paradoxus, and murmur of aortic insufficiency

c. Risk factors include hypertension, connective tissue disease, pregnancy, arterio-atherosclerosis, and cigarette use

6. Cocaine-induced chest pain may present with severe, sharp, pressure-like or squeezing substernal pain

a. Associated symptoms include euphoria, mydriasis, hyperstimulation, paranoia, delusions, followed by depression, nausea, vomiting, and muscle twitching

b. Complications include myocardial ischemia and infarction, arrhythmias, respiratory failure, and circulatory collapse

E. Pain from disorders of the gastrointestinal system can mimic cardiovascular symptomatology

1. Gastroesophageal reflux presents with burning, substernal pain which is related to consuming a large meal, lying down or bending over; pain is usually relieved by ingestion of antacid or food (see section on GASTROESOPHAGEAL REFLUX DISEASE)

2. Esophageal spasm often is substernal, radiating to neck, shoulder, arm and relieved by nitroglycerin

F. Other gastrointestinal problems such as cholecystitis, peptic ulcer disease, and pancreatitis sometimes resemble cardiac pain, but often they can be distinguished by their association with eating and their relief from antacids; however, remember that 10% of patients with acute myocardial infarction state that their chest pain is relieved by antacids

G. Chest pain may be due to psychiatric or mental health disorders

1. Patients with psychogenic problems often describe pain as generalized, constantly present and aggravated by any effort

a. Associated symptoms include dyspnea, fatigue, and other somatic symptoms

b. Common in childhood and may be similar to pain described by an adult in the child's family

2. Patients with panic disorders often have chest pain which is accompanied by intense fear, tachypnea, palpitations, diaphoresis, trembling, nausea, dizziness, and chills or hot flashes

IV. Diagnosis/Evaluation

A. History (Length of history will depend on patient's clinical presentation; perform a rapid history for any patient with a suspected emergent condition such as MI or dissecting abdominal aortic aneurysm)

1. Determine whether onset was sudden, gradual, recurrent, or new

2. Ask patient to describe the pain's location, regions of radiation, quality, intensity, and duration

3. Determine the quantity of pain, possibly on a scale from 0 to 10 with 10 being the worst pain ever experienced and 0 indicating no pain which is the ultimate goal

4. Inquire about aggravating factors such as exercise, stress, food intake, movement, coughing

5. Inquire about relieving factors such as rest, use of nitroglycerin, antacids, intake of food

6. Ask about associated symptoms such as dyspnea, hemoptysis, fever, chills, sputum production, exanthem, diaphoresis, dizziness, syncope, nausea, diarrhea

7. Determine whether patient has a coexistent viral illness or if other members of the household have a viral disease
8. Explore stress-related factors in the patient's school, work or home environments
9. Ask about risk factors for ischemic heart disease
10. Explore past medical history
11. Inquire about family history of chest pain and cardiovascular disease

B. Physical Examination
1. Observe general appearance of patient, assessing for level of distress and anxiety
2. Measure vital signs. Take blood pressure in both arms (dissecting abdominal aneurysm presents with discrepancy in readings between arms); if unable to detect, use Doppler and/or take thigh pressure to assess presence and compare with arm pressures
3. Inspect skin for pallor, cyanosis, jaundice, or herpetic rash
4. Examine eyes, including funduscopy
5. Auscultate carotid pulse for bruits
6. Assess neck for lymphadenopathy, thyromegaly, midline trachea, jugular venous distention, bruits
7. Perform a complete examination of the heart, noting extra heart sounds, murmurs, clicks, rubs, or irregular irregularities
8. Examine chest wall for herpes lesions and signs of trauma
9. Palpate chest wall noting tenderness and swelling
10. Auscultate lungs for equal breath sounds, a pleural rub, and crackles and wheezes
11. Auscultate abdomen for bowel sounds and bruits
12. Palpate abdomen for tenderness and masses (particularly in the right upper quadrant and epigastrium), organomegaly, bounding pulses, and ascites
13. Palpate for femoral pulses (with absent pulses suspect dissecting abdominal aortic aneurysm)
14. Assess lower extremities for cyanosis, diminished pulses, unilateral swelling, and other signs of phlebitis
15. Patients who present with pain that changes with movement should have a musculoskeletal and neurological exam performed, focusing on focal tenderness, muscular weakness, and motor and sensory deficits

C. Differential Diagnosis: All conditions listed under pathogenesis should be included in the differential diagnosis; generally, pain should be considered cardiovascular and life threatening until proven otherwise
1. The type of pain pattern is helpful at arriving at a diagnosis
   a. Pain brought on by exertion and relieved with rest suggests angina pectoris or psychogenic pain (psychogenic pain, however, usually is accompanied by a myriad of noncardiac symptoms such as headache, hyperventilation)
   b. Pain which worsens upon deep inspiration or cough suggests a pleural, pericardial or chest wall source; focal tenderness along with pain on inspiration suggests costochondritis
   c. Pain relieved by leaning forward and aggravated by lying supine suggests pericarditis
   d. Pain with a sudden onset and dyspnea suggests pneumothorax or pulmonary edema (PE); lean towards diagnosis of PE if patient has a risk for thrombophlebitis or has had a recent fracture
   e. Sudden onset of tearing pain in a hypertensive patient suggests dissecting aneurysm
   f. Pain occurring with eating suggests angina or esophageal, biliary, pancreatic, and peptic disease
2. Age and sex of the patient can also help narrow the differential diagnosis: Women less than 40 years of age without risk factors for coronary disease rarely have a cardiac problem; conversely, always first consider a cardiac problem in men >30 years with significant family history or risk factors
3. Risk factors provide important information to arrive at a diagnosis
4. Quality, location, radiation, and intensity of pain are nonspecific symptoms and are usually not helpful in arriving at a diagnosis

D. Diagnostic tests are based on the information collected in the history and physical examination; not every patient needs a routine chest x-ray and electrocardiogram (ECG)
   1. Consider pulse oximetry to assess for either oxygen desaturation or oxygen saturation in patients with suspected cardiac and pulmonary problems
   2. Order an ECG in the following cases: patients with suspected MI, angina pectoris, pericarditis and patients with significant risk factors
   3. Echocardiography is helpful in diagnosing mitral valve prolapse, pericarditis, and to assess for wall motion and ejection fraction
   4. Consider ordering a chest x-ray in the following cases:
      a. Suspected chest trauma such as rib fractures
      b. Suspected pulmonary diseases such as pneumonia or tuberculosis
      c. Suspected pneumothorax or pulmonary embolus
      d. A widened mediastinum may be seen in aortic dissection
   5. Computed tomography with contrast, transesophageal echocardiography, and aortic angiography are diagnostic tests for aortic dissection
   6. Consider CPK with isoenzymes and cardiac catheterization for patients with suspected urgent cardiac problems
   7. Consider exercise stress testing for diagnosing problems of cardiac exertion when patient has transient or exertional pain that is not urgent but may be emergent
   8. Thallium scintigraphy, cardiac untrasonography, and cardiac angiography are other tests to detect cardiac problems
   9. Consider a lung scan or ventilation scan for a patient with suspected PE
   10. Consider gram stain of sputum for suspected pulmonary infections and acid-fasts stains for suspected tuberculosis
   11. An acid perfusion (Bernstein) test or more invasive tests such as esophageal manometry, barium x-ray studies, and endoscopy may be helpful in diagnosing specific gastrointestinal problems

V. Plan/Management

   A. Relief of pain is based on the etiology

   B. Treatment of musculoskeletal problems such as costochondritis is usually symptomatic (see sections within MUSCULOSKELETAL topic)
      1. Apply local heat
      2. Prescribe nonsteroidal anti-inflammatory drugs such as ibuprofen (Motrin) 400-800 mg every 4-8 hours

   C. Treatment of pulmonary problems
      1. Pneumonia (see section on PNEUMONIA)
      2. Pulmonary embolus requires hospitalization and intravenous anticoagulation; typically patient is then placed on long-term anticoagulation
      3. Carefully assess vital signs and watch for mediastinal shift in patients with a pneumothorax
         a. A small, stable pneumothorax without evidence of respiratory compromise requires only observation for several days until stabilization and resolution
         b. Hospitalization and insertion of chest tubes is needed for a large, expanding tension pneumothorax

   D. Treatment of cardiac pain (also see section on ISCHEMIC HEART DISEASE)
      1. Hospitalization and immediate referral to cardiologist is required for myocardial infarction and aortic dissection
      2. Pericarditis is treated with aspirin, non-steroidal anti-inflammatory drugs, or for severe cases, corticosteroids; hospitalization is required for patients with signs of cardiac tamponade

363

3. Mitral valve prolapse
   a. No specific treatment is indicated for most patients, except for reassurance about a good prognosis
   b. The major therapeutic dilemma is whether to recommend antibiotic prophylaxis for infective endocarditis when certain invasive procedures are performed
      (1) Patients with MVP who have mitral regurgitation and/or thickened leaflets should have prophylaxis (see procedure for prophylaxis of bacterial endocarditis in section on RHEUMATIC HEART DISEASE)
      (2) Prophylaxis is also recommended for patients with MVP who have a murmur of mitral regurgitation, but not in those who have only a click
      (3) If there is uncertainty about the diagnosis of mitral regurgitation refer to cardiologist
   c. Patients with severe mitral regurgitation may require valve surgery
   d. Patients with annoying arrhythmias may benefit from a beta-blocker such as atenolol (Tenormin)

E. Treatment of abdominal problems (see section on GASTROINTESTINAL PROBLEMS)

F. Patient Education
   1. To avoid cardiac neurosis carefully explain to the patient or parents that a thorough history and physical exam revealed no abnormality
   2. Allow time for the patient to express concerns and questions
   3. Teach risk factors for cardiac and ulcer disease and strategies to reduce risks

G. Follow up is variable depending on diagnosis and patient's condition

Congestive Heart Failure Associated with Left Ventricular Dysfunction

I. Definition: Inability of the heart to pump blood at a rate sufficient to meet the metabolic needs of the peripheral tissues

II. Pathophysiology: Injuries to the heart predispose the individual to heart failure; exhaustion of the compensatory hemodynamic and neurohormonal mechanisms actually cause the signs and symptoms of the syndrome

   A. As the heart's ability to pump is reduced, several cardiac compensatory mechanisms occur as follows:
      1. The heart may attempt to compensate by dilating to increase cardiac output via the Frank-Starling mechanism
      2. Ventricular hypertrophy develops to handle the greater preload (end-diastolic volume) and hyperplasia develops to maintain cardiac output by increasing contractility or contractile mass
      3. Initially, these two mechanisms provide improvement in symptoms but over time the heart decompensates and functioning is compromised

   B. Neurohormonal systems are also triggered secondary to the stress response with the decreased efficiency of the heart's pumping:
      1. Plasma renin activity, ACTH, aldosterone, and plasma arginine vasopressin (ADH) levels are increased resulting in systemic vasoconstriction and sodium and water retention which if excessive leads to increased atrial pressure and/or pulmonary congestion

2. Increased sympathetic tone occurs with increased levels of epinephrine and norepinephrine which initially improves cardiac output and blood pressure, but eventually increases oxygen demand and accelerates myocardial cell death as well as causes excessive increases in ventricular preload and afterload (dynamic resistance against which the heart contracts)

C. The underlying injury to the heart may be due to ventricular systolic dysfunction, diastolic dysfunction, or both
1. Left-ventricular systolic dysfunction (most common) is due to decreased myocardial contractility which results in decreased cardiac output and left ejection fraction <35-40%. Common causes are the following:
   a. Dilated cardiomyopathies, viral cardiomyopathies, cor pulmonale
   b. Reduction in contractile muscle mass (e.g., myocardial infarction)
2. Ventricular diastolic dysfunction is due to disturbances in the relaxation properties of the heart or restriction in ventricular filling; underlying pathologic processes include myocardial ischemia, hypertrophy, hyperplasia, and fibrosis; common causes are the following:
   a. Pericardial disease (e.g., pericarditis, pericardial tamponade)
   b. Mitral or tricuspid valve stenosis
   c. Increased ventricular stiffness (e.g., hypertrophic cardiomyopathy, amyloidosis, sarcoidosis)
3. Several conditions are associated with both systolic and diastolic dysfunction such as ventricular hypertrophy, hyperplasia, and myocardial ischemia; myocardial infarction is the most common potentially reversible cause of heart failure

D. Major causes of congestive heart failure (CHF) (listed in order of frequency)
1. Ischemic heart disease
2. Hypertension (less common today because of improvements in diagnosing and treating)
3. Cardiomyopathy

E. Myocarditis is an uncommon cause but should be considered in young patients with acute onset of symptoms and unexplained heart failure

F. Patients with previously compensated heart failure may decompensate as a result of any of the following factors:
1. Lack of compliance with drugs or treatment regimes
2. Uncontrolled hypertension
3. Cardiac arrhythmias
4. Inadequate therapy
5. Endocrine disorders (thyrotoxicosis)
6. Pulmonary infection
7. Pulmonary embolism
8. Excessive intake of fluids and/or dietary sodium
9. Stress
10. Anemia
11. Liver and renal disease
12. Sleep apnea or general sleep disturbances
13. Alcoholism and cocaine use

III. Clinical Presentation

A. Although cardiovascular deaths have declined, mortality due to heart failure has risen over the past three decades; mortality rate is approximately 50% within 5 years of diagnosis

B. Signs and symptoms can develop gradually or abruptly as occurs with acute heart failure; acute heart failure can be grouped clinically into acute cardiogenic pulmonary edema, cardiogenic shock, and acute decompensation of chronic left heart failure

C. In left-ventricular systolic dysfunction, signs and symptoms are not reliable indicators of cardiac functioning; patients with severely impaired ventricular performance may be asymptomatic, particularly if heart failure developed gradually; nonetheless, common signs and symptoms are presented in the following table

SIGNS AND SYMPTOMS OF VENTRICULAR SYSTOLIC DYSFUNCTION			
Symptoms			
Dyspnea on exertion	Hemoptysis	Bloating	Weakness
Orthopnea	Abdominal Pain	Constipation	CNS symptoms
Paroxysmal nocturnal dyspnea	Anorexia	Exercise intolerance	Nocturia
Cough	Nausea	Fatigue	
Signs			
Bibasilar rales	Peripheral edema		Tachycardia
S$_3$ gallop	Jugular venous distention		Pallor
Cheyne-Stokes respirations	Hepatomegaly Hepatojugular reflex		Cyanosis

D. Diastolic dysfunction occurs in about 30-40% of all cases; it is characterized by the following:
   1. Normal systolic ejection fraction
   2. Presentation ranges from no symptoms to dypsnea, pulmonary edema, signs of right heart failure (abdominal complaints, peripheral edema), and exercise intolerance

E. Patients are often classified by their level of disability according to the New York Heart Association (see table that follows)

NEW YORK HEART ASSOCIATION FUNCTIONAL CLASSIFICATION	
Functional Class	**Descriptive Findings in Patients with Cardiac Disease**
I	No physical limitation in activity
II	Slight limitation in ordinary physical activity, resulting in fatigue, palpitations, dyspnea or angina
III	Marked limitation in activity; patients are comfortable at rest, but ordinary activity leads to symptoms
IV	Symptoms are present at rest; any activity leads to increased discomfort

IV. Diagnosis/Evaluation

   A. History
      1. Specifically ask about previous heart disease
         a. Coronary artery disease and atherosclerosis
         b. Myocardial infarction
         c. Hypertension
         d. Valvular disease
         e. Myopathies
      2. Ask about difficulty with breathing
         a. Ask how far patient can walk without developing shortness of breath (SOB)
         b. Ask about waking at night with SOB
         c. Ask how many pillows patient needs to sleep comfortably
         d. Ask about awakening with a cough
      3. Inquire about type, frequency, duration, and self-treatment of chest pain
      4. Inquire about amount of weight gain; ask whether gain was rapid over a few days or more gradual over weeks
      5. Question about other associated symptoms such as edema, abdominal complaints, palpitations, fatigue
      6. Inquire about risk factors for coronary heart disease

7. Ask about personal and family history of cardiovascular, thyroid, hepatic, and renal diseases
8. Explore possibility of patient having sleep apnea (e.g., snoring in sleep)
9. Obtain a thorough history of medication use
10. Explore sexual function, cognitive function, coping behaviors, and social support

B. Physical Examination; elevated jugular venous pressure and a third heart sound are most specific findings and often diagnostic in individuals with compatible symptoms
1. Observe patient's overall appearance, noting whether patient is in distress when sitting or walking
2. Check capillary refill
3. Quickly assess respiratory status
4. Inspect skin for color, moisture, and turgor
5. Carefully measure vital signs, noting decreased blood pressure, tachycardia, tachypnea
6. Measure weight at every visit
7. Perform a complete eye examination with funduscopy
8. Palpate thyroid
9. Observe neck for vein distention and hepatojugular reflux
10. Perform a complete heart examination; CHF patients often have extra heart sounds, murmurs, increased second pulmonic heart sounds, and points of maximal impulses which have shifted to the left and downward
11. Perform a complete lung examination
12. Perform an abdominal examination, noting hepatomegaly and ascites
13. Assess extremities for edema and peripheral pulses
14. Perform a mental status examination as unexplained confusion sometimes occurs, especially in elderly patients

C. Differential Diagnosis: Heart failure is actually a syndrome, not a disease; it is important to determine the underlying causes of the heart failure. Nonetheless, the following conditions tend to mimic the signs and symptoms of heart failure or may occur concomitantly with CHF
1. Dyspnea
   a. Chronic obstructive pulmonary disease
   b. Asthma
   c. Ischemic nephropathy caused by bilateral renal artery stenosis
2. Chest pain (see section on CHEST PAIN)
   a. Pulmonary emboli
   b. Bacterial endocarditis
3. Edema
   a. Renal disease
   b. Liver disease
   c. Peripheral edema is often due to venous insufficiency

D. Diagnostic testing is to evaluate for alternative diagnoses, to get baseline information before therapy, to determine the type of cardiac dysfunction, to determine degree of ventricular impairment and prognosis (remember that physical signs are not highly sensitive for detecting heart failure); order the following even in the absence of physical findings:
1. Echocardiogram or radionuclide ventriculography to measure chamber size, wall thickness, wall mobility, and left-ventricular ejection fraction (EF). Also, echocardiogram should be ordered for patients suspected of valvular or pericardial disease or in patients in whom the cause of heart failure is uncertain
   a. EF less than 35-40% denotes heart failure but patients with EF ≥40% may still have heart failure due to valvular disease or diastolic dysfunction
   b. Differentiates diastolic from systolic dysfunction; diastolic dysfunction may have following abnormalities: left-ventricular hypertrophy, prolonged isovolumic relaxation time, prolonged deceleration time, abnormal pulmonary venous flow pattern

2. Electrocardiogram to uncover the following:
   a. Myocardial infarction (acute MI usually has ST-T wave changes, whereas chronic MI has Q waves)
   b. Arrhythmias which may be due to thyroid disease, or heart failure caused by either rapid or low ventricular rate
   c. Low voltage which accompanies pericardial effusion
   d. Left-ventricular hypertrophy which may be due to diastolic dysfunction
3. Chest x-ray to determine heart size and assess pulmonary congestion; also chest x-ray will uncover pulmonary infections such as pneumonia which may be precipitating factors
4. Blood count to eliminate anemia and infection which may contribute to the pathogenesis of CHF
5. Urinalysis to determine proteinuria which may be result of nephrotic syndrome or to determine red blood cells or cellular casts which may denote glomerulonephritis
6. Serum creatinine which if elevated, denotes volume overload due to renal failure
7. Serum albumin which if decreased may be related to increased extravascular volume
8. T_4 and TSH to detect failure aggravated by hypo/hyperthyroidism (only recommended if patient has atrial fibrillation, evidence of thyroid disease or is >65 years)
9. The following tests are helpful in many cases
   a. Electrolytes before drug therapy is initiated
   b. Liver function tests to determine if liver disease is a contributing factor
   c. Cardiac enzymes to rule out myocardial infarction
   d. Serum iron and ferritin to rule out anemia
   e. Noninvasive stress testing to detect ischemia, particularly for patients who are possible candidates for revascularization
10. Consider other studies (probably conferring with a cardiologist)
    a. Radionuclide angiography provides good images in patients who are obese and who have severe chronic lung disease; can detect segmental wall motion abnormalities and determine left and right ventricular EFs
    b. Cardiac catheterization is ordered in patients in whom the diagnosis of heart failure is still uncertain after noninvasive techniques or in patients whose heart failure is refractory to medical therapy
    c. Myocardial biopsy may be useful in young patients with sudden onset of heart failure in whom cardiomyopathy or myocarditis is suspected
    d. Routine Holter monitoring or signal-averaged electrocardiography for patients with arrythmias and syncope
    e. Magnetic resonance imaging is a promising tool for assessing ventricular function, mass, and structural abnormalities but its high cost precludes current routine use
    f. If access to positive emission tomography (PET) is available, it is an excellent way to assess cardiac muscle viability in relation to EF and wall motion problems

V. Plan/Management: Goals are to improve patient's quality of life by reducing symptoms, and to prolong survival

A. Hospitalize patients with any of the following:
   1. Pulmonary edema with marked pulmonary rales and signs/symptoms of hypoxia (elevate stretcher and provide oxygen in clinic)
   2. Cardiogenic shock with severe hypotension, oliguria, and/or mental health changes
   3. Clinical or ECG evidence of myocardial ischemia or infarction
   4. Oxygen saturation <90% which is not due to pulmonary diseases
   5. Anasarca (generalized infiltration of edema fluid into subcutaneous connective tissue)
   6. Severe, complicating medical illness such as pneumonia
   7. Symptomatic hypotension or syncope
   8. Heart failure which is nonresponsive to outpatient therapy
   9. Inadequate social support for safe outpatient management, particularly if patient is nonadherent to therapy

B. Patients should only be discharged from hospital when the following are present:
   1. Symptoms are adequately controlled
   2. All reversible causes of morbidity have been treated or stabilized
   3. Patients and caregivers have education and understanding of disease (see V.J. PATIENT EDUCATION)

C.   Prevention
       1.   Management of etiologic factors can prevent left ventricular remodeling and dysfunction that can lead to heart failure (see table)
       2.   It is imperative that comprehensive risk reduction strategies be initiated at time of diagnosis and be maintained; intensive cardiac rehabilitation can reverse or stabilize decline

PREVENTIVE INTERVENTIONS	
Etiologic Factor	**Intervention**
Hypertension	Life style modifications & antihypertensive drugs
Coronary artery disease	Smoking cessation, weight reduction, exercise, blood pressure control, reduction in lipid levels, aspirin prophylaxis
Valvular disease	Surgery
Left ventricular hypertrophy	Blood pressure control & ACE inhibitor
Myocardial infarction	ACE inhibitor and possibly beta blocker or nitrate

Adapted from Cohn, J.N. (1998). Preventing congestive heart failure. American Family Physician, 57, 1901-1904

D.   First step of management is to determine the etiology of CHF and treat. For example, treat hypertension, anemia, hyperthyroidism with medications; offer surgery for patients with valvular defects

E.   General principles of pharmacologic therapy
       1.   Therapy must be individualized and based on the degree of cardiac impairment and the severity of symptoms
       2.   Initially prescribe low doses and slowly titrate to maximum dosage recommendations; the larger doses are those shown to be effective in reducing mortality

F.   Patients with functional class I: patients in this class are usually asymptomatic or mildly symptomatic and have reduced ejection fraction (approximately <35-40%); even if patient has no signs and symptoms of fluid overload, prescribe an angiotensin-converting enzyme (ACE) inhibitor
       1.   Researchers have found that ACE inhibitors prevent further development of heart failure in this class and improve patient survival
       2.   Contraindication to a trial of ACE inhibitors in this functional class is significant hyperkalemia
       3.   Choose one of the following agents: Titrate slowly, but aim for highest maintenance dose
             a.   Captopril (Capoten): Begin with a low dose such as 6.25 mg TID for patients with normal blood pressure or 12.5 mg TID for patients with hypertension; Maintenance dose 25-50 mg TID (take 1 hour before meal)
             b.   Enalapril (Vasotec): Begin with 2.5 mg BID; Maintenance dose 10-20 mg BID
             c.   Lisinopril (Zestril): Begin with 2.5 mg QD; Maintenance dose 10-20 mg QD
             d.   Other FDA approved agents include fosinopril (Monopril), quinapril (Accupril), and ramipril (Altace)
                   (1)   Advantage is once-daily dosing
                   (2)   However, these drugs have no major clinical advantage over previously available agents
       4.   For the few patients in this class who have peripheral edema, mild jugular distention or mild symptoms of fluid overload begin a sodium restriction diet (see under patient education V.J.3)
       5.   Add a nonloop diuretic if there are signs and symptoms of volume overload (orthopnea, paroxysmal nocturnal dyspnea, S_3) or other evidence of salt and water retention despite salt restriction
             a.   Diuretics are effective in reducing symptoms in most cases of CHF but they do not prevent progression of CHF or prolong life
             b.   Start with a thiazide such as hydrochlorothiazide (Hydrodiuril). Initial dose is 25-50 mg QD/BID; maximum dosage of 100-200 mg (in mild cases, may even be able to prescribe every other day regimens)

G.   Patients with functional classes II to IV:
       1.   Prescribe ACE inhibitor (see dosages in V.F.3) unless there is a contraindication such as shock, angioneurotic edema, or significant hyperkalemia; If patient is tolerating drug, therapy should be long-term (probably lifelong)

2. If patient is not tolerating ACE inhibitor, consider an alternative regime with isosorbide dinitrate (Isordil) 5 to 10 mg TID and hydralazine (Apresoline) 10 mg QID as initial doses

    a. If patient tolerates initial doses, gradually increase isosorbide dinitrate to 40 mg TID and hydralazine to 75 mg QID

    b. To avoid nitrate tolerance, recommend a minimal 10-hour "nitrate-free" period at night

    c. Isosorbide dinitrate and hydralazine are particularly helpful in patients with hypertension or severe mitral regurgitation

3. When symptoms of dypsnea and fatigue persist with ACE inhibitor, consider using isosorbide dinitrate and hydralazine in conjunction with ACE inhibitor even though there is limited research to support this practice

4. Diuretics should be used in conjunction with ACE Inhibitor and need to be given indefinitely

    a. Be careful when using ACE inhibitor and diuretic concurrently as excessive diuresis reduces blood pressure and activates the neurohormonal system

        (1) Clinical signs of overdiuresis include postural hypotension, tachycardia, reduced jugular venous distention, prerenal azotemia, hyponatremia, hypokalemia, and hypomagnesemia

        (2) If overdiuresis occurs, withhold diuretic for 24-72 hours

        (3) It is important to reach the recommended dose of the ACE inhibitor; therefore slowly increase dosage of ACE inhibitor until maintenance level is reached and then reintroduce or slowly increase dosage of diuretic to relieve symptoms

    b. Start with a thiazide such as hydrochlorothiazide (Hydrodiuril). Initial dose is 25-50 mg QD/BID; maximum dosage of 100-200 mg

    c. When patients become resistant to thiazides either because there is significant renal failure (serum creatinine >2-4 mg/dL) or when there is severe heart failure, add metolazone (Zaroxolyn) 2.5-10 mg QD

    d. Alternatively, may need to change from thiazide therapy to loop diuretic when serum creatinine increases to 2-4 mg/dL or when clinical condition worsens

        (1) Prescribe furosemide (Lasix): begin with 20 mg and double dose as needed up to 160 mg/dL or more

        (2) Usually given as a single dose in the morning, but may give BID to patients with severe CHF; second dose should not be delayed into evening as this will result in sleep problems due to nocturia

        (3) For maximum absorption, drug should be given 1 hour before to 2 hours after meals

    e. Furosemide doses above 160-240 mg/dL are usually not needed; when patient is at high dosages without symptom relief add a modest dose of hydrochlorothiazide 25-50 mg/day, or metolazone 2.5-5 mg/day, or a potassium-sparing diuretic such as spironolactone (Aldactone) 25 mg QD/BID (usually, do not use spironolactone with ACE inhibitors)

    f. Patients in this functional class should be on a salt-restricted diet

    g. Nonsteroidal anti-inflammatory agents should be avoided in patients with heart failure

    h. Hypomagnesemia (serum magnesium level <1.6 mEq/liter) should be corrected

5. Digitalis glycosides increase left ventricular ejection fraction and exercise tolerance, but do not improve survival

    a. Digitalis glycosides should be added to the ACE inhibitor and diuretic regimen in patients with the following:

        (1) Dilated hearts and in whom the symptoms of heart failure appear to be due to a decreased inotropic state of heart muscle (ejection fraction <40-45% or the presence of an S_3 gallop)

        (2) Atrial fibrillation and rapid ventricular rates

        (3) Severe heart failure and in whom symptoms persist despite optimal doses of other medications

    b. Do not give to patients with diastolic dysfunction

    c. Digoxin (Lanoxin) is the recommended digitalis agent

        (1) The average dose is 0.25 mg QD; in older patients or patients with renal impairment, prescribe 0.125 mg QD

        (2) In approximately 5-7 days full digitalization will be achieved

d. Assess (order serum digoxin concentration) and treat patients for signs and symptoms of digitalis toxicity which are often associated with decreased potassium and magnesium levels
   (1) Slowing of heart rate
   (2) Anorexia, nausea, vomiting, and diarrhea
   (3) Neurologic symptoms such as fatigue, confusion, muscle weakness, and visual disturbances (halos around light or red-green vision)
   (4) If patient is digitalis-toxic, often withdrawal of digoxin is all that is needed
6. Amlodipine (Norvasc) was found to improve survival in patients with nonischemic dilated cardiomyopathy; other calcium channel blockers are **not** recommended for treatment of CHF; Dosage of amlodipine: initiate at 2.5-5 mg QD and can increase to 10 mg
7. Beta-blockers may have a role in treatment of CHF
   a. Carvedilol (Coreg) which has combined beta blocker and vasodilator activity is FDA approved for mild-to-moderate ischemic and nonischemic heart failure
      (1) Drug improves left ventricular function and symptoms
      (2) Starting dose is 3.125 mg BID with target dose of 25-50 mg BID depending on body weight; do not make adjustments in doses sooner than one to two weeks; reduce dose if pulse rate falls below 55
      (3) Advise patients to take with meals to decease rate of absorption and risk of orthostasis
      (4) To discontinue drug, taper downward over one to two weeks
   b. Prescribe beta-blockers for the following patients:
      (1) Those who are high risk after an acute myocardial infarction
      (2) Those with dilated cardiomyopathy
8. Angiotensin II-receptor antagonists promote physiologic responses similar to those of ACE inhibitors; at present these agents have not been sufficiently studied and are not approved for treating CHF but hold promise for the future
9. In patients with atrial fibrillation or a history of systemic or pulmonary embolism, prescribe warfarin to achieve a target range of international normalized ration of 2.0 to 3.0
10. Low dose dobutamine or milrinone infusion may help some patients with refractory heart failure

H. Consider revasculization and heart transplantation but only after intensive cardiac rehabilitation efforts have failed

I. Treatment of diastolic dysfunction (recommendations do not include therapy for hypertrophic cardiomyopathy because the pathophysiologic features and therapy significantly differ from other causes of diastolic dysfunction); goal of therapy is to lower elevated filling pressures without significantly reducing cardiac output; use one or a combination of the following:
   1. Initially prescribe small doses of diuretics or nitrates with careful monitoring; remember, however, that excessive diuresis can reduce stroke volume and cardiac output
   2. β-blockers enhance ventricular relaxation and improve compliance: Propranolol (Inderal LA) 80 mg QD, maximum dosage 160 mg; Alternatively, prescribe atenolol (Tenormin) 50 mg QD; maximum dosage of 100-200 mg QD
   3. Alternative therapy: Calcium Channel Blockers; Verapamil (Calan) 80-120 mg every 8 hours
   4. The role of ACE inhibitors is unclear; they have beneficial effects by directly improving ventricular relaxation and causing regression of hypertrophy
   5. Do not use digoxin as this drug will further increase the contractility and deplete cardiac muscle reserves
   6. Heart transplantation is an option in patients whose symptoms are refractory to optimal medical/surgical management

J. Patient Education
   1. Provide information on nature of heart failure, drugs, and dietary restrictions
   2. Encourage regular exercise such as walking or cycling for stable patients
   3. Teach patients to restrict dietary sodium to as close to 2 grams per day as possible; remind not to add salt to foods and to eliminate foods high in salt such as pickles, potato chips, and salt-cured meats. Patients with poorly compensated heart failure may require further reductions in salt intake to 500 mg or 1 gram
   4. Teach patients to monitor their weight as an indirect measure of fluid retention
   5. Advise patient to avoid excessive fluid intake; fluid restriction is not recommended unless patients have hyponatremia

6.   Advise patients to consume no more than one drink per day (one drink equals a glass of beer or wine, or drink with no more than 1 ounce of alcohol)
7.   Emphasize that patient should not smoke or chew tobacco
8.   Teach patient to recognize symptoms of worsening heart failure and what to do if these symptoms occur
9.   Inform patient and family of the prognosis so decisions and plans for the future can be made; discuss desires regarding resuscitation and encourage patient to complete a durable power of attorney or another form of advance directive
10.   Other life style modifications include weight reduction in obese patients and elimination of undue stress
11.   Instruct patient to eliminate or cautiously use drugs that precipitate CHF such as the following:
   a.   Nonsteroidal anti-inflammatory drugs
   b.   Antiarrhythmic agents such as disopyramide and flecainide
   c.   Glucocorticoids
   d.   Androgens
   e.   Estrogens
12.   Discuss sex, sexual difficulties, and coping strategies
13.   Remind patient of importance of obtaining vaccinations against influenza and pneumococcal disease

K.   Follow Up
1.   All patients who have been hospitalized should be evaluated by phone or office visit within one week of discharge to determine if they are stable and to check their understanding of and compliance with treatment plan
2.   Patients treated as outpatients:
   a.   Contact within 24 hours after visit
   b.   Then, schedule return visit for every 1-2 weeks until patient is symptom-free and dry weight is maintained
3.   After patient is symptom-free, schedule visits for every 3-6 months
4.   Certain laboratory monitoring must also be done after beginning drug therapy:
   a.   Order blood urea nitrogen, serum creatinine, and electrolyte levels initially, at 2 weeks, at 8 weeks, and then every 6 months if patient is stable
   b.   If patient is taking diuretics, order uric acid at 3 months and then annually
   c.   If patient is taking an ACE inhibitor, monitor urinalysis for protein monthly for 2-4 months and then annually
   d.   Although not routinely done, consider checking serum digoxin level in 2 weeks after beginning drug treatment or if suspicion of noncompliance or digitalis toxicity
5.   Teach patients to seek immediate medical care if they experience increasing tachycardia, palpitations, chest pain, and unexplained weight gain greater than 3-5 pounds

HYPERTENSION IN ADULTS

I.   Definition: systolic blood pressure (SBP) of ≥140 mm Hg, diastolic blood pressure (DBP) of ≥90 mm Hg, or taking antihypertensive medications

II.   Pathogenesis

A.   Approximately 90-95% of hypertensives have essential hypertension in which there is no identifiable etiology. Blood pressure remains elevated because of an increase in peripheral arterial resistance which may be related to either of the following:
1.   Inappropriate renal retention of salt and water
2.   Increased endogenous pressure activity

B.   Hypertension can be related to the following secondary causes:
1.   Polycystic kidneys
2.   Renovascular disease
3.   Aortic coarctation

4.　Cushing's syndrome
　　　5.　Pheochromocytoma
　　　6.　Use of oral contraceptives and chronic alcohol abuse

III.　Clinical Presentation

　　A.　Approximately 50 million Americans have hypertension; the elderly, African Americans, and less educated and lower socioeconomic individuals have increased rates

　　B.　Disease typically appears between ages 30-55

　　C.　Environmental factors such as obesity, psychogenic stress, high fat and sodium intake, oral contraceptives, and large alcohol intake may increase blood pressure levels

　　D.　BP fluctuations have a reasonably predictive circadian pattern; in untreated hypertensives, BP rises in morning when awakening and declines by approximately 10-20% during sleep

　　E.　Most patients are asymptomatic but some have varying degrees of target organ disease (TOD) which may not appear until 10-20 years of disease progression; higher levels of both SBP and DBP are related to increased risks of morbidity, disability, and mortality due to cardiac, renal, and cerebral diseases

　　F.　"White coat" hypertension is blood pressure that is intermittently elevated and increases only in the health care provider's office

　　G.　Classification of adult blood pressure is based on the impact of risk; classification is for persons who are not taking antihypertensive medications and who have no acute disease (see following table)
　　　1.　Classification is based on average of 2 or more readings taken at each of 2 or more visits following an initial screening
　　　2.　When systolic and diastolic pressures fall into different categories, the higher category should be selected to classify the individual's blood pressure stage

CLASSIFICATION OF BLOOD PRESSURE FOR ADULTS AGE 18 AND OLDER*			
Category	Systolic (mm Hg)		Diastolic (mm Hg)
Optimal†	<120	and	<80
Normal	<130	and	<85
High-normal	130-139	or	85-89
Hypertension			
Stage 1	140-159	or	90-99
Stage 2	160-179	or	100-109
Stage 3	≥180‡	or	≥110§

*In addition to classifying stages of hypertension on the basis of average blood pressure levels, clinicians should specify presence or absence of target organ disease and additional risk factors.
†Optimal blood pressure with respect to cardiovascular risk is below 120/80 mm Hg. However, unusually low readings should be evaluated for clinical significance.
‡If greater than 210, treat as hypertensive emergency.
§If greater than 120, treat as hypertensive emergency.

Adapted from "The Sixth Report of the Joint National Committee on Detection, Evaluation, and Treatment of High Blood Pressure -- 1997". National Institutes of Health, National Heart, Lung, and Blood Institute, 1997. NIH Publication No. 98-4080.

　　H.　Malignant hypertension can occur and is characterized by severe headaches, visual impairment (double vision, blurring), papilledema and retinal hemorrhages or exudates

I. Prevalence of isolated systolic hypertension (ISH) increases after the age of 60 years
   1. ISH is SBP of 140 mm Hg or greater with a DBP <90 mm Hg
   2. Borderline isolated systolic hypertension is likely to progress to definite hypertension and has been linked to cardiovascular disease
   3. Among the elderly, SBP is a better predictor of events such as coronary heart disease, stroke, heart failure, renal disease than is DBP

IV. Diagnosis/Evaluation

   A. History
      1. Ask about the duration and levels of elevated blood pressure as well as successes/failures or side effects of previous treatment regimes
      2. Inquire about symptoms which suggest secondary hypertension such as palpitations, sweating, dizziness, abdominal and back pain
      3. Question about symptoms of cardiovascular disease, cerebrovascular disease, peripheral vascular disease, renal disease, diabetes, dyslipidemia, gout, sexual dysfunction
      4. Inquire about weight control, physical activities, tobacco use
      5. Explore diet including sodium intake, alcohol use, caffeine, and intake of cholesterol and saturated fats
      6. Ask about patient and family histories of hypertension, premature coronary heart disease (CHD), stroke, cardiovascular disease (CVD), diabetes, dyslipidemia, and renal disease
      7. Obtain a complete medication history including over-the-counter medications, herbal remedies, illicit drugs, oral contraceptives, steroids, nonsteroidal anti-inflammatory drugs, decongestants, appetite suppressants, cyclosporine, erythropoietin, tricyclic antidepressants, and monoamine oxidase inhibitors
      8. Explore psychosocial and environmental factors that may impact on blood pressure control

   B. Physical Examination
      1. Obtain two or more blood pressure measurements separated by 2 minutes with patient supine or seated and after standing for 2 minutes (obtain blood pressure in contralateral arm to verify measurement)
         a. Measurements should begin after at least 5 minutes of rest; patients should refrain from smoking and caffeine ingestion for at least 30 minutes prior to measurement
         b. Bladder of cuff should encircle at least 80% of arm
      2. Consider using an automated noninvasive ambulatory blood pressure monitoring device in the following situations:
         a. Patients with "white-coat" hypertension
         b. To evaluate drug resistance
         c. To evaluate nocturnal pressure changes
         d. Episodic hypertension
         e. Hypotensive symptoms associated with antihypertensive medications or autonomic dysfunction
         f. Carotid sinus syncope and pacemaker syndrome (ECG monitoring needed as well)
      3. Self-measurement of blood pressure may provide valuable information; validated electronic devices or aneroid sphygmomanometers are recommended; finger monitors are inaccurate
      4. Measure height, weight, waist circumference
      5. Perform a funduscopic exam, noting arteriolar narrowing, arteriovenous nicking, hemorrhages, exudates or papilledema
      6. Assess neck for distended veins, carotid bruits and thyromegaly
      7. Perform a complete heart exam, noting tachycardia, shift in point of maximal impulse (PMI), precordial heave, clicks, murmurs, arrhythmias and third and fourth heart sounds
      8. Perform complete lung exam, noting rales and evidence of bronchospasm
      9. Perform complete abdominal exam, noting bruits, enlarged kidneys, masses and abnormal aortic pulsation
      10. Assess extremities for abnormal peripheral arterial pulsations, bruits, and edema
      11. Perform a complete neurologic exam
      12. In the elderly patient with increased blood pressure measurements, perform the Osler maneuver because elderly may have pseudohypertension due to excessively sclerosed large arteries (see following table)

OSLER MANEUVER

▲ Palpate the radial or brachial artery

▲ Inflate the B/P cuff above the systolic pressure (at this point no pulsations can be palpated)

▲ Determine whether the artery is palpable even though it is pulseless

▲ A positive Osler Maneuver occurs when the artery is palpable; a negative Osler Maneuver occurs when the artery is nonpalpable

C. Differential Diagnosis
1. Important to correctly identify patients who are truly hypertensive rather than pseudohypertensive as seen above or who appear to be hypertensive because of faulty B/P measurements
2. Important to eliminate secondary causes of hypertension; clues to presence of secondary cause are the following:
    a. Hypertension presenting for first time in individuals <25 years of age in the absence of family history or in older adults >60 years of age (essential hypertension most typically presents between 30-55 years of age)
    b. Sudden occurrence of severe hypertension at any age which is not due to antihypertensive medication withdrawal
    c. Compliant patients whose blood pressure does not lower with antihypertensive medications
    d. The following characteristic symptom complexes from secondary causes can occur in association with hypertension (see table below)

SIGNS AND SYMPTOMS OF CERTAIN DISEASES ASSOCIATED WITH ELEVATED BLOOD PRESSURE

✦ Polycystic kidneys: Lassitude, edema, abdominal or flank masses

✦ Renovascular disease: Retinopathy and a lateralizing abdominal bruit

✦ Coarctation of the aorta: Diminished femoral pulses, precordial murmur, and discrepant leg and arm blood pressure measurements

✦ Cushing's syndrome: Central obesity, hirsutism, purple striae, and ecchymosis

✦ Pheochromocytoma: Paroxysmal complaints of headache, perspiration, palpitations, and dizziness

D. Diagnostic Tests
1. Before beginning therapy order the following: urinalysis, complete blood count, blood glucose (fasting, if possible), potassium, calcium, creatinine, cholesterol (total and high density lipoprotein) and triglyceride levels, and electrocardiogram
2. Consider creatinine clearance, urinary microalbumin determination, 24-hour urinary protein, blood calcium, uric acid, glycosolated hemoglobin, thyroid-stimulating hormone, and echocardiogram
3. In selected patients, consider examination of structural alterations in arteries by ultrasound, measurement of ankle/arm index, and plasma renin activity/urinary sodium determination

V. Plan/Management: Goals are to maintain arterial pressure below 140 mm Hg SBP and 90 mm DBP and lower if tolerated while concomitantly controlling the other modifiable cardiovascular risk factors

A. Treatment regimens for hypertension are based on stage of blood pressure and risk stratification (see following tables)

CARDIOVASCULAR RISK STRATIFICATION		
Major Risk Factors		
Smoking Age older than 60 years Diabetes mellitus	Dyslipidemia Sex (men and postmenopausal women)	Family history of cardiovascular disease: women under age 65 or men under age 55
Target Organ Damage/Clinical Cardiovascular Disease (TOD/CCD)		
Heart Diseases ♦ Left ventricular hypertrophy ♦ Angina/prior myocardial infarction ♦ Prior coronary revascularization ♦ Heart failure	Stroke or transient ischemic attack Nephropathy Peripheral arterial disease Retinopathy	

Adapted from National High Blood Pressure Education Program, National Institutes of Health, National Heart, Lung, and Blood Institute. (1997). The Sixth Report of the Joint National Committee on Detection, Evaluation, and Treatment of High Blood Pressure (NIH Publication no. 98-4080). Bethesda, MD: US Government Printing Office.

RISK STRATIFICATION AND TREATMENT*				
Blood Pressure	Category	Risk Group A (No Risk Factors; No TOD/CCD)[†]	Risk Group B (At Least 1 Risk Factor, Not Including Diabetes; No TOD/CCD)	Risk Group C (TOD/CCD and/or Diabetes, With or Without Other Risk Factors)
130-139/85-89	High normal	Lifestyle modification	Lifestyle modification	Drug therapy[§]
140-159/90-99	Stage 1	Lifestyle modification (up to 12 months)	Lifestyle modification[‡] (up to 6 months)	Drug therapy
≥160/≥100	Stages 2 and 3	Drug therapy	Drug therapy	Drug therapy

*Lifestyle modification should be adjunctive therapy for all patients recommended for pharmacologic therapy.
[†]TOD/CCD indicates target organ disease/clinical cardiovascular disease.
[‡]For patients with multiple risk factors, clinicians should consider drugs as initial therapy plus lifestyle modifications.
[§]For those with heart failure, renal insufficiency, or diabetes.

Adapted from National High Blood Pressure Education Program, National Institutes of Health, National Heart, Lung, and Blood Institute. (1997). The Sixth Report of the Joint National Committee on Detection, Evaluation, and Treatment of High Blood Pressure (NIH Publication no. 98-4080). Bethesda, MD: US Government Printing Office.

B. Lifestyle modifications are helpful in lowering blood pressure and can reduce other risk factors for premature cardiovascular disease
1. Counsel patients to stop smoking (see section on SMOKING CESSATION)
2. Weight reduction is effective in reducing blood pressure in individuals who are >10% above ideal weight (see section on OBESITY)
3. Moderation of alcohol intake can reduce blood pressure: Counsel patients to limit their daily intake to 1 oz of ethanol (2 oz of 100 proof whiskey, 10 oz of wine, or 24 oz of beer); women and lighter weight people should limit daily intake to 0.5 oz
4. Counsel patients to increase aerobic physical activity (30-45 minutes most days of week)
5. Moderation of dietary sodium is important in individuals who are sensitive to changes in dietary sodium chloride (e.g., African-Americans and elderly); Counsel patients to reduce sodium chloride to less than 100 mmol/day (<6 gm sodium chloride or <2.4 gm sodium). Remember 2 gm of sodium equals approximately 1/2 teaspoon of salt
6. Counsel patients to maintain normal plasma concentrations of potassium (approximately 90 mmol/day), calcium, and magnesium, preferable from food sources
7. Counsel patients to reduce dietary saturated fat and cholesterol intake (see section on NUTRITION IN ADULTHOOD FOR DASH DIET or DIETARY APPROACHES TO STOP HYPERTENSION)

C.   An algorithm is helpful to follow; begin pharmacological therapy if patient's blood pressure is in stages 2 and 3, if patient has intermediate and high risk factors, or if lifestyle modifications do not lower blood pressure to <140/90 mm Hg (see algorithm that follows)

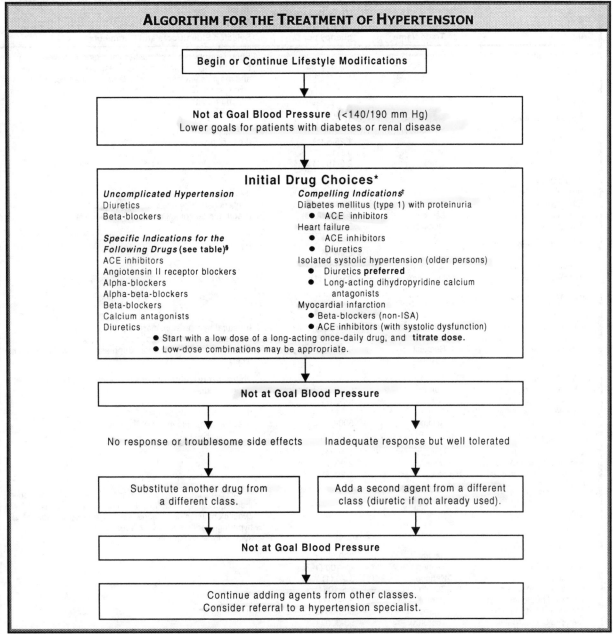

ALGORITHM FOR THE TREATMENT OF HYPERTENSION

Begin or Continue Lifestyle Modifications

Not at Goal Blood Pressure (<140/190 mm Hg)
Lower goals for patients with diabetes or renal disease

Initial Drug Choices*

Uncomplicated Hypertension
Diuretics
Beta-blockers

Specific Indications for the Following Drugs (see table)§
ACE inhibitors
Angiotensin II receptor blockers
Alpha-blockers
Alpha-beta-blockers
Beta-blockers
Calcium antagonists
Diuretics

Compelling Indications†
Diabetes mellitus (type 1) with proteinuria
   • ACE inhibitors
Heart failure
   • ACE inhibitors
   • Diuretics
Isolated systolic hypertension (older persons)
   • Diuretics **preferred**
   • Long-acting dihydropyridine calcium antagonists
Myocardial infarction
   • Beta-blockers (non-ISA)
   • ACE inhibitors (with systolic dysfunction)

• Start with a low dose of a long-acting once-daily drug, and **titrate dose.**
• Low-dose combinations may be appropriate.

Not at Goal Blood Pressure

No response or troublesome side effects

Inadequate response but well tolerated

Substitute another drug from a different class.

Add a second agent from a different class (diuretic if not already used).

Not at Goal Blood Pressure

Continue adding agents from other classes.
Consider referral to a hypertension specialist.

*Unless contraindicated. ACE indicates angiotensin-converting enzyme; ISA, intrinsic sympathomimetic activity.
†Based on randomized controlled trials.
§See table CONSIDERATIONS FOR SELECTING THE INITIAL ANTIHYPERTENSIVE DRUG in V.E.2.

Adapted from National High Blood Pressure Education Program, National Institutes of Health, National Heart, Lung, and Blood Institute. (1997). The Sixth Report of the Joint National Committee on Detection, Evaluation, and Treatment of High Blood Pressure (NIH Publication no. 98-4080). Bethesda, MD: US Government Printing Office.

D. General guidelines for pharmacological therapy (see table on oral antihypertensive drugs)

ORAL ANTIHYPERTENSIVE DRUGS*

Drug	Trade Name	Usual Dose Range, Total mg/day* (Frequency per Day)	Selected Side Effects and Comments*
Diuretics (partial list)			Short-term: Increase cholesterol and glucose levels; biochemical abnormalities: decrease potassium, sodium, and magnesium levels, increase uric acid and calcium levels; rare: blood dyscrasias, photosensitivity, pancreatitis, hyponatremia
Chlorthalidone (G)†	Hygroton	12.5-50 (1)	
Hydrochlorothiazide (G)	Hydrodiuril	12.5-50 (1)	
Indapamide	Lozol	1.25-5 (1)	(Less or no hypercholesterolemia)
Metolazone	Mykrox	0.5-1.0 (1)	
	Zaroxolyn	2.5-10 (1)	
Loop diuretics			
Bumetanide (G)	Bumex	0.5-4 (2-3)	(Short duration of action, no hypercalcemia)
Ethacrynic acid	Edecrin	25-100 (2-3)	(Only nonsulfonamide diuretic, ototoxicity)
Furosemide (G)	Lasix	40-240 (2-3)	(Short duration of action, no hypercalcemia)
Torsemide	Demadex	5-100 (1-2)	
Potassium-sparing agents			Hyperkalemia
Amiloride hydrochloride (G)	Midamor	5-10 (1)	
Spironolactone (G)	Aldactone	25-100 (1)	(Gynecomastia)
Triamterene (G)	Dyrenium	25-100 (1)	
Adrenergic inhibitors			
Peripheral agents			
Guanadrel	Hylorel	10-75 (2)	(Postural hypotension, diarrhea)
Guanethidine monosulfate	Ismelin	10-150 (1)	(Postural hypotension, diarrhea)
Reserpine (G)**	Serpasil	0.05-0.25 (1)	(Nasal congestion, sedation, depression, activation of peptic ulcer)
Central alpha-agonists			Sedation, dry mouth, bradycardia, withdrawal hypertension
Clonidine hydrochloride (G)	Catapres	0.2-1.2 (2-3)	(More withdrawal)
Guanabenz acetate (G)	Wytensin	8-32 (2)	
Guanfacine hydrochloride (G)	Tenex	1-3 (1)	(Less withdrawal)
Methyldopa (G)	Aldomet	500-3,000 (2)	(Hepatic and "autoimmune" disorders)
Alpha-blockers			Postural hypotension
Doxazosin mesylate	Cardura	1-16 (1)	
Prazosin hydrochloride (G)	Minipress	2-30 (2-3)	
Terazosin hydrochloride	Hytrin	1-20 (1)	
Beta-blockers			Bronchospasm, bradycardia, heart failure, may mask insulin-induced hypoglycemia; less serious: impaired peripheral circulation, insomnia, fatigue, decreased exercise tolerance, hypertriglyceridemia (except agents with intrinsic sympathomimetic activity)
Acebutolol§‡	Sectral	200-800 (1)	
Atenolol (G)§	Tenormin	25-100 (1-2)	
Betaxolol§	Kerlone	5-20 (1)	
Bisoprolol fumarate§	Zebeta	2.5-10 (1)	
Carteolol hydrochloride‡	Cartrol	2.5-10 (1)	
Metoprolol tartrate (G)§	Lopressor	50-300 (2)	
Metoprolol succinate§	Toprol-XL	50-300 (1)	
Nadolol (G)	Corgard	40-320 (1)	
Penbutolol sulfate‡	Levatol	10-20 (1)	
Pindolol (G)‡	Visken	10-60 (2)	
Propranolol hydrochloride (G)	Inderal	40-480 (1)	
	Inderal LA	40-480 (2)	
Timolol maleate (G)	Blocadren	20-60 (2)	
Combined alpha- and beta-blockers			Postural hypotension, bronchospasm
Carvedilol	Coreg	12.5-50 (2)	
Labetalol hydrochloride (G)	Normodyne, Trandate	200-1,200 (2)	
Direct vasodilators			Headaches, fluid retention, tachycardia
Hydralazine hydrochloride (G)	Apresoline	50-300 (2)	(Lupus syndrome)
Minoxidil (G)	Loniten	5-100 (1)	(Hirsutism)

(continued)

Oral Antihypertensive Drugs* (continued)

Drug	Trade Name	Usual Dose Range, Total mg/day* (Frequency per Day)	Selected Side Effects and Comments*
Calcium antagonists			
Nondihydropyridines			Conduction defects, worsening of systolic dysfunction, gingival hyperplasia (Nausea, headache)
Diltiazem hydrochloride	Cardizem SR	120-360 (2)	
	Cardizem CD, Dilacor XR, Tiazac	120-360 (1)	
Verapamil hydrochloride	Isoptin SR, Calan SR	90-480 (2)	(Constipation)
	Verelan, Covera HS	120-480 (1)	
Dihydropyridines			Edema of the ankle, flushing, headache, gingival hypertrophy
Amlodipine besylate	Norvasc	2.5-10 (1)	
Felodipine	Plendil	2.5-20 (1)	
Isradipine	DynaCirc	5-20 (2)	
	DynaCirc CR	5-20 (1)	
Nicardipine	Cardene SR	60-90 (2)	
Nifedipine	Procardia XL, Adalat CC	30-120 (1)	
Nisoldipine	Sular	20-60 (1)	
ACE inhibitors			Common: cough; rare: angioedema, hyperkalemia, rash, loss of taste, leukopenia
Benazepril hydrochloride	Lotensin	5-40 (1-2)	
Captopril (G)	Capoten	25-150 (2-3)	
Enalapril maleate	Vasotec	5-40 (1-2)	
Fosinopril sodium	Monopril	10-40 (1-2)	
Lisinopril	Prinivil, Zestril	5-40 (1)	
Moexipril	Univasc	7.5-15 (2)	
Quinapril hydrochloride	Accupril	5-80 (1-2)	
Ramipril	Altace	1.25-20 (1-2)	
Trandolapril	Mavik	1-4 (1)	
Angiotensin II receptor blockers			Angioedema (very rare), hyperkalemia
Losartan potassium	Cozaar	25-100 (1-2)	
Valsartan	Diovan	80-320 (1)	
Irbesartan	Avapro	150-300 (1)	

*These dosages may vary from those listed in the *Physicians' Desk Reference* (51st edition), which may be consulted for additional information. The listing of side effects is not all-inclusive, and side effects are for the class of drugs except where noted for individual drugs (in parentheses); clinicians are urged to refer to the package insert for a more detailed listing.

†(G) indicates generic available.

‡Has intrinsic sympathomimetic activity.

§Cardioselective.

**Also acts centrally.

Adapted from National High Blood Pressure Education Program, National Institutes of Health, National Heart, Lung, and Blood Institute. (1997). The Sixth Report of the Joint National Committee on Detection, Evaluation, and Treatment of High Blood Pressure (NIH Publication no. 98-4080). Bethesda, MD: US Government Printing Office.

1. Selection of specific drug should be individualized (see table under V.E.)
2. Start with a low dose of the initial drug and slowly titrate upwardly; in **patients with Stage 3 hypertension and those in risk group C** the following modifications should be made:
   a. Give drug therapy with minimal delay
   b. May need to add a second and third drug after a short interval if control is not achieved
   c. **Patients with SBP≥200 mm Hg and average of DBP ≥120 mm Hg** may require initial therapy with more than one drug and may need hospitalized if symptoms or target organ damage is present (see V.K. for hypertensive crises)
3. For the low and medium-risk patient: if blood pressure is still uncontrolled after 1-2 months of drug therapy, the next dosage level should be prescribed
4. For chronic maintenance, use 24-hour formulations to cover morning surge in B/P, for smooth persistent control, and to enhance adherence
5. Combinations of low doses of agents from different classes may provide additional efficacy and reduce likelihood of dose-dependent adverse effects (see table on combination drugs that follows)

COMBINATION DRUGS

Drug	Trade Name
Beta-adrenergic blockers and diuretics	
Atenolol, 50 or 100 mg/chlorthalidone, 25 mg	Tenoretic
Bisoprolol fumarate, 2.5, 5, 0r 10 mg/hydrochlorothiazide, 6.25 mg	Ziac*
Metoprolol tartrate, 50 or 100 mg/hydrochlorothiazide, 25 or 50 mg	Lopressor HCT
Nadolol, 40 or 80 mg/bendroflumethiazide, 5 mg	Corzide
Propranolol hydrochloride, 40 or 80 mg/hydrochlorothiazide, 25 mg	Inderide
Propranolol hydrochloride (extended release), 80, 120, or 160 mg/hydrochlorothiazide, 50 mg	Inderide LA
Timolol maleate, 10 mg/hydrochlorothiazide, 25 mg	Timolide
ACE inhibitors and diuretics	
Benazepril hydrochloride, 5, 10, or 20 mg/hydrochlorothiazide, 6.25, 12.5, or 25 mg	Lotensin HCT
Captopril, 25 or 50 mg/hydrochlorothiazide, 15 or 25 mg	Capozide*
Enalapril maleate, 5 or 10 mg/hydrochlorothiazide, 12.5 or 25 mg	Vaseretic
Lisinopril, 10 or 20 mg/hydrochlorothiazide, 12.5 or 25 mg	Prinzide,
	Zestoretic
Angiotensin II receptor antagonists and diuretics	
Losartan potassium, 50 mg/hydrochlorothiazide, 12.5 mg	Hyzaar
Calcium antagonists and ACE inhibitors	
Amlodipine besylate, 2.5 or 5 mg/benazepril hydrochloride, 10 or 20 mg	Lotrel
Diltiazem hydrochloride, 180 mg/enalapril maleate, 5 mg	Teczem
Verapamil hydrochloride (extended release), 180 or 240 mg/trandolapril, 1, 2, or 4 mg	Tarka
Felodipine, 5 mg/enalapril maleate, 5 mg	Lexxel
Other combinations	
Triamterene, 37.5, 50, or 75 mg/hydrochlorothiazide, 25 or 50 mg	Dyazide, Maxide
Spironolactone, 25 or 50 mg/hydrochlorothiazide, 25 or 50 mg	Aldactazide
Amiloride hydrochloride, 5 mg/hydrochlorothiazide, 50 mg	Moduretic
Guanethidine monosulfate, 10 mg/hydrochlorothiazide, 25 mg	Esimil
Hydralazine hydrochloride, 25, 50, 0r 100 mg/hydrochlorothiazide, 25 or 50 mg	Apresazide
Methyldopa, 250 or 500 mg/hydrochlorothiazide, 15, 25, 30, or 50 mg	Aldoril
Reserpine, 0.125 mg/hydrochlorothiazide, 25 or 50 mg	Hydropres
Reserpine, 0.10 mg/hydralazine hydrochloride, 25 mg/hydrochlorothiazide, 15 mg	Ser-Ap-Es
Clonidine hydrochloride, 0.1, 0.2, or 0.3 mg/chlorthalidone, 15 mg	Combipres
Methyldopa, 250 mg/chlorothiazide, 150 or 250 mg	Aldochlor
Reserpine, 0.125 or 0.25 mg/chlorthalidone, 25 or 50 mg	Demi-Regroton
Reserpine, 0.125 or 0.25 mg/chlorothiazide, 250 or 500 mg	Diupres
Prazosin hydrochloride, 1, 2, or 5 mg/polythiazide, 0.5 mg	Minizide

*Approved for initial therapy.

Adapted from National High Blood Pressure Education Program, National Institutes of Health, National Heart, Lung, and Blood Institute. (1997). The Sixth Report of the Joint National Committee on Detection, Evaluation, and Treatment of High Blood Pressure (NIH Publication no. 98-4080). Bethesda, MD: US Government Printing Office.

    a.   Combination of ACE inhibitor and calcium antagonist reduces proteinuria and results in less pedal edema than when calcium antagonist is used alone

    b.   Metolazone and a loop diuretic provide additive effects when used in patients with renal failure

6.   Drug interactions may be helpful or deleterious (see table on Drug Interactions)

7.   Some agents may cause adverse reactions; direct-acting smooth-muscle vasodilators, central alpha$_2$-agonists, and peripheral adrenergic antagonists are usually not used as the initial monotherapy

DRUG INTERACTIONS

Class of Agent	Increase Efficacy	Decrease Efficacy	Effect on Other Drugs
Diuretics	• Diuretics that act at different sites in the nephron (e.g., furosemide + thiazides)	• Resin-binding agents • NSAIDS • Steroids	• Diuretics raise serum lithium levels. • Potassium-sparing agents may exacerbate hyperkalemia due to ACE inhibitors
Beta-blockers	• Cimetidine • Quinidine • Food	• NSAIDS • Withdrawal of clonidine • Agents that induce hepatic enzymes, including rifampin and phenobarbital	• Beta-blockers may mask and prolong insulin-induced hypoglycemia. • Heart block may occur with nondihydropyridine calcium antagonists. • Beta-blockers increase angina-inducing potential of cocaine.
ACE inhibitors	• Chlorpromazine or clozapine	• NSAIDS • Antacids • Food decreases absorption (moexipril)	• ACE inhibitors may raise serum lithium levels. • ACE inhibitors may exacerbate hyperkalemic effect of potassium-sparing diuretics.
Calcium antagonists	• Grapefruit juice (some dihydropyridines) • Cimetidine or ranitidine (hepatically metabolized calcium antagonists)	• Agents that induce hepatic enzymes, including rifampin and phenobarbital	• Cyclosporine levels increase[†] with diltiazem hydrochloride, verapamil hydrochloride, mibefradil dihydrochloride, or nicardipine hydrochloride (but not felodipine, isradipine, or nifedipine). • Nondihydropyridines increase levels of other drugs metabolized by the same hepatic enzyme system, including digoxin, quinidine, sulfonylureas, and theophylline. • Verapamil hydrochloride may lower serum lithium levels.
Alpha-blockers			• Prazosin may decrease clearance of verapamil hydrochloride.
Central alpha$_2$-agonists and peripheral neuronal blockers		• Tricyclic antidepressants • Monoamine oxidase inhibitors • Sympathomimetics or phenothiazines antagonize guanethidine monosulfate or guanadrel sulfate • Iron salts may reduce methyldopa absorption	• Methyldopa may increase serum lithium levels. • Severity of clonidine hydrochloride withdrawal may be increased by beta-blockers. • Many agents used in anesthesia are potentiated by clonidine hydrochloride.

[†]This is a clinically and economically beneficial drug-drug interaction because it both retards progression of accelerated atherosclerosis in heart transplant recipients and reduces the required daily dose of cyclosporine.

Adapted from National High Blood Pressure Education Program, National Institutes of Health, National Heart, Lung, and Blood Institute. (1997). The Sixth Report of the Joint National Committee on Detection, Evaluation, and Treatment of High Blood Pressure (NIH Publication no. 98-4080). Bethesda, MD: US Government Printing Office.

E. Selecting the initial agent for therapy
1. Diuretics and beta-blockers are chosen first if there are no indications for another type of drug because of the numerous randomized controlled trials which found that these drugs were effective in reducing morbidity and mortality
2. However, there are compelling and specific indications for various agents in certain conditions (see table CONSIDERATIONS FOR SELECTING THE INITIAL ANTIHYPERTENSIVE DRUG)

CONSIDERATIONS FOR SELECTING THE INITIAL ANTIHYPERTENSIVE DRUG*

Indication	Drug Therapy
Compelling Indications Unless Contraindicated	
Diabetes mellitus (type 1) with proteinuria	ACE I
Heart failure	ACE I, diuretics
Isolated systolic hypertension (older patients)	Diuretics (preferred), CA (long-acting DHP)
Myocardial infarction	Beta-blockers (non-ISA), ACE I (with systolic dysfunction)
May Have Favorable Effects on Comorbid Conditions	
Angina	Beta-blockers, CA
Atrial tachycardia and fibrillation	Beta-blockers, CA (non-DHP)
Cyclosporine-induced hypertension (caution with the dose of cyclosporine)	CA
Diabetes mellitus (types 1 and 2) with proteinuria	ACE I (preferred), CA
Diabetes mellitus (type 2)	Low-dose diuretics
Dyslipidemia	Alpha-blockers
Essential tremor	Beta-blockers (non-CS)
Heart failure	Carvedilol, losartan potassium
Hyperthyroidism	Beta-blockers
Left ventricular hypertrophy	ACE I, diuretics, beta-blockers
Migraine	Beta-blockers (non-CS), CA (non-DHP)
Myocardial infarction	Diltiazem hydrochloride, verapamil hydrochloride
Osteoporosis	Thiazides
Preoperative hypertension	Beta-blockers
Prostatism (BPH)	Alpha-blockers
Renal insufficiency (caution in renovascular hypertension and creatinine ≥265.2 mmol/L {3 mg/dL})	ACE I
May Have Unfavorable Effects on Comorbid Conditions‡	
Bronchospastic disease	Beta-blockers§
Depression	Beta-blockers, central alpha-agonists, reserpine§
Diabetes mellitus (types 1 and 2)	Beta-blockers, high-dose diuretics
Dyslipidemia	Beta-blockers (non-ISA), diuretics (high-dose)
Gout	Diuretics
2° or 3° heart block	Beta-blockers,§ CA (non-DHP)§
Heart failure	Beta-blockers (except carvedilol), CA (except amlodipine besylate, felodipine)
Liver disease	Labetalol hydrochloride, methyldopa§
Peripheral vascular disease	Beta-blockers
Pregnancy	ACE I,§ angiotensin II receptor blockers§
Renal insufficiency	Potassium-sparing agents
Renovascular disease	ACE I, angiotensin II receptor blockers
Demographic Factors and Effects	
African American	Diuretics and calcium antagonists are recommended
Elderly	Thiazides or beta-blockers plus thiazides are recommended; also consider long-acting dihydropyridine calcium antagonists

*ACE I indicates angiotensin-converting enzyme inhibitors; BPH, benign prostatic hyperplasia; CA, calcium antagonists; DHP, dihydropyridine; ISA, intrinsic sympathomimetic activity; MI, myocardial infarction; and non-CS, noncardioselective.
‡These drugs may be used with special monitoring unless contraindicated.
§Contraindicated.

Adapted from National High Blood Pressure Education Program, National Institutes of Health, National Heart, Lung, and Blood Institute. (1997). The Sixth Report of the Joint National Committee on Detection, Evaluation, and Treatment of High Blood Pressure (NIH Publication no. 98-4080). Bethesda, MD: US Government Printing Office.

    F.   Either of the following two approaches is recommended when response to the initial drug is inadequate
        1.   Add a second drug from another class if patient is tolerating initial drug
            a.   If diuretic was not selected initially, choose it as second-step drug because its addition should enhance the effects of other drug
            b.   If addition of second agent controls BP, consider withdrawing first agent
        2.   Substitute an agent from another class if the patient is having significant adverse effects or no response

G. Step-down therapy
   1. After BP is controlled for at least 1 year, consider decreasing dosage and number of drugs
   2. Regular followup visits are needed because BP levels often rise when drug regimens are altered, particularly in patients who do not make lifestyle changes

H. Overview of classes of antihypertensive agents
   1. Diuretics:
      a. Advantages: inexpensive, effective, have additive and synergistic effects with other drugs, and in small doses have few adverse effects
      b. Disadvantages: in higher doses have adverse effects such as impaired glucose tolerance, increased lipids, electrolyte imbalance; approximately 15-30% of patients become hypokalemic on hydrochlorothiazide; the following should be considered in patients with hypokalemia
         (1) Monitor magnesium levels (magnesium deficiency is often associated with hypokalemia)
         (2) Prescribe K+ supplement such as K-Dur 20 mEq tablets (take one tablet at breakfast and one at dinner) or a K+ sparing diuretic
      c. Types:
         (1) Thiazides: More effective than loop diuretics except in patients with serum creatinine >221 mmol/L (2.5 mg/dL)
         (2) Loop diuretic: Use in patients with renal impairment
         (3) Potassium sparing agents
            (a) Avoid or reverse hypokalemia from other diuretics; may cause hyperkalemia, particularly when combined with an ACE inhibitor or potassium supplement
            (b) Avoid when serum creatinine is >221 mmol/L (2.5 mg/dL)
   2. Beta -blockers
      a. Beta-blockers are classified as either with intrinsic sympathomimetic activity (ISA) or without ISA; both types are equally effective, but those without ISA were found to reduce nonfatal myocardial infarctions (MI), sudden death, and total mortality from MIs
      b. Beta-blockers are somewhat less effective in treating black and elderly patients
      c. May cause depression and fatigue in some patients
      d. Use cautiously with calcium channel blockers
   3. Alpha blockers
      a. Usually not used as a first agent
      b. Cause postural effects; need to titrate based on standing blood pressure; start first dose at bedtime; start low and titrate slowly
      c. Beneficial in patients with benign prostatic hypertrophy
   4. Central alpha agonists
      a. No longer widely used because they depress central nervous system, cause fatigue, lethargy, and cognitive impairment
      b. Helpful in patients with panic attacks; methyldopa is drug of choice for hypertension in pregnancy
   5. Peripheral acting adrenergic antagonists: Rarely used, adverse reactions include postural hypotension, impotence, diarrhea, weight gain, and depression (reserpine)
   6. Calcium antagonists
      a. Mechanism of action
         (1) Verapamil and to lesser extent, diltiazem, reduce heart rate, slow ventricular conduction, and depress contractility (may reduce sinus rate and produce heart block)
         (2) Dihydropyridines have little effect on contractility and conduction but are good peripheral vasodilators (may cause dizziness, headache, flushing, edema, and tachycardia)
      b. Controversial research found that short-acting formulations (nifedipine) given immediately after MI increased mortality; another study found that short-acting calcium channel blockers increased risk for MI in a national sample of women; best to use long-acting formulations

7. ACE Inhibitors
   a. Some authorities, but not Joint National Committee on Blood Pressure VI, believe that in the absence of specific indications for another drug, ACE inhibitors are a good initial antihypertensive medication
   b. Effective as monotherapy in patients with left ventricular dysfunction, after MI, in type 1 diabetes; not effective as monotherapy in African American patients unless used with a diuretic
   c. Few side effects except may cause ticklish dry cough, particularly in older, female, white or Oriental patients, and patients with congestive heart failure
   d. Avoid or use with caution in combination with potassium supplements, salt substitutes, or potassium-sparing diuretics; may need to adjust doses if used with hypoglycemic agents
   e. A short-acting agent such as captopril (Capoten) may be useful as initial drug to determine effectiveness and patient's reactions; for chronic maintenance switch to long-acting agent
8. Angiotensin II receptor blockers: Main advantage over ACE inhibitors is the lack of undesirable side effects, specifically cough and angioedema; modestly increases potassium levels

I. Special situations
   1. Women on oral contraceptives and those taking estrogen replacement should have their BP measured more frequently after starting medications
   2. Older persons
      a. Elderly exhibit orthostatic falls in BP and thus should have measurements done in standing as well as seated or supine position
      b. Drugs that increase postural changes in BP (peripheral adrenergic blockers, alpha-blockers, and high dose diuretics) or drugs that cause cognitive dysfunction (central alpha$_2$-agonist) should be used with caution
      c. Starting dose in elderly should be half that used by younger patients
      d. Thiazide diuretics or beta-blockers in combination with thiazides or long-acting dihydropyridine calcium antagonists are recommended
   3. Patients with renal insufficiency with greater than 1 gram per day of proteinuria should be treated with goal of 125/75 mm HG; those with less proteinuria should have goal of 130/85 mm Hg; ACE inhibitors are often recommended
   4. Patients with diabetes should have target BP goal of 130/85 mm Hg

J. Resistant hypertension: BP which cannot be reduced below 140/90 mm Hg in patients adhering to adequate and appropriate triple-drug regimen which includes diuretic and drugs prescribed at almost maximum dosage or SBP which cannot be reduced below 160 mm Hg in older patients with isolated systolic hypertension
   1. Consider the following: pseudoresistance (white collar hypertensive, incorrect measurement techniques), volume overload (renal damage, excess salt intake, inadequate diuretic therapy), drug-related causes (drug interactions, drug actions), associated conditions (sleep apnea, chronic pain, increased alcohol intake, insulin resistance, chronic pain)
   2. Always consider nonadherence to therapy whenever BP is not controlled
   3. Refer to specialist if goal blood pressure cannot be achieved

K. Hypertensive Crises
   1. Emergencies: situations which require immediate BP reduction to prevent or limit target organ damage (hypertensive encephalopathy, intracranial hemorrhage, unstable angina, MI, heart failure, pulmonary edema, aneurysm, eclampsia)
   2. Urgencies: situations in which it is desirable to reduce BP within a few hours (upper levels of stage 3 hypertension, hypertension with optic disk edema, progressive target organ complications)
   3. Crisis therapy is not required when there is an absence of symptoms or when there is no new or progressive target organ damage
   4. Parenteral drugs should be used for emergencies; oral doses of loop diuretics, beta-blockers, ACE inhibitors, alpha$_2$-agonists or calcium antagonists can be used for urgencies

5. Do not excessively and rapidly reduce BP as this may precipitate renal, cerebral or coronary ischemia or cardiogenic shock; try to reduce mean arterial BP by no more than 25% (within minutes to 2 hours) then toward 160/100 in 2 to 6 hours
6. Do NOT administer sublingual fast-acting nifedipine because serious adverse effects have been reported

L. Follow Up
   1. See following table for follow up based on initial set of blood pressure measurements

RECOMMENDATIONS FOR FOLLOW UP BASED ON INITIAL SET OF BLOOD PRESSURE MEASUREMENTS FOR ADULTS AGE 18 AND OLDER		
Initial Blood Pressure (mm Hg)*		
Systolic	**Diastolic**	**Followup Recommendations†**
<130	<85	Recheck in 2 years
130-139	85-89	Recheck in 1 year‡
140-159	90-99	Confirm within 2 months‡
160-179	100-109	Evaluate or refer to source of care within 1 month
≥180	≥110	Evaluate or refer to source of care immediately or within 1 week depending on clinical situation

*If systolic and diastolic categories are different, follow recommendations for shorter time followup (e.g., 160/86 mm Hg should be evaluated or referred to source of care within 1 month).
†Modify the scheduling of followup according to reliable information about past blood pressure measurements, other cardiovascular risk factors, or target organ disease.
‡Provide advice about lifestyle modifications.

Adapted from National High Blood Pressure Education Program, National Institutes of Health, National Heart, Lung, and Blood Institute. (1997). The Sixth Report of the Joint National Committee on Detection, Evaluation, and Treatment of High Blood Pressure (NIH Publication no. 98-4080). Bethesda, MD: US Government Printing Office.

2. Patients treated with lifestyle modifications should be seen after 3-6 months; when their blood pressure is stabilized, they should be seen every 6-12 months
3. Patients who are started on pharmacological therapy should be seen every 1-2 months until their BP is stable; then, they should be seen every 6-12 months (patients in initial 2 & 3 hypertensive stages should be seen more frequently); remember that many ACE Inhibitors, angiotension blocking agents, and calcium antagonists do not peak until 3-4 weeks
4. Patients with emergent and urgent hypertension should be seen within 24 hours
5. When changing medication dosages, follow up should be within 1-3 months
6. Elderly patients, patients with TOD, patients with co-morbidities, and patients with a history of emergent or urgent hypertensive episodes should be followed more closely

ISCHEMIC HEART DISEASE: ASYMPTOMATIC CORONARY ARTERY DISEASE, ANGINA PECTORIS, AND MYOCARDIAL INFARCTION

I. Definitions

   A. Ischemic heart disease (IHD) or coronary heart disease (CHD): heart disease that occurs as a result of inadequate oxygen and blood supply to the myocardium due to atherosclerotic coronary artery disease; it has many clinical expressions, ranging from the asymptomatic preclinical phase to acute myocardial infarction and sudden death

B. Coronary artery disease (CAD): refers to atherosclerotic narrowing of the major epicardial coronary arteries

C. Angina pectoris: a clinical syndrome characterized by chest, neck, arm, or back discomfort that is associated with physical exertion and due to reversible myocardial ischemia resulting from significant underlying CAD

D. Myocardial infarction; acute process of myocardial ischemia associated with sufficient severity and duration that can potentially result in permanent irreversible myocardial damage

II. Pathogenesis

A. Ischemic heart disease (IHD) or coronary artery disease (CAD) is due to blockages made up of fats, platelets, and other debris in the large and medium-sized arteries serving the heart

B. Angina pectoris (AP) is due to myocardial ischemia which occurs when the cardiac work and myocardial oxygen demand exceed the ability of the coronary arteries to supply oxygenated blood

C. In unstable angina, artery blockages may be large, ruptured or have a lesion; a blood clot or thrombus may form around the damage which can be so large that blood flow is impeded or completely blocked

D. Myocardial infarction (MI) occurs when an atherosclerotic plaque completely blocks a major coronary artery or branch or when plaque ruptures with a thrombus extending out from the plaque to occlude the coronary lumen which leads to irreversible necrosis and cellular death

E. Risk factors for development of ischemic heart disease:
1. Hypertension
2. Hyperlipidemia
3. Diabetes mellitus
4. Cigarette smoking
5. Family history of premature CAD (individual whose father died of CAD before the age of 60)
6. Other possibilities include: oral contraceptives, personality type, sedentary living, obesity (particularly with a truncal distribution), stress, and high stored iron levels

F. Recent research indicates a possible role of other factors in the development of coronary artery disease
1. Infection with *Chlamydia pneumonia*, a common intracellular pathogen, has been linked with CAD; reinfection with the pathogen may trigger the onset of acute MI
2. Infection with *Helicobacter pylori* may increase inflammation and have a role in development of IHD
3. Homocysteine, an amino acid, has been linked with increased risks of IHD
4. Elevated fasting triglyceride levels have been associated with coronary risk particularly if there are other underlying risk factors
5. Cardiovascular disease has been associated with pathogenic low-density lipoprotein modification due to oxidation damage by free radicals

III. Clinical Presentation

A. Ischemic heart disease IHD)
1. Although ischemic heart disease (IHD) has declined by 20% over the last 20 years, it still is the leading nontraumatic cause of disability and death in US
2. Men die earlier from IHD than women, but after age 60 one in 4 women as well as men die of IHD; although the mortality rates have been falling from the 1960s, the rate of decline has been slower among women than men since 1979
3. IHD due to atherosclerosis is characteristically silent until critical stenosis, thrombosis, aneurysm or embolus develop

4. Signs and symptoms develop gradually as the atheroma extends in the vessels; fatigue, intermittent claudification, and mild angina on exertion are often the initial complaints

B. Angina Pectoris
1. Typical anginal chest pain is described as tightness, pressure, or aching and is often located in the substernal area, radiating down one or both arms for 5 minutes or less, precipitated by exercise or emotional stress and relieved by rest or nitroglycerin; associated symptoms include dyspnea, nausea, gas, sweating, weakness and palpitations
2. Course/type of anginal symptoms (see table that follows)

TYPE OF ANGINA	
Stable	No change in frequency, severity or duration of anginal episodes during the preceding 6 weeks
Progressive	Increase in frequency, severity or duration of anginal episodes during the last 6 weeks but not enough to require hospitalization
Unstable	Three principal presentations 1. Angina occurring at rest and usually prolonged >20 minutes occurring within one week of presentation 2. Marked limitations of ordinary physical activity (walking 1-2 blocks on level and climbing one flight of stairs) or inability to carry on any physical activity without discomfort; onset within 2 months of initial presentation 3. Previously diagnosed angina that is changing so that it is occurring with increasing severity, frequency, or duration and often occurring at rest; less likely to resolve with treatment and may begin to be resistant to efficacy of nitroglycerin

3. Patients with stable angina have a relatively good prognosis with an annual mortality rate of <4%; these patients are excellent candidates for reversal through risk reduction and lifestyle modifications

C. Myocardial Infarction
1. Evidence of acute congestive heart failure, a new or worsening mitral regurgitation murmur or systemic hypotension suggests high risk for death or nonfatal MI
2. Patients with acute MI often have severe ischemic discomfort which lasts more than 20-30 minutes and is not relieved by rest or sublingual nitroglycerin
3. Approximately 25% of all MIs in the United States are clinically unrecognized either because they are silent or have an atypical presentation such as discomfort in arm, neck, back, or jaw without chest pain
4. Postinfarction angina, congestive heart failure, arrhythmias, and arterial embolus are common complications

IV. Diagnosis/Evaluation (anyone who presents with a possible myocardial infarction should have a brief, directed history and physical examination, and a 12-lead electrocardiogram (ECG))

A. The following history should be done at intervals with urgent needs addressed first; place patient on cardiac monitor and give oxygen while history and physical are done if MI is suspected
1. Ask patient to describe any pain according to the following eight features: quality of discomfort, location, duration, severity, precipitants, factors providing relief, length of pain episodes
2. Ask about associated symptoms such as nausea, vomiting, shortness of breath, lightheadedness, diaphoresis
3. To classify severity of angina, ask about frequency duration and severity of chest pain (prolonged, episodes of severe pain suggest high-risk unstable angina)
4. To eliminate heart failure as a diagnosis, ask about orthopnea, paroxysmal nocturnal dyspnea, and peripheral edema
5. Question about previous cardiac disease, particularly any prior MI
6. Inquire about history of risk factors for CAD
7. Explore medication history

B. Physical Examination
1. Observe general appearance, noting signs of distress such as dyspnea, pallor, diaphoresis, weakness, confusion
2. Measure vital signs
3. Measure fat distribution by obtaining a waist to hip ratio
4. Perform a complete eye examination including funduscopy
5. Examine neck for jugular venous distention, thyromegaly, and bruits
6. Perform a complete heart exam; physical findings suggestive of ischemic heart disease include the following;
    a. Third or fourth heart sound
    b. Murmur
7. Assess peripheral pulses
8. Perform a complete exam of the lungs
9. Examine abdomen for organomegaly
10. Assess extremities for edema, peripheral pulses, cyanosis, and clubbing

C. Differential Diagnosis: Four main conditions mimic acute MI and need to be eliminated
1. Acute pericarditis (presents with pericardial friction rub)
2. Aortic dissection (asymmetry of pulses and blood pressures in both arms)
3. Spontaneous pneumothorax (absent breath sounds)
4. Pulmonary emboli (pleuritic chest pain, tachypnea, wheezing, and hemoptysis)
5. See section on CHEST PAIN for other conditions

D. Diagnostic Tests
1. There are no specific laboratory tests that are particularly helpful in diagnosing CAD (risk factor screening via a good history is the most helpful in uncovering asymptomatic CAD)
    a. For individuals free of symptoms of CAD, total cholesterol levels should be drawn every 5 years
    b. Order other tests to detect CAD on an individual basis; the most commonly ordered tests are the following: fasting glucose levels, chest x-ray, electrocardiogram (ECG)
    c. Exercise treadmill test (ETT) or graded exercise test (GXT) can be used to screen for occult CAD in asymptomatic subjects and is helpful for a patient who wishes to begin an exercise program
2. For patients with suspected CAD, order a 12-lead electrocardiogram (ECG); look for Q waves which indicate prior myocardial damage and the presence of ST-T wave changes (elevation or depression) and deep symmetrical T-wave inversion in multiple precordial leads which suggests ischemia; ECG is normal in approximately 25% of patients with angina
3. For patients with suspected CAD, order chest x-ray which provides information about heart size and heart failure; helpful in ruling out pulmonary edema, pleural effusions, and aortic aneurysm
4. For some patients, the next tests to order are the cardiac catheterization and coronary arteriography which are the gold standards of diagnosis of CAD but are invasive and have risks
    a. Measure extent of left ventricular dysfunction (ejection fraction)
    b. Measure amount of CAD present (number of coronary arteries with significant CAD)
    c. Order in the following cases: patients with unstable angina who fail to respond to medical therapy, patients with suspected CAD and signs and symptoms of CHF which may have a reversible cause
5. For patients with suspected CAD whom the clinician prefers to defer cardiac catheterization, order an exercise or functional test
    a. Exercise thallium and exercise MUGA (radionuclide angiography) are equivalent for prognostic data
    b. The dipyridamole thallium test is better for patients who are unable to exercise on a treadmill
    c. MUGA scan and two-dimensional echocardiogram can help determine the presence and extent of left ventricular damage but cannot distinguish an acute MI from an old healed MI; therefore, PET scan can be used to determine viability and extent of ischemia versus infarcted tissue

6. For patients with suspected acute myocardial infarction order serial determinations of the serum enzyme creatinine kinase (CK) and its isoenzyme (CK-MB)
   a. In acute MI, CK rises within 6-8 hours and CK-MB rises within 4-6 hours, peak values for both enzymes are reached within 18-24 hours, and levels return to normal within 36-72 hours
   b. Measure CK and CK-MB initially and then every 8 hours for 24 hours; 3 consecutive negative CK and CK-MB levels exclude diagnosis of MI
   c. Order lactate dehydrogenase (LDH) enzyme levels in patients who present 12-24 hours after symptom onset and have negative total CK and CK-MB; LDH enzyme levels begin to rise within 24-48 hours, peak at 4-6 days, and return to normal by 7-10 days
7. Recently some authorities suggest ordering troponin-T which is more sensitive as a marker of myocardial damage than CK-MB

V. Plan/Management

A. Primary prevention of the major modifiable risk factors for CAD should be implemented as follows:
   a. Goal of complete cessation of smoking (see section on SMOKING CESSATION)
   b. Lipid management with primary goal of low density lipids (LDL) <100 mg/dL and secondary goals of high density lipids (HDL) >35 mg/dL and triglycerides (TG) <200
      (1) Start American Heart Association Step II Diet in all patients: <7% of calories from saturated fat, ≤30% of calories from total fat, and <200 mg/d cholesterol; many experts recommend that ≤22% of calories should be from total fat
      (2) See table below for recommended drug therapy (also see section on DYSLIPIDEMIA)

RECOMMENDED DRUG THERAPY - LIPID MANAGEMENT*

LDL <100 mg/dL	LDL 100 to 130 mg/dL	LDL >130 mg/dL	HDL <35 mg/dL
No drug therapy	Consider adding drug therapy to diet, as follows:	Add drug therapy to diet, as follows:	Emphasize weight management and physical activity. Advise smoking cessation. Stress management and soy products in diet may be beneficial. If needed to achieve LDL goals, consider niacin, statin, fibrate.
	Suggested drug therapy		
	TG <200 mg/dL	TG 200 to 400 mg/dL	TG >400 mg/dL	
	Statin Resin Niacin	Statin Niacin	Consider combined drug therapy (niacin, fibrate, statin)	
	If LDL goal not achieved, consider combination therapy.		

*LDL = low-density lipoprotein; HDL = high-density lipoprotein; TG = triglycerides

Source: Smith, S.C., Blair, S.N., Criqui, M.H., et al. (1995). Preventing heart attack and death in patients with coronary disease, American Heart Association Medical/Scientific Statement, Consensus Panel Statement. Circulation, 92, 2-4

   c. Encourage regular exercise with the minimum goal of 30 minutes 3-4 times per week of moderate-intensity activity (walking, jogging, cycling, or other aerobic activity) supplemented by an increase in daily lifestyle activities such as walking breaks at work, gardening, household work
   d. Maintenance of ideal body weight: start intensive diet and appropriate physical activity intervention in patients >120% of ideal weight for height, particularly emphasize need for weight loss in patients with hypertension, elevated triglycerides, or elevated glucose levels (see section on OBESITY)

e. Antiplatelet agents/anticoagulation
   (1) Initiate aspirin 80-325 mg/d if not contraindicated
   (2) For post-MI patients not able to take aspirin; prescribe warfarin to reach International Normalized Ratio of 2-3.5
   (3) Recent study found that combination of low-dose warfarin and 75 mg/d of aspirin was more effective than either alone in primary prevention of IHD (further research is needed before this regime can be applied in clinical setting)
   (4) Clopidogrel bisulfate (Plavix) is FDA approved for reduction of atherosclerotic events in patients with recent MI, recent stroke, or established peripheral arterial disease
f. Consider estrogen-replacement therapy in all postmenopausal women; individualize this recommendation based on other health risks (see section on MENOPAUSE for recommended estrogen-replacement therapies)
g. Control blood pressure with goal of ≤140/90 mm Hg (see section on HYPERTENSION)
h. Medications (ACE-inhibitors, beta-blockers) are recommended for patients after an MI (see V.L.)
i. Other preventive therapies are still investigational
   (1) Combination of high dose vitamin E (400 IU/day), beta carotene (10,000-25,000 IU/day), and vitamin C (1,000-1,500 mg/day) is becoming a standard of care in some health care facilities
   (2) Supplementation of folic acid 0.4 mg per day to reduce homocysteine levels and prevent IHD
   (3) For patients with ischemic heart disease and co-morbidities of diabetes or hypertensive, supplemental vitamin C intake is sometimes recommended
   (4) Fish consumption; eating some fish every week
   (5) Progesterones may have a protective effect in IHD by inhibiting smooth muscle cell proliferation
   (6) Antibiotics such as azithromycin were found to prevent infection with *Chlamydia pneumoniae* which accelerated atherosclerosis in rabbits

B. Treatment of **infrequent anginal attacks in the patient with stable angina**
1. Correct treatable conditions such as hypertension, anemia, valvular disease, hyperthyroidism, and heart failure
2. Prescribe nitroglycerin (Nitrostat), 1 tablet (0.3-0.4 mg) sublingually or nitroglycerin spray (nitrolingual) 1-2 sprays onto or under tongue (do not inhale)
   a. Instruct patient to sit down before taking
   b. Tell patient to wait 3 minutes before taking another dose
   c. Instruct patient to call 911 if pain is not relieved after 3 doses or if doses must be taken more often than every 30-60 minutes
   d. Remind patient to keep tablets no longer than 3-4 months after opening the bottle and to keep in same brown bottle from which supplied
   e. Teach patients to not carry nitroglycerin bottle in pockets, especially on hot days (potency will be greatly reduced)
   f. Instruct patient that nitroglycerin is not an analgesic and that repeated use is not harmful or addictive; instruct to take the nitroglycerin at onset of pain
3. Prophylactic sublingual nitroglycerin or lingual aerosol nitroglycerin spray can be prescribed; instruct patient to take tablet or spray, wait 5-10 minutes and then proceed with activity such as exercise or sexual intercourse

C. **When the anginal attacks become more regular and predictable (i.e., every day) in patients with stable, angina pectoris,** nitrates, β-blocking agents or calcium channel blockers can be prescribed on a chronic basis (each of the drug classes will be described in further detail in sections D, E, and F that follow)
1. Initially patients should be prescribed either a β-blocker or a nitrate (β-blockers are becoming the most recommended initial therapy)
2. Increase the dose of initial drug until response is achieved or patient reaches maximum dosages

3. Calcium channel blockers are prescribed to patients whose symptoms persist despite treatment with nitrates and β-blockers and to select patients (see table on ANTIANGINAL DRUGS)

4. If initial therapy fails, either add a second drug (β-blockers and nitrates work well in combination) or substitute a drug; be careful in combining a β-blocker with a negative inotropic calcium channel blocker such as verapamil or diltiazem

5. Selection of which antianginal treatment option depends on specific patient characteristics (see following table)

ANTIANGINAL DRUGS FOR PATIENTS WITH AND WITHOUT CONCOMITANT DISEASE

| | | | Calcium Channel Blockers | | |
Concomitant Disease	Long-acting Nitrate	β-blocker	Dihydropyridine	Diltiazem HCL	Verapamil HCL
None	+++	+++	++	+++	+++
Hypertension	+	+++	+++	+++	+++
Recent MI	+++	+++	Avoid	Avoid	+
Reduced LV function	+++	++	Avoid*	Avoid	Avoid
COPD	+++	Avoid	+++	+++	+++
PVD	+++	+++	+++	+++	+++
Type 1 diabetes	+++	+	+++	+++	+++
Type 2 diabetes	+++	++	+++	+++	+++
Chronic renal disease	+++	+	+++	+++	+++
Sinus bradycardia or AV block	+++	Avoid	+++	Avoid	Avoid

*Amlodipine may be used
+++very effective, ++ moderately effective, + effective
AV, atrioventricular; COPD, chronic obstructive pulmonary disease; LV, left ventricular; MI, myocardial infarction; PVD, peripheral vascular disease

Adapted from Thadani,U. (1997). Management of patients with chronic stable angina at low risk for serious cardiac events. American Journal of Cardiology, 79(12B), 24-30.

D. β-blocking agents decrease heart rate and contractility
1. Advantages: efficacy in angina prophylaxis and cardioprotective effects after a myocardial infarction
2. Disadvantages: may cause serious side effects, cannot be prescribed in certain patients (see table above for ANTIANGINAL DRUGS)
3. Patients who have constant, effort-induced angina or chest pain which develops consistently with walking a certain distance are ideal candidates for β-blockers
4. Prescribe one of the following:
   a. Atenolol (Tenormin): Initially 50 mg once daily, may increase after one week to 100 daily which can be given in one or two divided doses
   b. Nadolol (Corgard): Initially 40 mg daily; increase if needed at 3-7 day intervals with usual maintenance dose of 40-80 mg daily and maximum dose of 240 mg daily

E. Long-acting nitrates are vasodilators and are widely used
1. Advantages: efficacy, multiple delivery routes, reasonably well tolerated, some products are inexpensive
2. Two relative contraindications to long-acting nitrates are a history of migraine or cluster headaches and demonstrated orthostatic hypotension
3. Isosorbide dinitrate (Isordil Titradose) is a good choice for ambulatory patients: start with 5-20 mg every 4-6 hours orally; Maintenance dose is 10-40 mg every 6 hours; allow a daily dose free interval of at least 14 hours; Alternatively, use isosorbide mononitrate (Ismo) 20 mg upon awakening and then 20 mg 7 hours later
4. Nitroglycerin 2% ointment (Nitrobid ointment) may be preferable : Apply using applicator, usually to chest and occlude; initially 1/2 inch every 8 hours, and increase by 1/2 inch with each successive dose if needed; maximum dose is 5 inches every 4 hours
5. Nitroglycerin patch (Transderm-Nitro patch) is convenient but expensive: Initially one 0.2 mg/hr or 0.4 mg/hr patch for 12-14 hrs/day; remove for 10-12 hours/day

6. The absorption of the drug when using both the patch and ointment is dependent on the site used (i.e., epidermal thickness, vascularity and amount of hair); instruct patient to use on upper body and alternate sites
7. Although most patients experience headaches initially, the headaches can usually be relieved with acetaminophen and usually abate after 1-2 weeks

F. Calcium channel blockers which dilate coronary arteries, prevent coronary vasospasm, and produce vasodilation are another option
   1. Advantages: prevent attacks, effectively treat attacks, useful in patients with coronary artery spasm, usually well tolerated, and may have a possible antiatherogenic effect
   2. Disadvantages: nuisance side effects such as constipation and peripheral edema, may have serious side effects; do not have cardioprotective effects after a myocardial infarction
   3. Amlodipine (Norvasc): Initially 5 mg QD; may increase to 10 mg QD; few side effects
   4. Nifedipine (Procardia XL) is the most potent vasodilator of this group of agents: initially 30-60 mg daily in three divided doses (take HS to reduce side effects). Titrate over 7-14 days with a maximum dose of 120 mg/day (use this drug cautiously in patients taking digitalis)
   5. Diltiazem HCl (Cardizem CD): Initially 120-180 mg once daily; titrate at 7-14 day intervals with maximum 480 mg daily (do not prescribe in patients who have an abnormal atrioventricular conducting system)
   6. Verapamil HCl (Calan): Initially 80 mg every 6-8 hours, Increase daily or weekly with maximum daily dose of 480 mg (do not use in patients with left ventricular failure, sinus bradycardia or heart block)

G. Percutaneous transluminal coronary angioplasty (PTCA) and coronary artery bypass surgery are options for patients with stable angina who cannot be controlled with medications

H. **Patients with unstable angina** are usually hospitalized and aggressively treated by cardiologists: Typically, β-blockers, heparin and intravenous nitroglycerin are prescribed; calcium channel blockers are used as second-line drugs

I. Patients who present with signs and symptoms of **acute myocardial infarction** need immediate transport to the hospital
   1. Intravenous thrombolytic therapy reduces mortality substantially if administered within the first 4-6 hours (or longer) after an acute myocardial infarction
   2. While awaiting transport to hospital, patients should be quickly assessed and kept quiet on bedrest
      a. Administer oxygen 2-4 liters by nasal prongs (in certain cases arterial blood gases should be obtained first)
      b. Give aspirin with minimum loading dose of 162-325 mg; if an enteric-coated aspirin is the only preparation available, the tablet should be chewed or crushed
         (1) There are no longer any absolute contraindications to use aspirin except allergy; there are relative contraindications such as those who have risk of hemorrhagic stroke
         (2) Continue aspirin therapy 75-160 mg/d at least for 30 days

J. Patients with acute myocardial infarctions are typically treated by cardiologists
   1. Reperfusion therapy with thrombolytic agents is the standard of care and recommended for all eligible patients within 30-60 minutes of arrival at the emergency department; reperfusion therapy may be beneficial in patients regardless of time of onset (see the following table for criteria for thrombolytic therapy)

ELIGIBILITY/EXCLUSION CRITERIA FOR THROMBOLYTIC THERAPY FOR ACUTE MI

1. **Eligibility Criteria:**

   Clinical

   Chest pain or chest-pain-equivalent syndrome consistent with AMI ≤12 hours from symptom onset with:

   ECG
   - ≥1 mm ST elevation in ≥2 contiguous limb leads
   - ≥2 mm ST elevation in ≥2 contiguous precordial leads
   - ≥ New bundle branch block

   Cardiogenic Shock

   Emergency catheterization and revascularization if possible; consider thrombolysis if catheterization not immediately available

2. **Contraindications:**

   Absolute Contraindications: Require consideration of other reperfusion strategy, such as PTCA or CABG
   - Altered consciousness
   - Active internal bleeding
   - Known spinal cord or cerebral arteriovenous malformation or tumor
   - Recent head trauma
   - Known previous hemorrhagic cerebrovascular accident
   - Intracranial or intraspinal surgery within 2 months
   - Trauma or surgery within 2 weeks, which could result in bleeding into a closed space
   - Persistent blood pressure >200/120 mmHg
   - Known bleeding disorder
   - Pregnancy
   - Suspected aortic dissection
   - Previous allergy to a streptokinase product (but not a contraindication to use of other thrombolytic agents)

   Relative Contraindications:
   - Active peptic ulcer disease
   - History of ischemic or embolic cerebrovascular accident (CVA)
   - Current use of oral anticoagulants
   - Major trauma or surgery >2 weeks, <2 months
   - History of chronic, uncontrolled hypertension (diastolic >100 mmHg), treated or untreated
   - Subclavian or internal jugular venous cannulation

Source: National Heart Attack Alert Program Coordinating Committee 60 Minutes to Treatment Working Group. (1995). Emergency Department: Rapid Identification and Treatment of Patients with Acute Myocardial Infarction. National Institutes of Health Publication No. 95-3278.

    2.   During the acute phase, β-blocker and ACE inhibitor along with aspirin and thrombolytic therapy should be given if there are no contraindications; nitrates may be given to relieve pain

K. **Post myocardial infarction care** is based on the condition of the patient; initial plan is usually done in conjunction with a cardiologist
   1. A thorough patient education program is usually started in the hospital and followed after discharge; program should include nature of disease, cardiac drugs, modification of risk factors, and guidelines for resumption of employment, sexual activities, and physical exertion; patients should be encouraged to join a formalized cardiac rehabilitation program
   2. At 3-6 weeks, a stress test is usually ordered to determine risk stratification including functional capacity, to provide guidelines on when to return to work, and to assess which patients are in the moderate-risk group and need further diagnostic testing with coronary arteriography and possibly CABG or PTCA

L. Prophylaxis with medications is usually prescribed for the postinfarction patients; although still investigational, a recent study found that a combination of a β-blocker and ACE inhibitor was more efficacious than monotherapy
   1. β-blockers reduce the risk of mortality and reinfarction; particularly beneficial in higher-risk patients with electrical or mechanical complications, patients with a prior MI, and patients with compensated heart failure
      a. Prescribe timolol maleate (Blocadren) 10 mg BID with maximum of 30 mg daily or propranolol HCl (Inderal LA) initially 80 mg daily with maximum of 240 mg daily in divided doses

       b.   Increase β-blockers to amount required to produce significant attenuation of heart rate and blood pressure response to exercise without causing significant side effects

       c.   β-blockers should be administered within hours post-MI and therapy should continue for at least 2-3 years

2. Alternatively an angiotensin converting enzyme (ACE) inhibitor may be given; found to reduce mortality risks after acute MI, particularly in patients with anterior MI, those with an ejection fraction <40, and those with prior history of heart failure symptoms; prescribe one of following:

       a.   Captopril (Capoten) 3 days post-MI start with 6.25 mg, gradually increase to 12.5 mg TID, then increase to 25 mg TID

       b.   Enalapril (Vasotec) initially 2.5 daily and gradually increase to maintenance dose of 10 mg BID

       c.   Ramipril (Altace) initially 1.25-2.5 mg BID and increase to usual maintenance of 5 mg BID

       d.   Prescribe for 4-6 weeks; if patient has <40% left ventricular ejection fraction or symptoms of congestive heart failure, ACE inhibitor should be continued for at least 3 years

3. Routine use of calcium channel blockers is not usually recommended; amlodipine (Norvasc) 5-10 mg daily may be beneficial in patients with severe chronic heart failure and an ejection fraction <30%

4. Anticoagulant therapy

       a.   Aspirin therapy is recommended unless allergic (dosage is controversial and may range from 80-325 mg daily)

       b.   Warfarin is recommended for certain patients: low left ventricular ejection fraction, a large anterior MI, a left ventricular clot, or atrial fibrillation; continue warfarin for 3 to 6 months or longer and then restart aspirin therapy

5. Sublingual nitroglycerin should be used as needed; long-acting nitrate therapy may be needed in patients with residual ischemia or significant left ventricular dysfunction

M. Follow Up

1. Frequency of return visits varies depending on the severity of the disease

2. Patients should be encouraged to enroll in a formal or home cardiac rehabilitation program

3. Patients with stable angina should be seen every 2-6 months and have a repeat ECG and stress testing every 1-2 years

4. Patients who have experienced an MI and who are stable, should be seen in 3-6 weeks after hospitalization for an exercise stress test and in 3 months for a repeat ECG

5. Patients with PTCA or CABG should have stress test done in 3-6 months and then every 2 years if normal

6. Patients should be taught the signs and symptoms of unstable angina and be instructed to seek care if they occur

PRESYNCOPE/SYNCOPE

I. Definitions:

   A. Presyncope: Sensation of dizziness, lightheadedness and an impending loss of consciousness

   B. Syncope: Sudden transient loss of consciousness with concurrent loss of postural tone with spontaneous recovery

II. Pathogenesis

    A. Usually due to any mechanism that decreases cerebral blood flow; results in decreased delivery of oxygen and nutrients to brain

    B. Pathophysiologic abnormalities underlying syncope
        1. Reflex-mediated vasomotor instability associated with a decrease in vascular resistance and/or venous return
            a. Conditions are usually benign and include vasovagal episodes, situational syncope, orthostatic hypotension, drugs, carotid sinus disorder, and psychiatric illnesses
            b. Vasovagal episodes or simple faint are most common cause of presyncope/syncope
        2. Cardiac causes associated with decreased cardiac output or obstruction of blood flow within heart or pulmonary circulation
            a. Electrical etiology such as arrhythmias and heart block
            b. Mechanical etiology such as idiopathic hypertrophic subaortic stenosis, valvular diseases, myxoma, myocardial infarction, and aortic dissection
        3. Neurologic causes such as cerebrovascular diseases, subclavian steal syndrome, seizures, and migraines
        4. Metabolic causes such as hypoglycemia, hypoxia, and hyperventilation; these disorders usually lead to somnolence and coma rather than syncope

    C. Most common causes are vasovagal episodes, heart disease and arrhythmias, orthostatic hypotension and seizures

    D. Approximately 48% of all patients who have syncope have an unexplained cause

III. Clinical Presentation of Important Causes of Presyncope/ Syncope; elderly are at the greatest risk for most causes of syncope

    A. Vasovagal syncope or the common faint (psychological activation of the autonomic system which causes an intense vagal drive)
        1. Results in transient decrease in cardiac output
        2. Often precipitated by fear, anxiety, alcohol, a large meal, or prolonged standing
        3. Symptoms occur in the standing or seated position
        4. Typically patient has prodromal symptoms such as nausea, warmth, lightheadedness, weakness, diaphoresis, constriction of visual fields, epigastric discomfort and a sensation of impending faint
        5. At first, patient has increased heart rate, but then becomes bradycardic
        6. In recovery stage the patient may have weakness, lightheadedness, fatigue but no confusion or signs of injury; usually after the episode, the patient remembers the event and does not have loss or bowel and bladder
        7. Occasionally, hypotension and hypoperfusion are so profound that cerebral hypoxia and seizure activity occur, but there is no loss of consciousness

    B. Situational syncope occurs after micturition, defecation, cough, or swallowing and is associated by a sudden loss of consciousness; often occurs in the elderly population.

    C. Orthostatic hypotension is common particularly in the elderly
        1. Reflex vasoconstriction and increase in heart rate fail to occur when the patient stands, leading to inadequate cerebral perfusion
        2. Defined as systolic blood pressure fall of 20 mm Hg or more on standing
        3. Possible etiologic factors
            a. Condition may be idiopathic; often this type occurs after patient has been exposed to a warm environment
            b. Medications such as diuretics and autonomic blocking agents
            c. Blood loss often due to a gastrointestinal bleed
            d. Dehydration

D. Drug-induced syncope is most likely when patients are taking nitrates, vasodilators, β-blockers, anti-Parkinson drugs, antidepressants, analgesics, and central nervous system antidepressants

E. Carotid sinus hypersensitivity
   1. Occurs primarily in elderly patients who have underlying atherosclerotic disease
   2. Condition is associated with pressure on carotid sinus which can occur with tumors and tissue scars in neck

F. Psychological distress often involves circumoral numbness and digital paresthesia
   1. Patients often have a history of generalized anxiety disorder, panic disorder, somatization, or depression
   2. Estimated that up to 20% of patients presenting with syncope have psychiatric illness

G. Typical presentation of syncope due to cardiac disease
   1. Symptoms often worsen on standing and improve with lying down; although patients with arrhythmias may have symptoms when supine
   2. May have generalized weakness, fatigue, and pallor; some patients are asymptomatic
   3. Syncope may be the presenting symptom in older patients with acute myocardial infarction

H. Arrhythmia often present with brief loss of consciousness, lack of prodrome, and palpitations

I. Subclavian steal syndrome
   1. Occlusion of proximal subclavian artery leading to reversal of flow in the adjacent vertebral artery, during arm exercise
   2. Blood flow is redirected from brain and ischemic symptoms develop
   3. Syncope occurs with arm exercise

J. Cerebrovascular disease
   1. Results from hypoperfusion of the vertebrobasilar vascular system
   2. Patients usually have visual, auditory, or vestibular symptoms

K. Seizures may have signs and symptoms of blue face, frothing at mouth, and disorientation after the event which are not common with other types of syncope

IV. Diagnosis/Evaluation (see also section on VERTIGO)

A. History; it is important to determine whether patient has a cardiac disease with a possible poor prognosis or a more benign condition
   1. Ask patient to briefly describe in own words the sensation he/she experiences.
   2. If possible obtain a description of the episode and events preceding the episode from a witness
   3. Differentiate feelings of fainting from vertigo, imbalance, fatigue, weakness, or anxiety; specifically ask the following types of questions:
      a. Is there a sensation of movement or rotation? (vertigo)
      b. Is the sensation similar to when you get out of bed too quickly? (orthostatic hypotension)
      c. Does it feel like you can't keep your balance? (disequilibrium)
   4. Ascertain that patient did not actually loose consciousness which may indicate an emergent problem
   5. Ask about frequency of syncopal or near syncopal episodes, even though frequency does not correlate well with specific causes
   6. Ask about duration of episode; brief duration is more common with vestibular disorders
   7. Inquire about associated symptoms such as hearing loss, heart palpitations, neurological problems
   8. Determine if sensation occurs after exertion and when one arises to sitting or standing position, which suggests cardiac disease
      a. Disequilibrium occurs primarily when one is standing or walking
      b. Benign positional vertigo often occurs with a change of position or when lying down

9. Determine precipitants such as cough with loss of consciousness (post-tussive syncope), emptying of distended bladder (postmicturition syncope), warm, crowded environment (simple faint), or shaving or tight collar (carotid sinus hypersensitivity)
10. Ask about symptoms occurring after episode; disorientation after an event is most common in patients who have seizures
11. Inquire about past medical history including history of cardiac disease or risk factors, trauma, infection, seizures, thyroid disease, metabolic problems, anxiety and medication/drug use

B. Physical Examination
   1. Vital signs should include check for orthostatic hypotension (see following table)

DETERMINING ORTHOSTATIC HYPOTENSION
• Measure in lying position first.
• After patients stands for 2-5 minutes, measure again.
• Normally, systolic pressure falls no more than 10 mm, diastolic pressures rises 2-5 mm, and heart rate increases 5-20 beats (if there is no increase in heart rate, consider a cardiac problem).

   2. Measure blood pressure in both arms; differences in pulse intensity and blood pressure (more than 20 mm Hg) in two arms suggests aortic dissection and subclavian steal syndrome
   3. Perform careful cardiac examination noting forceful left ventricular impulse, murmurs, or arrhythmias
   4. Auscultate neck for carotid bruits
   5. Perform thorough neurological examination.
   6. Dizziness simulation tests such as following:
      a. Valsalva maneuvers
      b. Carotid sinus massages help to determine autonomic impairment; tests should be done cautiously in facilities where cardiac monitoring and emergency equipment are available; if patient has bruits or history of cardiac or cardiovascular disease, massage should be performed by a specialist
   7. Determine if hyperventilation evokes symptomatology by asking patient to breathe rapidly for 1-3 minutes
   8. Other special tests:
      a. Ask patient to flex and extend arm at least 10 times to reproduce symptoms of subclavian steal syndrome
      b. Ask patient to flex and extend neck to reproduce symptoms of vertebrobasilar insufficiency
   9. Complete psychiatric examination is often needed

C. Differential Diagnosis: One way to sort out the many causes of dizziness is to differentiate the sensations the patient experiences into 3 categories:
   1. Presyncope/syncope: feeling of lightheadedness or feeling that one is about to faint
   2. Vertigo: Sensation of abnormal movements of the body or surroundings (see section on VERTIGO)
   3. Disequilibrium or imbalance due to multiple sensory deficits: Sensation of feeling drunk, seasick, or unsteady on one's feet; subtle, enduring symptom that one cannot quite keep balance and might fall
      a. Patient often has frequent falling, near-falling, or bumping into things
      b. Typically, the patient is elderly with peripheral neuropathy from alcohol or diabetes or has a combination of visual, hearing, sensory, and motor impairments

D. Diagnostic Tests; routine laboratory testing is not recommended; instead, laboratory testing should be done based on results of history and physical examination
   1. Electrocardiogram (ECG) should be core of the workup for most patients
   2. Consider pregnancy testing in women of child-bearing age, especially those for whom tilt table or electrophysiologic testing is being considered

3. Tilt-testing may be frightening to the patient and some patients, especially the elderly, may not be able to tolerate
   a. Upright tilt testing at 60 degrees for 45 minutes is ordered in patients in whom cardiac causes of syncope have been excluded who have infrequent syncopal episodes
   b. Tilt-table testing with isoproterenol is recommended for patients with negative results on passive tilt-table test who have a high pretest probability of neurally mediated syncope
4. Order 24-hour Holter monitor or prolonged ambulatory continuous-loop ECG recordings (patient activates a system when a syncopal episode occurs) in following cases
   a. Patients with normal heart who have frequent episodes of syncope
   b. Patients who have heart disease or an abnormal ECG or symptoms suggestive of arrhythmias
5. Echocardiogram is useful for detecting suspected heart disease such as valve dysfunction
6. Exercise stress testing is important in patients experiencing exertional syncope
7. Intracardiac electrophysiologic studies are needed when symptoms are suggestive of cardiac syncope, but no abnormality is uncovered with noninvasive tests
8. Computerized tomography (CT) scan or magnetic resonance imaging (MRI) is warranted if intracranial abnormalities (patient has focal neurologic signs) are suspected
9. Electroencephalogram (EEG) may be indicated to detect seizure disorder
10. Order carotid and transcranial Doppler ultrasonography for patients with bruits and who experience drop attacks (sudden loss of postural tone without a clear-cut loss of consciousness)
11. Lung ventilation-perfusion is reserved for patients with suspected pulmonary embolism
12. Consider other tests such as fasting blood glucose, hematocrit/hemoglobin, electrolytes, toxicology screens, thyroid function tests, and stool for occult blood based on patient symptomatology

V. Plan/Management

A. Admit to hospital the patients with known serious cardiovascular disease or new findings of cardiovascular disease, significant ECG changes, and patients who have chest pain; consider hospitalization for patients with disabling episodes of syncope, patients who have symptoms suggestive of coronary disease or pulmonary embolus, patients who have sudden loss of consciousness with injury, rapid pulses, or exertional syncope, and patients >70 years of age

B. Depending on etiological factors, consultation with a specialist is often needed; surgical procedures are considered for some conditions such as valvular and cerebrovascular diseases

C. Simple faint may resolve rapidly by elevating patient's feet and legs

D. Patients with recurrent, disabling episodes of vasovagal syncope may benefit from the following:
   1. Medications such as β-blockers [Atenolol (Tenormin) 25-50 mg/day] or anticholinergic agents (Transdermal scopolamine, one patch every 2-3 days)
   2. If symptoms are not relieved by first-line drugs, consider the following:
      a. Fludrocortisone acetate (Florinef) 0.1 to maximum of 0.3 mg/day; contraindicated in patients with congestive heart failure
      b. Fluoxetine (Prozac) 10 mg/day
   3. Measures to expand volume such as increased salt intake, custom-fitted counter pressure support garments from ankle to waist
   4. Atrioventricular pacing can be considered in patients with clinically important bradycardia in response to upright tilt testing

E. Orthostatic hypotension
   1. Prevention
      a. Wear elastic stocking
      b. Change positions slowly
      c. Sleep with head of bed elevated

        d.   Exercise legs before standing

        e.   Eat multiple small meals

        f.   Avoid alcohol

        g.   Avoid hot environments and hot showers or baths

    2.   Treatment: medications in V.D. may be prescribed if symptoms are more disabling

F.   Advise patient not to drive automobiles until symptoms are resolved; refer to laws in each state for health care providers' responsibilities in reporting condition

G.   Follow up is variable depending on diagnosis

PERIPHERAL ARTERIAL DISEASE (PAD)

I.   Definition: A disorder of the larger arteries involving the accumulation of fatty streaks, fibrous plaques, and complicated lesions in focal areas of the intima (lining of the arteries) that affects the lower extremities due to decreased blood flow

II.   Pathogenesis

    A.   The major cause of peripheral arterial disease (PAD) is atherosclerosis

    B.   Lesions of atherosclerosis are classified as fatty streaks, fibrous plaques, and complicated lesions

        1.   Fatty streaks (earliest lesions of atherosclerosis) are accumulation of lipid-filled smooth-muscle cells as well as tissue macrophages and fibrous tissue in focal areas of the intima; fatty streaks appear in all children by age 10

        2.   Fibrous plaques are elevated areas of intimal thickening and represent the most characteristic lesion of advancing atherosclerosis; appear in men before women, in the aorta before the coronary arteries

        3.   Complicated lesions are calcified fibrous plaques containing various degrees of necrosis, thrombosis, and ulceration; these are the lesions usually associated with symptoms

    C.   Even though atherosclerosis is a generalized disease developing in most people as part of aging, fatty streaks tend to localize at bends, branches, and bifurcations of the blood vessel

    D.   Patients with claudication have systemic atherosclerosis and are at risk for fatal and nonfatal myocardial infarction and stroke

    E.   Diabetes mellitus, hypertension, dyslipidemia, and use of tobacco are among the factors that predispose to the development of atherosclerosis

        1.   Tobacco use is believed to be the single most important cause of PAD

        2.   The major lipid risk factors for PAD are elevated low-density lipoprotein (LDL) cholesterol and triglyceride levels, and low high-density lipoprotein (HDL) cholesterol

III.   Clinical Presentation

    A.   Atherosclerosis in the coronary and cerebrovascular beds is the leading cause of death in the US in persons over age 65

    B.   PAD primarily affects the large conduit arteries and is a highly prevalent disorder

        1.   Between 5% and 10% of the adult population over the age of 55 in the US is affected

        2.   Most frequently occurs in elderly males

    C.   The development of the disease is a slow process, and formation of collateral vessels compensates for obstruction in the affected vessels

D.   When collateral circulation is adequate, only minimal symptoms are present; as collateral channels become progressively lost, symptoms occur

E.   The earliest manifestation of impaired arterial circulation is usually intermittent claudication, or muscle pain in the leg precipitated by exercise and relieved by rest (while standing)

F.   If the walking distance required to produce the pain varies substantially from day to day or if the patient must sit or lie down for more than a few minutes to obtain relief, a nonvascular cause for the pain (such as spinal stenosis) should be suspected

G.   Patients usually present with unilateral or bilateral disease and describe cramping pain in the calf, hip, thigh, or buttocks when walking a particular distance
1.   Buttock, hip, and thigh pain occurs in patients with aortoiliac disease
2.   Calf pain occurs in persons with femoral-popliteal disease

H.   Limitations in the ability to walk have a very detrimental impact on quality of life since both leisure and work activities are often severely disrupted

I.   Important physical findings are the following
1.   Decreased or absent pulses distal to the obstruction, the presence of bruits over the narrowed artery, and muscle atrophy
2.   Impotence from inability to maintain a stable erection
3.   Atrophic skin with hair loss, brittle nails
4.   Abnormal pallor on elevation of the extremity, rubor on dependency, and delayed capillary refill

J.   Complaints of pain at rest as well as with exercise suggests more advanced ischemia; patient usually reports that pain is relieved by getting out of bed and walking

IV.   Diagnosis/Evaluation

A.   History
1.   Inquire about onset and duration of symptoms
2.   Ask if leg pain occurs with exercise or if it is present with rest
3.   Ask patient how far he/she can walk before developing cramping pain and which muscle groups are involved (calf, thigh, hips, buttock)
4.   In males, ask if impotence is present
5.   Ask patient if dangling legs over the side of the bed or getting up and walking relieves pain (in arterial disease, the response should be "yes")
6.   Ask if hair on toes, lower legs has been lost
7.   Obtain tobacco use history and interest in smoking cessation
8.   Obtain past medical history; ask patient if he/she has been diagnosed with diabetes mellitus, high blood pressure, dyslipidemia
9.   Inquire regarding present medications

B.   Physical Examination
1.   Complete vascular exam should be done including blood pressure, palpation of peripheral pulses, and auscultation for bruits
2.   Observe for presence of hair on toes and anterior tibial areas; note skin texture (poor perfusion results in thin, parchment-like skin)
3.   Check for dependent rubor (a sign of severe ischemia), ischemic lesions (always examine areas between toes), and gangrenous areas

C.   Differential Diagnosis
1.   Diabetic neuropathy
2.   Arterial embolism

D. Diagnostic Tests
1. Obtain Ankle Brachial Index (ABI) to determine degree of arterial occlusive disease
2. Doppler ultrasonography can detect and evaluate blood flow through selected vessels (arteries tested usually include the common femoral, superficial femoral, popliteal, dorsalis pedis, and posterior tibial artery of the involved extremity)
3. Other vascular testing should be done by specialist to whom patient is referred

---

PROCEDURE FOR DETERMINING ANKLE BRACHIAL INDEX (ABI)

✦ Position the patient supine with the extremities at the level of the heart and the knee slightly bent
✦ Place a Doppler probe (transducer) on the long axis of the vessel angled at 45-60° (use posterior tibial artery or dorsalis pedis)
✦ Obtain systolic brachial pressures in both arms
✦ Place blood pressure cuff just above the ankle
✦ To obtain the systolic pressure in the leg, inflate the cuff 20 to 30 mm Hg beyond the last audible Doppler arterial signal and hold the probe at an angle of 45 to 60 degrees over the artery
✦ The systolic pressure is defined as the pressure at which the first audible Doppler signal returns
✦ If measurement needs to be repeated, deflate the cuff for at least one minute before reinflation
✦ To calculate the ABI, divide the ankle systolic pressure by the higher of the two systolic pressures obtained from the brachial arteries in both arms

---

INTERPRETATION OF ABI

ABI	Interpretation
>1	Normal with no evidence of arterial occlusive disease
0.9 - 1.0	Some authorities consider this normal; others consider this indicative of minimal disease
0.5 - <0.9	Significant arterial occlusive disease; patients often have exercise claudication
<0.5	Severe disease; patients often have pain at rest

V. Plan/Management

A. Primary objectives of claudication treatment are to reduce cardiovascular mortality and improve walking ability

B. All patients require aggressive risk-factor modification
1. Effective therapies that can alter risk must include tobacco cessation interventions for patients who use tobacco
    a. Nicotine patch therapy in smokers with cardiovascular disease has been proven to be safe in a number of studies
    b. Use of nicotine replacement therapies has not been shown to accelerate adverse limb events or worsen ischemic symptoms in PAD patients
    c. Bupropion (Zyban) is another pharmacologic option for smoking cessation and is not nicotine-based
    d. See section on TOBACCO USE AND SMOKING CESSATION for details regarding intervention strategies using both pharmacologic therapies and counseling
2. Effective pharmacologic therapies for patients who are candidates include antiplatelet aggregation agents, antihypertensives, and lipid lowering agents

C. Improvement of walking impairment can be achieved in most patients with aggressive use of an exercise rehabilitation program
1. Emphasize to patient that spontaneous improvement in walking ability without intervention of some type does not occur; walking on a regular basis is essential for relief of disability
2. Ideally, all patients with impaired exercise capacity should be referred to an exercise rehabilitation program that involves both treadmill testing and functional status measurement (most often via questionnaire) [The Walking Impairment Questionnaire is used to assess abilities in area of walking, including distances, speed, and stair-climbing-- see Regensteiner et al., 1990, in the reference list for more details]

3. The most effective mode of exercise rehabilitation to treat claudication is treadmill walking exercise in a supervised program
4. Home-based walking programs are much less successful, but may be the only option for some patients
5. Walking programs should include the following components
   a. A five minute warm-up period to increase the heart rate slowly, promote flexibility, and allow for stretching of the large muscle groups used for walking
   b. Initially, the patient should aim to walk for about 5 to 10 minutes before stopping to rest for a few minutes; gradually, the length of time spent in walking should be increased so that the patient is walking for about 35 minutes out of a 50 minute period (35 minutes spent in walking and 15 minutes spent in resting) [**Note**: The warm-up and cool-down periods are not included in the 50 minute period]
   c. Patient should be instructed to continue walking for as long as possible (even though leg pain is experienced) before stopping to rest with the goal of walking more and resting less
   d. A five minute cool-down period should be included at the end of the session to allow the heart rate to return to baseline values and to continue stretching the large muscle groups
   e. The program should last for a lifetime; exercise must be maintained for the benefit to be maintained
6. Patients should be provided frequent feedback and evaluation to encourage continued participation whether they are enrolled in a formal walking rehabilitation program or a home-based program

D. Instruct patient in proper foot care

E. Refer patients with significant arterial occlusive disease to an expert for management with either drug therapies which may relieve or improve claudication in some patients or for surgical revascularization, if indicated

F. Follow Up
1. In patients with minimal disease, frequent follow up may be needed to evaluate response to risk modification strategies
2. In patients with significant arterial occlusive disease, follow up should be with specialist to whom patient was referred

DEEP VENOUS THROMBOSIS

I. Definition: Acute formation of blood clots in the deep venous system of the lower extremities

II. Pathogenesis

A. Etiology of deep venous thrombosis is unknown, but the triad of stasis, injury to the vascular intima, and altered blood coagulability are central to the process

B. Deep venous thrombosis (DVT) appears to occur as blood clots in the tibial veins progress proximally to involve the popliteal, femoral, and even the iliac veins

III. Clinical Presentation

A. Major risk factors for DVT include stroke, cancer, orthopedic surgery, femoral fracture, major surgery of all types, acute myocardial infarction, prolonged bed rest, and childbirth

B. Old age is also a significant risk factor for DVT with the underlying cause probably related to inactivity

C.   Use of oral contraceptives is also associated with DVT, although the current oral contraceptives contain considerably less estrogen than in previous years

D.   Most patients present with pain, tenderness, and swelling of the affected extremity; however, swelling alone may be the only presenting symptom while others are asymptomatic

E.   The incidence of thrombi in the calves is higher than that in the thighs with thrombi in the thighs alone being least common

F.   Pulmonary embolism occurs in almost 40% of patients when the thigh veins are involved; the risk of pulmonary embolism is minimal when only the calf veins are involved

G.   Pulmonary embolism kills quickly, with up to 90% of those affected dying within the first few hours

H.   The prevention of pulmonary embolism is the primary reason why diagnosis and treatment of venous thrombosis is urgent

IV.   Diagnosis/Evaluation

A.   History
1.   Inquire about onset and duration of symptoms (usually pain, tenderness, and swelling of the involved extremity)
2.   Inquire about risk factors for DVT such as recent surgery, previous phlebitis, prolonged inactivity, use of oral contraceptives
3.   Inquire regarding recent injury to the affected leg

B.   Physical Examination
1.   Examine the affected extremity for tenderness on palpation, warmth, and swelling, presence of palpable cord (**Note**: In superficial thrombophlebitis, but not in DVT, thrombosed vein is often palpable)
2.   Palpate femoral, popliteal, post-tibial, and pedal pulses, comparing sides
3.   **Note:** It is virtually impossible to distinguish DVT from other processes on the basis of history and physical examination alone

C.   Differential Diagnosis
1.   Cellulitis
2.   Trauma
3.   Popliteal (Baker's) cyst
4.   Congestive heart failure; renal failure (bilateral edema would be present)

D.   Diagnostic Tests
1.   Should be ordered by the specialist to whom patient is referred
2.   Most commonly ordered tests are venous ultrasonography and impedance plethysmography

V.   Plan/Treatment

A.   DVT requires referral/hospitalization for anticoagulation therapy

B.   Follow Up: By specialist to whom patient was referred

LEG ULCERS

I. Definition: Chronic slow-to-heal lesion of the lower extremity between knee and ankle due to vascular disease

II. Pathogenesis

    A. Many possible causes but most are due to venous disease, arterial insufficiency, or neuropathy, alone or in combination. At least 20 percent of patients with venous ulcers may also have co-existing lower extremity arterial disease

    B. Minor trauma usually occurs at the site of eventual ulcer formation

III. Clinical Presentation of Most Common Types

    A. Chronic venous insufficiency: most common cause of leg ulcers between knee and ankle
        1. May follow a deep venous thrombophlebitis with disruption in the normal superficial-to-deep flow of blood
        2. Patient usually has long history of swelling of the affected leg with minor trauma to the site of ulcer
        3. Arterial circulation to the legs may be normal; varicosities may or may not be present; medial leg just above the medial malleolus is area most often involved
        4. Brown or brown-red hemosiderin pigmentation is often seen in skin surrounding ulcer; eczematous changes may be present
        5. Ulcer is usually superficial with shaggy borders and with exudate covering the base of the ulcer
        6. Patient usually complains of aching discomfort when the leg is dependent with pain relief when the leg is elevated

    B. Arterial insufficiency: the second most common cause of leg ulcers (with venous insufficiency, accounts for the great majority of leg ulcers)
        1. Ulcers usually begin with trauma and thus are located in areas where trauma most likely to occur (pressure sites, bony prominence, toes)
        2. Ulcers are usually quite painful and have a "punched out" defect with a sharply demarcated border
        3. Surrounding skin is likely to have hair loss and be atrophic
        4. Patient usually complains of severe pain exacerbated by elevation or exertion and relieved by dependency and rest

    C. Neuropathic/diabetic ulcers:
        1. Characteristic location is an area of pressure (heels, toes)
        2. Ulcers have appearance similar to those of arterial insufficiency ulcer ("punched out" appearance)
        3. Ulcer is fairly insensitive, although there may be tingling, burning sensation that increases at night and decreases with exercise

D. The following table compares physical findings in leg ulcers:

COMPARISON OF THREE COMMON TYPES OF LEG ULCERS		
	Venous	**Arterial**	**Neuropathic/Diabetic**
Location	Gaiter area of leg*	Pressure sites	Pressure sites
Lesion features	Shallow, partial thickness with irregular borders	Punched-out	Punched-out
Surrounding skin	Hyperpigmented, thickened, with dermatitis	Hair loss, not hyperpigmented	Hair loss, not hyperpigmented
Palpation findings	Non-pitting, tender, tight edema; peripheral pulses may be normal	Peripheral pulses decreased, capillary refill time increased	Altered sensation of touch, vibration, peripheral pulses decreased

*An area between the foot and upper calf, that extends from about 2.5 cm below malleoli to the point at which calf muscles become prominent posteriorly

IV. Diagnosis/Evaluation

A. History
1. Ask about onset, location, duration, and progress of lesion (slow or rapid development)
2. Ask if the ulcer is painful, and if elevating the leg increases or decreases the pain
3. Ask if leg edema is prominent at the end of the day
4. Ask about exercise: Does it make the pain better or worse?
5. Obtain past medical history including medication history; ask about previous surgeries, trauma, history of previous ulcers and prior episodes of DVT
6. Ask about treatments tried (topical antiseptics and topical corticosteroids can impair normal wound healing)
7. Inquire about tobacco use and interest in smoking cessation
8. Ask about lifestyle, employment, and how the wound has affected quality of life

B. Physical Examination
1. Examine leg when patient is standing or dangling leg
2. Evaluate for femoral, popliteal, dorsalis pedis, and posterior tibial pulses; test for light touch and vibratory sensation; check capillary refilling time; observe for dependent rubor
3. Examine the ulcer looking for characteristics of location, size, lesion features (color, drainage, odor), appearance of surrounding skin, and findings on palpation
4. To measure ulcer, place plastic sandwich bag over ulcer, trace with magic marker, discard side of bag that came in contact with ulcer; use tracing for future comparison (area is a better measure of wound size than diameter because it accommodates for irregularity)

C. Differential Diagnosis
1. Neoplasms (e.g., Kaposi's sarcoma, metastatic tumor)
2. Trauma
3. Infection (bacterial, fungal)

D. Diagnostic Tests
1. Culture and sensitivity of wound (**Note:** In the absence of clinical signs of infection, cultures are often misleading indicating colonization instead of true infection. Many authorities recommend wound punch biopsies instead of traditional swab cultures)
2. Consider CBC with sed rate, blood glucose level
3. Doppler studies to assess vascular status
4. Ankle brachial index (ABI) to rule out significant arterial occlusive disease (see PERIPHERAL ARTERIAL DISEASE section for technique of performing ABI)
5. Radiographs of ulcer site whenever osteomyelitis is suspected

V. Plan/Management

A. Patients with arterial ulcers and neuropathic/diabetic ulcers must be referred for expert evaluation and management

B. Guidelines for hospital admission of patients with chronic skin ulcers are contained in the following table; patients should be immediately referred for treatment

CRITERIA FOR HOSPITALIZATION	
◆ Suspected systemic infection	◆ Deep venous thrombosis
◆ Extensive regional infection	◆ Extensive leg edema
◆ Metabolic derangements	◆ Multiple ulcers
◆ Severe anemia/malnutrition	◆ Large (2-3 cm) or deep ulcers
◆ Acute arterial occlusion	◆ Poor social support or neglect

C. Management of small, shallow venous ulcer that meet the following criteria can be accomplished in outpatient setting with compliant patient with good support
1. There is no evidence of infection at the site and the patient is afebrile
2. At least 50% of the ulcer base contains pale pink to beefy red tissue
3. Patient's nutritional status is adequate
4. Edema is minimal
5. None of the conditions identified in the table above are present

D. The following approaches to management are usually effective
1. Wound debridement may need to be accomplished using mechanical, enzymatic, or autolytic methods
2. Would cleansing should be done with saline or water. Avoid soaps
3. Topical dressing selection is based on wound drainage and periwound skin

Minimum drainage	Hydrocolloid dressing
Highly exudative	Calcium alginate
Dry wound base	Hydrogel dressing

    a. If periwound skin is particularly fragile or has dermatitis, a foam dressing or hydrogel is indicated
    b. Avoid emollients or topical antibiotics. They contribute to stasis dermatitis
4. Edema control during wound healing may need to be accomplished via application of compression wraps
    a. Unna boots (zinc oxide-impregnated bandage) and/or flexible cohesive bandages
    b. Fitted compression stockings are generally required for life thereafter
5. Wounds that do not demonstrate improvement after 4-6 weeks of treatment require biopsy for histology and quantitative bacteriology and patient should be referred to a wound care specialist for management

E. Follow Up: Should be weekly until healing is assured

VARICOSE VEINS

I. Definition: Dilated, superficial, tortuous blood vessels that occur in the lower extremities

II. Pathogenesis

A. Either incompetence of the valves or weakness of the venous wall itself causes dilatation of the vein lumen and subsequent valve inadequacy

B. A self-perpetuating cycle ensues of venous reflux leading to further dilation and valve failure

C. Eventually, the superficial veins widen, elongate, and become tortuous

D. Factors that increase intraluminal vein pressure such as pregnancy, obesity, and wearing of constricting garments may also play a role in varicose vein development

III. Clinical Presentation

A. Varicosities most often involve the veins of the greater saphenous system and its tributaries; thus, occurrence is usually in the medial and anterior thigh, calf, and ankle regions

B. The presenting symptoms of varicose veins is variable and often bears little relationship to the severity of the varicosities

C. Occur twice as frequently in women as in men and occurs most often in the 20-40 year age group

D. Typically, patients complain of local aching, a feeling of heaviness, or burning pain in the area of the varicosities that is worse at the end of the day and after prolonged standing

E. Mild edema of the ankles that is worse in summer and at the end of the day may also be present

F. Infrequently, pruritus due to stasis dermatitis may occur in the region of a severe and chronic varix, but this is unusual with uncomplicated varicose veins

G. Ulceration due solely to varicose veins in extremely rare; ulceration almost always implies problems with the deep venous system

H. Large varices may be subject to trauma and bleeding; much more commonly, however, the distended vein will thrombose, leading to superficial phlebitis

I. Subcutaneous varicose veins (Sunburst varices) are not truly varicose veins, but are dilations of subcutaneous venous plexuses that are spider-like in arrangement and appearing purplish in color

IV. Diagnosis/Evaluation

A. History
    1. Inquire about onset, location, and presence of any symptoms such as pain, feeling of heaviness, and edema after standing for several hours
    2. Inquire about what makes condition better or worse
    3. Determine if cosmetic concerns are a high priority

B. Physical Examination
    1. Note the extent and location of the varicosities
    2. Observe for signs of pathology of the deep venous system (thrombophlebitis, stasis changes, ulceration, and swelling)

C. Differential Diagnosis
  1. Arterial insufficiency
  2. Orthopedic problems
  3. Joint problems
  4. Neurologic problems

D. Diagnostic Tests: None indicated with typical presentation of uncomplicated varicose veins

V. Plan/Management

A. All patients can benefit from proper elastic support stockings of medium weight and periodic elevation of the extremity during the day
  1. Stockings can be below the knee, but should be obtained from a surgical company such as Jobst; department and drug store stockings are usually unsatisfactory
  2. Ace wraps are not recommended because they are cumbersome, cosmetically unattractive, and patient compliance is usually poor

B. Obese patients need to be encouraged to lose weight (see section on OBESITY)

C. Prolonged standing should be avoided as much as possible

D. Women should be advised to avoid constricting panty girdles, tight garters or other garments which may constrict superficial venous return at the thigh level

E. Patients may be referred for sclerotherapy, a simple office procedure; several treatments are often necessary

F. Indications for referral for surgery include persistent symptomatic varicose veins after conservative treatment (above) has been tried; patient desire for removal because of cosmetic reasons, or episodes of superficial thrombophlebitis

G. Follow Up: None indicated

REFERENCES

ACCP Consensus Committee on Pulmonary Embolism. (1998). Opinions regarding the diagnosis and management of venous thromboembolic disease. Chest, 113, 499-504.

Albert, C.M. (1998). Fish consumption and risk of sudden cardiac death. JAMA, 279, 23-28.

American College of Cardiology/American Heart Association Task Force on Practice Guidelines (Committee on Evaluation and Management of Heart Failure). (1995). Guidelines for the evaluation and management of heart failure. Journal of American College of Cardiology, 26, 1376-1398.

American College of Emergency Physicians. (1995). Clinical policy for the initial approach to adults presenting with a chief complaint of chest pain, with no history of trauma. Annals of Emergency Medicine, 25, 274-299.

Aronow, W.S. (1997). Treatment of congestive heart failure in older persons. Journal of the American Geriatrics Society, 45, 1252-1258.

Atrial Fibrillation Investigators. (1994). Risk factors for stroke and efficacy of antithrombotic therapy in atrial fibrillation: Analysis of pooled data from five randomized controlled trials. Archives of Internal Medicine, 154, 2254.

Barloon, T.J., Bergus, G.R., & Seabold, J.E. (1997). Diagnostic imaging of lower limb deep venous thrombosis. American Family Physician, 56(3), 791-801.

Benditt, D.G., et al., (1996). Tilt table testing for assessing syncope. Journal of American College of Cardiology, 28, 263-275.

Bowen, J. (January, 1998). Dizziness: A diagnostic puzzle. Hospital Medicine, 39-44.

Brewster, D.C. (1995). Evaluation of arterial insufficiency of the lower extremities. In A.H. Goroll, L. A. May, & A.G. Mulley, Jr. (Eds). Primary care medicine. Philadelphia: Lippincott.

Brown, D.J., & Goodman, J. (1998). A review of vitamins A, C, and E and their relationship to cardiovascular disease. Clinical Excellence for Nurse Practitioners, 2, 10-22.

Brewster, D.C. (1995). Evaluation of peripheral venous disease. In A.H. Goroll, L. A. May, & A.G. Mulley, Jr. (Eds). Primary care medicine. Philadelphia: Lippincott.

Burke, M. (1995). Dizziness in the elderly: Etiology and treatment. Nurse Practitioner, 20,(12), 28-35.

Campbell, R.W.F., Wallentin, L., Verheught, F.W.A., et al. (1998). Management strategies for a better outcome in unstable coronary artery disease. Clinical Cardiology. 21, 314-322.

Cardiac Rehabilitation Guideline Panel. Cardiac rehabilitation. AHCPR Pub. No. 96-0672. Rockville, MD: Agency for Health Care Policy and Research, Public Health Services, US Department of Health and Human Services.

Chrzanowski, D.D. (1998). Managing atrial fibrillation to prevent its major complication: Ischemic stroke. Nurse Practitioner, 23(5), 26-42.

Cohn, J.N. (1998). Preventing congestive heart failure. American Family Physician, 57,1901-1904

Colledge, N.R., et al. (1996). Evaluation of investigations to diagnose the cause of dizziness in elderly people: A community-based controlled study. British Medical Journal, 313, 788-792.

Creager, M.A. (1997). Clinical assessment of the patient with claudication: The role of the vascular laboratory. Vascular Medicine, 2, 231-237.

Driscoll, D., Allen, H.D., Atkins, D.L., Brenner, J., Dunnigan, A., Franklin, W., Gutgesell, P., et al. (1994). Guidelines for evaluation and management of common congenital cardiac problems in infants, children, and adolescents: A statement for healthcare professionals from the Committee on Congenital Cardiac Defects of the Council on Cardiovascular Disease in the Young, American Heart Association. Circulation, 90, 2180-2188.

Dumas, M.A. (1997). Atrial fibrillation in primary care.The American Journal for Nurse Practitioners, 7-10, 36.

Engstrom, J.W., & Aminoff, M.J. (1997). Evaluation and treatment of orthostatic hypotension. American Family Physician, 56, 1378-1384.

Ennis, W.J., & Meneses, P. (1995). Leg ulcers: A practical approach to the leg ulcer patient. Ostomy/Wound Management, 41:7A, 52-62.

Epperly, T.D., & Fogarty, J.P. (1996). Syncope. In M.B. Mengel & L.P. Schwiebert (Eds.). Ambulatory medicine: The primary care of families (2nd ed.). Stamford, CT: Appleton & Lange.

Falanga, V. (1997). Venous ulceration. In Krasner, D., & Kane D. Chronic wound care. Wayne, PA: Health Management Publications.

Fleet, R.P., & Beitman, B.D. (1997). Unexplained chest pain: When is it panic disorder? Clinical Cardiology, 20, 187-194.

Freed, L.A., Eagle, K.A., Mahjoub, ZA., et al. (1997). Gender differences in presentation, management, and cardiac event-free survival in patients with syncope. American Journal of Cardiology, 80, 1183-1187.

Gavras, I., Manolis, A., & Gavras, H. (1997). Drug therapy for hypertension. American Family Physician, 55, 1823-1834.

Gilligan, D.M., Ellenbogen, K.A., & Epstein, A.E. (1996). The management of atrial fibrillation. The American Journal of Medicine, 101, 413-421.

Ginsberg, J.S., Merli, G.J., & Young, M.A. (1998, January). New options for deep vein thrombosis. Patient Care, 91-100.

Goldsmith, S.R., & Dick, C. (1993). Differentiating systolic from diastolic heart failure: Pathophysiologic and therapeutic considerations. The American Journal of Medicine, 95, 645-655.

Golzari, H., Cebul, R.d., & Bahler, R.C. (1996). Atrial fibrillation: Restoration and maintenance of sinus rhythm and indications for anticoagulation therapy. Annals of Internal Medicine, 125, 311-323.

Goroll, A.H., May, L.A., & Mulley, A.G. (1995). Evaluation of chest pain. In A.H. Goroll, L.A. May, & A.G. Mulley (Eds.), Primary care medicine (3rd ed.), Philadelphia: Lippincott.

Gupta, S., & Camm, A.J. (1997). Chronic infection in the etiology of atherosclerosis--the case for Chlamydia pneumoniae. Clinical Cardiology, 20, 829-836.

Gutgesell, H.P., Barst, R.J., Humes, R.A., Franklin, W.H., & Shaddy, R.E. (1997). Common cardiovascular problems in the young: Part I. Murmurs, chest pain, syncope, and irregular ryhthms. American Family Physician, 56, 1825-1830.

Heart Failure Guideline Panel. (1994). Heart failure: Evaluation and care of patients with left-ventricular systolic dysfunction. AHCPR Pub. No. 94-0612. Rockville, MD: Agency for Health Care Policy and Research, Public Health Services, US Department of Health and Human Services.

Hennekens, C.H., Albert, C.M., Godfried, S.L., Gaziano, J.M., & Buring, J.E. (1996). Adjunctive drug therapy of acute myocardial infarction--Evidence from clinical trials. The New England Journal of Medicine, 335, 1660-1667.

Hennekens, C.H., Dyken, M.L., & Fuster, V. (1997). American Heart Association scientific statement. Aspirin as a therapeutic agent in cardiovascular disease. Circulation, 96, 2751-2753.

Hiatt, W.R. (1997). Current and future drug therapies for claudication. Vascular Medicine, 2, 257-262.

Hill, B., & Geraci, S.A. (1998). A diagnostic approach to chest pain based on history and ancillary evaluation. Nurse Practitioner, 23(4), 20-37.

Hirsh, J. & Fuster, V. (1994). Guide to anticoagulant therapy Part 2: Oral anticoagulants. Circulation, 89, 1469-1480.

Hirsch, A.T., Treat-Jacobson, D., Lando, H.A., & Hatsukami, D.K. (1997). The role of tobacco cessation, antiplatelet and lipid-lowering therapies in the treatment of peripheral arterial disease. Vascular Medicine, 2, 252-256.

Hobbs, J. (1996). Chest pain. In M.B. Mengel & L. P. Schwiebert (Eds.), Ambulatory medicine: The primary care of families (2nd ed.), Stamford, Connecticut: Appleton & Lange.

Hoefnagels, W.A.J., Padberg, G.W., Overweg, J., van der Velde, E.A., & Roos, R.A.C. (1997). Transient loss of consciousness: The value of the history for distinguishing seizure from syncope. Journal of Neurology, 238, 39-43.

Holloway, G.A. (1997). Arterial ulcers: Assessment, classification and management. In Krasner, D., & Kane, D. Chronic wound care. Wayne, PA: Health Management Publications.

Homocysteine Lowering Trialists' Collaboration. (1998). Lowering blood homocysteine with folic acid based supplements: Meta-analysis of randomised trials. British Medical Journal, 316, 894-898.

Hupert, N., & Kapoor W. N. (March 15, 1997). Syncope: A systematic search for the cause. Patient Care, 136-152.

Jeppesen, J., et al. (1998). Triglyceride concentration and ischemic heart disease: An eight-year follow-up in the Copenhagen Male Study. Circulation, 97, 1029-1036.

Kaplan, N.M., & Gifford, R.W. (1996). Choice of initial therapy for hypertension. JAMA, 275, 1577-1580.

Kapoor, W.N. (1997). Syncope. In L. Dornbrand, A.J. Hoole, & R.H. Fletcher (Eds.), Manual of clinical problems in adult ambulatory care (3rd ed.). Philadelphia: Lippincott-Raven.

Katz, J.R., Krafft, P., & Fox, K. (1996). Assessing a murmur, saving a life: Current trends in the management of hypertrophic cardiomyopathy. Nurse Practitioner, 21(11), 62-75.

Kearon, C., Julian, J.A., Math, J.M., Newman, T.E., & Ginsberg, J.S. (1998). Noninvasive diagnosis of deep venous thrombosis. Annals of Internal Medicine, 128, 663-677.

Klatsky, A.L., Armstrong, M.A., & Friedman, G.D. (1997). Red wine, white wine, liquor, beer, and risk for coronary artery disease hospitalization. American Journal of Cardiology, 80, 416-420.

Kroenke, D. (August, 1996). Dizziness: A focused 5-minute workup. Consultant, 1715-1721.

Lee, W.S., et al. (1997). Progeserone inhibits arterial smooth muscle cell proliferation. Nature Medicine, 3,1005-1008.

Linzer, M., Yang, E.H., Estes III, N.A.M., Wang, P., Vorperian, V.R., & Kapoor, W.N. (1997). Diagnosing syncope: Part 1: Value of history, physical examination, and electrocardiography. Annals of Internal Medicine, 126, 989-996.

Linzer, M., Yang, E.H., Estes III, N.A.M., Wang, P., Vorperian, V.R., & Kapoor, W.N. (1997). Diagnosing syncope: Part 2: Unexplained syncope. Annals of Internal Medicine, 127, 76-86.

Mayrovitz, H.N., Delgado, M., & Smith, J. (1998). Compression bandaging effects on lower extremity peripheral and sub-bandage skin blood perfusion. Ostomy wound management 44(3), 56-67.

McGuckin, M., Stineman, M.G., Goin, J.E, & Williams, S.V. (1997). Venous leg ulcer guideline. Philadelphia: University of Pennsylvania Press.

Medical Research Council's General Practice Research Framework. (1998). Thrombosis prevention trial: Randomised trial of low-intensity oral anticoagulation with warfarin and low-dose aspirin in the primary prevention of ischaemic heart disease in men at increased risk. Lancet, 351, 233-241.

Michels, K.B., et al., (1998). Prospective study of calcium-channel blocker use, cardiovascular disease, and total mortality among hypertensive women. The Nurses' Health Study. Circulation, 97, 1540-1548.

Muhlestein, J.B., et al. (1998). Infection with Chlamydia pneumoniae accelerates the development of atherosclerosis and treatment with azithromycin prevents it in a rabbit model. Circulation, 97, 633-636.

National Heart Attack Alert Program Coordinating Committee 60 Minutes to Treatment Working Group. (1995). Emergency department: Rapid identification and treatment of patients with acute myocardial infarction. National Institutes of Health Publication No. 95-3278.

National High Blood Pressure Education Program, National Institutes of Health, National Heart, Lung, and Blood Institute. (1997). The Sixth Report of the Joint National Committee on Detection, Evaluation, and Treatment of High Blood Pressure (NIH Publication no. 98-4080). Bethesda, MD: US Government Printing Office.

Ninia, J.G. (1998). New approaches to varicose and telangiectatic leg veins. The Female Patient, 23, 10-15.

Pasceri, V. et al. (1998). Association of virulent Helicobacter pylori strains with ischemic heart disease. Circulation, 97, 1675-1679.

Psaty, B.M., Smith, N.L., Siscovick, D.S., Koepsell, T.D., Weiss, N.S., Heckbert, S.R. Lemaitre, R.N., Wagner, E.H., & Furberg, C.D. (1997). Health outcomes associated with antihypertensive therapies used as first-line agents: A systematic review and meta-analysis. JAMA, 277, 739-745.

Rapaport, E., & Gheorghiade, M. (1996). Pharmacologic therapies after myocardial infarction. American Journal of Medicine, 101(suppl 4A), 4A-61S-4A-69S.

Regensteiner, J.G. (1997). Exercise in the treatment of claudication: Assessment and treatment of functional impairment. Vascular Medicine, 2, 238-242.

Regensteiner, J.G., Steiner, J.F., Panzer, R.J., & Hiatt, W.R. (1990). Evaluation of walking impairment by questionnaire in patients with peripheral arterial disease. Journal of Vascular Medicine Biology, 2, 142-152.

Rich-Edward, J.W., Manson, J.E., Hennekens, C. H., & Buring, J.E. (1995). The primary prevention of coronary heart disease in women. New England Journal of Medicine, 332, 1758-1766.

Ross, B.S., King, J.M., & Fischer, R.G. (February 16, 1998). Therapeutic options for congestive heart failure. Drug Topics, 102-109.

Salonen, J.T., Nyyssonen, K., & Korpela, H. (1992). Association of myocardial infarction with dietary and body iron. Circulation, 86, 803-811.

Sibbald, R.G. (1998). Venous leg ulcers. Ostomy wound management 44(9), 62-64.

Sibbald, R.G. (1998). An approach to leg and foot ulcers: A brief overview. Ostomy wound management 44(9), 28-35.

Sieggreen, M. (1997, March). Limb and life: Principles of leg ulcer management. Advance for Nurse Practitioners, 17-26.

Simpson, R.J. (1997). Atrial fibrillation. In L. Dornbrand, A.J. Hoole, & R.H. Fletcher (Eds.), Manual of clinical problems in adult ambulatory care (3rd ed.). Philadelphia: Lippincott-Raven

Smith, S.C., Blair, S.N., Criqui, M.H., et al. (1995). Preventing heart attack and death in patients with coronary disease, American Heart Association Medical/Scientific Statement, Consensus Panel Statement. Circulation, 92, 2-4.

Solomon, A.J., & Gersh, B.J. (1998). Management of chronic stable angina: Medical therapy, percutaneous transluminal coronary angioplasty, and coronary artery bypass graft surgery. Annals of Internal Medicine, 128, 216-223.

Sorrentino, M.J. (1997). Drug therapy for congestive heart failure: Appropriate choices can prolong life. Postgraduate Medicine, 101, 83-94

Spencer, K.T. & Lang, R.M. (1997). Diastolic heart failure: What primary care physicians need to know. Postgraduate Medicine, 101, 63-78.

Stanton, M.S. (1998). Atrial fibrillation. In R.E. Rakel (Ed.), Conn's current therapy 1998. Philadelphia: Saunders.

Thadani, U. (1997). Management of patients with chronic stable angina at low risk for serious cardiac events. American Journal of Cardiology, 79(12B), 24-30.

Unstable Angina Guideline Panel. (1994). Unstable Angina: Diagnosis and Management. AHCPR Pub. No. 94-0602. Rockville, MD: Agency for Health Care Policy and Research, Public Health Services, US Department of Health and Human Services.

Vantrimpont, P., Rouleau, J.L., Wun, C-C, et al. (1997). Additive beneficial effects of beta-blockers to angiotensin-converting enzyme inhibitors in the Survival and Ventricular Enlargement (SAVE) study. Journal of American College of Cardiology, 29, 229-236

White, W.B. (1996). A chronotherapeutic approach to the management of hypertension. American Journal of Hypertension, 9, 29S-33S.

Whitehall, T.A. (1997). Role of revascularization in the treatment of claudication. Vascular Medicine, 2, 252-256.

Wolfe, P.A., & Singer, D.E. (1997). Preventing stroke in atrial fibrillation. American Family Physician, 56, 2242-2250.

Zalenski, R.J., McCarren, M., Roberts, R., Rydman, R.J., Jovanovic, B., Das, K., Mendez, J., El-Khadra, M., Fraker, L., & McDermott, M. (1997). An evaluation of a chest pain diagnostic protocol to exclude acute cardiac ischemia in the emergency department. Archives of Internal Medicine, 157, 1085-1091.

CHAPTER 12

Gastrointestinal Problems

ACUTE ABDOMINAL PAIN IN ADULTS

I.   Definition: Recent onset of severe abdominal pain

II.   Pathogenesis

    A.   Major mechanisms of abdominal pain include obstruction of a hollow viscus, capsular distention, peritoneal irritation, mucosal ulceration, vascular insufficiency, altered bowel motility, nerve injury, abdominal wall injury, and referral from an extraabdominal site

    B.   Types of abdominal pain can be helpful in determining the cause
        1.   Visceral pain is deep, dull, crampy, poorly localized, and originates from a solid or hollow viscus
        2.   Parietal pain is sharp, well localized, and originates from inflammation of the parietal peritoneum
        3.   Referred pain is pain that is experienced at a distance from the disease process and is explained by the embryologic origins of the structures involved

III. Clinical Presentation

    A.   Location of pain may provide clues to common causes of abdominal pain from both intraabdominal and extraabdominal sources

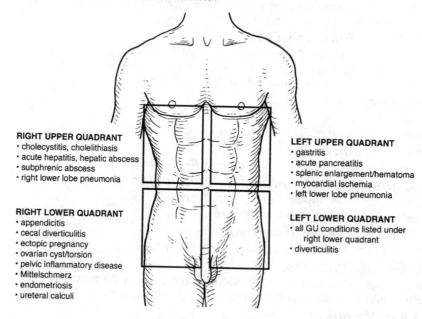

DIFFUSE PAIN or VARIABLE LOCATION
- hemolytic crisis (sickle cell disease)
- gastroenteritis
- peritonitis
- endocrinologic disorders
  (diabetic ketoacidosis, Addison's disease, hyperparathyroidism)
- intestinal obstruction

RIGHT UPPER QUADRANT
- cholecystitis, cholelithiasis
- acute hepatitis, hepatic abscess
- subphrenic abscess
- right lower lobe pneumonia

LEFT UPPER QUADRANT
- gastritis
- acute pancreatitis
- splenic enlargement/hematoma
- myocardial ischemia
- left lower lobe pneumonia

RIGHT LOWER QUADRANT
- appendicitis
- cecal diverticulitis
- ectopic pregnancy
- ovarian cyst/torsion
- pelvic inflammatory disease
- Mittelschmerz
- endometriosis
- ureteral calculi

LEFT LOWER QUADRANT
- all GU conditions listed under right lower quadrant
- diverticulitis

EPIGASTRIC or MIDLINE
- abdominal aortic aneurysm
  (may also present as back, flank, or hip pain, or as diffuse pain)
- cardiac disease (may be confused with pain from reflux disease)
- peptic ulcer (gastric or duodenal)

Figure 12.1. Location of Pain: Clues to Diagnosis.

B. Obstruction may occur in the bowel, biliary tree, and ureters with the severity of the pain dependent on both the speed of onset and the degree of distention
    1. Pain due to an acute obstruction is usually colicky and wavelike in nature; patients are restless, frequently shifting positions, and lack peritoneal signs
    2. Obstruction of the small bowel is greatest when the obstruction is jejunal and the patient may be comfortable between bouts of pain; obstruction of the large bowel may result in constipation; large bowel obstruction is generally less painful and distention is usually greater than is seen with small bowel obstruction
    3. Obstruction of the cystic duct by a stone produces acute pain, which is fairly steady and unremitting; in acute cholecystitis, the pain is typically in the right upper quadrant or epigastrium, radiating to the scapular region, and associated with nausea and vomiting (see CHOLECYSTITIS)
    4. Obstruction within the urinary tract can present as abdominal pain; the pain usually begins in the back and flank and radiates into the lower abdomen and groin; hematuria is frequently present

C. Peritoneal irritation can cause severe pain due to the rich innervation of the parietal peritoneum; suggests that a condition requiring surgical intervention is present
    1. An inflamed appendix is a common cause of peritoneal pain
    2. With peritoneal irritation, rebound tenderness is prominent on physical examination because pain is accentuated by pressure changes in the peritoneum

D. Vascular disorders such as acute arterial insufficiency or dissection or rupture of an abdominal aortic aneurysm may present with severe abdominal pain; with an abdominal aneurysm, a pulsating mass may be palpated in the epigastrium

E. Mucosal ulceration or inflammation of the gastrointestinal tract is usually accompanied by pain; with duodenal ulcer disease, the pain is usually burning or aching and is not usually severe unless there is perforation or penetration into the pancreas
    1. Gastroenteritis which produces inflammation of the mid or lower intestine can disturb motility and absorption
    2. Fever, nausea, vomiting and diarrhea are often associated with gastroenteritis and bowel sounds are frequently hyperactive

F. Altered bowel motility predominates in functional bowel disorders such as irritable bowel syndrome most often causing chronic, rather than acute abdominal pain

G. Capsular distention of the well-innervated capsule surrounding organs such as the liver causes a constant, aching abdominal pain; pain due to splenic capsular distention as may occur with blunt trauma is located in the left upper quadrant and with subdiaphragmatic peritoneal irritation, pain may radiate to the ipsilateral shoulder

H. Nerve injury from irritation such as occurs with herpes zoster, an extraabdominal source, produces pain via irritation of the nerve root that supplies an abdominal dermatome

I. Traumatic injury to the abdominal muscle wall can produce pain that is constant, aching, and made worse with movement or pressure on the abdomen

J. Referral of pain from an extraabdominal source such as the chest, particularly with conditions such as lower lobe pneumonia, may present as abdominal pain; an acute inferior myocardial infarction may present as upper abdominal pain, with nausea and vomiting

K. Lower abdominal pain may occur in women with sexually transmitted diseases, ectopic pregnancies, disorders of the ovaries, or other pelvic pathology; depending on the cause of the pain, patient may also experience vaginal discharge, bleeding, or irregular menses

IV. Diagnosis/Evaluation: Determine if patient has an emergent problem BEFORE proceeding with the complete evaluation (Patient should be examined promptly for evidence of obstruction, peritoneal irritation, vascular compromise, or cardiopulmonary disease)

    A.   History
1. Determine onset, location, and quality of pain
2. Ask patient to rate pain on scale of 1 to 10; ask if pain interferes with sleep
3. Ask if pain has changed since onset (progression of pain)
4. Determine if pain is referred to or radiates to other sites
5. Ask about aggravating and relieving factors
6. Ask about associated symptoms of vomiting, diarrhea, constipation or urogenital symptoms (see Clinical Presentation on previous page for clues to possible causes). Ask regarding associated fever or chills
7. In women, obtain a gynecologic history including dates of last two normal menstrual periods, type of contraception used, whether sexually active, condom use, and timing of last intercourse
8. Obtain past medical history, surgical history, and medication history
9. Obtain social history including alcohol and tobacco use

    B.   Physical Examination
1. Determine if patient is febrile; assess for orthostatic hypotension
2. Observe general appearance for pallor, perspiration, restlessness, signs of peritonitis, toxicity
3. Perform a complete exam focusing on possible extraabdominal sources of the abdominal pain
4. To examine the abdomen, position patient with hips flexed; observe for surgical scars and distension; auscultate for bowel sounds; palpate abdomen, beginning in non-painful region
    a. Determine areas of localized tenderness, masses, liver and spleen size
    b. Assess for rigid abdomen, guarding, rebound tenderness, presence of abdominal bruits, CVA tenderness (see following table ASSESSING FOR REBOUND TENDERNESS)
    c. Assess for positive Murphy's sign (pain and "inspiratory arrest" when patient takes a deep breath while examiner applies pressure in area of gallbladder, a sign that suggests cholecystitis)
    d. Assess for positive obturator and psoas signs (see techniques in Figures 12.2 and 12.3)
    e. Assess for hernias
5. Percuss the liver span and assess for fluid wave (**Note:** Percussion tenderness is a very sensitive sign of peritoneal irritation)
6. Percuss the back for costovertebral angle tenderness
7. Perform pelvic exam on women to evaluate cervix, assess for cervical motion tenderness (CMT), adnexal tenderness or abnormal masses
8. Perform digital rectal exam to assess for occult bleeding, to obtain stool for occult blood to evaluate for fecal impaction, prostate enlargement, tenderness and hemorrhoids

ASSESSING FOR REBOUND TENDERNESS
After thorough exam of the abdomen, evaluate for peritoneal irritation as follows
✦ Using the flat of your hand, press on the area identified by the patient as most painful
✦ Press sufficiently to depress the peritoneum. The patient will experience pain with this maneuver
✦ Keep pressing with a constant pressure and, as the patient adjusts to the constant pressure over a 30 to 60 second period, the pain lessens in intensity and may even subside
✦ Then, without warning, remove your hand suddenly to just above skin level
✦ Observation of the patient's face may be the best index of a complaint of pain and peritoneal irritation

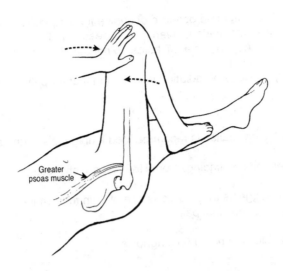

Figure 12.2. Psoas Sign.

With the patient in the supine position, instruct him/her to lift the right thigh against the resistance of the examiner's hand which is placed just above the patient's knee. Increased pain with the maneuver is a positive test, indicating irritation of the psoas by an inflamed appendix

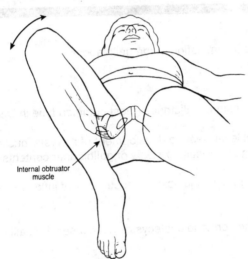

Figure 12.3. Obturator Sign.

Passively flex the right hip and knee and internally rotate the leg at the hip, stretching the obturator muscle. Right-sided abdominal pain is a positive sign, indicating irritation of the obturator muscle by an inflamed appendix

    C.   Differential Diagnosis
        1.   Many causes of acute abdominal pain
        2.   Need to rule out all emergent conditions

    D.   Diagnostic Tests
        1.   CBC, differential, and platelet count (an elevated WBC [>12,000 μL] suggests inflammation or infection)
        2.   Amylase, lipase if pancreatitis is suspected
        3.   Liver enzymes if hepatic or biliary disease is suspected
        4.   Urinalysis for both men and women, and urine HCG for women of childbearing age
        5.   Consider obtaining DNA probe for gonorrhea and chlamydia, based on patient history
        6.   Other laboratory tests may be ordered based on history and physical examination
        7.   Abdominal ultrasound or computed tomography
            a.   If conditions such as ovarian torsion, ectopic pregnancy, or pelvic abscess are suspected, transvaginal ultrasonography is more sensitive than transabdominal

b. CT scan is the procedure of choice for diagnosing such conditions as appendicitis, abscess formation, diverticular disease, and enlargement of the pancreas
    (1) Appendiceal CT takes 15 minutes to perform and results are available in one hour
    (2) Dose of radiation is less than that for pelvic CT

V. Plan/Management

    A. Consultation with a specialist is recommended if diagnosis is unclear and the patient is unstable

    B. Management depends on findings from H&P, diagnostic tests, and specialist recommendations

    C. Recent research suggests that judicious use of pain medication may enable a more accurate evaluation of acute abdominal pain

    D. Follow up is variable depending on diagnosis

CHOLECYSTITIS

I. Definition: Acute or chronic inflammation of the gallbladder

II. Pathogenesis

    A. Pathogenesis of cholesterol gallstones (most common type in US) is multifactorial

    B. High bile cholesterol levels lead to development of a crystal nucleus, stone growth, delayed gallbladder emptying with resultant stasis of gallbladder contents

    C. Symptoms develop from mechanical obstruction, local inflammation, or a combination of these factors

    D. Pain occurs when the hormone cholecystokinin causes the gallbladder to contract against an obstructing stone

III. Clinical Presentation

    A. Gallstones are more common in obese persons and in women

    B. Gallstones frequently develop during pregnancy but usually do not become symptomatic until after delivery

    C. Pain is usually colicky, located in the right upper quadrant with radiation to the flanks and occasionally the right shoulder

    D. Pain of classic acute cholecystitis occurs within one hour after eating a large meal, lasts for several hours, and is followed by a residual aching that can last for days

    E. May be associated with anorexia, nausea, and fever, and less often with vomiting

    F. Most patients report a prior episode

    G. Symptoms may be minimal in the elderly

IV. Diagnosis/Evaluation

    A. History
        1. Question about onset, duration, location, radiation of pain; and if pain is severe and persistent
        2. Ask about presence of associated symptoms and provocative and palliative factors; specifically ask if pain is precipitated by heavy meal and aggravated by deep inspiration
        3. Question regarding prior episodes of similar symptoms
        4. If female, ask if pregnant during past year
        5. Obtain past surgical and medical history
        6. Obtain medication history

    B. Physical Examination
        1. Determine if febrile
        2. Examine abdomen for right upper quadrant abdominal tenderness and involuntary guarding, indicative of early peritoneal inflammation
        3. Check for Murphy's sign (increased pain and tenderness on inspiration during palpation of right upper quadrant)
        4. An enlarged gallbladder may be palpable in right upper quadrant

    C. Differential Diagnosis
        1. Peptic ulcer disease
        2. Pancreatitis
        3. Irritable bowel syndrome
        4. Appendicitis

    D. Diagnostic Tests
        1. Obtain CBC with differential and chemistry profile to determine if liver chemistries are elevated
        2. Order right upper quadrant ultrasound to confirm the presence of gallstones
            (Note: Test has a sensitivity >95% in detecting stones in the gallbladder)

V. Plan/Management: Consultation with a specialist is indicated for evaluation, possible hospitalization

CONSTIPATION

I. Definition: Diminished frequency of defecation, incomplete evacuation, or stools that are too hard or too small

II. Pathogenesis

    A. Fecal continence is defined as the ability to control defecation voluntarily and requires normal contractions of the anal sphincters, normal sensory receptors in the rectum and anus to identify the rectal contents as liquid, solid, or gaseous, and a normal rectal reservoir

    B. Movement of a fecal bolus into the rectum stimulates several automatic, coordinated reflexes
        1. The lower colon, including the rectum, contracts and the internal sphincter relaxes
        2. The external sphincter initially contracts, but the initial contraction is followed by a total inhibition of both the external and internal sphincters
        3. Intraabdominal pressure is voluntarily increased (Valsalva maneuver), the pelvic floor descends and stool is expelled

    C. Defecation can be delayed until it is convenient
        1. Retention of stool over prolonged periods of time can result in a stretching of the rectal wall and the subsequent development of megarectum
        2. When the whole colon is dilated and full of stool, the condition is referred to as megacolon

D. Common causes of constipation are the following
1. Ignoring urge to defecate
2. Inadequate ingestion of fluids and fiber in diet
3. Sedentary lifestyle
4. Medications
5. Metabolic and endocrine disorders
6. Neurologic diseases
7. Colonic and anorectal disorders

E. Constipation is **most commonly functional** with no underlying pathology

III. Clinical Presentation

A. Constipation accounts for 2.5 million health care visits per year

B. The most common cause of chronic constipation in adults is failure to initiate defecation

C. In elderly patients, chronic disease, medications, decreased mobility, poor dietary habits, and decreased fluid intake contribute to development of constipation
1. Constipation affects as many as 26% of men and 34% of women ≥65 years of age
2. Estimates are that up to 75% of residents in nursing homes use laxatives for bowel regulation

D. Despite the high incidence of constipation, only a small minority of adults with constipation have a significant abnormality

E. Abdominal pain, pain with defecation, blood in stools, diarrhea alternating with hard stools, weight loss, and depression may be associated with constipation

IV. Diagnosis/Evaluation

A. History
1. Determine what the patient means by constipation (Is it small stools, infrequent stools, a feeling of fullness, or difficulty/pain with passing stools?)
2. Assess stooling pattern, dietary intake, and activity level
3. Determine if any recent changes in pattern (acute or chronic process)
4. Inquire about current medications and laxative use
5. Obtain past medical and surgical history; determine if there is a family history of colon cancer

B. Physical Examination
1. Determine if there is a weight loss
2. Assess abdomen for tenderness, masses
3. Rectal exam for anal fissures, hemorrhoids, or irritation; obtain stool for guaiac
4. Check for fecal impaction, especially in elderly patients with a history of chronic constipation

C. Differential Diagnosis
1. Partial bowel obstruction (tumor)
2. Irritable bowel syndrome
3. Rectal fissures
4. Hypothyroidism

D. Diagnostic Tests: Stool for occult blood x 6 and other appropriate tests if underlying causes (metabolic/endocrine/gastrointestinal tract disorder) suspected

V. Plan/Management

    A. Retrain in proper bowel habits
        1. Never ignore urge to defecate, even though it may not be convenient
        2. Allow adequate time for bowel movements; learn to sit on toilet and relax
        3. Capitalize on the gastrocolic reflex by establishing a routine for bowel movements that coincides with after having eaten a meal such as breakfast

    B. Increase daily fluid intake (1.5-2.0 liters per day)

    C. Increase dietary fiber with bran cereal, raw fruits and vegetables, whole wheat breads, oats, barley

    D. Skip orange juice in the morning and eat a whole orange instead

    E. Choose cereals with 5 or more grams of fiber per serving

    F. Increase activity level using easy, no-cost approaches such as parking as far away from the store as possible; using the restroom at work that is on another floor; walking to do errands that are just a few blocks away

    G. Continue these measures for at least one month before effects on bowel function are determined

HOW MUCH FIBER DO ADULTS NEED?

Adults need about 20-35 grams of fiber in their diet each day

Increase fiber intake gradually over a 2 week period to reduce abdominal discomfort sometimes associated with high fiber intake!

There is no Recommended Dietary Allowance (RDA) for daily intake of fiber, but most experts agree that the above intake of fiber is appropriate

FIBER CONTENT OF SELECTED FOODS

Fruits

Food	Amount	Fiber (grams)	Food	Amount	Fiber (grams)
apple (with skin)	1 medium	3	orange	1 medium	3
banana	1 medium	2	orange juice	3/4 cup	<1
blueberries	1/2 cup	2	pear (with skin)	1 medium	4
grapes	1/2 cup	1	strawberries	1 cup	4

Vegetables, raw

Food	Amount	Fiber (grams)	Food	Amount	Fiber (grams)
carrots	1 medium	2	lettuce, romaine	1 cup	1
celery	1 stalk	<1	tomato	1 medium	2

Vegetables, cooked

Food	Amount	Fiber (grams)	Food	Amount	Fiber (grams)
broccoli	1/2 cup	2	spinach	1/2 cup	2
potato, baked (with skin)	1 medium	4	zucchini	1/2 cup	1

Legumes, cooked

Food	Amount	Fiber (grams)	Food	Amount	Fiber (grams)
baked beans	1/2 cup	3	kidney beans	1/2 cup	3

(continued)

FIBER CONTENT OF SELECTED FOODS (CONTINUED)

Breads, grains, and pasta

Food	Amount	Fiber (grams)	Food	Amount	Fiber (grams)
bagel	1 medium	1	white bread	1 slice	<1
brown rice (cooked)	1/2 c	2	whole wheat bread	1 slice	2
wheat germ	1 tablespoon	1			

Breakfast Cereals

Food	Amount	Fiber (grams)	Food	Amount	Fiber (grams)
bran flakes	3/4 cup	5	oatmeal, cooked	3/4 cup	3
cornflakes	3/4 cup	1	raisin bran	3/4 cup	5

Snack Foods

Food	Amount	Fiber (grams)	Food	Amount	Fiber (grams)
peanuts, dry roasted	1/4 cup	3	popcorn, air popped	1 cup	1

H.   Adults over 50 with constipation representing a change from a usual pattern and for all ages who are unresponsive to general measures (above) OR all ages with positive fecal occult blood test or weight loss need referral to a specialist for evaluation

I.   If general measures fail, may try the following alternatives:
1.   Bulk-forming agents: Psyllium (Effersyllium), methylcellulose (Citrucel), and polycarbophil (Fibercon)
   a.   Start with 1 tbsp daily and increase to 3 tbsp
   b.   Must drink plenty of fluids for product to work (**Note:** 16 oz water with each dose)
   c.   Must be used on regular basis, can be used long term
2.   Stool softeners: Docusate sodium (Colace) and docusate calcium (Doxidan)
   a.   Can be used for short-term constipation only (few days to 2 weeks)
   b.   Do not use in chronic constipation
3.   Osmotic agents: Nonabsorbable sugar lactulose (Cephulac) available as 10 g/15 mL syrup
   a.   Adults: 15-30 mL/day
   b.   Not recommended as a first-line treatment because it is expensive, but it is particularly useful in elderly patients and is the agent of choice in patients with hepatic failure
4.   Agents such as milk of magnesia can be used occasionally (every 2-3 weeks) to treat constipation in otherwise healthy adults

J.   Follow Up: Unnecessary unless there is failure to improve which may indicate serious underlying cause and need for referral

DIARRHEA

I.   Definition: A change in bowel habits characterized by increased stool volume, looseness, and frequency

II.   Pathogenesis

    A.   Pathophysiology of diarrhea involves one or a combination of three basic mechanisms
        1.   Increased fluid secretion
        2.   Decreased water absorption
        3.   Abnormal intestinal motility

    B.   Diarrhea that is produced via increased fluid secretion can be caused by inflammation (such as occurs with viral and bacterial infections) and enterotoxins (such as are produced with *Staphylococcus aureus* infection)

    C.   Damage to the bowel mucosa (such as occurs with some infectious agents or inflammatory conditions such as inflammatory bowel disease and sprue [sprue is a malabsorption syndrome that causes inflammation of the bowel mucosa]) or the presence of poorly absorbable, osmotically active substances in the lumen (such as lactose in a lactase deficient patient) cause diarrhea via the mechanism of decreased reabsorption of fluid

    D.   Abnormal intestinal motility (such as occurs in irritable bowel syndrome and with the ingestion of such medications as erythromycin) can decrease contact time with the bowel mucosa, limiting reabsorption of fluids, and producing diarrhea

III.   Clinical Presentation

    A.   Most diarrheal illness is acute, lasts only a day or two and resolves spontaneously

    B.   By far the most common cause of **acute diarrhea** in adults is infection of the gastrointestinal tract by a variety of pathogens with viral etiologies being most common

    C.   Distinguishing features of commonly occurring infectious causes of acute diarrhea are summarized in the table that follows

COMMONLY OCCURRING INFECTIOUS CAUSES OF ACUTE DIARRHEA: DISTINGUISHING FEATURES

Infectious Agent	Mode of Transmission	Incubation Period	Associated Signs and Symptoms	Characteristics of Stool	Laboratory Examination of Stool	Important to Remember
Viral Rotaviruses and Norwalk virus	Fecal-oral; fomites may have a role	24-72 hours	Nausea, vomiting, abdominal cramps Fever	Watery No occult or gross blood	No WBCs in stool	By far the most common cause of acute diarrhea in both children and adults In children, rotavirus infection is more common; in adults Norwalk virus is more common Vomiting most prominent symptom in children; diarrhea most prominent in adults
Bacterial *Staphylococcus aureus*	Ingestion of food containing a preformed toxin produced by enterotoxicogenic staphylococci Food products most commonly involved are ham, poultry, filled pastries, egg/potato salads Contamination is via food handlers Not transmissible from person-to-person	Very short--30 minutes to 6 hours	Nausea, vomiting, abdominal cramps Fever is uncommon	Soft, but not watery No occult or gross blood	No WBCs in stool	Onset is abrupt Look for a common source pattern
Clostridium perfringens	Ingestion of food contaminated by the organism Once ingested, an enterotoxin is produced in the lower intestine of the host, producing symptoms Beef, poultry, Mexican-style foods are common sources Not transmissable from person-to-person	8-12 hours	Nausea, vomiting, moderate-to-severe mid-epigastric pain Fever is uncommon	Watery No occult or gross blood	No WBCs in stool	Onset is not as abrupt as in staphylococcal food poisoning because enterotoxin is not preformed, but is produced in host's intestine Look for a common source pattern Look for recent ingestion of foods served from steam tables
Campylobacter jejuni	Ingestion of contaminated food, including unpasteurized milk and untreated water OR by direct contact with fecal material from infected persons/animals Main vehicles of transmission: Improperly cooked poultry, untreated water, unpasteurized milk Person-to-person spread is not common	1-7 days	Nausea, vomiting, abdominal pain, malaise Fever	Watery Occult and gross blood	WBCs in stool Positive culture	Abdominal pain can mimic that produced by appendicitis Mild infection lasts 1-2 days with most patients recovering in <7 days Outbreaks in child care centers are uncommon

(continued)

424

COMMONLY OCCURRING INFECTIOUS CAUSES OF ACUTE DIARRHEA: DISTINGUISHING FEATURES--CONTINUED

Infectious Agent	Mode of Transmission	Incubation Period	Associated Signs and Symptoms	Characteristics of Stool	Laboratory Examination of Stool	Important to Remember
Salmonella	Major modes: Ingestion of food of animal origin, including poultry, red meat, eggs, and unpasteurized milk Other modes: Ingestion of contaminated water, contact with infected animals such as pet turtles/reptiles Direct person-to-person transmission (fecal-oral) are less common than other modes	6-72 hours; usually <24 hours	Nausea, vomiting, abdominal cramping Fever	Watery Occult and gross blood	WBCs in stool Positive culture	Most likely to occur in children <5 (peaks in first year of life) and adults >70 Outbreaks of this infection are rare in day care centers Report all confirmed cases to local public health department
Shigella	Ingestion of contaminated food or water and homosexual transmission most common routes in adults Fecal-oral transmission is most common route in children Feces of infected humans are source of infection No animal reservoir known	1-7 days; usually 2-4 days	Abdominal pain Fever	Watery Occult blood No gross blood	WBCs in stool Positive culture	Most common in children 1-4 years of age Important problem in child care centers in US Report all confirmed cases to the local health department
Escherichia coli (enterotoxigenic) [ETEC]	One of at least 5 different groups of diarrhea-producing strains of *E. coli* Most commonly from food or water contaminated with human or animal feces Most common cause of "travelers' diarrhea," acquired by travelers to developing countries	10 hours to 6 days	Abdominal cramps Usually no fever	Watery No occult or gross blood	No WBCs (usually); can be present Positive culture	The enterotoxin that is produced by the organism promotes fluid secretion in the small bowel which results in a watery diarrhea History of recent travel to a developing country is important epidemiologic information
Protozoal *Giardia*	Main route of spread is fecal-oral transfer of cysts from feces of an infected person Many common source outbreaks are traced to contaminated drinking water Humans are principle reservoir but organism can infect animals such as dogs, cats, beavers	1-4 weeks	Abdominal pain associated with flatulence, distention, and anorexia Passage of foul-smelling stools No fever	Soft, watery No occult or gross blood	Positive stool for O & P (see IV.D.3 DIAGNOSTIC TESTS)	Most often represents an acute presentation of chronic or recurrent diarrhea

D. Drugs such as laxatives, antibiotics, caffeine, magnesium containing antacids and alcohol also cause diarrhea

E. Chronic diarrhea (lasting at least 2 weeks or frequent recurrences after initial attack) also often presents in primary care settings

F. Some of the more common causes of chronic diarrhea along with their associated signs and symptoms are listed here:
1. Irritable bowel syndrome: recurrent abdominal pain, diarrhea alternates with constipation; the most common of the motility disorders causing chronic diarrhea (see IRRITABLE BOWEL SYNDROME section for a discussion of this condition)
2. Inflammatory bowel diseases: destruction of the bowel wall compromises absorption of electrolytes; characterized by bloody stools, abdominal pain, fever, and extraintestinal manifestations involving skin, joints, liver, and heart
3. Malabsorption of fat or carbohydrate
    a. With fat malabsorption, there are foul, bulky, greasy stools and the signs and symptoms are those associated with the resultant caloric and vitamin deficiencies (weight loss, ecchymosis, glossitis, peripheral neuropathy)
    b. With carbohydrate malabsorption, patients report bloating, abdominal cramps and diarrhea after intake of dairy produces
4. Chronic laxative abuse can also cause diarrhea; occurs often in patients with bulimia

IV. Diagnosis/Evaluation

A. History
1. Determine if acute or chronic process; recent relatively sudden onset of non-bloody diarrhea in otherwise healthy persons is usually due to infectious causes and likely to be self-limited
2. Question regarding stool volume, frequency, and consistency; ask if stool contains blood, mucus
3. Ask about the presence of associated signs and symptoms including abdominal pain, vomiting, fever, malaise
4. Ask about intake of fluids and urine output
5. Obtain past medical history and medication history
6. Question regarding similar illness in others. Viral etiology likely when secondary cases develop in household suggesting person-to-person spread rather than one-time exposure to a common food or drink
7. Ask appropriate questions to identify if patient is at risk of being HIV positive

B. Physical Examination
1. Determine if patient is febrile and assess cardiovascular status (pulse, blood pressure; check for postural changes, a reflection of significant volume depletion)
2. Weigh patient and determine if there has been a weight loss (more of an issue in the elderly and in chronic diarrhea)
3. Examine abdomen for tenderness, rigidity, abnormal tympany, bowel sounds, liver/spleen enlargement
4. Perform rectal exam for tenderness, masses; obtain stool for occult blood

C. Differential Diagnosis: Diarrhea is a symptom. Refer to common causes of acute and chronic diarrhea under section III. above

D. Diagnostic Tests
1. If no systemic signs and symptoms and duration 24-48 hours, no lab studies indicated
2. Obtain stool culture if any of the following are present:
    a. Fever over 24 hours
    b. Diarrhea persistent over several days with no improvement
    c. Family or close population outbreak
    d. Stool positive for blood (either occult or gross)
    e. Gram's stain of stool positive for WBCs

3. If *Giardia* is suspected
   a. Obtain stool specimens on 3 separate days for O&P (excretion of organism is intermittent)
   b. Identification of either trophozoite or cysts on direct smear examination is diagnostic
   c. Detection of *G. lamblia* antigens in stool specimen by enzyme immunoassay (EIA) is also diagnostic; enzyme immunoassay techniques for antigen detection in stool specimens are available commercially and have greater sensitivity than microscope detection
   d. Examination of duodenal contents for trophozoites via commercially available string test (Entero-test) is also diagnostic

V. Plan/Management

A. Management of acute diarrhea involves identification of causes that need specific treatment and restoring and/or maintaining hydration status while waiting for the resolution of the symptoms
   1. See TREATMENT OF ACUTE DIARRHEA CAUSED BY COMMONLY OCCURING INFECTIOUS AGENTS in the table that follows
   2. Whether or not the cause of the diarrhea is determined, supportive therapy should be instituted immediately to rehydrate (if necessary) and maintain hydration status in the patient

TREATMENT OF ACUTE DIARRHEA CAUSED BY COMMONLY OCCURRING INFECTIOUS AGENTS

Infectious Agent	Pharmacologic Management	Counseling and Control Measures
Viral Rotavirus Norwalk virus	✓ No specific antiviral therapy is available	✓ Emphasize importance of good hand washing ✓ Advise to clean all surfaces where diapering is done with chlorine-based disinfectants ✓ Infected children should be excluded from child-care centers until diarrhea resolves
Bacterial *Staphylococcus aureus*	✓ Antibiotics are not recommended	✓ Proper cooking and refrigeration of food helps prevent the disease ✓ Persons with staphylococcal infections should be excluded from handling food
Clostridium perfringens	✓ Antibiotics are not recommended	✓ *C. perfringens* should not be allowed to proliferate in food (beef, poultry, gravies, and Mexican-style foods are common sources) ✓ Foods should never be held at room temperature to cool, but should be refrigerated promptly, and reheated thoroughly before serving ✓ Foods should not be kept in warming devices or serving tables for long periods of time
Campylobacter infections	✓ Erythromycin, given early in the course of infection, shortens duration of illness and prevents relapse * Dose: 250 mg PO QID x 5-7 days ✓ Ciprofloxicin is an alternative agent * Dose: 500 mg BID x 5-7 days	✓ Persons who prepare food should practice frequent handwashing, wash surfaces that have been exposed to raw poultry, and thoroughly cook poultry ✓ Pasteurization of milk and chlorination of water supplies are essential ✓ Infected food handlers who are asymptomatic need not be excluded from work if proper personal hygiene measures are maintained ✓ Outbreaks are uncommon in child care centers
Salmonella infections (nontyphoidal)	✓ Antimicrobial therapy is not indicated for uncomplicated gastroenteritis caused by nontyphoidal *Salmonella* species because it can prolong excretion of the organism ✓ Treatment of patients at an increased risk of invasive disease such as persons with HIV infection and patients with severe colitis is recommended. Consult specialists for treatment recommendations	✓ Emphasis should be on good hand-washing and personal hygiene ✓ There must be proper sanitation in food processing and preparation; **infected persons should be excluded from handling food** ✓ Eggs and other foods of animal origin should be cooked thoroughly before ingestion ✓ Raw eggs as well as food containing raw eggs should not be eaten ✓ Handwashing when handling pet turtles and other reptiles is important ✓ Outbreaks of *Salmonella* infection are rare in child care centers ✓ Vaccination for typhoid is recommended only for international travelers ✓ Report all cases of *Salmonella* infection to local public health department so that proper investigation of outbreak can be conducted

(continued)

427

TREATMENT OF ACUTE DIARRHEA CAUSED BY COMMONLY OCCURRING INFECTIOUS AGENTS (CONTINUED)

Infectious Agent	Pharmacologic Management	Counseling and Control Measures
Shigella	✓ To shorten course and prevent further spread, may treat with trimethoprim-sulfamethoxazole * Dose: 1 DS tab BID x 5 days ✓ Intestinal motility patterns are considered important in recovery from infection, therefore anti-diarrhea drugs should not be given	✓ Emphasis should be on good hand-washing and personal hygiene, particularly among workers in group care settings such as child care and group living facilities ✓ There must be proper sanitation in food processing and preparation; **infected persons should be excluded from handling food** ✓ Prevention of contamination of food by flies during preparation and serving ✓ Insuring that water supply is not contaminated is important ✓ Outbreak of Shigella infection must be reported to the local health department for investigation

Escherichia coli infection (entero-toxigenic) [ETEC], major cause of Travelers' Diarrhea	✓ May treat with trimethoprim-sulfame-thoxazole
	  * Dose: 1 DS tab, BID x 3 days
	✓ Ciprofloxicin is an alternative agent
	  * Dose: 500 mg BID x 3 days
		✓ When traveling in developing countries or in any area where water supply is questionable, drink only bottled water
		✓ Avoid all raw fruits and vegetables that may not have been properly washed (unless can peel and eat)

Protozoal *Giardia*	✓ Drug of choice is metronidazole
	  * Dose: 250 mg TID x 5 days
	✓ Alternative drug is furazolidone
	  * Dose: 100 mg QID x 7-10 days
	✓ In pregnant women, panomycin is recommended for treatment of symptomatic infections. Consult PDR for dosing recommendations
		✓ Emphasize sanitation and personal hygiene, especially in group care settings
		✓ Hand washing after diaper changes and after personal toilet use by workers cannot be overemphasized; persons with diarrhea (both workers and children) should be excluded from day care until problem resolves
		✓ Adequate filtration of municipal water supply prevents water-borne outbreaks in metropolitan areas
		✓ Boiling of water by campers, backpackers will eliminate cysts; drinking from streams is risky
		✓ Treatment of asymptomatic carriers is not recommended except for prevention of household transmission by toddlers to pregnant women
		✓ Outbreaks in day care centers require reporting to local public health department for epidemiological investigation

B. Supportive therapy should focus on attaining and maintaining adequate hydration status through appropriate fluid intake
   1. Water or sports drinks may be used for hydration as well as the commercial rehydration products such as Pedialyte and Rehydralyte
   2. Patients may also like products such as Pedialyte Freezer Pops
   3. Normal diet should be resumed as soon as the patient can tolerate it; special diets are no longer recommended as they are not calorie dense enough, and lack adequate amounts of protein and fat

C. The following anti-diarrheal agents are available and may be used in selected cases where there are no contraindications

ANTI-DIARRHEAL AGENTS FOR ACUTE DIARRHEA

Agents	Medication	Dosage
Antimotility agents	Loperamide (Immodium), available as 2 mg caps	4 mg initially, then 2 mg after each unformed stool. Maximum 16 mg/day; use for 2 days
	Immodium A-D (OTC), available as 1 mg/5mL syrup and 2 mg caplets	4 mg initially, then 2 mg after each unformed stool. Maximum 8 mg/day; use for 2 days
	Lomotil, available as 2.5 mg tabs and liquid, 2.5 mg/5 mL	2 tabs QID (maximum 20 mg/day) for 2-3 days
Adsorbents	Kaolin-pectin mixture (Kaopectate) liquid	30-120 mL after each loose stool
Antisecretory agents	Bismuth subsalycilate, available as 262 mg chewable tabs and 262 mg/15 mL liquid	2 tabs or 30 mL Q 30-60 minutes (Maximum 8 doses/day)

D.   Patients with chronic diarrhea require treatment of the underlying cause
    1.   Refer to sections on HIV/AIDS and IRRITABLE BOWEL SYNDROME for management of patients with these conditions
    2.   If *Giardia* is suspected, obtain appropriate diagnostic tests
    3.   If a medication that the patient is taking is producing the diarrhea, change medication if possible
    4.   If inflammatory bowel disease or a malabsorption syndrome such as sprue or lactase deficiency is suspected, refer to a specialist for management

E.   Follow Up: In 48 hours if diarrhea has not resolved

DYSPHAGIA IN ADULTS

I.   Definition: Difficulty in swallowing due to neuromuscular or anatomic pathology involving the esophagus

II.   Pathogenesis

    A.   A lack of movement of the contents within the esophagus (and sometimes the oropharynx) indicates the presence of a motor disorder or an obstruction from either an intrinsic or extrinsic source

    B.   All dysphagia is caused by motor impairment or mechanical obstruction of the esophagus either intrinsically from narrowing due to such causes as tumors, stricture, webs, and rings or extrinsically through compression of the esophagus from such causes as mediastinal tumors and vascular anomalies

III.   Clinical Presentation

    A.   Transfer dysphagia (also called oropharyngeal dysphagia) is a motor disorder usually caused by neurologic or neuromuscular disease and most often presents with difficulty initiating swallowing (choking and regurgitation are prominent)
    1.   Particularly common among very elderly
    2.   Important causes are stroke, tumor, degenerative diseases
    3.   Medications with central effects (benzodiazepines, L-dopa) may also compromise swallowing mechanism
    4.   Patients with neuromuscular etiologies have more difficulty with liquids, have nasal regurgitation, choking, and aspiration as compared with patients with mechanical obstruction of the pharynx/upper esophagus who have more difficulty with solids

    B.   Achalasia is the most common cause of motor dysphagia
    1.   Slowly progressive motor disorder characterized by loss of peristaltic activity in distal esophagus
    2.   Lower esophageal sphincter also fails to relax properly causing an obstruction at the esophagogastric junction
    3.   Substernal chest pain often is present (reported in up to 80% of patients)
    4.   Difficulty with swallowing both solids and liquids is reported with very cold liquids often provoking symptoms
    5.   Repeated swallowing and performing the Valsalva maneuver may help propel food and fluids into stomach

    C.   Scleroderma can cause both a decrease in lower esophageal tone and a lack of propulsive motor activity in the esophagus
    1.   Approximately 75% of these patients have esophageal involvement of some type
    2.   Reflux is more common in these patients than is dysphagia which can be helpful in distinguishing it from other motor disorders

D. Mechanical obstruction produces characteristic signs and symtoms
   1. More difficulty swallowing solids than liquids; with time, difficulty for liquids may also be present (dysphagia is a late sign of mechanical obstruction, and lumen must be reduced by approximately 40% before the person is symptomatic)
   2. Duration of symptoms is relatively short (less than 1 year) for malignancy as compared with benign causes of obstruction
   3. Most persons with tumor are over age 50 and report marked weight loss
   4. Patients with stricture due to severe esophagitis usually have a long-standing history of reflux

E. A history of dysphagia always indicates esophageal disease and thus an extensive evaluation must be undertaken to determine the cause

IV. Diagnosis/Evaluation

A. History: Focus on differentiating a motor disorder from a mechanical obstruction
   1. Determine duration and progression of symptoms
      a. Is dysphagia new?
      b. Is it chronic and recurrent with some intervening periods of swallowing that are relatively normal?
      c. Was the onset fairly short and is the condition progressing?
      d. **Note:** Gradual onset, slow progression and chronic course suggest a motor disorder whereas a more rapid onset and progressive course suggest an obstruction
   2. Question regarding swallowing difficulty -- is it for solids, liquids, or both; ask if there is temperature sensitivity, especially to cold substances
      a. With motor disorders, there is equal difficulty with solids and liquids, symptoms are aggravated by cold substances (liquid or solid) and passage of bolus is assisted with repeated swallowing and Valsalva maneuver
      b. With mechanical obstruction, there is more difficulty with solids than liquids, cold substances have no effect, and swallowing a bolus is not helped by Valsalva maneuver or repeated swallowing
   3. Ask if there is choking, regurgitation of fluid into the nose and if the difficulty with swallowing seems to be localized in the suprasternal area or if it is lower in the chest
   4. Ask if there is pain on swallowing (odynophagia)
   5. Determine if reflux is a problem
   6. Ask if there has been weight loss
   7. Obtain past medical history related to neurological disease, chronic reflux disease, esophagitis
   8. Obtain a good medication history to determine if medications are playing a role in the condition

B. Physical Examination
   1. Examine the skin for pallor, signs or scleroderma (sclerodactyly, telangiectasia, calcinosis) and hyperkeratotic palms and soles (rarely found, but suggests esophageal carcinoma)
   2. Examine mouth for lesions, pharynx for masses
   3. Palpate for enlarged lymph nodes in neck; palpate for thyroid enlargement
   4. Perform abdominal exam for masses, tenderness, enlargement of liver/spleen
   5. Perform rectal exam to obtain stool for occult blood
   6. Neurological examination should include testing of tremor, rigidity, and cranial nerves (gag reflex, palatal movement, and tongue protrusion)

C. Differential Diagnosis: Many causes that can be divided into motor and obstructive categories
   1. Motor diseases include the following: Transfer dysphagia, myasthenia gravis, multiple sclerosis, Parkinson's disease, amyotrophic lateral sclerosis, achalasia, scleroderma, diffuse esophageal spasm
   2. Obstructing diseases/lesions include the following: tumor, goiter, carcinoma, stricture, webs and rings, foreign body

D. Diagnostic Tests
    1. Barium swallow is the first test that should be done in the diagnostic evaluation (particularly important if mechanical obstruction is suspected; sensitivity of this test in detecting motor disorders is not high)
    2. Upper GI endoscopy and biopsy are indicated when mechanical obstruction is suspected and malignancy is a concern
    3. Manometry allows the actual function of the esophageal muscle to be observed and useful when motor disease is suspected or if barium swallow is inconclusive; however, manometry often fails to give conclusive data
    4. Consultation with a specialist is recommended prior to and after any diagnostic testing is undertaken

V. Plan/Management

  A. Regardless of etiology and pending definitive diagnosis, an adequate caloric intake that can be swallowed with a minimum of difficulty should be advised
    1. Liquid or soft diets work best if mechanical obstruction is suspected
    2. If motor disturbances are suspected, small amounts that are eaten slowly work best

  B. Patient should be referred to a specialist for management

  C. Follow up should be done by specialist

GASTROESOPHAGEAL REFLUX DISEASE (GERD)

I. Definition: Reflux of gastric contents into the esophagus resulting in a symptomatic condition

II. Pathogenesis

  A. The lower esophageal sphincter allows for the flow of food between the esophagus and the stomach and several structures at the esophagogastric junction operate to maintain an antireflux barrier

  B. The sphincter mechanism at the lower end of the esophagus is composed of both the intrinsic smooth muscle of the distal esophagus and the skeletal muscle of the crural diaphragm

  C. Transient relaxation of this sphincter mechanism (involving the simultaneous relaxation of the lower esophageal sphincter and crural diaphragm) is the major mechanism of gastric reflux
    1. A neural reflex mediated through the brain stem is responsible for transient relaxation of the smooth muscle of the distal esophagus
    2. Mechanism of relaxation of the crural diaphragm has not been established

  D. Recently, hiatal hernia has once again emerged as an important factor in the pathogenesis of GERD
    1. Most patients with moderate-to-severe reflux disease have hiatal hernia
    2. This condition may promote reflux in a number of ways

  E. Pathologic reflux differs from physiologic reflux in both frequency and volume of refluxed material

  F. Excessive reflux overwhelms the intrinsic mucosal defense mechanisms producing symptoms and signs of esophageal inflammation

III. Clinical Presentation

  A. Ten percent of adults suffer daily heartburn and 30% of adults have symptoms monthly; heartburn typically occurs postprandially

B. Classic presenting symptom is burning substernal pain that radiates upward; the mechanism of the pain is unclear, but is thought to be related to the stimulation of chemoreceptors or to distention of the esophagus

C. Antacids usually relieve the pain and heartburn; stress may make the condition worse

IV. Diagnosis/Evaluation

A. History
1. Inquire about onset, progression and duration of the most prominent presenting symptom -- heartburn
2. Determine if heartburn aggravated by meals and relieved by sitting up or antacids
3. Determine if patient smokes
4. Diagnosis can be made on basis of history alone if patient is under age 45, has history of heartburn, has no dysphagia, recent weight loss, or blood loss

B. Physical Examination
1. Determine if patient is overweight
2. Perform abdominal exam for masses, tenderness
3. Check for occult blood in stool

C. Differential Diagnosis
1. Cardiac chest pain
2. Esophagitis/esophageal motility/structural disorders
3. Peptic ulcer disease
4. Esophageal tumor

D. Diagnostic Tests
1. Usually none indicated
2. In patients with atypical presentations (dysphagia, weight loss, blood loss) referral to a specialist for endoscopy is recommended

V. Plan/Management

A. Patients with typical symptoms of uncomplicated GERD with no alarm symptoms (dysphagia, weight loss, blood loss) can be treated empirically

B. Goals of management for GERD are the following:
1. To modify risk factors
2. To inhibit acid production
3. To promote gastric contractility

C. Phase I therapy should be used for all patients. This involves the following lifestyle changes to reduce the incidence of reflux and to neutralize stomach acid
1. If obese (see section on OBESITY to determine degree of obesity), should be counseled to lose weight; even 10 pound loss can decrease symptoms
2. Stop smoking; a crucial change since smoking reduces esophageal sphincter tone
3. Elevate head of bed or sleep on wedge-shaped bolster
4. Eat smaller meals, and do not eat for 2-3 hours prior to bedtime
5. Reduce fat in diet so that no more than 30% of calories come from fat
6. Avoid foods that produce symptoms such as chocolate, citrus fruits, mints, coffee, alcohol
7. Use antacids on an as-needed basis

D. Approximately 25% of patients are effectively treated using Phase I therapy

E. Phase II therapy should be instituted for patients who fail Phase I therapy and who have mild to moderate disease (Phase I therapy must be continued in all patients and Phase II therapy added)
1. H_2 receptor antagonists (see section on PEPTIC ULCER DISEASE; for drugs and dosages, same total daily dose should be used)

2. Dosing note: In reflux disease BID dosing is recommended. The first dose in the AM to inhibit acid production after breakfast and lunch; the second dose about 1 hour after the evening meal

F. An alternative medication to use in Phase II therapy is a prokinetic agent such as cisapride (Propulsid) which may be effective in decreasing symptoms in up to half of patients with mild-to-moderate disease
   1. Drug has selective prokinetic effects (it increases lower esophageal sphincter tone, improves esophageal peristalsis, and promotes gastric emptying)
   2. Dosing of cisapride is 10 mg taken 15 minutes before meals and at bedtime
   3. **Revised Propulsid labeling issued in June 1998** warns that serious cardiac arrythmias including ventricular tachycardia, ventricular fibrillation, torsades de pointes, and QT prolongation have been reported in patients taking Propulsid

G. Proton pump inhibitors such as omeprazole (Prilosec) [dosed at 20 mg/day] and lansoprazole (Prevacid) [dosed at 30 mg/day] should be reserved for the treatment of patients with moderate to severe disease because of concerns about potential carcinogenesis and interference with the cytochrome P-450 system

H. Refer all patients with dysphagia, recent weight loss, or blood loss to a specialist for management

I. Follow Up
   1. Re-evaluate patient after 1-2 weeks; if symptoms are controlled, institute full course of treatment which is 8 weeks
   2. After 8 weeks of therapy at full dosing, instruct patient to reduce dosage to the lowest possible level that provides relief (usually one dose a day or one dose every other day, taken before bedtime)
   3. Most patients require low-dose maintenance therapy indefinitely because of the recurrent nature of the problem
   4. If patient remains symptomatic after completion of 8-week therapeutic trial with drugs from two different classes (i.e., symptoms are not controlled **even** with treatment), referral to gastroenterologist is appropriate

HEMORRHOIDS

I. Definition: Dilated, possibly thrombosed or prolapsed, perirectal veins, often causing painful swelling at the anus

II. Pathogenesis

A. Anal cushions, part of the normal anatomy of the anal canal, become displaced through an unknown mechanism

B. Prolapse of a vascular anal cushion through the anal canal results in entrapment by the internal anal sphincter and the result is hemorrhoid formation

C. Prolapse may be initiated by:
   1. Shearing force from passage of large firm stool
   2. Increase in venous pressure from congestive heart failure or pregnancy
   3. Straining that occurs with lifting or defecation

D. In most cases of hemorrhoids, however, no definite cause can be identified

III. Clinical Presentation

    A. Classic symptom is bleeding, which is usually painless, and anal discomfort

    B. Occurs most often in persons over age 50; uncommon in persons under 25 except women who have been pregnant

    C. Rectal itching, pain or burning may be present

IV. Diagnosis/Evaluation

    A. History
       1. Inquire about onset, duration of symptoms -- pain, itching, burning; occurrence of bleeding
       2. Ask about past medical history of hemorrhoids, recent pregnancy, liver disease, anorectal surgery, or chronic constipation

    B. Physical Examination
       1. Inspect anal area and perform digital rectal exam
       2. Anoscopy is recommended in severe cases

    C. Differential Diagnosis
       1. Hypertrophic anal papilla, seen with anal fissure, Crohn's Disease
       2. Anal tags
       3. Prolapse of rectal mucosa (much more common in elderly)
       4. Anorectal abscess
       5. Perianal tumors
       6. Perianal thrombosis

    D. Diagnostic Tests: None indicated; consider hematocrit

V. Plan/Management

    A. For mild hemorrhoidal symptoms, advise
       1. High fiber diet and bulk-forming agents (see section on CONSTIPATION)
       2. Use of witch hazel pads (Tucks) or gel (Tucks Gel) both OTC products that are applied up to 6 x day
       3. Sitz baths 1-2 x day

    B. For moderate hemorrhoidal symptoms, advise that recommendations under V.A. be followed
       1. Use of the following can also be recommended
          a. Anusol HC-1 ointment (OTC); apply 3-4 x/day for 7 days
          b. Preparation H ointment (OTC); apply up to 4x/day
          c. Topical ointments are most effective applied with a finger cot inside the anus
       2. Note that ointments applied correctly are much more effective than suppositories

    C. For severe hemorrhoidal symptoms, refer patient for excision of the involved hemorrhoid; internal hemorrhoids can be effectively treated using injection sclerotherapy

    D. Follow Up: None needed unless persistence, recurrence of symptoms

VIRAL HEPATITIS

I.   Definition: An inflammatory process of the liver caused by infection by one of the five distinct viruses (A, B, C, D, and E); other causes of hepatitis are not considered here

II. Pathogenesis

    A.   Hepatitis A (HAV): RNA virus which is classified as a member of the picornavirus group; replication appears to be limited to the liver; only one serotype of HAV has been recognized in humans

    B.   Hepatitis B (HBV): DNA-containing hepadenavirus; important components include HbsAg, hepatitis B core antigen, and hepatitis B e antigen

    C.   Hepatitis C (HCV): Small, single-stranded RNA virus of the Flavivirus family; multiple HCV genotypes exist

    D.   Hepatitis D (HDV): Small particle consisting of an RNA genome and a delta protein antigen, both of which are coated with hepatitis B surface antigen; requires HBV as a helper virus; cannot produce infection in absence of HBV

    E.   Hepatitis E (HEV): Single-stranded RNA virus that is structurally similar to a calicivirus

III. Clinical Presentation

    A.   Hepatitis A
       1.   In US, HAV infection is endemic with periodic outbreaks occurring in certain groups such as Native Americans, Alaskan natives, Hispanic communities
       2.   **Mode of transmission** is primarily through fecal-oral route; spreads readily in households and child care centers, with risk of spread in such centers increasing with the number of children who wear diapers
       3.   Common source **outbreaks** from food and water contaminated with human sewage also occur
       4.   Unlike other infectious diseases that spread in child care centers, children who are infected are either asymptomatic or have very mild, nonspecific symptoms; adult contacts of infected children who themselves become infected, on the other hand, usually are symptomatic
       5.   Illness is self-limited and includes jaundice, anorexia, nausea, vomiting, malaise, and fever
       6.   When acquired during infancy and early childhood, infections are likely to be mild without jaundice; adult infections are likely to be quite severe
       7.   Viral shedding and the contagious period last 1-3 weeks, with the infected person being most contagious 1-2 weeks before the onset of illness; risk of transmission diminishes and is minimal in the week after onset of jaundice (if present)
       8.   **Incubation period** is 15-50 days, with an average of 25-30 days
       9.   **Chronic infection does not occur**
       10. **Diagnosis**: Anti-HAV IgM appears early in the disease, diminishes after several weeks; Anti-HAV IgG develops and usually persists for life. (Thus, Anti-HAV IgM is a marker of acute infection, while anti-HAV IgG persists throughout life and is a reliable marker of past infection)
       11. Presence of serum anti-HAV IgG in unvaccinated persons indicates lifelong immunity to HAV
       12. Children vaccinated with HAV only rarely have detectable anti-HAV IgM titers

    B.   Hepatitis B
       1.   Approximately 300,000 persons are infected with HBV each year with most infected persons acquiring the disease as adolescents or adults

2. **Transmission** occurs via contact with infected blood or body fluids such as semen, cervical secretions, wound exudates, and saliva

3. **Modes of transmission** include
   a. Transfusion of blood or blood products (rare in US today)
   b. Needle-sharing
   c. Percutaneous or mucous membrane exposures to blood or body fluids
   d. Heterosexual and homosexual activity
   e. Vertical transmission (during perinatal period)
   f. More than 30% of infected persons do not have a readily identifiable risk factor
   g. Not transmitted via fecal-oral route

4. The primary reservoir for infection is the HBV chronic carrier (defined as person with serum HBsAg-positive for 6 months or more)

5. Hepatitis B causes a spectrum of illness ranging from an asymptomatic seroconversion, to acute illness with anorexia, nausea, malaise, and jaundice, to fatal hepatitis

6. Arthralgias, arthritis, and a macular skin eruption can also occur as part of the illness

7. Asymptomatic infection is most common in young children

8. Age of the person at initial HBV infection is the major determinant of chronicity; chronic HBV infection is much more likely to develop after prenatal or perinatal exposure than after exposure later in life

9. To illustrate the effect of age on chronic disease, chronic HBV infection develops in
   a. Up to 90% of infants infected by perinatal transmission
   b. Thirty percent of children 1-5 years of age
   c. Five to ten percent of older children, adolescents, and adults

10. **Incubation period** is 45-160 days, with an average of 120 days

11. **Diagnosis**: During acute illness, two detectable factors in serum are hepatitis B surface antigen (HBsAg) and antibody to the viral core proteins (Anti-HBc); when the patient recovers, HBsAg usually disappears and evidence of surface antibody (anti-HBs) can be found; the finding of coexistent anti-HBs and anti-HBc indicates a state of recovery; the e antigen (HBeAg) can also be detected during the acute phase; the presence of HBeAg in conjunction with HBsAg in the serum indicates a more serious prognosis than the presence of HBsAg alone (see INTERPRETATION OF THE HEPATITIS B PANEL table)

INTERPRETATION OF THE HEPATITIS B PANEL

Tests	Results	Interpretation
HBsAg anti-HBc anti-HBs	negative negative negative	susceptible
HBsAg anti-HBc anti-HBs	negative negative or positive positive	immune
HBsAg anti-HBc IgM anti-HBc anti-HBs	positive positive positive negative	acutely infected
HBsAg anti-HBc IgM anti-HBc anti-HBs	positive positive negative negative	chronically infected
HBsAg anti-HBc anti-HBs	negative positive negative	four interpretations possible*

* 1. May be recovering from acute HBV infection
  2. May be distantly immune and test not sensitive enough to detect very low level of anti-HBs in serum
  3. May be susceptible with a false positive anti-HBc
  4. May be undetectable level of HBsAg present in the serum and the person is actually a carrier

(continued)

Laboratory Diagnosis of Chronic Hepatitis B and C

Hepatitis B	HBsAg. If positive, obtain IgM anti-HBc to differentiate acute hepatitis B (IgM anti-HBc is positive) from chronic hepatitis B (IgM anti-HBc is negative). Chronic hepatitis B is also defined by 2 HBsAg-positive tests separated by at least 6 months
Hepatitis C	Anti-HCV. Verify a positive test with a supplemental assay such as RIBA or nucleic acid detection of HCV RNA, depending on the clinical situation

For More Information about Hepatitis B including guidelines for the management of the hepatitis B carrier, contact the Hepatitis B Coalition, 1573 Selby Avenue, St. Paul, MN 55104,

Source: Immunization Action Coalition. (1997.) Basic facts about adult hepatitis B. St. Paul, MN: Author

C. Hepatitis C
1. Prevalence of HCV infection among all age groups is estimated at 1.8%; accounts for 21% of cases of acute viral hepatitis and 60% of cases of chronic viral hepatitis in US each year
2. **Mode of transmission** is primarily through parenteral exposure to blood and blood products
3. Highest seroprevalence rates of infection (60-90%) occur in those with repeated exposure to blood or blood products such as IV drug users or patients with hemophilia (**Note**: Current risk of HCV infection following blood transfusion is about 0.1%)
4. Much lower rates (1-10%) are found among persons with inapparent parenteral exposures such as persons with high-risk sexual behaviors and sexual/household contacts of infected person
5. Other body fluids contaminated with infected blood can be source of infection with intranasal cocaine users having high rates of infection believed to be related to epistaxis and shared equipment
6. For most infected children and adolescents, no specific source can be identified
7. Signs and symptoms are often indistinguishable from those of hepatitis A or B infection
8. Acute disease is most often mild in adults and asymptomatic in children with jaundice occurring in only about 25% of those infected
9. Approximately 65-70% of patients develop chronic hepatitis with 20% developing cirrhosis
10. All persons with HCV antibody and/or HCV-RNA in their blood are considered to be contagious
11. **Incubation period** ranges from 2 weeks to 6 months with an average of 6-7 weeks
12. **Diagnosis**: Two types of tests are available for diagnosis of HCV (see following table)

DIAGNOSTIC TESTS FOR HCV

Antibody-based tests
- ⇨ Include an enzyme-linked immunosorbent assay (ELISAII) and Recombinant immunoblot assay (RIBA)
- ⇨ Diagnosis using antibody assays involves an initial screening enzyme immunoassay (EIA)
  - ✦ Positive results are confirmed by a recombinant immunoblot assay (RIBA)
  - ✦ Both assays detect IgG antibody; no IgM assays are currently available
  - ✦ Within 5-6 weeks after onset of illness, 80% of patients will be positive for serum anti-HCV antibody

PCR and branched chain DNA (bDNA) assays for HCV
- ⇨ Are able to identify HCV sooner after infection than the antibody based tests
- ⇨ Compared with antibody-based tests, HCV RNA testing
  - ✦ Is more sensitive
  - ✦ Provides a better marker for effectiveness of treatment
  - ✦ Is much more expensive
  - ✦ Is best used for follow-up to help distinguish active from past infection in patients who are anti-HCV positive

Note: Tests for detecting HCV antigen have not yet been developed

D. Hepatitis D
1. Prevalence of HDV in the US is highest among parenteral drug users, hemophiliacs, and immigrants from endemic areas of the world
2. Occurs as either a **coinfection** with HBV (e.g., following inoculation with blood or secretions that contain both agents) or as a **superinfection** in established chronic HBV infection

3. **Mode of transmission** is via blood or blood products, injection drugs, or sexual contact providing HBV also is present
4. Transmission from mother to newborn is uncommon
5. Hepatitis D resembles hepatitis B in terms of when symptoms appear and period of infectivity
6. Hepatitis D can cause hepatitis only in persons with acute or chronic HBV infection
7. **Incubation period** for HDV superinfection is approximately 2-8 weeks; when both viruses (B and D) infect simultaneously, incubation period averages 120 days and ranges from 45-160 days
8. **Diagnosis**: Diagnosis of hepatitis D is made by detecting anti-HDV antibody in the serum

E. Hepatitis E
1. Occurs predominantly in India, South Central Asia, and the Middle East, but also occurs in the Western Hemisphere, including the US (rare)
2. **Mode of transmission** is the fecal-oral route
3. Causes an acute illness with jaundice, malaise, anorexia, abdominal pain, arthralgias, and fever
4. Occurs more commonly in adults than children and is most serious when it occurs in pregnant women
5. **Period of communicability** is unknown, but probably continues for at least 2 weeks after the acute phase
6. **Chronic infection does not occur**
7. **Incubation period** ranges from 15-60 days, with an average of 40 days
8. **Diagnosis**: Serologic testing for hepatitis E is not available; diagnosis rests on excluding other causes of viral hepatitis

F. The following table contains a comparison of the 5 forms of viral hepatitis

COMPARISON OF FIVE FORMS OF VIRAL HEPATITIS			
Form	Primary Route of Transmission	Incubation Period	Chronicity
Hepatitis A	Fecal-oral, contaminated food/water	15-50 days	None
Hepatitis B	Blood/body fluids	45-160 days	Yes
Hepatitis C	Blood/blood products	14-180 days	Yes
Hepatitis D	Blood/body fluids	45-160 days	Yes
Hepatitis E	Fecal-oral	15-60 days	None

G. All five types of viral hepatitis are similar in their clinical expression and therefore cannot be readily distinguished by clinical features

H. Clinical features include the following:
1. Fatigue, lassitude, anorexia, nausea, dark urine, low grade fever, right upper abdominal discomfort, myalgia, and arthralgias
2. Only a minority of persons who are infected develop jaundice
3. Many infected persons are asymptomatic

I. The characteristic laboratory abnormalities are elevated aminotransferase levels that are high early in the prodromal period, peak before jaundice is maximal, and fall slowly during the convalescent period
1. Aspartate aminotransferase (AST) and alanine aminotransferase (ALT) levels are typically 500-2000 IU/L
2. ALT is usually higher than AST (in alcoholic hepatitis, the reverse is usual)
3. Alkaline phosphatase is only modestly elevated
4. Degree of hyperbilirubinemia is variable

     5.   Urinary bile usually precedes jaundice

     6.   Increase in prothrombin time is uncommon; if present suggests severe illness

     7.   WBC count is usually low-normal, and blood smear may show a few atypical lymphocytes

  J.   Serologic testing determines the specific etiologic diagnosis

IV.   Diagnosis/Evaluation

  A.   History
     1.   Question about onset and duration of symptoms (usual symptoms are general fatigue, malaise, joint and muscle pain, loss of appetite, nausea, vomiting, diarrhea, and low-grade fever; tenderness of right upper quadrant and jaundice may also occur)
     2.   Ask about darkened urine, light-colored stools
     3.   Inquire about similar illness in household contacts
     4.   Ask about sexual behaviors and similar illness in sexual partners
     5.   Ask about history of blood transfusions, IV drug use, alcohol abuse
     6.   Inquire about occupation
     7.   Obtain travel history, especially travel to Asia or Africa where hepatitis B is especially common
     8.   Obtain past medical history and medication history

  B.   Physical Examination
     1.   Examine skin, mucous membranes, and sclera for jaundice
     2.   Perform abdominal exam to determine size, surface characteristics, and tenderness of liver; determine if spleen is enlarged

  C.   Differential Diagnosis: Noninfectious causes of hepatitis including medications, acute alcohol induced injury

  D.   Diagnostic Tests
     1.   If acute hepatitis is suspected, order appropriate diagnostic tests recommended above based on type of hepatitis that is suspected (many insurance carriers will not pay for "hepatitis panels")
     2.   Serologic features of viral hepatitis are summarized in the following table:

SEROLOGIC FEATURES OF VIRAL HEPATITIS		
Form of Infection	**Serologic Markers**	**Interpretation**
Hepatitis A	IgM anti-HAV	Acute disease
	IgG anti-HAV	Remote infection and immunity
Hepatitis B	HBsAg	Acute or chronic disease
	HBeAg	Active replication (If persists beyond first 3 months, likelihood of chronic infection increases; thus more important to test for in chronic disease)
	IgM anti-HBc	Positive in acute infection; negative in chronic infection
	Anti-HBs	Remote infection and immunity
Hepatitis C	Anti-HCV	Acute, chronic, or resolved disease
Hepatitis D	HBsAg and anti-HDV	Acute disease
	● IgM anti-HBc positive	Co-infection
	● IgG anti-HBc positive	Superinfection
Hepatitis E	None commercially available	
Anti-HAV, antibody to hepatitis A virus; anti-HCV, antibody to hepatitis C virus; anti-HDV, antibody to hepatitis D virus; HBeAg, hepatitis B e antigen; HBsAg, hepatitis B surface antigen; anti-HBc, antibody to hepatitis B core antigen; anti-HBs, antibody to HBsAg		

     3.   If HBsAg is present, testing for HBeAg is needed to determine whether active viral replication is present
     4.   Testing for anti-HDV should be done in all persons with chronic hepatitis B to rule out coexisting hepatitis D

5. If all test results are negative, follow up testing for anti-HCV is appropriate because of delay in appearance of antibody

6. CBC, total and direct bilirubin, prothrombin time, liver function tests, urinalysis should be obtained also

7. All persons with chronic hepatitis should have liver biopsy to determine extent of disease

V. Plan/Management

A. Hepatitis usually resolves spontaneously over 4-8 weeks

B. For acute infections for all types of viral hepatitis (A, B, C, D, E), provide symptomatic treatment for symptoms such as myalgia, nausea, vomiting, and pruritus

C. Bed rest, special diets, vitamin supplements are not required

D. If patient on hepatotoxic drugs, those should be discontinued until recovery has occurred

E. Interferon alpha is the only treatment that has been shown to be effective in treatment of chronic hepatitis infection in adults

VI. Control measures: Hepatitis A

A. Improved sanitation and personal hygiene (especially good hand washing) are the keys to controlling spread of the virus

B. Postexposure prophylaxis for household and sexual contacts: Give 0.02 mL/kg of immune globulin (IG) as soon as possible after exposure (use of IG more than 2 weeks after last exposure in not indicated) **and** give HAV vaccine in dosage and schedule under VI.E. below

C. Newborn infants of infected mothers: If mother's symptoms began 2 weeks before or 1 week after delivery, give IG (0.02 mL/kg) to newborn (**Note:** Perinatal transmission is rare)

D. When there is an index case in a child care center:
1. Report all child care associated hepatitis A cases to local health department
2. Stress importance of good hygiene to prevent fecal-oral spread
3. Children and adults with acute hepatitis should be excluded from child care until one week after onset of illness
4. For use of immune globulin (IG) in child care facilities, consult Red Book (1997) for details of management

E. Hepatitis A vaccine: Havrix and Vaqta, both with pediatric and adult formulations are now available in the US
1. Havrix for children 2-18 years of age has two formulations, one for a 2 dose and the second for a 3 dose schedule
2. Vaqta for children 2-18 years of age is given in a 2 dose schedule only
3. Children ≥19 and adults receive a 2 dose schedule of either Havrix or Vaqta

F. Hepatitis A vaccine should be given to the following groups:
1. International travelers
2. Children ≥2 years living in communities with high endemic rates/periodic outbreaks
3. Patients with chronic liver disease
4. Homosexual and bisexual men
5. Users of injection/illicit drugs
6. Persons with occupational risk of exposure
7. Any healthy person at least 2 years of age at discretion of health care provider (examples, child care center staff/attendees, custodial care workers, hospital workers, food handlers)

VII.   Control Measures: Hepatitis B

A.   **All infants** should receive hepatitis B vaccine as part of their routine immunizations in childhood (series of 3 doses is required for optimal antibody response); all children who have not received the vaccine previously should be immunized by or before 11 or 12 years of age [see IMMUNIZATIONS section]
1.   Susceptibility testing before vaccination is not recommended in children and adolescents
2.   Testing for previous infection should be considered in adults in high-risk groups

B.   Prenatal screening for HBsAg can prevent perinatal transmission (for care of infant whose mother is HBsAg-Positive, consult Red Book (1997), pp. 256-257, as these children do need special care including HBIG within 12 hours after birth)

C.   Prevention of HBV transmission to medical personnel is possible through use of universal precautions for blood and body fluids; nonetheless, all health care workers and others with occupational exposure to blood are at high risk and should be immunized

D.   Consult Red Book (1997) for complete listing of other high-risk groups who should receive pre-exposure hepatitis B immunization

E.   Recommendations for Hepatitis B prophylaxis after percutaneous or permucosal exposure are contained in the following table

RECOMMENDED POSTEXPOSURE PROPHYLAXIS FOR PERCUTANEOUS OR PERMUCOSAL EXPOSURE TO HEPATITIS B VIRUS, UNITED STATES			
Vaccination and Antibody Response Status of Exposed Person	Treatment When Source Is		
	HBsAg[1] Positive	HBsAg Negative	Source Not Tested or Status Unknown
Unvaccinated	HBIG[2] x 1; initiate HB vaccine series[3]	Initiate HB vaccine series	Initiate HB vaccine series
Previously vaccinated: Known responder[4]	No treatment	No treatment	No treatment
Known non-responder	HBIG x 2 or HBIG x 1 and initiate revaccination	No treatment	If known high-risk source, treat as if source were HBsAg positive
Antibody response unknown	Test exposed person for anti-HBs[5] 1. If adequate,[4] no treatment 2. If inadequate,[4] HBIG x 1 and vaccine booster	No treatment	Test exposed person for anti-HBs 1. If adequate,[4] no treatment 2. In inadequate,[4] initiate revaccination

[1]Hepatitis B surface antigen [2]Hepatitis B immune globulin; dose 0.06 mL/kg intramuscularly [3]Hepatitis B vaccine [4]Responder is defined as a person with adequate levels of serum antibody to hepatitis B surface antigen (i.e., anti-HBs ≥10 mIU/mL); inadequate response to vaccination defined as serum anti-HBs <10 mIU/mL [5]Antibody to hepatitis B surface antigen
Source: Centers for Disease Control. (1997). Immunization of health care workers. MMWR, 46, No. RR-18.

VIII.   Control measures: Hepatitis C

A.   Should be managed with the universal precautions for blood and body fluids as in Hepatitis B

B.   Because a high percentage of persons with Hepatitis C develop chronic liver disease, referral to specialist for management is indicated

IX.   Control measures: Hepatitis D

A.   Transmission is similar to that of HBV, so universal precautions for blood and body fluids should be observed

B.   Cannot be transmitted in the absence of HBV, so prevention of HBV is key to prevention

C.   Immunoprophylaxis not available

X.   Control measures: Hepatitis E

    A.   Immunoprophylaxis not available

    B.   Prevention through good sanitation and hygiene

XI.   Follow Up

    A.   Variable depending on type of hepatitis

    B.   Hepatitis A and E do not have a chronic stage, so generally resolve without any long-term effects (Hepatitis E only found in developing countries and rarely in the US at this time)
        1.   Make sure IG prophylaxis is given as described above
        2.   Emphasize control measures to prevent spread
        3.   Recheck patient after 2 weeks to evaluate condition

    C.   Hepatitis B, C, D should be referred for management because of development of high rate of chronic hepatitis

ABNORMAL LIVER FUNCTION TESTS

I.   Definition: Elevations in serum values of liver chemistries in asymptomatic patients

II.   Pathogenesis:

    A.   Although these tests are referred to as "liver function tests," they are not a true assessment of liver function but rather markers of hepatic injury

    B.   Liver function tests provide information on three liver functions: cellular integrity, protein synthesis, and excretory function
        1.   Alanine aminotransferase (ALT) and aspartate aminotransferase (AST) are measures of cellular integrity
        2.   Prothrombin time (PT) and albumin level reflect the liver's synthetic capacity
        3.   Bilirubin, gamma-glutamyl-transpeptidase (GGT) and alkaline phosphatase (ALP) measure hepatic excretory function

    C.   **Evaluation of cellular integrity**: ALT and AST are enzymes found in many tissues and cellular injury causes these enzymes to leak into the interstitial space and plasma
        1.   Serum levels are elevated not only with hepatocellular injury, but also with such conditions as myocardial infarction and musculoskeletal injury
        2.   Highest elevations are seen in toxin or drug induced, viral or ischemic hepatitis
        3.   To confirm that elevated aminotransferases are hepatic in origin, a GGT level should be obtained [should also be elevated]
        4.   Alanine Aminotransferase (ALT)
            a.   High concentrations are located in liver, especially the periportal area; found in muscle to a lesser extent
            b.   A more specific marker of hepatocellular damage than AST as elevated ALT level is more likely to reflect damage to liver than to other organ systems
            c.   (**Note**: Determination of creatine phosphokinase [CPK] levels can exclude brain and muscle injury as the source of abnormal levels)
            d.   Isolated measures not as useful as serial measures because levels change rapidly
        5.   Aspartate Aminotransferase (AST)
            a.   Predominantly found in liver, cardiac and skeletal muscle, and the kidney
            b.   Levels become elevated when injury to hepatocyte occurs, particularly to mitochondria
        6.   An AST:ALT ratio >2 is highly correlated with damage from alcohol ingestion

D. **Evaluation of protein synthesis**: Measurement of the hepatic synthetic function is done through measurement of serum albumin level and prothrombin time (Protime) [a reflection of hepatic synthesis of Factors I, II, V, VII, and X]

1. Albumin is the most abundant serum protein with about 12 g synthesized by the liver each day
2. Albumin synthesis can be affected by such factors as decreased dietary protein intake, increased alcohol consumption, trauma, and conticosteroids
3. Elevated Protime can be due to deficiency of one of the Factors, but can also be due to vitamin K deficiency
   a. To differentiate between hypovitamin K and liver disease, administer vitamin K, 10 mg IM and recheck Protime in 24 hours
   b. If the Protime improves by at least 30%, hepatic synthetic function is intact

E. **Evaluation of excretory function**: Alkaline Phosphatase (ALP), bilirubin, and gamma-glutamyl-transpeptidase (GGT) are markers of cholestatic injury/hepatic excretory function

1. Alkaline Phosphatase has origin in multiple tissues including bone, liver, placenta, intestine, and leukocytes, with more than 80% derived from liver and bone
   a. In late pregnancy, level can double and still be considered normal
   b. Can be normally elevated in childhood/adolescence as it is a measure of osteoblastic activity in bone
   c. Elevations of this enzyme to a degree greater than transaminase elevation is consistent with cholestatic injury (intra- or extrahepatic biliary obstruction)
   d. If the Alkaline Phosphatase is the only abnormality on the LFT screen, consider a GGT (described below) to help differentiate liver versus bone as the source
2. Bilirubin is elevated in patients with cholestasis and liver damage
   a. Humans produce about 4 mg/kg/day of bilirubin with the majority attributable to red blood cell breakdown
   b. Small contribution comes from degradation of heme containing proteins in the liver and destruction of erythroid cells when erythropoiesis is ineffective
   c. Total bilirubin levels reflect both direct and indirect bilirubin
   d. Pathway of bilirubin metabolism
      (1) About 80% of bilirubin is derived from breakdown of RBCs in the reticuloendothelial system
      (2) Bilirubin is then transported to liver for further metabolism bound to albumin
   e. After arriving in liver, three phases of metabolism occur
      (1) First, uptake-dissociation from albumin takes place
      (2) Second, there is conjugation-addition of one or two molecules of glucuronic acid
      (3) Third, excretion-via bile occurs (the rate limiting step)
   f. Indirect bilirubin (unconjugated) is insoluble in water, but is lipid soluble allowing for diffusion across membranes
   g. Direct bilirubin (conjugated) is bilirubin conjugated to glucuronic acid, which is water soluble and allows for intestinal excretion in bile
   h. An excess of unconjugated bilirubin implies a problem in bilirubin metabolism at level of conjugation or any of the other steps
   i. Specifically, this means overproduction of bilirubin
   j. Direct (conjugated) hyperbilirubinemia is most often due to hepatobiliary disease; indirect (unconjugated) is often due to hemolytic syndromes and Gilbert's syndrome, an inherited defect that causes mild elevations of the indirect bilirubin fraction [other LFTs are usually normal]
3. Gamma-glutamyl-transpeptidase (GGT) is found in liver, kidney, pancreas, heart, and brain
   a. Function of enzyme remains unclear but serves as tool in correlation of hepatobiliary disease with abnormal serum alkaline phosphatase (ALP); parallels the activity of ALP, except in the presence of bone disease
   b. A sensitive indicator of hepatic disease (elevated in >95% of all diseases involving liver)
   c. Particularly sensitive to damage caused by drugs and chemicals

           d.   Isolated elevation of GGT is a sensitive screening test for excess alcohol use
           e.   GGT may also be increased in thyrotoxicosis, renal failure, post MI, pancreatitis,
                 diabetes, and prostate cancer

III.   Clinical Presentation

       A.   Patient may be asymptomatic and abnormal laboratory findings were unanticipated (abnormal
             LFTs occur in 1-6% of an asymptomatic population)

       B.   Variable presentation depending on the underlying cause

IV.   Diagnosis/Evaluation

       A.   History
             1.   Inquire about any symptoms such as anorexia, weight loss, malaise
             2.   Ask about alcohol and drug use
             3.   Obtain detailed medication history (always ask about use of vitamins, dietary supplements,
                   herbs)
             4.   Ask about previous medical history including any previous acute illnesses that could have
                   been hepatitis, surgical history for any gastrointestinal problems, history of blood
                   transfusions
             5.   Obtain detailed sexual history
             6.   Question patient about household/work exposures to chemicals such as carbon
                   tetrachloride, vinyl chloride

       B.   Physical Examination: Focus should be on searching for evidence of liver disease
             1.   Skin exam for spider angioma, palmar erythema, jaundice
             2.   Sclera for icterus
             3.   Abdominal exam, checking for ascites, right upper quadrant tenderness, hepatomegaly,
                   splenomegaly
             4.   Complete other parts of the exam as necessary

       C.   Diagnostic Testing
             1.   If history and physical examination are normal, and patient is completely asymptomatic,
                   repeat testing is the first step with the addition of ancillary tests to confirm liver damage; as
                   part of the repeat blood draw, consider testing for hepatitis B and C
                   a.   Consultation with a specialist at this point may be helpful in order to determine if
                         imaging studies are indicated
                   b.   Note: Serum ALP and GGT levels are often abnormal if tumors, granulomas, or
                         cholestasis are present, which would indicate need for imaging studies
             2.   If history and physical examination are abnormal, refer patient to a specialist for imaging
                   studies, with ultrasound usually being the first choice

       D.   Differential Diagnosis: Many conditions/diseases affect cellular integrity, protein synthesis, and
             excretory function; common causes of elevation are contained in the tables that follow

┌───┐
| **MOST COMMON CAUSES OF ELEVATED ALT AND AST** |
├───┤
| ◆ Alcoholic hepatitis |
| ❖ Most common cause |
| |
| ◆ Viral hepatitis |
| ❖ With acute infections, levels may be more than 1,000 IU/liter |
| ❖ Bilirubin also elevated in viral hepatitis |
| |
| ◆ Cytotoxic drugs |
| ❖ Commonly used drugs that can cause toxicity include acetaminophen, NSAIDs, |
| phenytoin, sulfonamides, rifampin, and imipramine |
└───┘

V.   Plan/Management

    A.   Diagnostic testing as outlined above is the first step in management

    B.   If no underlying cause is found, and the patient remains completely asymptomatic, observation for 3 to 6 months for progressive symptoms and liver dysfunction may be appropriate
       1.   Further laboratory testing should be done at the end of this period of observation
       2.   If abnormalities in liver function tests persist, referral to a specialist is indicated

    C.   Follow up: Should be done by specialist to whom patient was referred

ABDOMINAL HERNIAS

I.   Definition: Protrusion of an abdominal viscus or part of a viscus through the abdominal wall

    A.   Incarcerated hernias are hernias that cannot be reduced and the contents of the hernial sac cannot be returned to the peritoneal cavity

    B.   Strangulated hernias are hernias which occur when the blood supply to the viscera lying within the hernial sac is obliterated or cut off

II.   Pathogenesis

    A.   A hernia is a defect in the normal musculofascial continuity of the abdominal wall and is either congenital or acquired

    B.   Acquired hernias may occur from any condition that increases intraabdominal pressure such as obesity, chronic cough, ascites, chronic constipation with straining, and lifting heavy objects

    C.   Distinction between congenital and acquired hernias is often unclear as hernias can be acquired because of a congenital predisposition
       1.   Distinction has little implication for management
       2.   Distinction may be very important when work-related injury is claimed

III.   Clinical Presentation

   A.   The symptoms of reducible hernias are related to the degree of pressure of contents rather than to size

   B.   Most patients with reducible hernias are asymptomatic or complain of only mild pain, whereas patients with strangulated hernias have colicky abdominal pain, nausea, vomiting, abdominal distention, and hyperperistalsis

   C.   Inguinal hernias are classified as direct (portions of the bowel and/or omentum protrude directly through the floor of the inguinal canal and emerge at the external inguinal ring) or indirect (pass through the internal abdominal ring, traverse the spermatic cord through the inguinal canal and emerge at the external inguinal ring) [see Figure 12.4]
      1.   Approximately 75% of abdominal hernias are inguinal; most common type of hernia in both genders but occurs more frequently in men
      2.   Indirect hernias are more common in younger persons since they are due to a congenital defect in which the processus vaginalis remains patent
         a.   However, the incidence of inguinal hernias increases with advancing age and are approximately four times more common after age 50 years than before
         b.   Indirect hernias often enter the scrotum
      3.   Direct hernias occur mainly in the middle and later years of life and are due to a weakness in the abdominal structures. Direct hernias usually reduce and rarely enter the scrotum
      4.   Symptoms of both direct and indirect hernias include a dull ache in the groin and a bulge localized in the groin or extended into the scrotum (referred to as a complete hernia); in women a complete hernia may enter the labia major as a labial hernia

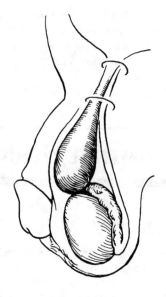

Figure 12.4. Hernia.

Source: Judge, R.D., Zuidma, G.D., & Fitzgerald, F.T. (Eds.). (1989). Clinical diagnosis. Boston: Little, Brown, & Company, p. 381. Reprinted by permission.

   D.   Femoral hernias: Protrusion of omentum through the femoral canal
      1.   Second most common abdominal hernia in both women and men; rare in children
      2.   Occurs 3-5 times more commonly in females than males
      3.   Incidence increases with age and with increased pressure produced by pregnancy and straining
      4.   Risk of strangulation is high
      5.   In women, may have signs of intestinal obstruction

446

E. Incisional hernias: Protrusion of bowel and/or omentum through a surgical incision
   1. Risk factors are post-operative wound infection, dehiscence, malnutrition, obesity, and smoking
   2. Bulge can usually be seen through incision
   3. If not repaired immediately, an intestinal obstruction can develop

F. Umbilical hernias: Protrusion of bowel and/or omentum through the umbilical ring
   1. Also occurs in middle-aged multiparous women, patients with cirrhosis and ascites, chronically ill patients and elderly patients
   2. Infrequently, patient may have vague, intermittent pain and tenderness

G. Epigastric hernias: Protrusion of fat or omentum through the linea alba between the umbilicus and the xiphoid
   1. Most common in men between the ages of 20-50
   2. Presents as small, painless subcutaneous mass

IV. Diagnosis/Evaluation

A. History
   1. Inquire about circumstances and time of onset of hernia
   2. Ask about presence of **alarm markers**: acute onset of colicky abdominal pain, nausea, vomiting (suggests entrapment/strangulation in person with known hernia)
   3. Inquire about groin pain and swelling
   4. Determine whether patient can reduce hernia
   5. Ask about aggravating and alleviating factors (worse with standing, straining, coughing?)

B. Physical examination is directed at determining type of hernia, distinguishing hernias from other causes of inguinal swelling/pain, and identification of hernias that require no therapy, those that should be referred for elective surgery, and those for which emergency surgery is indicated
   1. Patients with reducible hernias should be examined in both standing and supine positions
   2. Carefully inspect abdomen and groin, with and without patients performing Valsalva maneuver
   3. With hernias that are not reducible, assess for discoloration, edema, elevated temperature, tenderness, and signs of bowel obstruction
   4. Do not try to reduce strangulated hernias, because reduction can cause gangrenous bowel to enter the peritoneal cavity
   5. Examination for inguinal hernias involves the following:
      a. In men, if a suspected hernia is not visible the examiner's finger should gently invaginate the scrotum and advance toward the head and laterally into the inguinal canal to the external inguinal ring; then the patient should cough or strain and the examiner should feel for a bulge at the examining finger (see Figure 12.5)
      b. With a direct hernia, when the finger is inserted through the external canal a bulge will be felt striking the side of the finger
      c. With an indirect hernia, when the finger is inserted through the external canal, the bulge will be felt at the finger tip when the patient coughs
      d. In females, it is more difficult to establish the diagnosis of inguinal hernia; locate the external inguinal ring by identifying the inguinal ligament and os pubic; place hand over inguinal ring and palpate for bulge when patient coughs
   6. Femoral hernias are more difficult to diagnose
      a. The external opening of the femoral canal can be located just medial to the femoral artery and deep to the inguinal ligament
      b. Ask patient to cough and palpate for swelling and impulse within the femoral canal
   7. To detect umbilical and incisional hernias, inspect abdomen while patient lifts head from a supine position while bearing down to tense abdominal wall
   8. Check the groin area for lymphadenopathy and other masses that are unchanged with position or Valsalva; groin pain but no mass suggests a musculoskeletal etiology

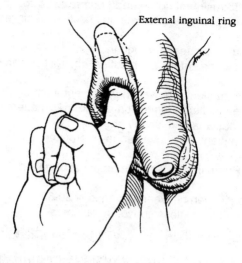

Figure 12.5. Technique of Examination for Inguinal Hernia.

Source: Judge, R.D., Zuidma, G.D., & Fitzgerald, F.T. (Eds.). (1989). <u>Clinical diagnosis</u>. Boston: Little, Brown, & Company, p. 383. Reprinted by permission.

    C.   Differential Diagnosis
         1.   Inguinal hernias (see sections on HYDROCELE and VARICOCELE)
              a.   Hydrocele
              b.   Varicocele
              c.   Spermatocele
              d.   Epididymal cysts
              e.   Epididymitis
              f.   Testicular tumor
              g.   In children, undescended testes
         2.   Femoral hernias
              a.   Enlarged lymph node
               b.   Lipoma
              c.   Direct inguinal hernia
              d.   Saphenous varix
               e.   Psoas abscess
          3.   Other causes of groin pain/swelling include muscle strain, inguinal adenopathy, and hip arthritis
         4.   Incisional, umbilical, and to a lesser extent, epigastric hernias are usually not confused with other conditions

    D.   Diagnostic Tests: Often none needed, may order ultrasound if uncertain about abdominal mass

V.   Plan/Management

    A.   Patients with asymptomatic, easily reducible inguinal hernia can be managed with watchful waiting
         1.   Elective surgery should be considered in younger patients
         2.   Obviously, should signs of incarceration develop, the patient should be referred for surgery

    B.   Patients with symptomatic, reducible inguinal hernia should be referred for elective repair

    C.   Patients with nontender incarcerated inguinal hernia of recent onset, with no signs of inflammation/obstruction, can be referred to a specialist for an attempt at reduction before referral to surgeon

    D.   Patients with reducible femoral hernias should be referred for immediate elective repair because of high rate of strangulation

E. Umbilical hernias in adults must be referred for repair because there is a high risk of incarceration and strangulation

F. Patients with small neck incisional hernias should undergo immediate repair

G. Factors associated with hernia formation should be corrected, if possible

H. Patients who are managed conservatively should receive detailed instruction about symptoms of incarceration and strangulation

I. Follow Up: Return visits will usually occur after surgery; for patients who do not undergo immediate surgery follow up is only needed for problems

ASCARIASIS (ROUNDWORM)

I. Definition: An intestinal parasitic infection caused by *Ascaris lumbricoides*, a large roundworm of humans

II. Pathogenesis

A. Adult worms live in small intestine of humans; ova are excreted in the stool and incubate in soil for 2-3 weeks in order for embryo to form and become infectious

B. Ingestion of infective eggs from soil that is contaminated leads to infection

C. Ingestion occurs from eating food that is unwashed or drinking water contaminated by human feces

D. Interval from ingestion of eggs and development of egg-laying adult worms is about 8 weeks

III. Clinical Presentation

A. Most commonly occurs in the tropics, in areas of poor sanitation, and in areas where human waste is used for fertilizer

B. Worldwide, most common nematode parasite of humans; in US, second only to pinworms in prevalence

C. Most infections are either asymptomatic infections or so mild that the infected person does not present for treatment

D. May cause nausea, vomiting, anorexia, weight loss, fever, irritability, diarrhea, and abdominal cramping

E. Larvae in the lungs may cause cough and wheezing

F. Adult worms may be vomited or passed in the stool

G. Eosinophilia is common

IV. Diagnosis/Evaluation

A. History
   1. Question about anorexia, nausea, vomiting, weight loss, fever, irritability
   2. Ask about pica
   3. Inquire if cough, fever (lung migration) present
   4. Ask if adult worm found in stool

B. Physical Examination
1. Measure weight
2. Perform abdominal exam for tenderness, masses
3. Obtain stool for occult blood

C. Differential Diagnosis
1. Asthma, pneumonia
2. Poor nutrition
3. *Giardiasis*

D. Diagnostic Tests
1. If worm is visualized, none needed
2. Three stool specimens for O&P

V. Plan/Treatment

A. Consult the following table for treatment recommendations

DRUGS FOR TREATMENT OF ASCARIASIS (ROUNDWORM)		
Drug of Choice		**Adult Dosage**
Mebendazole	OR	100 mg BID x 3 days
Pyrantel pamoate	OR	11 mg/kg x 1 dose (Maximum 1 g)
Albendazole		400 mg x 1 dose
In pregnant women, benefits and risks should be considered		

B. In cases of partial or complete intestinal obstructions by worms, piperazine citrate solution (75 mg/kg/day, not to exceed 3.5 g) may be given through a gastrointestinal tube

C. Sanitary disposal of feces should be emphasized

D. Follow Up
1. Not essential
2. Re-examination of stools 3 weeks after therapy to determine treatment efficacy may be helpful

PINWORM INFESTATION (ENTEROBIASIS VERMICULARIS)

I. Definition: An intestinal parasitic infection caused by *Enterobius vermicularis*, a white, threadlike worm for whom humans are the only hosts

II. Pathogenesis

A. Worms live primarily in the cecum and adjacent bowel

B. Adult gravid females, which are about 1 cm in length, migrate to perianal area to deposit eggs on perianal skin and then die

C. Infection would be self-limited at that point were it not for re-infestation

D. Transmission occurs via various routes, but primarily through fecal-oral route with worm eggs transmitted by fingers and via fomites such as toys, bedding, and toilet seats

E. Infection must be acquired from others by ingesting the ova

F. Incubation period from ingestion of egg until an adult worm migrates to perianal area is about 1-2 months

G. Eggs are fairly hardy and can remain infective in an indoor environment for 2-3 weeks; however, most eggs die within a day

III. Clinical Presentation

A. Occurs worldwide and commonly in family clusters; incidence appears to have declined over past few decades

B. Prevalence rates are highest in preschoolers, in school-aged children, in mothers of infected children, and in the institutionalized

C. Perianal pruritus with secondary excoriation and dermatitis is common; rarely, pruritus vulvae occurs

D. Restlessness, insomnia, and loss of weight and appetite may occur

E. Bruxism or teeth grinding is not due to pinworms, contrary to popular opinion

F. In general, pinworms cause no serious problems

IV. Diagnosis/Evaluation

A. History
   1. Inquire about time of and circumstances surrounding onset of symptoms
   2. Ask if anal pruritus is present
   3. In females, question about genital irritation
   4. Ask if others in household have similar symptoms

B. Physical Examination
   1. Focus on exam of anus; may be excoriated from scratching
   2. In females, also examine for genital irritation

C. Differential Diagnosis
   1. Poor hygiene
   2. Chemical irritants, such as bubble bath

D. Diagnostic Tests: Technique for detection follows

USING CELLOPHANE TAPE TO DETECT PINWORM EGGS

✔ Instruct patients in the following technique
   ✗ First thing in the morning, either immediately before or immediately after arising, is the best time to obtain specimen
   ✗ Using cellophane tape that is transparent, apply the tape to the perianal skin
   ✗ Cover tape with specimen with a second piece of tape and place in plastic bag for transport to office/lab
✔ Technician affixes specimen to slide (using more tape if necessary)
   ✗ Slide is then scanned under low power for eggs (eggs are 50 x 30 μg, oval, flat on one side, and thin-shelled)
     ✦ A single specimen usually detects 50% of infestations
     ✦ Three tests will detect 90%
     ✦ Five tests will detect almost 100%

V.   Plan/Treatment

    A.   Consult the following table for treatment recommendations

    B.   No unusual cleaning or hygienic measures are required, but the following common sense recommendations should be followed
        1.   Keep nails trimmed short as eggs may lodge under nails with scratching
        2.   Wash hands frequently, and always on arising, before eating, and after toileting
        3.   Morning showers will wash away any eggs deposited during the night
        4.   Application of bland ointment such as petroleum jelly to the perianal area may help with dispersion of eggs

    C.   There is a high incidence of reinfections particularly in child care centers and schools; repeated infections should be treated the same as initial one

DRUGS FOR TREATMENT OF PINWORMS	
Drug of Choice	**Adult Dosage**
Pyrantel pamoate OR	11 mg/kg x 1 dose (Maximum 1 g) Repeat in 2 weeks
Mebendazole OR	100 mg x 1 dose Repeat in 2 weeks
Albendazole	400 mg x 1 dose Repeat in 2 weeks
In pregnant women, benefits and risks should be considered	

    D.   Families may need to be treated as a group

    E.   Follow Up: None indicated

VISCERAL LARVA MIGRANS (HOOKWORM)

I.   Definition: An intestinal parasitic infection caused by *Ancylostoma duodenale* and *Necator americanus*, two worms with similar life cycles

II.   Pathogenesis

    A.   Larval penetration into skin, usually soles of feet, palms of hands, occurs via contact with contaminated soil

    B.   Eggs pass out with the stools of infected persons and hatch into larvae that become infective for humans; contact with contaminated soil for 5-10 minutes results in skin penetration

    C.   Larvae are carried by the circulation to the lungs and eventually arrive in their final habitat, the small intestine

    D.   Incubation period is about 4-6 weeks

III. Clinical Presentation

A. Humans are the major reservoir and the disease is prevalent in rural, tropical and subtropical areas where soil is contaminated with human waste

B. Intense pruritus can occur at the site of larvae penetration into skin; a papulovesicular eruption lasting for 1-2 weeks also commonly occurs

C. Abdominal pain with diarrhea and eosinophilia may occur about 1 month after onset of infection

D. Chronic infection can result in anemia secondary to blood loss

E. Pulmonary infiltration with cough and wheezing can occur in heavily infected individuals

F. Many infected persons who are otherwise healthy are often asymptomatic

IV. Diagnosis/Evaluation

A. History
   1. Inquire about episodes of intense pruritus of feet, palms of hands, and buttocks in recent past
   2. Inquire about presence of papulovesicular rash on area of skin where initial penetration was likely
   3. Inquire about transitory chest symptoms (cough, wheezing)
   4. Inquire about abdominal pain, diarrhea, and weight loss

B. Physical Examination
   1. Examine skin for erythematous papular vesicular lesions that may be excoriated from scratching. Usually located on feet, hands, or upper thighs (from sitting in sand, dirt)
   2. Abdominal exam for masses, tenderness
   3. Chest exam for wheezing

C. Differential Diagnosis
   1. Asthma, pneumonia
   2. Poor nutrition
   3. *Giardia*

D. Diagnostic Tests:
   1. Stool for O & P x 3
   2. Microscopic examination of stools that reveal hookworm eggs in feces is diagnostic
   3. Potassium iodide saturated with iodine can be used to better visualize the eggs in the fecal smear

V. Plan/Management

A. Consult the following table for treatment recommendations

DRUGS FOR TREATMENT OF HOOKWORM INFECTION		
Drug of Choice		**Adult Dosage**
Mebendazole	OR	100 mg BID x 3 days
Pyrantel pamoate	OR	11 mg/kg (Maximum 1 g) x 3 days
Albendazole		400 mg x 1 dose
In pregnant women, benefits and risks should be considered		

B.	Sanitary disposal of human waste to prevent contamination of the soil is of paramount importance, particularly in endemic areas; wearing shoes is also helpful

C.	Follow Up
1.	A repeat stool exam should be performed 2 weeks posttreatment
2.	If positive, re-treatment is indicated

IRRITABLE BOWEL SYNDROME

I.	Definition: Chronic, benign gastrointestinal disorder characterized by abdominal pain, bloating, and disturbed defecation in the absence of structural or biochemical abnormalities with no inflammatory component and no underlying identifiable organic cause

II.	Pathogenesis

A.	Considered a functional disorder which by definition is a disorder in which symptoms are not explained by structural or biochemical abnormalities

B.	Symptoms characteristic of irritable bowel syndrome (IBS) are believed to result from disturbances in intestinal motility and enhanced visceral sensitivity

C.	While the symptoms of IBS do have a physiologic basis, a physiologic mechanism **unique** to IBS has not been identified

D.	Psychosocial factors have an important role in modulating the illness experience and thereby affecting the clinical outcome

III.	Clinical Presentation

A.	Irritable Bowel Syndrome (IBS) is a common malady occurring in about 15% of the population, with symptoms most often appearing during late teens, early adulthood

B.	Women are affected more often than men (2:1); IBS accounts for 50% of all referrals to gastroenterologists

C.	Most common presentation is that of abdominal pain and bloating along with altered bowel habits with either diarrhea or constipation predominating

D.	Pattern of symptoms varies from person to person but symptoms are generally mild to moderate with little disability

E.	Symptoms are most often intermittent, though some patients have daily problems and a small percentage of patients are refractory to treatment, with pain that is disabling

F.	The symptom-based diagnostic classification system known as the *Rome criteria* can be helpful in evaluating patients and are contained in the following table

---

SYMPTOMS OF IRRITABLE BOWEL SYNDROME USED AS DIAGNOSTIC CRITERIA

Continuous or recurrent abdominal pain or discomfort for at least a 3 month period that is
- ✦ Relieved with defecation and/or
- ✦ Associated with a change in frequency of stooling and/or
- ✦ Associated with a change in consistency of stool

PLUS

Two or more of the following that occur at least a quarter of the time
- ✦ Altered stool frequency (more than 3 bowel movements/day or fewer than 3 bowel movements/week)
- ✦ Altered stool passage (straining, urgency, feeling of incomplete evacuation)
- ✦ Altered stool form (lumpy/hard or loose/watery)
- ✦ Feeling of abdominal distension or bloating
- ✦ Passage of mucus

Adapted from Drossman, D.A. (1995). Diagnosing and treating patients with refractory functional gastrointestinal disorders. Annals of Internal Medicine, 123, 688-697.

IV.   Diagnosis/Evaluation

    A.   History
        1.   Ask about onset, duration, location, and severity of abdominal pain and changes over time
        2.   Ask questions relating to diagnostic criteria outlined above
            a.   Has the abdominal pain/discomfort been present for at least 3 months on a continuous or recurrent basis?
                (1)   Is pain relieved with defecation?
                (2)   Is pain associated with a change in frequency of stool?
                (3)   Is pain associated with change in consistency of stool?
            b.   Regarding stooling quality and pattern, ask the patient if two or more of the following are present at least 25% of time
                (1)   Is there altered stool frequency?
                (2)   Is there altered stool form, that is lumpy and hard or loose and watery?
                (3)   Is there altered stool passage?
                (4)   Is there passage of mucus?
                (5)   Is there a feeling of bloating or distension?
        3.   If diarrhea is present, question about blood in diarrhea, awakening in night because of diarrhea (if positive response to either question, points to inflammatory bowel disease rather than IBS)
        4.   Question about weight loss (significant weight loss should not occur with IBS)
        5.   Inquire if any stresses occurred at time the disorder appeared or intensified
        6.   Obtain diet history to determine usual diet and eating patterns
        7.   Ask about drug/alcohol use/present medications used
        8.   Ask detailed questions about previous diagnostic evaluations by other health care providers
        9.   Ask about treatments tried and results
        10.   Ask about the impact of the disorder on daily functioning
        11.   In women, take menstrual history

    B.   Physical Examination
        1.   Determine if weight loss has occurred
        2.   Perform abdominal exam for tenderness (usually present in left lower quadrant), guarding, rigidity, abnormal bowel sounds, masses, liver or spleen enlargement
        3.   Perform rectal exam for tenderness, masses; stool for occult blood
        4.   **Note:** The physical exam serves mainly to exclude other diagnoses and to reassure the patient

    C.   Differential Diagnosis
        1.   Ulcerative colitis
        2.   Crohn's disease
        3.   Lactose intolerance

4. Diverticulitis
5. Gastroenteritis
6. Psychiatric disorder

D. Diagnostic Tests
1. CBC and sedimentation rate
2. Fecal occult blood x 6
3. Stool for O&P x 3
4. Stool for culture, leukocytes, and fecal fat
5. If symptoms are severe, or diagnosis is uncertain, sigmoidoscopy and barium enema are necessary or colonoscopy if >50 years of age

V. Plan/Management

A. For patients with typical presentation (no significant weight loss, no occult blood in stool, no abnormal physical findings) symptomatic treatment with consideration to both physiologic and psychosocial factors should be offered with the plan being to evaluate the patient's response in 3-6 weeks

B. Approach to management should be guided by individual patient characteristics that can be determined by evaluating the patient response to several key questions

---

KEY QUESTIONS TO ASK IN THE EVALUATION OF PATIENTS WITH IBS

Is there a pain history?
Does the patient have a long-standing pattern of pain behaviors, such as frequent headaches, back pain, dysmenorrhea that treatment has been sought for?
✔ If yes, the patient's prognosis is poorer than if response is "no"

What is the patient's understanding of the condition?
Ask "What do you think is causing your symptoms?" and "What do you hope I can do for you?"
✔ Patient's who are not satisfied by negative findings
✔ who are convinced there must be an organic basis for symptoms
✔ who are unrealistic in their expectations for treatment
✔ will continue to seek new diagnostic tests and treatments

Does the patient understand and accept the fact that stress may play a contributing role?
✔ Persons who have a tendency to deny or minimize the psychological effect of stressful life events more often seek care than do those who have insight into the role that mood disturbances have on symptoms such as gastrointestinal pain
✔ Those with insight are often able to manage the condition on their own (**Note:** Estimates are that up to 70% of persons with IBS do not seek medical attention)

Does that patient have abnormal illness behavior?
✔ Patients who are eager to adopt the "sick role," who relentlessly search to validate the existence of disease, and who place responsibility for "cure" on the health care provider have abnormal illness behavior which interferes with optimal management

Is the family's involvement associated with emotional support and oriented toward recovery and health?
✔ Families who pay undue attention to the condition as a mechanism for avoiding family problems that arise need counseling

What is the reason for this visit or referral?
Ask "What led you to come into see me at this time?"
✔ Clarify the reason that patient is seeking help at this time as he/she has had the symptoms for a while (in most cases)

What are the patient's coping mechanisms?
✔ Factors that promote health and buffer the effects of stress need to be identified as these are associated with improved outcomes

---

Adapted from Drossman, D.A. (1995). Diagnosing and treating patients with refractory functional gastrointestinal disorders. Annals of Internal Medicine, 123, 688-697.

C. Establishment of an effective patient-provider relationship based on patient education and reassurance is important
1. Use the KEY QUESTIONS in the above table to determine patient's understanding of illness and then to provide a thorough explanation of the disorder

2. Use the KEY QUESTIONS in the previous table to identify and respond to the patient's concerns and expectations and to set realistic and consistent limits

3. Use the KEY QUESTIONS in the previous table to determine why help is being sought at this time and if there is a hidden agenda such as drug-seeking, pending disability, or secondary gain

4. Recognize that research shows that 30-88% of patients with IBS have a positive response to treatment regardless of the treatment used; this demonstrates the value of an effective patient-provider relationship

D. Set realistic treatment goals in which the patient takes responsibility for own care
1. One approach is to use of a symptom diary for several weeks in which patient records symptom, date/time of occurrence, description of severity (scale of 1-10), factors associated with symptom (diet, activity, menses, stressful event, etc.); emotional responses (what person feels); thoughts and cognition (what person thinks)
2. Review diary with patient on each return visit as a way of evaluating his/her progress in "gaining control" of the condition

E. Severity of symptoms and degree of disability dictate treatment plan; most patients with IBS have mild to moderate symptoms and can be managed in primary care settings
1. For patients with predominant diarrhea,
   a. Increasing soluble fiber intake helps to bulk up the stool and improve quality of bowel movements (**Note:** Increasing fiber can cause bloating so recommend with caution)
   b. Use of antidiarrheal agents such as loperamide, 2-4 mg QID can be helpful
2. For patients with predominant constipation,
   a. Increase dietary fiber to 20-30 grams/day
   b. Laxative use should be strongly discouraged, but if laxatives must be used on an occasional basis, osmotic laxatives such as lactulose are preferred (see section on CONSTIPATION for dosing)
3. For patients with predominant pain or gas syndromes,
   a. Elimination of gas-forming foods may be helpful (lactose, legumes, broccoli, cauliflower, brussel sprouts, onions, cucumbers); if symptoms improve, these foods can be gradually reintroduced
   b. Dicyclomine (Bentyl), 10-20 mg TID or QID acts mainly on smooth muscle and may have fewer side effects than nonselective anticholinergic agents

F. Discuss with all patients modifications in lifestyle that can improve symptoms
1. Stress reduction is important, and can be accomplished via the use of relaxation tapes, books, or meditation taught by behavioral therapists
2. Biofeedback can sometimes help decrease stress and reduce gut hypersensitivity
3. Regular exercise can also reduce stress and increase feelings of well-being; can also improve bowel transit

G. For patients with IBS symptoms (particularly abdominal pain) that are moderate to severe and are associated with impaired quality of life and psychologic distress, consider prescribing antidepressants
1. Selective serotonin reuptake inhibitors (SSRIs) are the drug of choice because of their low side-effect profile and better safety compared with tricyclic antidepressants
2. Referral to a mental health specialist is recommended for patients suspected of having an associated psychiatric disorder or a history of abuse

H. Follow Up: In 3-6 weeks; then every 3-6 months

NAUSEA AND VOMITING

I.   Definition

    A.   Nausea: An unpleasant feeling in the throat or epigastric region alerting one that vomiting is imminent

    B.   Vomiting: The forceful expulsion of gastric contents through the mouth

II.   Pathogenesis

    A.   Three consecutive phases of emesis include nausea, retching, and vomiting

    B.   Vomiting is triggered by afferent impulses received in the vomiting center (VC) believed to be located in the medulla

    C.   Sensory centers such as the cerebral cortex, visceral afferents from the pharynx and gastrointestinal tract, and the chemoreceptor trigger zone (CTZ) are responsible for sending the impulses to the vomiting center

    D.   Once the VC is stimulated, efferent pathways to the salivation center, respiratory center, and the pharyngeal, GI, and abdominal musculature work in concert to produce vomiting

III. Clinical Presentation

    A.   Nausea and vomiting are among the most common symptoms that children and adults experience and may be associated with a variety of clinical presentations

    B.   May be evoked by disorders of the gastrointestinal tract and may also be caused by neurologic, endocrine, metabolic, psychogenic, iatrogenic, and toxic conditions

    C.   Common causes
        1.   Gastrointestinal mechanisms (examples of common causes only)
            a.   Acute gastroenteritis, both viral and bacterial
            b.   Peptic ulcer disease/gastritis
            c.   Motility disorders such as gastroparesis, drug-induced gastric stasis, irritable bowel syndrome
            d.   Intraabdominal emergencies such as appendicitis, obstruction, pancreatitis, cholecystitis
        2.   Central nervous system causes (examples of common causes only)
            a.   Motion sickness
            b.   Migraine headache
        3.   Systemic causes (examples of common causes only)
            a.   Pregnancy
            b.   Infections/food poisoning
            c.   Drug overdose
        4.   Iatrogenic causes: (examples)
            a.   Medications such as antibiotics, theophylline, digitalis, and antineoplastic agents
            b.   Bulimia

    D.   Vomiting rapidly produces dehydration in the debilitated and elderly

IV.   Diagnosis/Evaluation

    A.   History
        1.   Question about onset, duration, quantity and quality of vomitus (undigested food, blood)
        2.   Ask about timing of vomiting with respect to meals and presence of associated symptoms such as abdominal pain, diarrhea, dizziness, headache
        3.   Ask if systemic symptoms of fever and malaise are present
        4.   Ask about past medical history and medication history
        5.   Ask if others in household are ill to identify a common source cause

    B.   Physical Examination
        1.   Determine if febrile
        2.   Assess hydration status: Check for dry mucous membranes, decreased skin turgor, tachycardia, and oliguria
        3.   Assess cardiovascular status (pulse, blood pressure; check for postural hypotension)
        4.   Examine abdomen for tenderness, rigidity, abnormal tympany, bowel sounds, liver and spleen size
        5.   Perform rectal exam for tenderness, masses; stool for occult blood

    C.   Differential Diagnosis: Vomiting is a symptom.; see Pathogenesis for possible causes

    D.   Laboratory Tests
        1.   If no systemic signs and symptoms, and duration <24 hours, no lab studies indicated
        2.   If vomiting persists longer than 24 hours, consider following laboratory tests
             a.   Serum chemistries to document acid-base, electrolyte status
             b.   Glucose
             c.   HCG
             d.   Amylase
             e.   Drug levels, if indicated

V.   Plan/Management

    A.   Identification of most likely cause dictates therapy

    B.   Most episodes of nausea and vomiting are self-limiting and supportive therapy is all that is indicated

    C.   Nonpharmacologic interventions:

NONPHARMACOLOGIC INTERVENTIONS

- ✓ Discontinue solid foods
- ✓ Encourage clear liquids only (not milk) until at least 4 hours have passed without vomiting
- ✓ Start with 1 tbsp (15 cc) every 10 minutes
- ✓ If vomiting does not occur, double the amount each hour
- ✓ If vomiting does occur, allow stomach to rest briefly and then start again
- ✓ Key is to gradually increase amount of fluid until taking 8 oz every hour
- ✓ May use glucose-electrolyte solutions developed for infants/small children such as Pedialyte or Rehydralyte (May combine with flavored gelatin to make more palatable) or sports drinks such as Gatorade
- ✓ Resume regular diet as soon as tolerated (usually, 4 hours after vomiting stops)

    D.   Pharmacologic therapy is usually not indicated; however, for selected patients (for example, those with electrolyte disturbances, severe anorexia/weight loss, motion sickness, pregnancy, or with chemotherapy-induced nausea and vomiting) antiemetic therapy may be indicated
        1.   Emetrol (OTC): Do not dilute or take fluids 15 minutes before or after. Can be used in pregnancy: 15-30 mL at 15 minute intervals as needed
        2.   Promethazine (Phenergan) is the agent of choice for n/v from gastroenteritis: Available as 12.5, 25, 50 mg tabs and rectal supp; also available as syrup (6.25 mg/5 mL and 25 mg/5 mL). Dosing: 25 mg Q 8-12 hrs

3. Prochlorperazine (Compazine): Available 5, 10 mg tabs; 10, 15, 30 mg spanules; 5 mg/5 mL syrup; 2.5, 5, 25 mg rectal supp: Tabs/5-10 mg 3-4 times day. Dosing: Spanules/10mg Q 12 hrs; rectal supp/25 mg BID

4. Trimethobenzamide (Tigan) works well for gastroenteritis and motion sickness: Available as 100, 250 mg caps and rectal supp--adult/100, 200 mg; pediatric/100 mg. Dosing: 250 mg caps OR 200 mg rectal supp 3-4 x day

E. Follow Up: None needed unless failure to respond to nonpharmacologic or pharmacologic therapy

PEPTIC ULCER DISEASE

I. Definition: A circumscribed ulceration of the gastrointestinal mucosa occurring in areas exposed to acid and pepsin

II. Pathogenesis

A. The initial step in the development of a peptic ulcer is a mucosal defect

B. Once the defect occurs, the presence of both acid and pepsin are necessary for ulcer formation

C. In the majority of cases of both duodenal and gastric ulcer, infection with *Helicobacter pylori* produces damage to the mucosa and thus is causally related to ulcer development (**Note:** Most persons infected with *H. pylori* do not develop ulcers)

D. The second most common cause of peptic ulcer formation is damage to the mucosa caused by use of nonsteroidal anti-inflammatory drugs (NSAIDs); two mechanisms are involved:
1. NSAIDs damage the mucosa through a direct action
2. A systemic effect also occurs whereby endogenous prostaglandin synthesis is inhibited

E. Uncommon etiologies such as gastrinoma, mastocytosis, and annular pancreas account for some ulcer formation

F. A small minority of ulcers remain in the idiopathic category

III. Clinical Presentation

A. Peptic ulcer disease (PUD) affects approximately 10% of Americans and is a significant cause of morbidity and mortality

B. Historically, PUD has affected males and females in a 2:1 ratio, but recently the occurrence has been declining in young men and increasing in women

C. Duodenal ulcers (DU) have the following characteristics
1. Much more common than gastric ulcers
2. Rarely harbor malignancy
3. Associated with *H. pylori* infection in 95% of cases

D. Gastric ulcers (GU) have the following characteristics
1. About 2-4% of gastric ulcers harbor malignancy
2. Associated with *H. pylori* infection in most cases
3. NSAID related ulcers are more likely to be gastric than duodenal

E. Epigastric distress is the classic and most common symptom; if actual pain occurs, it is typically aching or burning

F.   Other dyspeptic symptoms such as nausea, vomiting, belching, and bloating also occur

G.   Classically, distress of duodenal ulcer occurs 1-3 hours after meal and may awaken patient from sleep in early morning. Pain is relieved by food, antacids, or vomiting (distress-food-relief pattern)

H.   In gastric ulcer, the presentation is more variable
   1.   A similar distress-food-relief pattern may exist
   2.   In other cases, food makes the discomfort worse or there is no change with food
   3.   Nausea, vomiting, anorexia, and weight loss are more common in GU than in DU

I.   The elderly and patients with NSAID-induced ulcers are often symptom free until bleeding or perforation occur

J.   Cigarette smoking increases gastric acid secretion thereby increasing the risk of occurrence and recurrence of DU and GU

K.   Cause and effect relationship between stress and ulcer development has not been demonstrated

L.   Diet has no role in causing ulcers, but certain foods exacerbate symptoms in some people; alcohol ingestion can cause acute gastritis and may interfere with healing

IV.   Diagnosis/Evaluation

   A.   History
      1.   Question about presence, location of distress/pain
      2.   If distress/pain are present, determine onset, duration, character of pain, and effect of food/antacids on pain
      3.   Ask about associated symptoms of nausea, vomiting, and heartburn
      4.   Question about presence of alarm markers: anorexia, early satiety, weight loss, gastrointestinal bleeding (black stools)
      5.   Obtain past medical history for associated diseases such as cirrhosis, pancreatitis, arthritis, COPD, hyperparathyroidism
      6.   Obtain social history, specifically, smoking, alcohol use, stress in family and at work
      7.   Ask about regular use of NSAIDs, oral corticosteroids
      8.   Inquire about PUD in first-degree relatives

   B.   Physical Examination
      1.   Perform abdominal exam for tenderness (specifically in epigastric area), rigidity, abnormal bowel sounds, masses, liver/spleen enlargement
      2.   Do rectal exam for tenderness, masses; obtain stool for occult blood

   C.   Differential Diagnosis
      1.   Neoplasm of the stomach
      2.   Pancreatitis
      3.   Diverticulitis
      4.   Nonulcer dyspepsia

   D.   Diagnostic Tests
      1.   All patients should receive the following tests to detect bleeding
         a.   Stool hemoccult
         b.   Hemoglobin/hematocrit
      2.   Management options outlined in V.A. (below) determine criteria for additional diagnostic testing
         a.   Option 1: Endoscopy if treatment failure
         b.   Option 2: Endoscopy for definitive diagnosis
         c.   Option 3: Test for *H. pylori* using serology, urea breath test, or endoscopic biopsy

V. Plan/Management

A. Three options are available for management of new-onset dyspepsia that is determined not to be related to NSAID ingestion (**Note:** if patient is taking NSAIDs regularly, this should be discontinued and the patient reassessed after several weeks)

    1. **Option 1**: A single, short term trial of empiric treatment with antisecretory drugs, either an H_2 receptor antagonist or proton pump inhibitor (see tables below)

        a. If symptoms fail to resolve after 2 weeks, the patient should receive a workup

        b. If symptoms resolve, the treatment should be continued for a total of 6-8 weeks and then discontinued; at that point, if symptoms recur, a workup should be performed

        c. This option is recommended for patients who are reliable and in settings where follow-up is certain

    2. **Option 2**: A definitive diagnostic evaluation should be conducted

        a. This option must **always** be followed for patients who present with **alarm markers** (anemia, anorexia, early satiety, weight loss, or gastrointestinal bleeding)

        b. This option must also always be followed for patients with new onset of dyspepsia who are over the age of 50

        c. Upper endoscopy is the diagnostic approach of choice

    3. **Option 3**: Noninvasive testing for *H. pylori*

        a. In patients who are positive for *H. pylori*, antibiotics should be given

        b. The cost effectiveness of empirical antibiotic administration (after confirming the presence of *H. pylori* but not of an ulcer), is unknown

        c. Patients with nonulcer dyspepsia have a variable response to antibiotics (**Note:** Only about 15-30% of *H. pylori* positive patients have underlying peptic ulcer)

        d. With this option, definitive workup is reserved for those patients whose symptoms recur after antibiotic therapy

B. Presently, empiric antibiotic therapy without *H. pylori* testing is discouraged for two reasons

    1. Prevalence of *H. pylori* is likely to be much less than 50%, particularly in younger patients with dyspepsia

    2. Wide-spread use of antibiotics carries risks of morbidity in the patient and development of antibiotic resistance among populations

C. Option 1: EMPIRIC TREATMENT WITH ANTISECRETORY DRUGS is described in the following table

---

EMPIRIC TREATMENT WITH ANTISECRETORY DRUGS

Treatment With H_2 Receptor Antagonists

Four agents presently available Equally effective when prescribed in equipotent doses All 4 agents are relatively expensive Can be given in split-dose, evening, or nighttime doses Fewer drug interactions with famotidine and nizatidine	Cimetidine (Tagamet) 800 mg daily at bedtime or 400 mg BID for up to 8 weeks Famotidine (Pepcid) 40 mg daily at bedtime or 20 mg BID for up to 8 weeks Nizatidine (Axid) 300 mg daily at bedtime or 150 mg BID for up to 8 weeks Ranitidine (Zantac) 300 mg daily at bedtime or 150 mg BID for up to 8 weeks

Proton-Pump Inhibitors

Two agents presently available Both are expensive Require activation in the acidic compartments of the stimulated parietal cell Thus, should not be given in fasting state or at bedtime **Most effective** when given 30 minutes **before meals**	Omeprazole (Prilosec), 20 mg QD, 30 minutes before a meal Lansoprazole (Prevacid), 15 mg QD, 30 minutes before a meal

D.   Option 3: Antibiotic treatment recommendations and tips for selection of treatment regimens are contained in the following tables

REGIMENS FOR *H. PYLORI* CURE: DRUG COMBINATIONS, DURATION OF TREATMENT, AND CURE RATES				
Medications	Dose	Frequency	Duration	Cure Rate
Bismuth Subsalicylate	2 tabs	All taken QID (With meals and at bedtime)	1 week	86-90%
Metronidazole	250 mg			
Tetracycline	500 mg			
Same drugs, dosing, and frequency			2 weeks	88-90%
Add omeprazole, 20 mg BID (before meals) to the above regimen			1 week	94-98%
Bismuth Subsalicylate	2 tabs	All taken QID (With meals and at bedtime)	1 week	75-81%
Metronidazole	250 mg			
Amoxicillin	500 mg			
Same drugs, dosing, and frequency			2 weeks	80-86%
Metronidazole	500 mg	BID (With meals)	1 week	87-91%
Clarithromycin	500 mg	BID (with meals)		
Omeprazole	20 mg	BID (before meals & Loading dose*)		
*Loading dose: 20 mg omeprazole TID given the day prior to beginning antibiotic therapy				
Amoxicillin	1 gram	BID (with meals)	1 week	86-91%
Clarithromycin	500 mg	BID (with meals)		
Omeprazole	20 mg	BID (before meals & Loading dose*)		
*Loading dose: 20 mg omeprazole TID given the day prior to beginning antibiotic therapy				

Adapted from: Soll, A.H. (1996). Consensus statement: Medical treatment of peptic ulcer disease: Practice guidelines. <u>JAMA,</u> <u>275</u>, 622-629.

FDA-APPROVED TREATMENT REGIMENS FOR *H. PYLORI* INFECTION
The following five combinations have been approved by the FDA for treatment of *H. pylori* infection (**Note:** The five are considered to be equally effective)

Regimen 1	Omeprazole 40 mg QD PLUS clarithromycin 500 mg TID x 2 weeks, FOLLOWED BY monotherapy with omeprazole 20 mg QD x 2 more weeks
Regimen 2	Ranitidine bismuth citrate (Tritec) 400 mg BID PLUS clarithromycin 500 mg TID x 2 weeks, FOLLOWED BY Ranitidine bismuth citrate 400 mg BID for 2 weeks
Regimen 3	Bismuth subsalicylate 525 mg QID PLUS metronidazole 250 mg QID AND tetracycline 500 mg QID x 2 weeks PLUS H$_2$ receptor-antagonist (dose as directed) x 4 weeks
Regimen 4	Lansoprazole, 30 mg BID PLUS amoxicillin, 1 g BID AND clarithromycin, 500 mg BID x 14 days
Regimen 5	Lansoprazole, 30 mg TID PLUS amoxicillin, 1 g TID x 14 days (**Note:** This regimen is only indicated for patients unable to tolerate clarithromycin or for infection with strains known to be clarithromycin resistant)

Source: Centers for Disease Control and Prevention, Bacterial and Mycotic Disease Division. (1998). [On-line]. Available: www.cdc.gov/ncidod/dbmd/hpylori.htm.

E.   Prevpac, a daily administration pack containing 2 Prevacid 30 mg caps, 4 amoxicillin 500 mg caps, and 2 clarithromycin 500 mg tabs, has recently become available to simplify triple therapy prescribing and dispensing. Patients should be prescribed 14 packs

TIPS FOR SELECTION OF TREATMENT REGIMEN: IMPORTANT CONSIDERATIONS	
Problem	**Solution**
Keep in mind the following:	
Antibiotic resistance is a problem ✗ **With** metronidazole and clarithromycin ✗ **Not with** bismuth, amoxicillin, or tetracycline	**Prior antibiotic exposure** predicts resistance in individual patients ✗ **Select** regimen based on medication history in the patient to reduce chance of resistance ✗ **Or** select antibiotics without resistance problems
Adverse effects associated with antibiotics ✗ **Rarely**, significant events such as pseudomembranous colitis or drug reactions occur ✗ **More commonly**, minor adverse events such as diarrhea with amoxicillin, nausea with metronidazole, metallic taste with metronidazole and clarithromycin, and black stools with bismuth can create problems	**Consider** the shorter treatment period of one week ✗ **Educate** the patient regarding what might occur in terms of adverse events
Poor patient compliance because of complex treatment regimens	**Educate** patient regarding importance of compliance ✗ **Anticipate** adverse events (as above)

F. Counsel all patients regarding the following lifestyle changes
   1. Patient should discontinue use of NSAIDs, unless use is absolutely necessary (see G. below)
   2. All patients who smoke should stop
   3. No dietary restrictions are necessary unless certain foods are associated with problems
   4. Alcohol should be used in moderate amounts (no more than 1-2 drinks/day) and with food
   5. Consider using stress reduction techniques which may improve the quality of life for some patients

G. Prevention of NSAID ulcers
   1. Consider preventive therapy for patients taking NSAIDs based on risk factors
   2. Patients with a prior history of ulcer disease, who are using NSAIDs with steroids or anticoagulants, or who have coexisting conditions that would seriously limit ability to cope with ulcer complications are appropriate candidates for preventive cotherapy with an antiulcer agent
   3. Misoprostol (Cytotec) is the only drug that is FDA approved for prevention of NSAID-induced ulcers
      a. Usual dose is 200 mg PO QID
      b. Diarrhea and abdominal cramps are common adverse reactions and limit patient compliance
      c. Start therapy with lower doses and advance to therapeutic level to limit these GI adverse effects which are usually transient
   4. There are no other approved therapies for patients who fail this therapy
   5. Nabumetone (Relafen) and etocolac (Lodine) may have a decreased risk of causing ulcers but the research is inconclusive

H. Follow Up
   1. Confirming cure is necessary in patients with history of complicated or refractory ulcers but remains controversial in patients with uncomplicated ulcers who remain asymptomatic
      a. Urea breath tests are a noninvasive way to establish cure, but false negatives occur about 10% of time
      b. Serum antibody titers of *H. pylori* can be measured with falling titers as evidence for eradication, but this method is not always reliable
      c. Repeat endoscopy and biopsy reliably confirm cure, but expensive and while necessary with complicated ulcers may not be justifiable to use in others
      d. If confirmation of cure is indicated, none of the above tests should be done until at least 1 month after treatment and preferably longer
   2. Patients who remain symptomatic after treatment outlined above should be referred to a specialist for management

REFERENCES

American Academy of Pediatrics. (1997). Red book: Report of the committee on infectious diseases (24th ed.). Elk Grove Village, IL: Author.

Bonis, P.A., & Norton, R.A. (1996). The challenge of irritable bowel syndrome. American Family Physician, 53, 1229-1236.

Brady, W.M. (1997). Controversies in diagnosis and treatment of hepatitis C. Postgraduate Medicine, 102 (5), 201-206.

Centers for Disease Control. (1997). Immunization of health care workers. MMWR, 46, RR-18.

Damianos, A.J., & McGarrity, T.J. (1997). Treatment strageties for Helicobacter pylori infection. American Family Physician, 55, 2765-2774.

DiPiro, J.T. (1998). Gastrointestinal disorders. In B.G. Wells, J.T. Dipiro, T.L. Schwinghammer, & C.W. Hamilton (Eds.), Pharmacotherapy handbook. Stamford, CT:Appleton & Lange.

Drossman, D.A. (1995). Diagnosing and treating patients with refractory functional gastrointestinal disorders. Annals of Internal Medicine, 123, 688-697.

Drossman, D.A., Whitehead, W.E., & Camilleri, M. (1997). Irritable bowel syndrome: A technical review for practice guideline development. Gastroenterology, 112, 2118-2137.

Fass, R., Hixson, L.J., Ciccolo, M.L., Gordon, P., Hunter, G., & Rappaport, W. (1997). Contemporary medical therapy for gastroesophageal reflux disease. American Family Physician, 35 (1), 205-212.

Graber, M.A. (1998). Dealing with acute abdominal pain: Part 1: Clues to the diagnosis. Emergency Medicine, 30(2), 74-100.

Greenberger, N.J. (1997). Update in gastroenterology. Annals of Internal Medicine, 127, 827-834.

Hillemeier, A.C. (1996). Gastroesophageal reflux: Diagnostic and therapeutic approaches. Pediatric Clinics of North America, 43(1), 197-210.

Hoofnagle, J.H., & Bisceglie, A.M. (1997). The treatment of chronic viral hepatitis. New England Journal of Medicine, 336, 347-355.

Immunization Action Coalition. (1997). Basic facts about adult hepatitis. St. Paul, MN: Author.

Johnson, D.A. (1997). Gastroesophageal reflux disease: Short-term management strategies. Consultant, 1329-1334.

Margolies, M.N. (1995). Approach to the patient with an external hernia. In A.H. Goroll, L.A. May, & A.G. Mulley, Jr. (Eds.), Primary care medicine. Philadelphia: Lippincott.

McColl, I. (1998). More precision in diagnosing appendicitis. New England Journal of Medicine, 338, 190-191.

Mittal, R.K., & Balaban, D.H. (1997). The esophagogastric junction. New England Journal of Medicine, 336, 924-932.

Perez, E.A., & Hallstone, H.A. (1998). Nausea and vomiting. In R.E. Rakel (Ed.), Conn's Current Therapy. Philadelphia: Saunders.

Richter, J.M. (1995). Evaluation of dysphagia and suspect esophageal chest pain. In A.H. Goroll, L.A. May, & A.G. Mulley, Jr. (Eds.), Primary care medicine. Philadelphia: Lippincott.

Romero, Y., Evans, J.M., Fleming, K.C., & Phillips, S.F. (1996). Constipation and fecal incontinence in the elderly population. Mayo Clinical Proceedings, 71, 81-92.

Rucker, L.M. (1997). Diarrhea and constipation. In L.M. Rucker (Ed.), Essentials of Adult Ambulatory Care. Baltimore: Williams & Wilkins.

Schaefer, D.C., & Cheskin, L.J. (1998). Constipation in the elderly. American Family Physician, 58, 907-914.

Soll, A.H. (1996). Consensus statement: Medical treatment of peptic ulcer disease. Practice guidelines. JAMA, 275, 622-629.

Stone, R. (1996). Primary care diagnosis of acute abdominal pain. Nurse Practitioner, 21(12), 19-27.

Theal, R.M., & Scott, K. (1996). Evaluating asymptomatic patients with abnormal liver function test results. American Family Physicain, 53, 2111-2119.

Verne, G.N., & Cerda, J.J. (1997). Irritable bowel syndrome: Streamlining the diagnosis. <u>Postgraduate Medicine, 102</u>, 197-208.

Wagner, J.M., McKinney, W.P, & Carpenter, J.L. (1996). Does this patient have appendicitis? <u>JAMA, 276</u>, 1589-1594.

Wald, A. (1998). Constipation. In R.E. Rakel (Ed.), <u>Conn's Current Therapy</u>, Philadelphia: Saunders.

CHAPTER 13

Genitourinary Problems

BENIGN PROSTATIC HYPERPLASIA

I.   Definition: Benign adenomatous hyperplasia of the periurethral prostate gland

II.   Pathogenesis

    A.   Enlarged prostate compresses on urethra, causing reduced or interrupted urinary flow, inability to empty bladder and increased frequency of urination

    B.   The etiology of benign prostatic hyperplasia (BPH) is uncertain but several factors appear to play a role
        1.   Increased 5α-dihydrotestosterone (DHT), the active form of testosterone
        2.   Increased estrogen
        3.   Stimulation of α-adrenergic nerve endings interfering with the opening of the bladder neck internal sphincter
        4.   Smoking may have a protective effect

III.   Clinical Presentation

    A.   Commonly seen in men over 50 years; approximately 90% of men older than 85 years have microscopic evidence of BPH; approximately 1/4 of males in U.S. will eventually require treatment for relief of symptoms of BPH

    B.   Most patients have a gradual worsening of the following symptoms:
        1.   Obstructive symptoms include a weak urinary stream, abdominal straining to void, hesitancy, intermittency, incomplete bladder emptying, and terminal dribbling
        2.   Irritative symptoms include frequency, nocturia, and urgency

    C.   Complications of BPH are variable:
        1.   Patients are often more susceptible to urinary tract infections
        2.   In long-standing BPH, urinary incontinence may be present
        3.   Severe prostate enlargement can block the urethra, causing acute urinary retention

IV.   Diagnosis/Evaluation

    A.   History
        1.   Determine onset and duration of symptoms
        2.   The American Urological Association (AUA) Symptom Index which is presented in the 1994 Agency for Health Care Policy and Research (AHCPR) Clinical Practice Guideline for BPH can be used for the initial assessment
            a.   The AUA Index is a self-administered 7-item questionnaire which rates the severity of symptoms on a scale from 0 (not at all) to 5 (almost always); items are then summed to obtain a total score
            b.   The questionnaire asks men to rate the following symptoms which they might have had over the past month: Sensation of not emptying their bladder after urination, occurrence of the need to urinate within 2 hours of last urination, episodes of having to start and stop during urination, difficulty postponing urination, weak urinary stream, occurrence of needing to push and strain to urinate, and the number of times got up from bed to urinate during the night
        3.   Ask about pain or discomfort as well as hematuria
        4.   Question about fevers and penile discharge
        5.   Possibly ask patient to record symptoms for a period of one week
        6.   Ask about recent onset of back or bone pain, anorexia, or weight loss which often accompanies malignancy
        7.   Obtain a complete medical history, specifically asking about genitourinary problems and surgeries, diabetes mellitus and neurological diseases
        8.   Ask about history of indwelling urinary catheter

9. Gather a complete medication history:
   a. Ask patients whether cold or sinus medications aggravate their symptoms
   b. Drugs such as anticholinergics can impair bladder contractility and sympathomimetics can increase outflow resistance

B. Physical Examination
   1. Perform a complete abdominal examination to detect a distended bladder, renal tenderness, or a mass
   2. Perform a digital rectal examination (DRE) to estimate the size of the prostate, to detect nodules or indurations that may be indicative of prostate cancer, and to evaluate anal sphincter tone (prostate size does not correlate well with complications of BPH)
      a. Normal prostate is about 2.5 x 3 cm in vertical and transverse diameters
      b. In BPH, the gland is often enlarged, firm, smooth, symmetrical, with an obliterated median sulcus
      c. In prostate cancer the gland may be asymmetric, nodular with a hard and fixed mass
   3. Consider watching the patient void to determine size and force of urinary stream (normally, a man should be able to empty bladder of 300 mL of urine in 12-15 seconds)
   4. Perform a focused neurologic examination to detect associated neurogenic diseases such as multiple sclerosis

C. Differential Diagnosis
   1. Other causes of bladder outlet obstruction
      a. Prostatic cancer (see IV.B.2.c. above)
      b. Urethral obstruction
      c. Vesical neck obstruction
   2. Impaired detrusor contractility related to a neurogenic, myogenic or psychogenic factors
   3. Detrusor instability/hyperreflexia from inflammatory or infectious conditions
      a. Cystitis
      b. Prostatitis
      c. Bladder cancer
   4. Any disease causing increased urinary frequency may mimic BPH such as diabetes mellitus, hypercalcemia or nocturnal diuresis of congestive heart failure

D. Diagnostic Tests
   1. The 1994 AHCPR Guidelines on BPH include the following recommended tests:
      a. Urinalysis to rule out urinary tract infection, hematuria, and glycosuria
      b. Creatinine to assess renal function; elevated levels suggests urinary retention or underlying renal disease which necessitates early referral to urologist
      c. Serum Prostate-Specific Antigen (PSA) is an optional test
         (1) Recent research found that digitally manipulating prostate does not elevate PSA levels; finasteride therapy, prostatic surgery and urethrocystoscopy can elevate PSA levels
         (2) Serum values of PSA increase in direct proportion to the volume of BPH, thus PSA levels may be as high as 10 µg/L without being indicative of prostate cancer
         (3) In the past it was believed that patients in whom the prostatic volume was not proportional to the PSA value, had a significant risk of prostatic cancer; the 1994 AHCPR guidelines, however, state that the serum PSA alone is not a reliable test for distinguishing men with BPH from those with early prostate cancer
         (4) DRE together with the serum PSA is the best strategy for detecting prostate cancer
   2. For patients with moderate-to-severe symptoms consider the following optional tests: Urinary flowrate, postvoid residual urine, and pressure-flow urodynamic studies
   3. According to some urologists, the gold-standard for diagnosing bladder outflow obstruction is a simultaneous measurement of intravesical pressure and urine flow rate done with urodynamic studies

4.   Transrectal ultrasonography is recommended for visualizing prostate lesions and staging suspected prostate cancer

5.   If invasive treatment may be administered, consider ordering a urethrocystoscopy

V.   Plan/Management

A.   The following types of patients should be treated surgically
     1.   Men with refractory urinary retention who have failed at least one attempt at catheter removal
     2.   Men who have recurrent urinary tract infections, recurrent gross hematuria, bladder stones, large bladder diverticula, or renal insufficiency clearly related to BPH

B.   The treatment of patients who have no absolute indications for surgery is usually based on severity of symptoms; however, the risks and benefits of all options should be carefully discussed with the patient

C.   Men with mild symptoms (AUA score ≤7) should be followed with a strategy of watchful waiting; probabilities of disease progression and development of complications are uncertain
     1.   Monitor patients' symptoms and clinical course annually
     2.   Discuss behavioral techniques to reduce symptoms
          a.   Limit fluid intake after dinner
          b.   Avoid certain medications (see following table)

MEDICATIONS THAT MAY WORSEN BPH SYMPTOMS		
Class	**Agents**	**Comments**
ANTICHOLINERGICS		
Antidepressants	**Highest effects:** amitriptyline (highest), amoxapine, clomipramine, protriptyline **Moderate effects:** bupropion, doxepin, imipramine, maprotiline, nortriptyline, trimipramine	Includes non-prescription and prescription medications which have anticholinergic properties; may worsen outflow obstruction
Antiparkinson agents	benztropine, trihexyphenidyl	
Antipsychotics	**Highest effects:** clozapine, mesoridazine, promazine, triflupromazine, thioridazine **Moderate effects:** chlorpromazine, chlorprothixene, pimozide	
Antispasmodics	anisotropine, atropine, belladonna alkaloids, clidinium bromide, dicyclomine HCl, glycopyrrolate, hexocyclium, isopropamide, L-hyoscyamine, mepenzolate bromide, methantheline bromide, methscopolamine bromide, oxyphencyclimine HCl, propantheline bromide, tridihexethyl chloride	
Cold preparations containing antihistamines	**Highest effects:** carbinoxamine, clemastine, diphenhydramine, methdilazine, promethazine, trimeprazine **Moderate effects:** azatadine, brompheniramine, chlorpheniramine, cyproheptadine, dexchlorphenir-amine, phenindamine, triprolidine	
α-ADRENERGIC AGONISTS	phenylpropanolamine pseudoephedrine	Includes cold preparations that contain decongestants
DIURETICS	**Thiazides:** chlorthalidone, hydrochlorothiazide **Thiazide-like:** indapamide, metolazone **Loop Diuretics:** bumetanide, furosemide, torsemide	These medications do not worsen outflow obstruction, but may make symptoms of polyuria and frequency more bothersome. Thus, they are generally safe for use in patients with BPH, but their influence on symptoms should be considered

Adapted from Hebel, S.K. (Ed.). (1996). <u>Drugs Facts and Comparisons.</u> St. Louis: Facts and Comparisons, Inc.

c. Consider other behavioral techniques which may or may not prove helpful:
   (1) Frequent voiding and double voiding (urinate, wait 3 minutes, and void again)
   (2) Avoidance of sudden diuresis which often occurs after drinking caffeine or alcohol
   (3) Avoidance of certain medications such as anticholinergics, tranquilizers, antidepressants
   (4) Performance of prostatic massage after intercourse

D. Carefully evaluate for complications; refer to urologist if complications exist or consider referral if patients have severe symptoms

E. Offer men with moderate and severe symptoms (AUA score ≥ 8) information on the benefits and harms of watchful waiting, alpha blocker therapy, finasteride therapy, and surgery (each option will be discussed in the following sections); Provide the patient with the pamphlet, Treating Your Enlarged Prostate: Patient Guide available from the AHCPR (call 800-358-9295)

F. Medications may reduce the size of the prostate and relieve symptoms (always perform digital rectal examination and obtain PSA level before initiating drugs)
   1. Alpha-adrenergic blockers are drugs of choice for men with smaller prostates (<40 grams and acute, mainly irritative symptoms)
      a. Drugs reduce symptoms and increase uroflow by decreasing bladder outlet resistance to urinary flow
      b. There is limited evidence that these drugs reduce complication rates or postpone the need for future surgery, but they should be considered a treatment option
      c. Prescribe one of the following long-acting agents; to avoid postural hypotension, both terazosin and doxazosin should be taken at bedtime and the dosages should be slowly increased; caution patients to carefully arise from bed at night and in the morning; terazosin and doxazin will lower blood pressure (BP) in hypertensive patients, but should not alter BP in normotensive patients
         (1) Terazosin (Hytrin)
            (a) Begin with small initial doses such as 1 mg for 3 days, 2 mg for 11 days, 5 mg for 7 days and 10 mg once daily, thereafter
            (b) Maximum dose is 20 mg/day
            (c) Most extensively studied drug for treatment of BPH
         (2) Doxazosin mesylate (Cardura)
            (a) Begin with 1 mg QD HS; double dose every 1-2 weeks if needed
            (b) Maximum dose is 8 mg/day
         (3) Tamsulosin HCl (Flomax)
            (a) Adverse effect profile associated with this drug is milder than that seen with other α-adrenergic blockers except that patient may have increased ejaculation problems
            (b) Drug is a more specific α-adrenergic blocker; preferentially binds to the α_{1c}-adrenergic receptor sites in the urinary tract but not as strongly to α_1-adrenergic receptor sites in cardiovascular tissue or elsewhere in the body
            (c) Has no cardiovascular side effects; offers no advantage to reducing B/P in hypertensive patients
            (d) Typically, prescribe 0.4 mg QD about 30 minutes before the same meal each day; does not require titration but may need to increase dosage to 0.8 if there is no response after 2-4 weeks
            (e) Do not crush, chew or open caps
            (f) Generally well-tolerated, but may cause abnormal ejaculation, rhinitis; initially may cause postural hypotension and dizziness

471

2. Finasteride (Proscar), a 5α-reductase inhibitor, is the drug of choice for men with relatively large prostates (>40 grams) and patients who have contraindications or failed treatment with alpha-adrenergic drugs
   a. It is effective in decreasing prostatic size, increasing peak urinary flowrate, and reducing symptoms
   b. Reduces growth of prostate by inhibiting conversion of testosterone to the more active dihydrotestosterone
   c. Prescribe 5 mg QD for at least 6 months; no titration is needed; inform patient that full response to therapy may take 6-12 months
   d. Drug is usually well tolerated, but 5% of men complain of sexual dysfunction
   e. Drug causes a 50% decrease in serum concentration of PSA; highest value that is normal in men taking finasteride is one-half that for men not receiving finasteride
3. Combination therapy with α-blocker and 5α-reductase inhibitor was no more effective than monotherapy in clinical studies
4. Other drugs used less often to treat BPH include the following: GnRH agonists, progestational antiandrogens, flutamide, and testolactone

G. Surgery is the most effective treatment for most men with severe symptoms
   1. Surgery has the best chance for relief of symptoms, but also has the greatest risks, even though most men have no problems with surgery
   2. The three most common surgical procedures follow:
      a. Transurethral resection of prostate (TURP): Special instrument is inserted into urethra and inside of prostate is partially removed
      b. Transurethral incision of the prostate (TUIP): Instrument makes one or two small incisions into prostate to reduce pressure on the urethra:
         (1) Used when the prostate is not enlarged
         (2) Less risk than TURP in certain cases
      c. Open prostatectomy involves an incision into the lower abdomen to remove part of the inside of the prostate; performed when the prostate is large; infrequently performed today

H. Newer treatments include the following
   1. Transurethral needle ablation (TUNA) and transurethral microwave therapy (TUMT) use heat for treatment; both have lower morbidity when compared with TURP, but are less effective
   2. Electrovaporization of the prostate (EVP) is a technical evolution of TURP; a roller electrode vaporizes the prostatic tissue which reduces bleeding
   3. Fiber optics combined with laser technologies can also reduce prostatic tissue
   4. Intraprostatic stents maintain urethral patency in patients who cannot tolerate TURP and who are not candidates for TUIP

I. Transurethral balloon dilation (TUBD) has a low efficacy rate but may reduce symptoms temporarily; it is reserved for patients who cannot tolerate medications or surgery

J. Hormonal therapy with leuprolide acetate (Lupron) and goserelin acetate (Zoladex) is used infrequently; hormonal therapy is expensive and associated with many side effects

K. Phytotherapy, the use of plants or plant extracts for medicinal use, is a controversial option
   1. Saw palmetto berry is the agent most extensively studied, but the results have been inconclusive
   2. Cholesterol-lowering agents such as β-sitosteryl glucoside have been tried based on the fact that prostatic secretions and the prostate gland contain cholesterol; one drug in this group, Harzol, was effective in a large, controlled study; however further research is needed before this drug and other phytotherapeutic agents are recommended

L. Follow Up
    1. Teach patient to assess for signs and symptoms of retention and obstruction
    2. Patients who opt for the "watchful waiting" strategy should be followed annually
    3. Patients on terazosin and cardura should be reevaluated in 4-6 weeks although some clinicians titrate medications every 1-2 weeks; typically, clinical response to these drugs is not seen for 4-6 weeks after beginning therapy
    4. Patients on tamsulosin should be reevaluated at 2-4 weeks for dosage adjustment if needed
    5. Patients on finasteride should be reevaluated at approximately 6 months to determine drug effectiveness
    6. Follow up for patients who have balloon dilation or surgery is at the discretion of the urologist and surgeon and dependent on the patient's progress

CHRONIC RENAL FAILURE

I. Definition: Renal insufficiency or a decrease in renal function that progresses over months to years; other important terms related to chronic renal failure (CRF) include the following:

    A. Azotemia: Excess of nitrogenous compounds in the blood

    B. Uremia or uremic syndrome: Toxic condition produced by increase of nitrogenous compounds and toxins

    C. End-stage renal disease (ESRD): Last stage of CRF in which the renal function has deteriorated to the point that dialysis is needed to sustain life

II. Pathogenesis

    A. Occurs with a decrease in glomerular filtration rate and a reduction in the clearance of certain solutes principally excreted by the kidneys
        1. Initially the functioning nephrons blunt the drop in total glomerular filtration rate
        2. Eventually glomerular hyperfiltration and hypertension lead to progressive glomerular sclerosis and overt proteinuria
        3. When serum creatinine rises above 2 mg/dL or creatinine clearance falls to 60 mL, progression to ESRD is imminent

    B. Major causes of chronic renal failure
        1. Hypertensive nephrosclerosis
        2. Chronic glomerulonephritis
        3. Diabetic nephropathy
        4. Interstitial nephritis due to analgesic excess, other drugs such as nonsteroidal antiinflammatory agents, lead exposure, vesicoureteral reflux or other factors that cause hydronephrosis in children, and hereditary disorders such as Alport's syndrome
        5. Polycystic kidney disease
        6. Hyperlipidemia is associated with progressive renal disease

III. Clinical Presentation

    A. Because CRF is usually a result of intrinsic kidney damage, the progression of CRF can be slowed but usually the damage is not reversible

    B. Patients with declining renal function are often asymptomatic until the very late stages of the disease, because of the compensatory ability of the remaining nephrons; often patients with CRF are discovered by accident with routine medical tests

C. In the first stage, decreased renal reserve with reduced glomerular filtration rate, symptoms are vague and difficult to recognize

D. In the second stage, renal insufficiency, patients may be asymptomatic but many have nocturia, hypertension, and mild anemia

E. In the third stage, renal failure, the following typically occurs:
1. Because patients with CRF sometimes have systemic diseases which involve the kidneys such as systemic lupus erythematous or other rheumatoid conditions, joint pain and skin changes may be early manifestations
2. Patients with intrinsic chronic disease of the kidneys may have early symptoms of flank pain, hematuria, and dysuria; foamy urine and peripheral edema may be the first sign of chronic glomerulonephritis
3. Other possible symptoms include fatigue, cold intolerance, anorexia
4. Hyperphosphatemia, hypocalcemia, hyperkalemia, metabolic acidosis, and worsening anemia usually develop

F. In the last stage, uremia, the following symptoms develop: pruritus, generalized malaise, lassitude, forgetfulness, loss of libido, nausea, weight loss, changes in sleep pattern, metallic taste in mouth, brown, dry tongue, hyperreflexia, altered behavior, and cognitive changes
1. May have fluid overload and the signs and symptoms that accompany congestive heart failure
2. Peripheral neuropathy may be present and includes the following symptoms: Restless leg syndrome, asterixis (flapping of the hands when the arms are extended and hands are in dorsiflexion), myoclonus, and loss of vibratory sense
3. Ultimately, the patient may develop the following: pale or yellow skin, uremic frost (rare today with use of dialysis), reversible hair loss, nail changes, coma, and seizures

G. Hypertension is a common problem in the majority of patients; uncontrolled hypertension as well as ingestion of nonsteroidal anti-inflammatory agents, or intercurrent diseases may hasten the course to end stage

H. Diagnosis is usually confirmed by a laboratory evaluation
1. An elevated blood urea nitrogen, high serum creatinine, metabolic acidosis with or without hyperkalemia, low calcium and high phosphate concentrations are characteristic
2. Usually patients have a profound anemia (normochromic normocytic)

IV. Diagnosis/Evaluation

A. History
1. Ask about symptoms related to abnormalities of the urinary tract such as dysuria, frequency, hesitancy, nocturia, urinary incontinence, and renal colic
2. Inquire about other associated symptoms such as nausea, vomiting, fatigue, itching, or restless legs
3. Obtain a complete medication history, particularly nonsteroidal anti-inflammatory agents and nephrotoxic antibiotics (aminoglycosides)
4. Obtain a thorough medical history, with particular emphasis on discovering the presence of a systemic illness that can cause renal failure such as hypertension, diabetes mellitus, collagen vascular disease, and HIV infection
   a. Ascertain that patient has not had recent radiocontrast induced x-rays
   b. Inquire about GI problems and hemorrhage, dehydration (diarrhea, vomiting, diuretic ingestion), and bleeding
5. Review family history for Alport's syndrome, renal disease, kidney disease, diabetes mellitus, or renal failure

B. Physical Examination
1. Measure vital signs including orthostatic blood pressure readings
2. Do a complete eye exam, including funduscopy
3. Observe skin for rashes

4. Auscultate neck for carotid bruits
5. Perform a complete cardiovascular examination
6. Auscultate lungs
7. Perform a complete abdominal examination; carefully palpate for enlarged kidneys
8. Pelvic or rectal examination should be done to evaluate for causes of lower urinary tract obstruction such as prostatic or cervical carcinoma
9. Examine lower extremities for edema
10. Because CRF is often related to systemic diseases, a complete physical examination may be needed, especially assessment of musculoskeletal and neurological systems

C. Differential Diagnosis:
1. Ascertain that the renal failure is not acute or involves conditions that can be treated; acute renal failure (ARF) is associated with the following:
    a. Blood urea nitrogen (BUN) is increased out of proportion to the increase in serum creatinine clearance
    b. Patients with ARF tend to be more symptomatic than patients with CRF
    c. Moderate to severe anemia, hypocalcemia, and hyperphosphatemia are more common in CRF than in ARF
    d. Certain clinical situations cause ARF and the damage can be reversed with proper treatment
        (1) Renal hypoperfusion is often caused by congestive heart failure, bleeding, or depletion of NaCl and water typically due to diuretic therapy
        (2) Urinary tract obstruction
        (3) Pyelonephritis
        (4) Acute tubular necrosis (ATN) following administration of x-ray contrast media, ingestion of certain drugs such as aminoglycosides, or intense physical effort in the heat
2. Important to determine cause of CRF
    a. Hypertensive nephrosclerosis is a common cause of chronic interstitial nephritis, particularly in African Americans; consider in persons with long history of poorly controlled hypertension in association with nonnephrotic-range proteinuria
    b. Consider ischemic renal disease in patients with significant history of cigarette smoking and evidence of extrarenal vascular disease; usually have asymmetrical kidneys on renal ultrasonography
    c. Consider diagnosis of diabetic nephropathy in patients with duration of 7-8 years of type 2 diabetes or 12-15 years of type 1 diabetes
    d. Obstructive nephropathy, polycystic kidney disease, and stone disease can be excluded by ultrasonography or computed tomography

D. Diagnostic Tests: Ordered to establish the severity and etiology of the renal failure and to determine the presence of complicating abnormalities
1. Order an urinalysis (UA)
    a. Glomerular disease is associated with RBCs, RBC casts, and proteinuria
    b. WBCs and casts may be found in interstitial nephropathies
    c. Multiple cellular elements such as RBCs, WBCs, and various casts suggest a collagen vascular disease
    d. Acute tubular necrosis is associated with gross or microscopic hematuria, pigmented granular casts and renal tubular cells
    e. Sterile pyuria is associated with renal tuberculosis
2. Order a 24-hour urine specimen to quantify proteinuria (adults normally excrete less than 160 g. of protein per day) and to calculate creatinine clearance (normal is 120 mL/min)
3. Determine renal size either with a simple x-ray of the abdomen, a renal ultrasound, or an intravenous pyelogram (IVP)
    a. If anatomic anomalies are suspected IVP is test of choice
    b. Renal ultrasound is often used to avoid radiocontrast-induced acute renal failure and provides information on kidney size, echogenicity, thickness of the cortex and the presence of obstruction

4. Order blood chemistries
   a. Blood urea nitrogen (BUN) (normal range, 11 to 23 mg/dL)
      (1) This test is dependent on renal blood flow, volume expansion and protein intake; as such it is not an ideal test for diagnosing CRF
      (2) Urea nitrogen may be elevated with dehydration and gastrointestinal bleeding
   b. Creatinine (normal range, 0.6 to 1.2 ml/dL)
      (1) Better indicator of CRF than BUN
      (2) Creatine is higher in persons with great deal of muscle mass
      (3) Creatinine is reduced when intake of red meat is low
      (4) A formula for estimating creatinine clearance is as follows: Cl_{cr} (mL/min) = $(140-Age)/(Serum_{cr} \times 72)$
   c. Electrolytes
5. Order CBC, serum iron level, total iron-binding capacity, and serum ferritin level; may need to also rule-out deficiency of vitamin B_{12} or folate (see section on MEGALOBLASTIC ANEMIA)
6. Diabetic patients should be followed for microalbuminuria by radioimmunoassay
7. In patients over age 40 with unexplained renal failure, order a urine electrophoresis to exclude the possibility of multiple myeloma
8. Renal biopsy is useful in diagnosing glomerulonephritis

V. Plan/Management

A. A nephrologist is usually involved in the initial plans and consulted regularly as the patient's condition changes

B. Institute mechanisms to slow the progression of the renal failure
   1. Eliminate offending agents such as discontinue medications (NSAIDs, antibiotics) or refer to surgeon for urinary obstruction
   2. Many of the immunologically mediated renal diseases may respond to corticosteroids, cytotoxic agents or plasmapheresis
   3. A low-protein diet is probably not beneficial with moderate renal impairment; for patients with severe renal impairment (GFR = 13-24 mL/min/1.73^2) a low protein diet of 0.6 g/kg/day may slow disease progression
      a. Adequate calorie intake (35-50 kcal/kg/day) must be maintained to avoid endogenous protein catabolism
      b. Follow patients carefully for evidence of malnutrition
      c. Nutritional goals are serum albumin >4 g/dL and transferrin >200 mg/dL
      d. Correction of lipid abnormalities may be important in slowing progression of disease (see section on HYPERLIPIDEMIA)
   4. Modify the dosage of many medications

C. Treat complications
   1. Sodium imbalance
      a. In early stages, do not restrict intake of sodium as this could accelerate renal damage
      b. In later stages when excretion of sodium and water becomes diminished, cautious sodium and fluid restrictions are necessary
         (1) Restrict sodium to 4 g daily
         (2) Intake of fluids should equal urine output and insensible losses
   2. Renal osteodystrophy and secondary hyperparathyroidism with altered calcium and phosphorus levels
      a. In early renal failure (serum creatinine 2-3 mg per dl) when serum phosphate is less than 5 mg dl, dietary phosphate restriction is sufficient (restrict ingestion of dairy products and cola-colored soft drinks)
      b. When the serum creatinine concentration rises to >4mg/dL, prescribe a calcium supplement such a calcium carbonate 500 mg BID/TID with meals to provide a source of calcium and to bind phosphate in the gut

     c.   Exogenous 1,25-dihydroxycholecalciferal [calcitriol (Rocaltrol)] with dosage range of 0.25-0.75μg/day should also be prescribed when creatinine level is >4mg/dL; frequent measurements of serum calcium levels are needed to detect hypercalcemia which may occur from exogenous active form of vitamin D

     d.   In past, aluminum hydroxide was used to prevent rise in serum phosphate level but because of problems with aluminum-induced bone disease, current recommendation is to use calcium carbonate only; however, if serum calcium level is >11mg/dL, aluminum hydrochloride should be initially used and then stopped as levels return to normal

         (1)   Prescribe (Basaljel) at a dose of 15 to 30 ml with meals three times a day

         (2)   Take antacids immediately after meals

         (3)   Avoid magnesium-containing antacids

3.   Metabolic acidosis is usually mild and does not need treatment in early stages

     a.   When the plasma bicarbonate concentration falls below 15 mEq/L, consider alkali supplements such as Shohl's solution or sodium bicarbonate tablets 600 mg BID and titrate bicarbonate to the 16-20 mEq/L range

     b.   Remove any external acid loads such as aspirin, vitamin C, or excess protein intake

     c.   Regularly monitor serum potassium and calcium levels as both may fall

4.   Hyperkalemia rarely occurs until late in CRF

     a.   Cautiously use drugs which predispose to potassium retention such as potassium-sparing diuretics, potassium supplements, beta-adrenergic blockers, NSAIDs

     b.   Avoid salt substitutes

     c.   Monitor potassium levels regularly as elevated levels can lead to electrocardiographic changes

     d.   Dietary potassium should be restricted to 60 mEq per day initially; restrict to 40 mEq/day when glomerular filtration rate falls below 20 ml/min

     e.   For severe hyperkalemia, a combination of furosemide, sodium polystyrene sulfonate (Kayexalate) and/or fludrocortisone acetate (Florinef) may be needed (consult nephrologist)

5.   Anemia of CRF is primarily due to a relative deficiency in erythropoietin (EPO)

     a.   Early in course of disease, suggest a multivitamin regimen that includes folate

     b.   Patients with severe debilitating anemia or patients with coronary artery disease of congestive heart failure are best candidates for treatment

     c.   Erythropoietin (EPO) treatment can be started at a dose of 20-30 U per kg administered subcutaneously three times a week, aiming for target hematocrit of 30-35%

         (1)   Monitor B/P because EPO can elevate blood pressure

         (2)   Monitor iron stores and administer supplemental iron as needed

     d.   Regularly measure blood pressure (BP) because BP sometimes increases with rising hematocrit

     e.   Prescribe oral ferrous sulfate, 325 mg/day to patients with iron deficiency

6.   Diabetic nephropathy

     a.   Patients need to be closely monitored for microalbuminuria and their blood glucose level should be tightly controlled

     b.   Patients with persistent microalbuminuria, should be started on angiotensin converting-enzyme (ACE) inhibitors regardless of whether they are hypertensive or not (see section on DIABETES MELLITUS

7.   Hypertension

     a.   Maintain a tight control of blood pressure with whatever antihypertensive agent is needed (see section on HYPERTENSION)

     b.   Goal for patients with renal disease is 125/75 mm Hg if proteinuria is >1 g/day and there are no contraindications

     c.   ACE inhibitors, calcium channel blockers, and diuretics are often recommended for hypertensive patients with renal diseases

8.   Congestive heart failure (see section on CONGESTIVE HEART FAILURE)

     a.   Loop diuretics such as furosemide or ethacrynic acid should be used when serum creatinine is > 4.0 mg/dl; metolazone (Mykrox) 2.5 to 5 mg QD or BID may be added if goals are not reached with loop diuretics

  b. Angiotensin-converting enzyme inhibitors such as captopril 12.5-25 mg BID/TID may help to preserve renal failure in addition to lowering blood pressure; ACE inhibitors must be used with caution in patients with late-stage CRF

9. Symptoms of itching, hiccups, and nausea

  a. Reducing protein intake may lessen symptoms

  b. Order prochlorperazine (Compazine) 5-10 mg PO QID prn for nausea

  c. Itching may be minimized with menthol or phenol lotion or capsaicin cream

10. Azotemia develops gradually and does not require treatment until the BUN exceeds 100 to 125 mg/dl; consider chronic dialysis or transplantation at this point

D. Follow up is dependent on severity of condition; patients in early stages of CRF should be seen every 1-4 months

ERECTILE DYSFUNCTION

I. Definition: Persistent inability to achieve and maintain a penile erection sufficient for satisfactory sexual intercourse; the term erectile dysfunction has replaced impotence because the latter has a pejorative connotation and encompasses other aspects of sexuality such as libido, orgasm, and ejaculation in addition to erectile function

II. Pathogenesis: Normal erectile function requires coordination of psychological, vascular, neurological, hormonal, and cavernosal factors; impairment of any of these factors may result in erectile dysfunction

A. Psychogenic factors may result in inhibitory sympathetic nervous system activity which can lead to erectile dysfunction

  1. Although only 10-20% of cases are due solely to psychogenic factors, many men have a psychogenic component secondary to an organic etiology

  2. Depression is related to erectile dysfunction; approximately 90% of severely depressed men report complete erectile dysfunction

B. Common organic causes

  1. Systemic disorders: hypertension, atherosclerosis, peripheral vascular disease, diabetes mellitus, renal failure

  2. Neurogenic disorders: Parkinson's disease, cerebrovascular accidents, multiple sclerosis

  3. Endocrine disorders: hypogonadism, thyroid diseases, hyperprolactinemia

  4. Penile disorders such as priapism, Peyronie's disease

  5. Medications: antihypertensives, antidepressants, antiandrogens, NSAIDs, benzodiazepines, gemfibrozil, digoxin, cimetidine, metoclopramide

  6. Alcohol, tobacco, recreational drugs

  7. Injuries:

    a. Radiation or surgery to the pelvis or retroperitoneum; perineal, pelvic, or nervous system trauma

    b. Erectile dysfunction due to bicycling and its deleterious effects on peripheral nerves may be higher than previously recognized

III. Clinical Presentation

A. Affects approximately 39% of 40-year-old males and 69% of 70 year-old males, but only about 1% of affected males of all ages seek treatment

B. Erectile dysfunction is associated with loss of self-esteem, poor self image, increased anxiety, issues of masculinity and affects interactions with families and associates

IV.   Diagnosis/Evaluation

   A.   History
      1.   Because many men will not mention erectile dysfunction unless directly questioned, begin history with a question such as, "Are you having any concerns or problems about sexual intimacy?"
      2.   After erectile dysfunction is identified, ask the patient what he thinks is causing the problem
      3.   Inquire about the onset, duration, and evolution of the problem; a gradual onset suggests an organic problem, whereas a sudden onset indicates a psychogenic origin unless the patient has experienced trauma or surgery
      4.   Determine if problem is intermittent or constant; intermittent problems are usually associated with psychogenic causes
      5.   Ask the patient how the disorder affects his life
      6.   Ask the patient to rate his current degree of erection on a scale of 1-10 with "10" the fullest erection he can ever recall
      7.   Determine whether the problem is failure to attain or maintain an erection; problems with initiating an erection indicate a neurologic, endocrinologic or psychogenic cause whereas problems with sustaining an erection suggest a vascular problem
      8.   Determine whether patient can achieve any degree of penetration
      9.   Inquire whether patient has nocturnal or morning erections; inability to have nocturnal/morning erections suggests an organic cause
      10.   Explore whether other sexuality problems exist such as changes in libido, difficulty having orgasms, premature ejaculation, or performance anxiety
      11.   Explore possible risk factors such as changes in medical status, injuries, surgery, and frequency of bicycling
      12.   Obtain a complete medication history
      13.   Question about alcohol, tobacco, and recreational drug use
      14.   Explore associated situational factors such as overwork, stressors, marital tensions, boring sexual routine
      15.   Question about previous attempts to manage the problem by the patient or another health care provider
      16.   Determine whether the patient has a partner
      17.   If patient has a partner, ask about the quality of the relationship and the health of the partner
      18.   If possible, involve the partner in the evaluation and encourage a joint discussion of how the problem is affecting the couple's relationship
      19.   A diary of the patient's erectile activity for 3-4 weeks may be helpful
      20.   The International Index of Erectile Function is a 15-item, self-administered questionnaire which can be used to assess erectile function prior to and during treatment (see Rozen, et al., 1997 in reference list)

   B.   Physical Examination
      1.   Observe general appearance, noting signs of depression and anxiety which may reveal a psychogenic cause
      2.   Measure vital signs with particular attention to blood pressure to uncover a vascular problem
      3.   Assess the distribution of facial, axillary, and pubic hair to check for hypogonadism
      4.   Palpate neck for thyromegaly to identify a thyroid problem
      5.   Examine breasts for gynecomastia and nipple tenderness to detect an endocrine problem
      6.   Perform a complete cardiovascular examination including peripheral pulses and auscultation for abdominal and inguinal bruits to detect a vascular cause
      7.   Inspect penis to detect deformities such as micropenis or hypospadias and signs of inflammation and infection
      8.   Palpate penis to uncover Peyronie's disease which involves corporeal plaques and thickening of the tunica albuginea
      9.   Examine testes for size, position, consistency, and abnormalities to detect a testicular problem

10. Perform a rectal exam to check for prostate hypertrophy, prostatitis, or malignancy
11. Perform a complete neurologic examination, including the following:
    a. Deep tendon reflexes and a sensory motor examination of the lower extremities
    b. Genital and perineal sensation
    c. Anal sphincter tone and the bulbocavernosus reflex which is performed by asking patient to squeeze the glans penis during a rectal examination (when the reflex is present, the anal sphincter contracts)

C. Differential Diagnosis: Premature ejaculation, sexual desire disorders, orgasmic disorders, and sexual arousal disorders are often confused with erectile dysfunction

D. Diagnostic Tests
    1. To identify hypogonadism, obtain a morning serum total testosterone; if level is <500 ng/dL, repeat the test and order the following additional tests:
       a. Serum prolactin level
       b. Serum gonadotropins (luteinizing hormone, follicle-stimulating hormone)
    2. Tests to exclude unrecognized systemic disease may be helpful and include the following: lipid profile, thyroid function tests, fasting blood sugar, urinalysis, complete blood count, and creatinine
    3. A noninvasive device such as the RigiScan Plus System can be used at home or in the office
       a. At home, patient sleeps with a portable monitor attached to the penis and device records nocturnal erectile activity
       b. At the office, the RigiScan Plus System can be used to detect patient's response to visual erotic stimulation
    4. A less sophisticated and costly test to determine presence and quality of nocturnal erections is the Snap-gauge band which is placed on base of penis at bedtime and examined in the morning for breakage of three plastic filaments
    5. To detect a vascular problem, a diagnostic test injection of prostaglandin E_1, phentolamine, and papaverine is given intracorporeally and the response of the penis is observed
    6. Duplex ultrasonography, penile angiography, penile biothesiometry, and nerve conduction may be needed; referral to an urologist is recommended for these tests

V. Plan/Management

A. Refer the patient to specialists in the following cases:
    1. Patients with certain systemic diseases such as multiple sclerosis and uncontrollable diabetes mellitus
    2. Patients with a suspected urologic problem such as Peyronie's disease or prostate cancer
    3. Patients whose problems fail to improve with standard primary care therapies

B. Treat the underlying cause of erectile dysfunction
    1. For example, if problems are due to bicycling, suggest changing body positioning, restricting riding intensity, and reducing the duration of the ride
    2. Encourage patient to quit smoking
    3. If possible, alter medications with adverse effects on erectile function
    4. Treat associated medical problems
    5. Age is positively correlated with dysfunction; advise patients that behavioral modifications such as slowing down the pace of foreplay may counteract the effects of aging

C. The contribution of psychological factors should always be considered; referral to a sex therapist and/or a psychologist/psychiatrist/counselor may be useful for both organic and psychogenic problems and is often used in conjunction with physical treatments

D. Several physical interventions are available
    1. The advantages and disadvantages of the options should be discussed with the patient and his partner
    2. As a general rule, the least invasive therapies and those with the fewest adverse effects should be tried first

E. Oral pharmacological therapies
   1. Sildenafil (Viagra) is a phosphodiesterase inhibitor
      a. Although this drug is expensive it has advantages over many of the other therapies; it permits discreet administration, is well-tolerated, and is not invasive
      b. Sildenafil enhances normal sexual response by preventing the inactivation of the potent second messenger molecules in the smooth muscle relaxation of erectile tissue; unlike other therapies, it augments rather than bypasses the normal erection process
      c. Absolutely contraindicated in patients taking medications that contain nitrates such as nitroglycerin; taken together with nitrates, viagra can cause significant hypotension; combination of viagra with inhaled nitrates such as amyl nitrates or "poppers" can be fatal
      d. Use cautiously in the following patients: patients with acute coronary ischemia, CHF, and patients on complicated, multidrug antihypertensives and other drugs such as cimetidine and erythromycin; half life may be prolonged in patients with liver or renal disease
      e. Advise patient to take medication 1 hour before anticipated sexual activity; however, viagra can be taken anywhere from 4 hours to 30 minutes before intercourse
      f. Dosage range is 25-100 mg/day; for most patients the recommended dose is 50 mg; available in 25, 50, 100 mg tabs
      g. No more than one dose per day is recommended
      h. Adverse effects include headache, indigestion, facial flushing, and visual abnormalities such as a bluish tinge to vision
   2. Yohimbine, an alpha-2 adrenoceptor (sympathetic) antagonist, is not recommended in the American Urological Association (AUA) guidelines, but recent studies have found it effective, particularly for patients with psychogenic problems
      a. Prescribe on a trial basis for 1 month at a dosage of 5.4 mg TID
      b. Usually well tolerated, but may cause mild blood pressure elevations, palpitations, nervousness, and irritability
   3. Trazodone HCl (Desyrel) is not recommended in the AUA guidelines because of lack of data supporting its effectiveness but it may have modest beneficial effects on nocturnal erections and psychogenic erectile problems
      a. Affects central serotonin and dopamine pathways and has adrenoceptor antagonistic effects
      b. Prescribe on a one-month trial at a dosage of 100 mg at HS (dosage ranges from 50-200 mg/day)
      c. Adverse effects include drowsiness, irritability, and rarely priapism
   4. Investigational drugs
      a. Phentolamine (Vasomax), a vasodilator, will soon be available in an oral form; presently this drug is given by penile injection
      b. Dopamine agents, serotoninergic drugs, apomorphine, and topical agents are drugs that may be used in the future
      c. Ginkgo biloba is sometimes used to improve sexual dysfunction caused by antidepressants
         (1) Initiate therapy at 50 mg BID and titrate upward (dose range is 50- 240 mg BID)
         (2) Patient may need to take for several weeks before an improvement occurs
         (3) Use cautiously with anticoagulants such as daily aspirin or coumadin

F. Intracavernosal or penile injection therapy
   1. Injection produces erections in approximately 5-20 minutes by relaxing the penile muscle tissue and allowing blood to become trapped in the penile shaft; erections last about 1 hour
   2. Approximately 90% of patients have a functional erection with penile injection therapy
   3. Local complications of all medications include hematomas and edema
   4. Inform patient of the possibility of a prolonged erection which must be treated promptly
      a. Priapism is an infrequent complication and usually occurs when patient increases dose on his own
      b. Priapism may cause irreversible cellular damage and fibrosis

c. An erection lasting for >4 hours is a medical emergency
d. Treatment of injection-induced priapism involves corporal aspiration of blood or intracorporeal injection of phenylephrine HCl; long-term management involves decreasing medication so that erection lasts no longer than 1 hour

5. Prostaglandin E$_1$ (alprostadil) [Caverject] is the drug of choice for initial penile injection therapy
   a. Determine optimal dose in office; on first trial, patient should stay in office until complete detumescence occurs
      (1) Initial dose is 2.5 mcg for vasculogenic, psychogenic or mixed etiology; initial dose is 1.25 mcg for neurogenic etiology
      (2) If no response to first dose occurs, may give 2nd dose after 1 hour; if partial response occurs, wait 24 hours before 2nd dose
      (3) Maintenance dose range is 5 mcg to 60 mcg with most patients having doses ranging between 10-20 mcg
   b. Inject drug into dorsolateral aspect of the proximal third of the penis; visible veins should be avoided; the side injected and the site of injection should be alternated
   c. The erection lasts about 30-60 minutes
   d. Recommended frequency is no more than 3 times weekly, with 24 hours between each dose
   e. Contraindications include myeloma, leukemia, deformity of penis or penile implant, sickle cell anemia or carrier state, and patients for whom sexual activity is inadvisable
   f. Needle for injection is very fine and causes little pain; an autoinjector is available for patients with needle phobia, poor vision, or suboptimal manual dexterity

6. If alprostadil fails other drugs such as papaverine, and phentolamine can be tried
   a. Papaverine causes less pain and is less expensive than alprostadil; however, it has increased risks of priapism and fibrosis
   b. Phentolamine is another, less frequently used drug

7. Combination therapies with papaverine and phentolamine or papaverine, phentolamine, and alprostadil may be beneficial

G. Intraurethral treatments are effective in about 40% of patients
1. Patient inserts an applicator into the distal urethra (about 1 inch) which allows for placement of the drug suppository, prostaglandin E$_1$ (alprostadil [MUSE])
2. Drug is absorbed into surrounding tissue called corpus spongiosum and relaxes the smooth muscle within the penis which allows blood to enter and become trapped into penis
3. Erection occurs within 5-10 minutes of insertion
4. Dosage is based on extent of patient's erectile dysfunction and his response to titration in the office; initial dose is 125 or 250 mcg
5. Available in four standard dosages of 125, 250, 500, and 1,000 mcg
6. Maximum is 2 suppositories per day
7. Adverse effects include local discomfort, urethral bleeding, dizziness, and hypotension; priapism is an uncommon adverse effect; partners may have vaginal burning or itching

H. Vacuum/constriction devices provide a nonpharmacologic and noninvasive method for producing an erection
1. A plastic cylinder is applied over the penis, creating a closed chamber; the cylinder is connected by tubing to a vacuum which withdraws air from around the penis and produces penile engorgement with blood; a constrictor ring is positioned as base of penis to trap the blood
2. Device is inexpensive, reversible, and well tolerated
3. Effective in approximately 95% of patients
4. Adverse effects are minimal and include edema and ecchymosis
5. Keeping the constrictor ring on for more than 30 minutes may cause permanent damage to the penis and is not recommended under any circumstances
6. Some patients dislike the mechanical nature of the devices and others are bothered by the lack of spontaneity in sexual relations

I. Surgery is recommended only after other treatments have failed
 1. Penile prosthesis surgery
   a. A semirigid malleable or hydraulic inflatable device is implanted into two sides of the penis, allowing erections as often as desired
   b. Inform patient of the possibility of infection, erosion, mechanical failure and the need for possible reoperation; also discuss that an implant will preclude use of other therapies in the future
   c. This therapy should not be used in patients with psychogenic erectile dysfunction unless a psychiatrist or psychologist participates in preoperative evaluation and agrees with the need for implantation
 2. Penile vascular surgery which includes both arterial revascularization and venous ligation procedures is investigational but may be an option in the future; optimal candidate is a young trauma patient with a vascular lesion

J. Hormonal replacement therapy is considered for patients with clearly documented hypogonadism
 1. Prior to beginning therapy it is important that a PSA level and a digital rectal examination be done to evaluate for possible prostate disease; testosterone may enhance prostatic hyperplasia and stimulate the growth of occult prostate cancer
 2. Intramuscular injections or transdermal formulations of testosterone are available
   a. Intramuscular injections of 200 mcg are given every 14-21 days
   b. Testoderm: Apply 5 mg patch every 24 hours to clean, dry area of arm, back, or upper buttocks
   c. Monitor liver function, hemoglobin, hematocrit, prostate specific antigen, cholesterol and lipids
   d. During therapy measure serum testosterone levels to determine attainment of therapeutic blood levels

K. Hyperprolactinemia is typically treated with bromocryptine or less commonly surgery is performed to remove tumors secreting prolactin

L. Patient Education
 1. With any pharmacological method, teach patients to use drugs as prescribed; to enhance performance patients may take drugs in higher doses and more frequently than advised which can lead to serious consequences
 2. With all physical therapies, it is important to provide an integrated educational plan which stresses the importance of the emotional and sexual relationship between the patient and his partner
 3. Caution patients with cardiovascular disease, particularly elderly patients, that there is a degree of risk with sexual intercourse like other forms of physical activity; intercourse increases heart rate and cardiac work load; patients should report any chest pain and cardiac symptoms
 4. Remind patients that therapies enhance sexual satisfaction but do not protect them against STDs, including HIV infection

M. Follow Up: Reevaluate patients approximately every 3 months

HEMATURIA

I. Definition: Presence of red blood cells (RBCs) in urine; typically, more than 3 RBCs per high-power field on microscopic examination of a centrifuged specimen is the criteria used to make the diagnosis of hematuria

II. Pathogenesis: RBCs can enter the genitourinary tract at any site from the glomerulus to the urethral meatus and the causes can be categorized as prerenal, renal, postrenal, or false

   A. Prerenal
       1. Coagulopathy such as hemophilia or thrombocytopenic purpura
       2. Drugs such as warfarin sodium, heparin sodium or aspirin
       3. Sickle cell disease or trait
       4. Collagen vascular disease such as systemic lupus erythematosus
       5. Wilm's tumor

   B. Renal
       1. Nonglomerular
           a. Pyelonephritis
           b. Polycystic kidney disease
           c. Granulomatous disease such as tuberculosis
           d. Malignant neoplasm
           e. Congenital and vascular anomalies
       2. Glomerular
           a. Glomerulonephritis
           b. Berger's disease
           c. Lupus nephritis
           d. Benign familial hematuria
           e. Vascular abnormalities such as vasculitis
           f. Alport's syndrome (familial nephritis)

   C. Postrenal
       1. Renal calculi
       2. Ureteritis
       3. Cystitis
       4. Prostatitis
       5. Benign prostatic hyperplasia
       6. Epididymitis
       7. Urethritis
       8. Malignant neoplasm

   D. False
       1. Vaginal bleeding
       2. Recent circumcision
       3. Hemoglobinuria
       4. Intake of certain foods such as beets, rhubarb, blackberries, fava beans
       5. Intake of certain medications such as quinine sulfate, phenazopyridine, phenytoin, phenindione, phenothiazine, rifampin, sulfasalazine
       6. Excretion of porphyrins

   E. Miscellaneous causes
       1. Strenuous exercise
       2. Fever
       3. Trauma
       4. Viral infections

F.   Hematuria may be a complaint in patients with factitious hematuria such as narcotic seekers complaining of kidney stones or individuals in families with Munchausen's disease

G.   Essential hematuria occurs when no definable cause can be found

III.   Clinical Presentation

A.   Hematuria may be gross (visible to naked eye) or microscopic (detected on dipstick or microscopic exam)

B.   Clinical manifestations are variable
1.   Hematuria may be painful or painless; painless hematuria is often associated with a malignancy
2.   Associated symptoms such as fever, edema, or dysuria may be present

C.   Common causes include the following:
1.   Infection, neoplasms, and benign prostatic hypertrophy are the most common diagnoses
2.   Patients >40 years are at increased risk for uroepithelial cancer (see following table for risk factors)

RISK FACTORS FOR MALIGNANCY
* Analgesic abuse such as acetaminophen, aspirin compounds
* Cigarette smoking
* Male gender
* Pelvic irradiation
* Occupational exposures: individuals working in printing, leather, rubber, and dye industries
* Cyclophosphamide use
* Family history of urologic cancer

IV.   Diagnosis/Evaluation

A.   History
1.   Question about timing and appearance of hematuria
a.   Hematuria seen at onset of urination often indicates bleeding in the urethra
b.   Terminal hematuria seen in the last few drops of urine often indicates the bladder neck or prostate as the source
c.   Hematuria seen throughout urination suggests that a lesion could be located anywhere from the upper urinary tract to the bladder
2.   Ask about associated symptoms:
a.   Colicky flank pain radiating to groin suggests a kidney stone
b.   Dysuria and frequency suggest cystitis, especially in females
c.   Hesitancy and dribbling suggest benign prostatic hypertrophy
d.   Hemoptysis, hematuria, and acute renal failure in an anemic patient suggests Goodpasture's syndrome
e.   Loin-pain and hematuria in a young women taking oral contraceptives may indicate small-vessel occlusive vascular disease
f.   In a systemic disease, fever, joint pains, and rash are typical manifestations
3.   Ask patient to describe any blood clots that have occurred
a.   Large, thick clots suggest the bladder as the bleeding source
b.   Specks or thin, stringy clots suggest the upper urinary tract as the source
4.   Determine whether hematuria is transient or persistent
a.   In persons <40 years, transient hematuria is common and seldom secondary to significant disease
b.   In persons >40 years, persistent and transient hematuria may be due to malignancy
5.   Ask whether the patient bruises easily or has extended bleeding after a minor cut or dental work (coagulopathy or bleeding dyscrasia may be present)
6.   In females, inquire about the last menstrual period

7. Obtain a complete medication history
8. Inquire about a history of pharyngitis with an impetiginous skin rash followed by hematuria, edema and hypertension (presentation of glomerulonephritis)
9. Ask about recent trauma and strenuous exercise
10. Question about risk factors for developing uroepithelial cancer (see preceding table)
11. Explore previous medical history, making certain to inquire about sickle cell disease and trait, previous urinary tract infections, metabolic and endocrine diseases, and surgeries
12. Inquire about exposure to tuberculosis
13. Explore patient's family history; kidney stone disease, Alport's syndrome and familial nephritis are common across generations of families

B. Physical Examination
1. Measure vital signs; elevated temperature suggests infection, neoplasm, or systemic disease; elevated blood pressure suggest glomerulonephritis
2. Observe skin for signs of exanthems, pallor, ecchymosis, or purpura
3. Examine for systemic infection such as tonsillar enlargement, lymphadenopathy, and exanthems
4. If Alport's syndrome is suspected, perform a hearing test as this syndrome is associated with hearing defects
5. Auscultate heart
6. Perform complete abdominal exam, noting tenderness, organomegaly, bladder distention, masses, or bruits
7. Assess for costovertebral angle tenderness which suggests pyelonephritis or urinary tract obstruction
8. Examine extremities for edema which may be associated with glomerulonephritis
9. In males, perform a prostate and rectal exam; a swollen, tender prostate suggests prostatitis; prostate nodule suggests prostatic carcinoma
10. In males, examine testes, spermatic cord, and vas deferens for tenderness and masses
11. In males, examine penis for condyloma acuminatum, meatal stenosis, foreign body
12. In females, perform a pelvic examination
    a. Inspect vulva and urethral meatus, noting signs of atrophic vaginitis, urethral caruncle, or urethral irritation
    b. Bimanual exam may uncover a uterine or ovarian mass which may secondarily involve the genitourinary tract

C. Differential Diagnosis
1. Essential hematuria is a diagnosis of exclusion
2. The majority of cases of hematuria will present with symptoms, signs, or laboratory test results that pinpoint a specific diagnosis
3. For those patients with asymptomatic, isolated hematuria for whom a cause cannot be identified always consider neoplasm, particularly in those >40 years of age

D. Diagnostic Tests
1. Always obtain urinalysis (UA) and a subsequent culture to confirm findings on the UA (best to obtain a freshly voided, morning specimen and examine it within 30 minutes); dipstick can give false-positive results and should always be used in conjunction with a microscopic examination
    a. Alkaline pH and positive nitrite and leukocyte esterase reactions suggest urinary tract infections
    b. Hematuria with pyuria but no bacteria suggest a sexually transmitted disease (chlamydia, gonorrhea), viral infection, or less commonly, tuberculosis
    c. Protein suggests glomerulonephritis
    d. If the dipstick test is negative for RBCs but the urine appears red, pigmenturia caused by endogenous substances that change color of urine is the likely cause
    e. Microscopic examination of urinary sediment can help determine the site of bleeding
        (1) RBC casts suggest glomerulonephritis
        (2) Crystals suggest renal calculi
    f. If exercise hematuria is suspected, patient should refrain from active participation in sports for at least 48 hours prior to urinalysis

2. Phase contrast microscopy is being used more frequently to determine the site of bleeding; this test is promising and is recommended early in the evaluation of hematuria after an infection has been excluded

3. If only isolated microscopic hematuria is demonstrated in the absence of bacterial infection a basic set of tests should be ordered:

   a. Order blood urea nitrogen and creatinine; elevated levels suggest obstruction by a renal calculi or renal insufficiency

   b. Order a complete blood count to document blood loss and presence of systemic involvement

   c. Order a 24-hour urine specimen for determination of the concentration of calcium and uric acid

   d. African American patients should be screened for sickle cell disease or trait

   e. Most authorities recommend that an intravenous pyelogram (IVP) should be included in this initial battery of tests before referral to a specialist

      (1) Most effective method to visualize anatomy of upper urinary tract; with the addition of a cystourethrogram, the lower urinary tract can be viewed as well

      (2) Has utility in evaluation of urolithiasis, renal tumors, renal trauma, benign prostatic hypertrophy, and carcinoma of bladder;

   f. Ultrasonography can be helpful if the patient is allergic to the dye used in IVP or has compromised renal function; diagnostic yield is similar to IVP

      (1) Test is noninvasive and can approximate size of kidney and reveal kidney stones, urinary tract obstruction and deformities

      (2) Also, helpful in differentiating a cystic from a solid mass

   g. Cystoscopy is recommended in patients >40 years who have negative urine cultures, IVP, or ultrasounds; cystoscopy is test of choice for evaluating patients with suspected carcinoma of the bladder

      (1) Lesions can be viewed directly and biopsies can be taken

      (2) A high-yield sample for cytology may also be obtained

   h. Urine cytology can detect transitional cell carcinoma of the bladder and collection system missed on IVP and cystoscopy

      (1) Three first-morning voidings urine specimens should be obtained on three separate days

      (2) Recommended in patients over >40 years of age, particularly those who are smokers with hematuria of nonglomerular origin

4. Order additional tests depending on the patient's presentation

   a. Order clotting studies (i.e., prothrombin time, partial thromboplastin time, platelet count, bleeding time) if a coagulopathy or a bleeding disorder is suspected

   b. Administer a purified protein derivative (PPD) and order urine culture for acid-fast bacillus when tuberculosis is a possibility

   c. In patients who have proteinuria in addition to hematuria order a 24-hour collection of creatinine and protein

   d. In patients <40 years, a 24-hour urine collection to exclude hyperuricosuria and hypercalciuria may be helpful

   e. Order erythrocyte sedimentation rate (ESR) for patients with suspected secondary glomerular disease such as endocarditis and systemic lupus erythematosus

   f. An immunologic survey consisting of titers of IgG, IgA, IgM, and IgE are helpful if Schönlein-Henoch purpura or glomerular disease is suspected

5. Consider additional testing

   a. Voiding cystourethrography can reveal congenital anomalies, stone formation or foreign bodies

   b. Computed tomography (CT) can delineate a small mass, but it is not cost-effective in most cases

   c. Magnetic resonance imaging is less sensitive than the CT scan for detecting complicated masses but is helpful in imaging other masses such as renal cysts

   d. Angiography is not usually performed, but is the only test to detect arteriovenous malformations and may be considered in patients with gross, painless hematuria after other studies have excluded carcinoma and other renal disease

   e. A biopsy is performed when no cause is apparent

V. Plan/Management

    A. Refer the following patients to a specialist:
        1. Patients with gross, painless hematuria throughout the voiding process
        2. Patients with risk factors for malignancy such as older age and smoking
        3. Patients with unexplained hematuria without characteristics of glomerular hematuria such as RBC casts, proteinuria, and with a nondiagnostic IVP
        4. Patients with urologic trauma

    B. Treat infections with appropriate antibiotics (see sections on URINARY TRACT INFECTIONS)

    C. Exercise-induced hematuria requires no treatment as it is self-limited

    D. Treatment of urinary stones
        1. Once ureteral obstruction is excluded and acute episode has passed, small stones which can be passed may be managed with hydration (maintain urine flow rate of 3-4 L/day) and analgesia; refer patients with large stones to specialist
        2. Patients can be considered for lithotripsy
        3. A low-purine diet and uricosuric agents may prevent recurrence of uric acid stones

    E. Follow Up
        1. Because patients who are treated for uncomplicated infections may also have underlying, noninfectious disorders such as a malignancies, close follow up is needed; repeat urinalysis 2-3 times in a 4-6 week period to determine that hematuria and all other signs and symptoms have abated
        2. Patients with a negative initial workup will need close monitoring; patients with possible undetected malignancy, particularly patients >40 years should have following: Urinalysis, urine cytologies, and cystoscopy at 3-6 month intervals
        3. Patients who may have glomerulonephritis should have blood pressure measurements, serum creatinine concentrations and urinalyses annually

URINARY INCONTINENCE IN ADULTS

I. Definition: Involuntary loss of urine

II. Pathogenesis: Results from pathologic, anatomic or physiologic factors

    A. Transient incontinence is a temporary condition which can be reversed and related to the following factors:
        1. Delirium, hypoxia, urinary tract infections, atrophic urethritis or vaginitis, recent prostatectomy, glycosuria, excessive urine production such as congestive heart failure, restricted mobility, psychological factors such as depression, or stool impaction
        2. Ingestion of certain medications such as sedatives, hypnotics, diuretics, anticholinergic agents, alpha-adrenergic agents, calcium channel blockers, alcohol, caffeine, or narcotics

    B. Stress incontinence is leakage of urine during activities that increase abdominal pressure such as coughing, sneezing, laughing or other physical activities
        1. In females, condition is due to hypermobility of the base of the bladder and urethra associated with poor pelvic support or infrequently by intrinsic urethral weakness from previous surgery or radiation
        2. In males, condition is due to an overflow from an underactive or acontractile detrusor associated with one of the following: prostate gland problems, urethral stricture, neurological problems or idiopathic detrusor failure

C. Urge incontinence is the inability to delay urination with an abrupt and strong desire to void and is due to bladder hyperactivity such as detrusor instability, detrusor hyperactivity or to an hypersensitive bladder which may be idiopathic or associated with any of the following:
1. Lower urinary tract problems such as carcinoma, infection, atrophic vaginitis-urethritis, obstruction
2. Central nervous system disorders such as stroke, multiple sclerosis, or Parkinson's disease
3. Drugs such hypnotics or narcotics

D. Overflow incontinence occurs with overdistension of the bladder due to the following:
1. Underactive or acontractile detrusor secondary to drugs, fecal impaction, or neurologic conditions such as diabetic neuropathy or low spinal cord injury
2. Bladder outlet or urethral obstruction secondary to prostatic hyperplasia, prostatic carcinoma or urethral stricture in men; cystoceles or uterine prolapse in women
3. Detrusor external sphincter dyssynergia associated with multiple sclerosis or spinal cord injury

E. Urge/stress mixed incontinence may occur and is caused by a combination of the above factors

F. Functional incontinence is mainly caused by factors outside the lower urinary tract such as dementia or immobility that hinder the patient from appropriate toileting

G. Some patients, particularly the elderly, have mixed types of incontinence

III. Clinical Presentation

A. Approximately 15-30% of all noninstitutionalized individuals older than 60 have urinary incontinence (UI); women have twice the prevalence of men

B. Incontinence often goes undetected, because fewer than 50% of affected patients report episodes to health care provider

C. Associated urinary symptoms are irritative (frequency, urgency, nocturia) or obstructive (hesitancy, weak stream, straining to void)

D. Urinary incontinence has social, psychological, and financial ramifications such as family burden due to home care, patient's embarrassment and stress due to odor and appearance, and enormous costs in caring for incontinent patients

E. Incontinence is often a major factor in the decision to place persons in nursing homes

F. Incontinence is associated with decubitus ulcers, urinary tract infections, sepsis, renal failure, and increased mortality

G. Stress incontinence is the most prevalent type of incontinence; common in women who have borne children and postmenopausal women

H. In urge incontinence, patients often have a sensation of bladder fullness with little warning before passage of urine

I. Overflow incontinence is characterized by frequent passage of small amounts of urine

IV. Diagnosis/Evaluation

A. History
1. Ask about onset of incontinence
2. Inquire about characteristics of UI such as stress, urge, dribbling
3. Ask about the amount and frequency of urine loss and daily voids
4. Ask about lower urinary tract symptoms such as dysuria, hesitancy, nocturia, frequency, hematuria, pain

5. Recent study found that the following single question was most helpful: "Do you consider this accidental loss of urine a problem that interferes with your day-to-day activities or bothers you in other ways?"
6. To determine severity, assess the number and types of protection used per day
7. Determine fluid intake such as drinking of caffeine-containing and/or other diuretic fluids
8. Question about changes in bowel habits
9. Ask about sexual function
10. Determine whether patient has changes in mental status, depression or difficulty with mobility
11. Explore types and results of previous treatments
12. Ask about use of pads, briefs or other protective devices
13. Complete past medical and medication history
14. Review of systems should focus on neurologic and genitourinary histories
15. Explore precipitants such as cough, surgery, childbirth, menopause, trauma, new onset of illness or new medications
16. Ask patient to complete a "voiding" record or diary to monitor the frequency, timing, amount of voiding, and factors associated with UI
17. With frail or functionally impaired persons, also ask about environmental factors such as access to toilets and social factors such as living arrangements and caregiver involvement

B. Physical Examination
1. Perform complete abdominal exam to detect masses, suprapubic tenderness or fullness
2. In a male, perform genital exam to detect abnormalities of the foreskin, glans, penis and perineal skin
3. In a female, perform a pelvic exam to assess perineal skin, pelvic prolapse (cystocele, uterine prolapse), pelvic mass, perivaginal muscle tone, atrophic vaginitis, and to estimate post-voiding residual (PVR) urine by abdominal palpation and percussion and/or bimanual examination; also assess the vaginal wall and urethra
4. Perform a rectal exam to assess for perineal sensation, resting and active sphincter tone, rectal mass, and fecal impaction; in men, also assess the consistency and contour of the prostate and check for bulbocavernosus reflex
5. Complete a neurological exam including deep tendon reflexes, soft and sharp sensation
6. Assess mental status
7. Perform a musculoskeletal exam to uncover secondary causes of incontinence such as occurs with functional incontinence due to weakness and problems ambulating
8. Measure postvoid residual urine volume (PVR):
   a. After patient has voided, catheterize patient (use Coudé tip catheters in men to ease insertion) or assess by pelvic ultrasound; ultrasound is best approach in men with suspected prostate obstruction
   b. PVR <50 mL is adequate bladder emptying; PVR >200 mL is inadequate emptying; PVRs between 50-200 mL are considered equivocal and test should be repeated
9. Consider additional tests
   a. Provocative stress testing can be performed
      (1) Ask patient to relax and then cough vigorously
      (2) Watch for urine loss from the urethra
   b. Marshall test
      (1) During pelvic exam, patient bears down or coughs with a full bladder
      (2) If the examiner can stop the observed stress incontinence by manually elevating and supporting the anterior vaginal wall, then the test is considered positive for anatomic stress incontinence
   c. Observe voiding to detect problems with hesitancy, dribbling or interrupted stream

C. Differential Diagnosis
1. Important to differentiate transient incontinence from other types of incontinence; transient incontinence usually has an acute onset with identifiable precipitating factors
2. Vaginal reflux is a common problem that is often misdiagnosed as UI; usually occurs in overweight children and adults

a.   Voided urine becomes trapped in vagina; later, as female stands and moves, the urine dribbles out of urethra

b.   Treatment is patient education on ways to avoid trapped urine in vagina
(1)   Spread legs wide apart when urinating
(2)   Reverse sitting position on toilet to spread labia may be helpful

3.   Important to differentiate between stress, urge, and overflow incontinence

D.   Diagnostic Tests
1.   Obtain a urinalysis (UA) to detect contributing conditions such as hematuria, pyuria, bacteriuria, glycosuria, and proteinuria (dipstick is acceptable for screening, but microscopic exam is usually needed)

2.   Order a urine culture if bacteria is detected from the UA

3.   Simple cystometry can be performed in the office as a substitute for the expensive, gold standard, cystometrography
a.   Catheter is inserted into bladder
b.   After bladder empties, the plunger is removed from a bayonet-tipped 50 mL syringe and tip is inserted into end of catheter
c.   50 mL of sterile water is poured into the open end of the syringe which is held 15 cm above the urethra
d.   Continue instilling water in 50 mL increments until patient experiences urge to urinate
e.   At this point, instill water in 25 mL increments until patient complains of severe urgency or until bladder contractions occur (contractions can be detected with rise and fall of fluid level in syringe)
f.   Severe urgency or bladder contractions <300 mL of bladder volume leads to diagnosis of urge incontinence

4.   In a patient suspected of having obstruction, noncompliant bladder, or urinary retention order blood urea nitrogen (BUN) and creatinine levels

5.   In patients with polyuria in absence of diuretic drugs, order fasting serum glucose levels and serum calcium levels

6.   In patients with hematuria and possible malignancy or recent onset of irritative voiding, perform urine cytology

7.   Consult specialist about further testing of patients who meet one of the following criteria:
a.   Uncertain diagnosis and trouble developing a treatment plan based on basic diagnostic tests
b.   Failure to respond to adequate therapeutic trial and thus a candidate for further treatment
c.   Presence of other comorbid conditions such as severe pelvic prolapse, prostate nodule

8.   Specialized tests are not routinely required to make diagnosis of UI but may be ordered and include urodynamic tests, endoscopic tests, cystoscopy, multichannel or subtracted cystometrography, urethral pressure profiles, urethral sphincter electromyography, and imaging tests of the upper tract and lower tract with and without voiding

V.   Plan/Management

A.   Refer patients with the following problems to a specialist: previous pelvic or anti-incontinence surgery, incontinence associated with recurrent urinary tract infections, prostate nodule or prostate assymetry, gross pelvic prolapse, neurologic abnormality, hematuria without infection, significant persistent proteinuria, failure to respond to treatment of presumptive diagnosis

B.   Treat any reversible cause of UI such as a urinary tract infection; important to quickly identify transient incontinence and treat appropriately

C.   Behavioral techniques are first-line options for patients with stress and urge incontinence; they are effective in reducing incontinence and have no reported side effects; patients with overflow UI do not benefit from behavioral intervention

1. Bladder training involves three components: education, scheduled voiding, and positive reinforcement
    a. Patients are required to resist or inhibit the sensation of urgency, to postpone voiding, and to void according to a schedule
    b. Initially the voiding schedule is set between 2-3 hours
    c. Treatment may continue for several months with frequent health care contacts
2. For patients not motivated or unable to do bladder training, try habit training. In habit training, a scheduled toileting is planned at regular intervals; unlike bladder retraining, there is no systematic plan to motivate the patient to delay voiding and resist the urge to void
3. For the dependent or cognitively impaired incontinent patient, prompted voiding which teaches patients to discriminate their incontinence status and to request toileting assistance from caregivers may be beneficial. Prompted voiding is often used as a supplement to habit training. Steps in prompted voiding are the following:
    a. Patient is regularly checked by caregiver and asked to verbally report if wet or dry
    b. Patient is asked to attempt to use toilet
    c. Patient is praised for dryness and trying to use toilet
4. Pelvic muscle exercises or Kegel exercises improve urethral resistance through active exercise of the periurethral and pelvic muscles
    a. First, teach the correct technique of contracting and differentiating the periurethral and pelvic muscles with palpation and verbal feedback to assure correct performance
    b. Teach to "draw in" muscles as if to control urination, but do not contract abdominal, buttock or inner thigh muscles
    c. Teach how to sustain contractions for up to 10 seconds followed by an equal period of relaxation
    d. Exercises should be done about 30-80 times a day for at least 6 weeks; may need to be done indefinitely
    e. Exercises are indicated for females with stress incontinence, males following prostatic surgery, females after multiple surgical repairs, and patients with urge UI
5. Vaginal cones may be used along with pelvic muscle training in women
    a. Patient uses cones that are of identical shape and volume but of increasing weight
    b. Women insert cone into vagina and rests cone on the superior surface of the perineal muscle
    c. Twice daily women try to retain cone by doing pelvic muscle exercise for up to 15 minutes
    d. As muscles get stronger, the weight of the cone is increased
6. Biofeedback can be used in conjunction with other behavioral therapies
7. Add physical, social and environmental devices to facilitate patient's toileting such as the following:
    a. Grab bars in the bathroom, elevated toilet seats, adequate lighting to bathroom
    b. Toilet supplements such as commodes and urinals
    c. Walkers or other mobility aids
    d. Chairs designed for easy rising
8. Dietary modifications may be helpful and include decrease or elimination of alcohol, sweetener substitutes, and caffeine consumption
9. Plan ways to eliminate constipation
    a. Encourage eating foods high in fiber and increasing exercise and activity
    b. Aggressively treat constipation as this alone could be primary factor of UI
10. Recommend double voiding to anyone with post voiding residual (PVR); urinate, wait 3 minutes, and void again (double voiding also reduces risk of urinary tract infections)
11. Pharmacologic treatment should be based on type of incontinence (see following table)

PHARMACOLOGIC TREATMENT FOR INCONTINENCE

Drugs for Urge Incontinence

Drug	Dosage	Side Effects	Comments
Anticholinergic and smooth muscle relaxant			
Oxybutynin (Ditropan)	2.5-5.0 mg TID/QID	Anticholinergic effects	First-line pharmacologic agent for treating detrusor overactivity
Tolterodine (Detrol)	2 mg BID	Anticholinergic effects, but less than oxybutynin	More expensive than oxybutynin; previously reserved for patients who cannot tolerate oxybutynin but gaining favor as a first-line agent
Anticholinergic agent			
Propantheline (Pro-Banthine)	7.5-30.0 mg, 3-5x/day	Anticholinergic effects, urinary retention, dry mouth, visual blurring	Effective for less impaired patients
Tricyclic agent			
Imipramine (Tofranil)	Initial: 10-25 mg QD/BID/TID. Max total daily dose: 25-100 mg	Nausea, insomnia	Research is limited on these drugs
Doxepin (Sinequan)	Initial: 10-25 mg QD/BID/TID. Max total daily dose: 25-100 mg	Fatigue, dizziness, blurred vision	
Drugs for Stress Incontinence			
α-Adrenergic agonist			
Phenylpropanol-amine*	25-75 mg in sustained release form BID	Anxiety, insomnia, headache	Use cautiously in patients with hypertension, hyperthyroidism, cardiac problems
Estrogen therapy			
Conjugated estrogen* (Premarin), progestin (Medroxypro-gesterone)	Estrogen: 0.3-1.25 mg/day orally or vaginally Progestin: 2.5-10.0 mg/day either continuously or intermittently	Risks include neoplasm and thromboembolism	May also benefit patients with urge incontinence
Tricyclic agent			
Imipramine (Tofranil)	10-25 mg QD/BID/TID	Nausea, insomnia, postural hypotension	Used as an alternative therapy for stress and urge incontinence

*Combined α-adrenergic agonist such as phenylpropanolamine and estrogen supplementation therapy may be effective when initial single drug fails; usual dose of phenylpropanolamine is 75 mg (in sustained release form) BID/TID

12. Consult specialist for patients with stress and urge incontinence who fail to respond to behavioral training and initial drug treatment

D. Treatment of overflow incontinence is intermittent (first choice), indwelling or suprapubic catheterization; before catheterization, an exhaustive evaluation should be undertaken to identify the cause of retained urine and to exclude conditions that require surgical or other interventions such as benign prostatic hyperplasia

E. Surgery is an option for patients with UI due to bladder neck or urethral obstruction, detrusor overactivity, intrinsic and sphincter deficiency, and urethral hypermobility in females; surgery is third-line treatment option for patients with urge or stress incontinence

F. Other techniques and devises may be beneficial; emphasize that any device which decreases urine outflow should be used cautiously; warn patient to never delay voiding >4 hours
    1. Penile clamps
    2. Pessaries are soft pieces of plastic or rubber that women put into their vaginas to hold up prolapsed bladders or uteri
        a. Patients must be individually fitted
        b. Teach patient how to insert and remove pessary
        c. Reinforce that patient should remove pessary each night and should reinsert it in the morning
        d. Pessary should be washed with soap and water prior to insertion
    3. An internal urinary-control insert (Reliance Urinary Control Insert) is a disposable, single-use device that is placed in urethra by the patients when they are at increased risk for stress incontinence such as during exercise
        a. After insertion, the patients inflate a 3-mL balloon
        b. Device is removed for voiding by deflating a small balloon that retains the device in the urethra
        c. Patient's urethra must be measured to assure the correct length of catheter
    4. A single-use foam patch (Impress) can be sealed over the urethral meatus and held in place with specific adhesive gel; patch is removed for voiding and replaced with new patch
    5. FemAssist is a reusable, silicone-domed cap that fits over the external urethral meatus and is secured by suction and ointment; device is removed before voiding and replaced afterwards; devices should be changed weekly
    6. UroMed Patch can be purchased OTC and is a small, disposable foam patch which is placed over the urinary opening where the adhesive forms a seal to reduce urine leakage; worn 2-3 hours at a time during the day and then replaced; can be worn throughout night
    7. Contigen Bard Collagen Implant
        a. Implant is injected into tissues surrounding the urethra to add bulk to tissues and to close the passage to prevent leakage
        b. An allergy test to bovine collagen must be performed before implantation
        c. Repeated injections are sometime required
    8. Electrical stimulation (research is inconclusive)
        a. A probe is placed in vagina or rectum and electrical stimulation which causes reflex contraction of the pelvic muscles is applied; stimulation can also be delivered transspinally
        b. Stimulation is typically performed at home once or twice daily for 1-2 hours to keep the pelvic floor muscles contracted
        c. This therapy should be used in conjunction with pelvic muscle exercises
    9. Absorbent pads or garments

G. Follow Up: Frequent contact via the phone or with office visits is needed to provide support and positive reinforcement

CYSTITIS AND PYELONEPHRITIS

I. Definition: Bacteria in urine which have the potential to injure tissues of the urinary tract and adjacent structures. Urinary tract infections (UTIs) are often classified as upper and lower tract infections

    A. Cystitis, infection of the bladder, is an example of a common lower tract infection

    B. Pyelonephritis is the main upper tract infection and involves infection of the renal parenchyma

II. Pathogenesis of cystitis and pyelonephritis

    A. In women, the major cause is invasion of the urinary tract by bacteria that have ascended the urethra from the introitus. Females have a short urethra which is in close proximity to the perirectal area making colonization possible

B. Currently, researchers are exploring whether there is a genetic link for women who are prone to frequent UTIs; studies are underway to develop a blood test to identify high-risk females

C. In males, cystitis and pyelonephritis are uncommon
 1. In the past, these problems were always considered the result of an underlying urologic abnormality; currently in young, healthy males with isolated cystitis, the literature suggests that infection may be due to endogenous bacteria without an underlying abnormality or related to a subclinical case of prostatitis
 2. In older man over age 50 years, a broad range of pathogens may be involved, and these infections are often related to structural abnormalities such as benign prostatic hypertrophy

D. Pathogens: Bacteria adhere to uroepithelial cells
 1. Gram negative bacilli are most common; 80-90% of community-acquired infections are due to *Escherichia coli*
  a. Other gram negative bacilli organisms include *Klebsiella pneumoniae* or *Proteus mirabilis*
  b. A wide range of gram-negative bacilli and other microorganisms may be causative agents in men; particularly in older men
 2. Gram-positive cocci account for 10-15% of community acquired infections; *Staphylococcus saprophyticus* is the second most common pathogen and often occurs in young, sexually active females
 3. In postmenopausal women *E. coli* infection is common, but other bacteria are also prevalent due to the increased pH of the vagina that occurs with estrogen deficiency
 4. In hospital settings, *E. coli* is less prevalent with Proteus, Klebsiella, Enterobacter, Pseudomonas, Staphylococci, and Enterococci species being more common

E. Risk factors in both genders
 1. Diabetes mellitus; not necessarily an increased risk for developing infection but often there is a disorder of bladder emptying which makes UTI more difficult to eradicate
 2. Urinary instrumentation and catheterization
 3. Obstruction of normal flow of urine resulting from calculi, tumors, urethral strictures
 4. Neurogenic bladder disease from strokes, multiple sclerosis, spinal cord injuries
 5. Vesicoureteral reflux as a result of a congenital abnormality or more often from bladder overdistention from obstruction

F. Risk factors in females
 1. Females with increased sexual activity, diaphragm and spermicide use, and failure to void after intercourse
 2. Pregnancy
 3. History of recent urinary infection
 4. Postponing urination or incomplete voiding in women
 5. Tampons and wiping from back to front after a bowel movement are **not** risk factors

G. Risk factors in males
 1. Homosexuality
 2. Lack of circumcision
 3. Having a sexual partner with vaginal colonization by uropathogens
 4. HIV infection with CD4+ T- lymphocyte counts of less than 200 per cubic millimeter
 5. Obstruction of normal flow resulting from prostatic hypertrophy and urethral strictures

III. Clinical Presentation

A. After puberty, the prevalence of UTIs increases significantly in females, but remains low in males

B. After age 65, UTIs are more common with an equal incidence in males and females

C. In the elderly, UTIs are the most common cause of sepsis; elderly patients may present with changes in mental status, decreased appetite, somnolence and mild fever

D. Cystitis
1. Onset is usually abrupt
2. Adults, particularly the elderly, may be asymptomatic
3. Typical symptoms include dysuria, urgency, frequency, nocturia, suprapubic heaviness or discomfort; fever is uncommon
4. Bacturia: 10^2 to >10^5 colony-forming units per milliliter of urine (cfu per ml.)

E. Pyelonephritis
1. Acute onset of chills, fever, flank pain, headache, malaise, costovertebral angle tenderness, and possibly hematuria
2. Often occurs concurrently or after a lower urinary tract infection
3. May be associated with renal calculi, ureteral obstruction, or neurogenic bladder.
4. Urine almost always has white blood cells; urine cultures >10^5 cfu per mL, usually have bacterial casts

IV. Diagnosis/Evaluation

A. History
1. Determine onset and duration of urinary symptoms
2. Ask about strength and character of urine stream when voiding, particularly in older men
3. Determine whether dysuria occurs during urination or after urine begins to pass over inflamed labia as with herpes simplex infections
4. Inquire about associated symptoms such as fever, chills, nausea, vomiting, diarrhea, constipation, abdominal and back pain, hematuria
5. Ask about onset, duration, and characteristics of vaginal or urethral discharge
6. Always query females about method of birth control and date of last menstrual period
7. Past medical history should include drug allergies, chronic diseases such as diabetes mellitus or multiple sclerosis, previous genitourinary problems
8. Ask patient to count number of previous UTIs and discuss successes and failures of previous treatments

B. Physical Examination
1. Assess vital signs, particularly noting elevated temperature and signs of orthostatic hypotension
2. Perform a complete abdominal exam to detect tenderness, a distended bladder, or a mass
3. Palpate back for costovertebral tenderness
4. In females may need to inspect perineum and do complete pelvic, speculum, and rectal exams
5. In males may need to inspect and palpate external genitalia and scrotum
6. In males perform a prostate and rectal exam
7. Consider performing a neurologic examination to detect neurogenic diseases such as multiple sclerosis

C. Differential Diagnosis
1. Males
   a. Gonococcal and nongonococcal urethritis in males (often asymptomatic, but may have mucoid or purulent urethral discharge)
   b. Prostatitis (a tender prostate on rectal exam is usually present)
   c. Epididymitis (testicular tenderness and erythema are present)
   d. Benign prostatic hypertrophy (symptoms include changes in urinary stream and nocturia)
   e. Prostatodynia (presents with perineal or back pain accompanied by unilateral testicular pain or dysuria; urinalysis and urine culture are negative)
2. Females
   a. Interstitial cystitis
      (1) Painful bladder condition which is most common between 20-60 years of age
      (2) Characterized by suprapubic pain which is relieved by bladder emptying
      (3) Involves inflammation of the bladder which may progress to ulcerations, fibrosis, and decreased bladder capacity

(4) Diagnosed with cystoscopy, urodynamic studies, and bladder biopsy
(5) There is no cure; the following treatments may be beneficial:
    (a) Oral medications such as pentosan polysulfate (Elmiron) 100 mg cap one hour before or 2 hours after meals with water, amitriptyline (Elavil), hydroxyzine (Atarax), nifedipine (Adalat), or cimetidine (Tagamet)
    (b) Intravesical therapies such as hydrodistention of the bladder
    (c) Intravesical instillation of dimethyl sulfoxide (DMSO)
(6) Surgery is the last option

    b. Urethral syndrome
      (1) Patient has irritative voiding symptoms with an absence of objective findings
      (2) There is no cure, treatment is symptomatic
    c. Vulvovaginitis (external dysuria, vulvar erythema, and vulvar lesions are often present)
    d. Vaginitis
      (1) Patients deny urinary urgency and frequency
      (2) Usually there are no WBCs or bacteria in the urine
      (3) Vaginal discharge, odor, and pruritis may be present
    e. Cervicitis (cervix will be abnormal on pelvic exam)

3. Both genders
    a. Urinary calculi (usually patient has severe pain and hematuria)
    b. Bladder outlet obstruction (changes in urinary stream occur)
    c. Renal tuberculosis (hematuria is common)
    d. Tumors and carcinoma (hematuria is common)

D. Diagnostic Tests
1. Urine collection
    a. Clean catch voided specimens are usually acceptable for adults
      (1) First morning specimen is the best voided specimen
      (2) If urine specimen is obtained later in the day, bladder should not be emptied for at least 2 hours and patients should avoid high fluid intake which would dilute sample
    b. Single in-and-out catheterization of the bladder should be done on patients who are unable to give a clean midstream urine specimen (i.e., elderly patients who are incontinent or demented)

2. Urinalysis
    a. Dipstick urinalysis: Findings of UTIs are the following:
      (1) Leukocyte esterase test is positive and denotes pyuria or WBCs in the urine; false positive esterase tests occur with kidney stones, tumors, urethritis, and poor collection techniques
      (2) Nitrites are positive with gram negative infections; false negatives occur with use of diuretics, inadequate levels of dietary nitrate or presence of bacteria that do not produce nitrate reductase (*Staphylococcus saprophyticus, Enterococcus, Pseudomonas*)
    b. Microscopic analysis: Examine urine sediment under high power (40X), to count WBCs and perform gram stain to identify type of bacteria
      (1) Significant pyuria is >2-5 leukocytes per high power field or if using a counting hemocytometer, 10 or more white blood cell/mm^3 is used as the criterion
      (2) Gram stain is done to identify whether bacteria are gram negative or positive and the shape and pattern of bacteria; it is not helpful to count bacteria on a gram stain

3. Urine culture and sensitivity (Urine C&S)
    a. The traditional standard for significant bacteriuria was 10^5 colony-forming units (cfu) of a uropathogen per mL of urine; today the criterion that is used is 10^2 in symptomatic females or 10^3 in symptomatic males
    b. Bacterial identification and determination of antibiotic susceptibilities or urine C&S is not necessary in most uncomplicated UTIs
    c. Bacterial identification or urine C&S is important in infections in males, females who have complicated UTIs, and females who are symptomatic but pyuria is absent

4. With systemic symptoms order CBC with differential and in severely ill and possibly, elderly patients order blood cultures; consider ordering erythrocyte sedimentation rate
5. In females with symptoms associated with sexually transmitted disease (STD), perform wet mount of vaginal secretions and order *N. gonorrhoea* (GC) cultures and chlamydia test; also can gram stain cervical secretions
6. In a male with a possible STD, gram stain urethral secretion and order GC culture and chlamydia tests
7. Other studies are usually not needed; consider additional tests such as renal ultrasound, voiding cystourethrogram, intravenous pyelogram (IVP), renal scan, renal biopsy, or cystoscopy in patients with repeat infections, slow resolution of symptoms, and atypical features such as persistent hematuria

V. Plan/Management (the treatment for females and males differ; treatment of isolated and recurrent infections in females will be discussed first)

A. Bacterial cystitis:
1. In females with uncomplicated UTIs (young, nonpregnant, non-diabetic women without structural problems or previous UTIs), urine cultures are generally not indicated before treatment
2. Choose either the 3-day or 7-day regimen or fosfomycin tromethamine (Monurol) in a single dose if patient has uncomplicated UTI (see following table for ANTIBIOTICS)
3. The 3-day antibiotic therapy is currently gaining favor as the most cost-effective regimen because it is less expensive and has less side effects than the traditional 7-10 day regimen; women at risk for recurrent or relapsing infections should be treated for 7-10 days

ANTIBIOTICS FOR TREATING CYSTITIS			
Trimethoprim/sulfamethoxazole (Bactrim)	160 mg/800 mg	1 DS tab	BID
Trimethoprim (Trimpex)	100 mg	1 tab	BID
Nitrofurantoin (Macrodantin)[†]	100 mg	1 tab	QID
Amoxicillin (Amoxil)[*]	500 mg	1 tab	TID
Lomefloxacin (Maxaquin)[**§]	400 mg	1 tab	QD
Norfloxacin (Noroxin)[**§‡]	400 mg	1 tab	BID
Fosfomycin tromethamine (Monurol)	3 g	1 sachet with 3-4 oz. of H_2O	Single dose

[*]Amoxicillin cure rates are lower because of increasing resistance of *E. coli*
[**]Avoid if possible, because the fluoroquinolones are expensive and have potential teratogenic effects
[†]Take with food
[§]Take with full glass of water
[‡]Take on an empty stomach

4. Order follow up urinalysis for any patient who is at risk for recurrent or relapsing infections (if urinalysis is abnormal order urine culture)
5. Phenazopyridine HCl (Pyridium) may be prescribed 100 mg TID for three days if the patient is experiencing bladder spasms; warn patient that urine will turn orange

B. Recurrent infections in females (Must repeat urine culture and sensitivity each time patient has symptoms)
1. Relapse (uncommon and caused by original infecting pathogen)
a. Occurs within two weeks of completion of therapy
b. Treat for 2-6 weeks longer
c. Seek occult source of infection or urologic abnormality; consider ordering tests of renal function (BUN & creatinine), an intravenous pyelogram (IVP) and referring to a specialist

2. Reinfection (cystitis) in premenopausal females: Most recurrent UTIs are due to reinfection with a new organism rather than a relapse of the same initial infection
   a. If patient has 2 or fewer UTIs in one year:
     (1) Recommend patient-initiated therapy for symptomatic episodes (give patient a written prescription which she may fill when symptoms occur)
     (2) Prescribe 3-day regimen (see preceding table on ANTIBIOTICS) based on patient's past culture results and clinical success
   b. If patient has greater than or equal to 3 UTIs in one year:
     (1) If UTIs occur only after intercourse recommend a single-dose antiobiotic after coitus such as trimethoprim/sulfamethoxazole 160 mg/800 mg (2 double strength tablets) or nitrofurantoin (Macrodantin) 200 mg
     (2) If UTIs are not related to intercourse, prophylactic antimicrobials should be used for 6 months after the infection has been eradicated
       (a) Urine cultures should be done every 1-2 months.
       (b) Extend prophylactic therapy to 1-2 years if reinfection occurs at end of 6-month period.
       (c) One of the following prophylactic antimicrobials should be prescribed for 6 months (may take daily or thrice weekly): Nitrofurantoin (Furadantin) 50 mg tablet HS; Trimethoprim/sulfamethoxazole (Bactrim) 40/200 mg tablets, half tablet of regular strength at HS; Cephalexin (Keflex) 250 mg tablet at HS
   c. Explore whether patient is using diaphragms, spermicides, and not voiding after intercourse which may be causing reinfections
3. Reinfections in perimenopausal women may occur due to residual urine after voiding which is associated with bladder or uterine prolapse and also due to lack of estrogen which changes vaginal microflow allowing increased colonization by *E. coli*
   a. Aforementioned antimicrobial prophylaxis may be beneficial
   b. Alternatively, prescribe topical estradiol cream (see section on ATROPHIC VAGINITIS for dosage)
   c. Oral intake of at least 300 mL/day of cranberry juice may prevent infections
   d. Teach patient to double void (urinate completely, wait 3 minutes, and then urinate again)
4. Vaccines to protect against recurrent *E. coli* infections are being studied

C. Pyelonephritis in females (consider consultation with a specialist)
1. Urine cultures are always indicated to definitively identify the invading organism and its antimicrobial sensitivity before treatment
2. Therapy and hospitalization are needed in all cases suggestive of bacteremia
3. Consider hospitalization for adults with pyelonephritis, particularly those who are pregnant, have a chronic disease, are vomiting, and who have a history of nonadherence to therapies
4. Close monitoring of female patients is needed if treated on an outpatient basis
5. Outpatient treatment is one of the following (modifications in the antibiotic should be made once the susceptibility profile is known)
   a. Trimethoprim-sulfamethoxazole (Septra) DS tablet BID for 14 days
   b. Ciprofloxacin (Cipro) 250-500 mg BID for 14 days
   c. Ceftriaxone (Rocephin) IM can be used on an outpatient basis in some patients
6. If the 2-week regimen fails, a longer course of 4-6 weeks should be considered because renal parenchymal disease is more difficult to eradicate than bladder mucosal infections
7. Patient's symptoms should improve within 12-48 hours; if not, consider consultation with a specialist and look for deeper infections (imaging studies are often done to exclude obstruction, calculi, and formation of intrarenal abscesses)
8. Schedule return visits or contact patient by phone in 12-24 hours
9. Follow up cultures should be ordered at 2 weeks and 3 months post-treatment
10. Consult specialist for patients who present with recurrences of pyelonephritis (recommended that these patients need further urologic investigation such as an excretory urography)

D. Treatment of uncomplicated bacterial cystitis in healthy males <50 years
   1. In the past all cases of bacterial cystitis in males were believed to be due to underlying structural problems such as prostatic hypertrophy; today, some, but not all experts, recommend that the first UTI can be treated with 7-10 day regimen of trimethoprim-sulfamethoxazole, trimethoprim or a fluoroquinolone (see preceding table on ANTIBIOTICS for dosages)
   2. Shorter treatments are not recommended
   3. Pretreatment and posttreatment urine cultures are recommended
   4. Some authorities recommend reculturing urine at 4-6 weeks as prostatitis may be a related cause

E. In males over age 50 years, a broad range of bacteria may be causing the infection
   1. Consider ordering renal function tests (blood urea nitrogen [BUN], creatinine) and consider urological consult and intravenous pyelogram (IVP)
   2. Prescribe extended 10-14 day course of one of antibiotics (see preceding table on ANTIBIOTICS)
   3. Always do urine culture prior to starting drug therapy and after therapy has been completed
   4. Because many men have relapse infection, a follow up visit in 4-6 weeks is recommended; consider ordering a segmented urine collection to detect bacterial prostatitis which often causes subsequent infections (see section on PROSTATITIS for procedure)
   5. May prescribe phenazophyridine HCl (Pyridium)100-200 mg TID for 3 days for bladder spasm

F. Persistent or recurrent bladder infections in males: Consult urologist

G. Pyelonephritis in males (consultation with a specialist is recommended)
   1. In men, pyelonephritis usually suggests a structural problem and is an indication for hospitalization, parenteral antibiotic therapy, and an IVP
   2. Close follow up is essential

H. Patient education may help prevent future recurrent infections
   1. Avoid a full bladder
   2. Do not postpone urinating or rush during urination
   3. High fluid intake at first signs of infection
   4. For women, void after intercourse
   5. For women, consider other types of birth control if using a diaphragm or spermicides

I. Asymptomatic bacteriuria
   1. Defined as reproducible growth of at least 10^5 cfu of the same species of bacteria per milliliter of urine in a patient who has no signs or symptoms of UTI (need 2 positive urine specimens collected over a period of time)
   2. Treatment is controversial: In pregnant women, patients with diabetes, and patients who are to have urologic surgery prescribe antimicrobial therapy in a similar fashion as other UTIs; a repeat culture should be done at 2 weeks posttreatment and if positive, the treatment regimen for relapse should be followed
   3. A more conservative approach is to rule out any underlying or predisposing pathology and then treat the first episode with antibiotics (based on the urine culture and sensitivity); do not treat subsequent episodes if the patent remains asymptomatic

J. Referral
   1. In women consider referral for upper tract illness, recurrent multiple infections, and infections with unusual organisms
   2. Consider referring all males with UTIs with exception of young, healthy men who do not have recurrent infections

K. Follow up is variable depending on age, gender, and condition of patient
1. For uncomplicated cystitis in females treated with 3-10 day regimen, no follow up or urine testing is needed
2. For cystitis in males, follow up urine culture is needed after treatment; some recommend following these patients with repeat urine testing and a segmented urine collection to detect prostatitis in 4-6 weeks
3. Reinfections need close follow up with urine cultures every 1-2 months
4. Patients with pyelonephritis should be contacted within 12-24 hours after treatment is begun; then, reschedule visits 2 weeks and 3 months post-treatment for urine cultures

PROSTATITIS

I. Definition: Inflammation or infection of the prostate gland; four common forms are acute bacterial, chronic bacterial, nonbacterial, and prostatodynia

II. Pathogenesis

A. May result from an ascending urethral infection, reflux of infected urine, extension of a rectal infection, or from hematogenous spread

B. Nonbacterial prostatitis has an unknown etiology and may be associated with an autoimmune process, an allergic reaction, neuromuscular dysfunction, or psychological factors

C. Extraprostatic causes of prostatodynia are suspected such as a disorder of the bladder outlet, detrusor hyperreflexia, or pelvic floor tension myalgia

D. Pathogens
1. Acute and chronic bacterial prostatitis: Gram-negative bacilli (predominantly *Escherichia coli*), *Enterobacter*, *Klebsiella*, *Pseudomonas* and *Proteus*
2. Nonbacterial prostatitis: *Gardnerella vaginalis*, Chlamydia species, *Ureaplasma urealyticum*, or mycoplasma

III. Clinical Presentation

A. Acute bacterial prostatitis
1. Least common type of prostatitis
2. Usually occurs in young and elderly, male adults
3. Characterized by systemic illness with fever, chills, and malaise
4. Acute onset of dysuria, frequency, inhibited urinary voiding, low back pain, suprapubic discomfort, and perineal pain is typical
5. May have painful sexual intercourse and pain when defecating
6. Initial, terminal, or less often, total hematuria may be present
7. May have significant edema that results in acute urinary retention
8. Urine specimens contain pyuria and bacteriuria

B. Chronic bacterial prostatitis
1. Occurs in older men
2. Systemic illness is not usually present
3. Characterized by exacerbations and remissions
4. Symptoms are varying degrees of bladder outflow obstruction such as dribbling, hesitancy, loss of stream volume and force
5. Hematuria, hematospermia or painful ejaculations may be present
6. Hallmark feature is recurrent urinary tract infections; patient is typically asymptomatic and urine is sterile between episodes

7. Many patients have stones in prostrate (prostatic calculi)
8. Infertility may occur
9. Urine specimens contain pyuria and bacteriuria

C. Nonbacterial prostatitis
1. Most common type of prostatitis; eight times more common than bacterial prostatitis
2. Usually patient has mild perineal pain, ejaculatory pain, dysuria, frequency, and urgency but no signs and symptoms of systemic illness
3. Penile discharge is common
4. Sequelae may be infertility
5. WBCs but <u>no</u> bacteria are detected in urine and expressed prostate secretion cultures

D. Prostatodynia
1. Presents as perineal or back pain accompanied by unilateral testicular pain, dysuria, hesitancy, decreased flow, or postvoid dribbling
2. Usually affects males between 22 and 56 years
3. There are no WBCs nor bacteria in the urine or expressed prostate secretions

E. All types of prostatitis can have dangerous sequelae and lead to urinary retention, renal parenchymal infection or bacteremia; chronic infection may produce prostatic stones

IV. Diagnosis/Evaluation

A. History
1. Ask about onset and course of illness
2. Inquire about associated symptoms such as urethral discharge, urethral meatal itching, fever, perineal pain, hematuria, hesitancy, decreased stream, painful ejaculation, incontinence, back pain, and weight loss
3. Ask patient about the number of previous urinary tract infections and the successes and failures of previous treatments
4. Ask if sexual partner is having symptoms such as dysuria
5. Explore whether the patient has had new sexual partners

B. Physical Examination
1. Observe general appearance for signs of systemic illness
2. Measure vital signs
3. Perform a complete abdominal exam; bladder distention may be present
4. Assess external genitalia and scrotum
5. Carefully and gently palpate prostate because vigorous massage can disseminate bacteria in the bloodstream, resulting in bacteremia
   a. Prostate often is tender, warm, swollen and boggy in acute bacterial prostatitis
   b. Although prostate may feel normal, it may be irregular and mildly tender in chronic bacterial, nonbacterial prostatitis, and prostatodynia

C. Diagnostic Tests
1. For patients with acute symptoms order a urinalysis and urine culture; diagnosis of acute prostatitis is based on clinical findings and a positive urinalysis and culture; do **not** collect segmented urine culture if acute prostatitis is suspected due to danger of septicemia
2. Obtain a segmented culture of urine and expressed prostatic secretions (not recommended for acute prostatitis)
   a. 10 mL of voided urine is collected and labeled VB_1 (first specimen of bladder voiding)
   b. Ask patient to void but stop in midstream and collect 50-100 mL of urine; VB_2 (classic midstream voiding)
   c. Massage prostate from each lateral lobe to the midline, about 6-7 times on each side; milk urethra to produce secretion; collect secretions on a swab, slide, or in a cup and label EPS (expressed prostatic secretion)

                    (1)   Do not collect EPS or the expressed prostatic secretion on a patient who is
                           suspected of having acute prostatitis
                    (2)   Instead, use the first (VB$_1$) and midstream (VB$_2$) specimens to guide
                           treatment
             d.   Then ask patient to void another 5-10 mL of urine; label VB$_3$ (voided urine post
                   prostatic massage)
             e.   Perform microscopic analysis of all specimens
                    (1)   If EPS has >10 white blood cells per high power field, suspect some type of
                           prostatitis
                    (2)   Lipid-laden macrophages are common in bacterial prostatitis
             f.   Order cultures on all specimens
                    (1)   Growth of bacteria in VB$_1$ and VB$_2$, but no growth in EPS and VB$_3$ suggests
                           cystitis
                    (2)   A 10-fold increase in EPS and VB$_3$ suggests bacterial prostatitis
                    (3)   WBCs in EPS and VB$_3$ but no growth of bacteria suggest nonbacterial
                           prostatitis
       3.   Consider initial sterilization of the urine before performing prostate massage if VB$_2$ is
             positive for bacteria
             a.   In this approach, use an antibiotic without appreciable prostatic tissue penetration
                   such as nitrofurantoin (Macrodantin) 100 TID/QID for 1-2 days until urine is
                   sterilized
             b.   Perform prostate massage and repeat culture of segmental samples (if patient has
                   prostatitis bacteria should be present in EPS and VB$_3$)
       4.   With chronic bacterial prostatitis evaluate renal function with blood urea nitrogen,
             creatinine, and consider ordering a intravenous pyelogram
       5.   With chronic bacterial prostatitis, consider transrectal ultrasound to discover prostrate
             calculi
       6.   In older men, consider ordering urine cytologies to rule out bladder malignancy
       7.   If prostatodynia is suspected, urodynamic testing is recommended

  D.   Differential Diagnosis
       1.   Acute prostatitis is usually apparent from the characteristic presentation
       2.   Chronic prostatitis often has a less clear presentation and may resemble other disorders
             a.   Nonbacterial prostatitis and prostatodynia
             b.   Benign prostatic hyperplasia (see section on BPH)
             c.   Urethral stricture
             d.   Bladder carcinoma
       3.   Nonbacterial prostatitis and prostatodynia often resemble the following
             a.   Cystitis (see section on CYSTITIS)
             b.   Nongonococcal urethritis (see section on URETHRITIS)

V.   Plan/Management

  A.   Treatment of acute bacterial prostatitis
       1.   Some patients require hospitalization and parenteral antibiotics; abscess is sometimes
             present and needs aggressive therapy
       2.   Initial empiric outpatient treatment is trimethoprim/sulfamethoxazole (Bactrim) 160/800 mg,
             one double strength tablet BID until the culture sensitivity report is available, treatment
             should last 4-6 weeks (some clinicians treat for 14-21 days)
       3.   Alternative therapy is norfloxacin (Noroxin) 400 mg tablets BID for 4-6 weeks
       4.   Symptomatic treatment may provide comfort such as bed rest and sitz baths for 20-30
             minutes for 2-3 times a day
       5.   For pain, prescribe analgesic or anti-inflammatory agent and a stool softener
       6.   Patients who fail to improve within 48 hours of antibiotic treatment, need referral to a
             urologist because of the likelihood of associated benign prostatic hypertrophy
       7.   If patient is over the age of 50 or has recurrent or persistent acute prostatitis, consider
             referral to urologist as acute prostatitis is often associated with benign prostatic
             hyperplasia and will often have a high recurrence rate

B. Chronic bacterial prostatitis is often difficult to cure
1. Prescribe 3-4 month course of double-strength trimethoprim-sulfamethoxazole (Bactrim) BID or norfloxacin (Noroxin) 400 mg tab BID or ciprofloxacin (Cipro) 500 mg tablets BID (duration of treatment is controversial, some clinicians treat for only 6 weeks)
2. Prescribe prophylactic drugs if infection persists: 1 regular tablet (80 mg trimethoprim/400 mg sulfamethoxazole [Bactrim]) HS for an indefinite period or nitrofurantoin (Macrodantin) 100 mg HS, indefinitely
3. Patients with refractory prostatitis should be evaluated for prostatic stones with an x-ray of kidneys, ureters, and bladder
4. Segmented cultures should be obtained 4-6 weeks after therapy is initiated
5. Other successful treatment strategies include local injection of antimicrobials (gentamicin and cephzolin) into the caudal prostate, and short-term intramuscular injections of kanamycin; surgery is a last resort

C. Nonbacterial prostatitis
1. Prescribe doxycycline (Vibramycin) 100 mg BID for 6 weeks. Alternative therapy is erythromycin (E-mycin) 250 mg QID for 6 weeks or trimethoprim-sulfamethoxazole (Bactrim) 1 DS tablet BID for 6 weeks (some clinicians treat for 14-21 days)
2. If relapse occurs after discontinuation of antibiotics, continue low-dose antimicrobial therapy indefinitely
3. If patient has no response to antibiotic therapy, discontinue medications and consider consultation with a urologist and one or more of the following therapies:
    a. Antispasmodic agent, oxybutynin (Ditropan) 5 mg BID/TID
    b. Alpha-adrenergic blocking drugs such as prazosin or alfuzosin
    c. Diazepam may be used alone or in combination with prazosin
    d. Anticholinergic agents to reduce irritative urinary symptoms
    e. A select group of patients have responded to a 28-day course of zinc sulfate
    f. Transurethral microwave thermotherapy
    g. Prostate massage, particularly after sexual activity

D. Prostatodynia
1. Referral to a urologist is recommended
2. Alpha-blocking agents may be helpful; prescribe prazosin (Minipress) 1mg HS for 7 days, followed by 1 mg BID for 7 days, and gradually increase to 2 mg BID
3. Other treatments include muscle relaxants, low-dose anxiolytic drugs, biofeedback, diathermy, or exercise

E. Patient education for all types of prostatitis
1. Sitz baths can be taken BID/TID for 20 minutes
2. Teach patients to avoid alcohol, coffee, or tea
3. Instruct patient to discontinue all over-the-counter drugs with anticholinergic properties such as antihistamine/decongestants

F. Follow Up
1. For bacterial prostatitis return in 4-6 weeks for urinalysis and culture of urine and expressed prostate secretions
2. For nonbacterial prostatitis and prostatodynia follow up will depend on patient's symptoms and response to therapy

EPIDIDYMITIS

I.   Definition: Inflammation of the epididymis

II. Pathogenesis: Pathogens apparently reach the epididymis through the lumen of the vas deferens from infected urine, the posterior urethra, or seminal vesicles

 A. In postpubertal boys and males under 35 years, infection is often sexually transmitted and 75% of cases are caused by *Neisseria gonorrhoea* or *Chlamydia trachomatis* (most common); underlying structural disorders are rare; in homosexual men *Escherichia coli* may be a pathogen

 B. Epididymitis may be nonsexually transmitted
  1. Typically caused by coliform or *Pseudomonas* species; in most cases of bacterial epididymitis, gram-negative rods are found but gram-positive cocci are also important pathogens
  2. Usually associated with urinary tract infections in men >35 years with urinary tract instrumentation, surgery, or anatomical abnormalities

 C. Uncommon causes are due to trauma or tuberculous epididymitis

III. Clinical Presentation

 A. Most common cause of acute scrotal pain in postpubertal males
  1. Usually patients have a history of sexual activity
  2. Sexually transmitted epididymitis usually is associated with urethritis

 B. Commonly, there is a gradual onset of unilateral testicular pain and tenderness, dysuria, and urethral discharge

 C. Fever occurs in approximately 50% of patients; nausea and vomiting is unusual

 D. Scrotum is tender on palpation and usually accompanied with a hydrocele and palpable swelling of the epididymis

 E. Uncommon complications include testicular necrosis, testicular atrophy, and infertility

IV. Diagnosis/Evaluation

 A. History
  1. Determine onset, duration, and course of symptoms
  2. Ask about scrotal pain, dysuria, urinary frequency and urgency, and color, amount and consistency of urethral discharge
  3. Inquire about possible associated symptoms such as fever, nausea, and vomiting
  4. Explore sexual history; ask about new sexual partners and if sexual partners have complained of dysuria or urinary frequency
  5. Question about previous urinary tract infections and treatments
  6. Inquire about previous genitourinary surgery, urinary tract instrumentation and anatomic abnormalities
  7. Inquire about recent trauma to testes

 B. Physical Examination
  1. Inspect scrotum, noting edema and erythema which are typical
  2. Palpate scrotum
   a. In epididymitis, testes are tender but the position, size, and consistency of testes is entirely normal
   b. Palpable swelling of epididymis is usually present

3. Passive elevation of testis may relieve pain in epididymitis (Prehn's sign)
4. Perform rectal exam (this exam may elicit prostatic tenderness and result in expression of urethral discharge)

C. Differential Diagnosis
1. Must differentiate testicular torsion which is an emergent condition from epididymitis (see following table)

DIFFERENTIATION OF EPIDIDYMITIS AND TESTICULAR TORSION		
	Epididymitis	Testicular Torsion
History		
Onset of pain	Gradual	Acute
Nausea and vomiting	Rare	50%
Voiding symptoms	50%	No
Urethral discharge	50%	No
Physical Examination		
Epididymal swelling only	Early	10%
Scrotal edema	Most	Most
Scrotal erythema	Most	Most
Fever	50%	Rare

2. Orchitis (patient usually has recently had parotitis)
3. Testicular tumor (usually not tender)
4. Trauma
5. Skin pathology such as insect bites or folliculitis

D. Diagnostic Tests
1. Obtain urinalysis (in about 20-95% of epididymitis cases there is pyuria compared to 0-30% in cases with testicular torsion)
2. Collect urine culture and sensitivity and gram-stained smear of uncentrifuged urine for gram-negative bacteria
3. In postpubertal boys or adult men who may have a sexually transmitted disease obtain the following:
   a. Gram-stained smear of urethral exudate or intraurethral swab specimen to detect urethritis (≥5 polymorphonuclear leukocytes per oil immersion field) and for presumptive diagnosis of gonococcal infection
   b. Culture of urethral exudate or intraurethral swab specimen or nucleic acid amplification test (either by first-void urine or intraurethral swab) for *N. gonorrhoeae* and *C. trachomatis*
   c. Collect first-void urine and examine for leukocytes if the urethral Gram stain is negative; culture and gram-stained smear of uncentrifuged urine should be collected
   d. Syphilis serology and HIV counseling and testing
4. In older men, a culture of expressed prostatic secretions should be obtained and a search should be made for an obstruction at the bladder outlet with tests such as an intravenous pyelography
5. Emergency testing for testicular torsion may be necessary when the onset of pain is sudden and severe or if there is uncertainty about the diagnosis; consult a specialist and consider ordering one of the following: Doppler ultrasound, scrotal ultrasound, or radionuclide scrotal imaging

V.   Plan/Management

    A.   For active heterosexual men <35 years of age, most likely cause is a sexually transmitted disease

        1.   For epididymitis most likely due to gonococcal of chlamydial infection, treat empirically based on clinical diagnosis before culture results are available with the following: doxycycline (Vibramycin) 100 mg PO BID for 10 days <u>and</u> ceftriaxone (Rocephin) 250 mg IM in a single dose

        2.   For epididymitis most likely caused by enteric organisms or in patients allergic to tetracyclines and/or cephalosporins, treat empirically with ofloxacin (Floxin) 300 mg PO BID for 10 days

        3.   Treat sexual partners if their contact with the index patient was within 60 days preceding onset of symptoms in the patient

        4.   Instruct patients to avoid sexual intercourse until they and their sex partners are cured or until treatment is completed and patients and partners are asymptomatic

    B.   In older men, treatment with a broad-spectrum antibiotic is also indicated. Prescribe trimethoprim-sulfamethoxazole (Septra) 1 double-strength tablet PO BID for 10 days or ciprofloxacin (Cipro) 250 mg PO BID for 10 days. If there is evidence of an underlying bacterial prostatitis, continue antimicrobial therapy for 4 weeks

    C.   Symptomatic treatment of bed rest, scrotal support, scrotal elevation, sitz baths, pain medication, and ice packs may be beneficial

    D.   Follow Up

        1.   For patients whose symptoms fail to improve within 3 days, reevaluate both the diagnosis and treatment

            a.   Swelling and tenderness that persist after antimicrobial therapy require comprehensive evaluation

            b.   Differential diagnosis includes tumor, abscess, infarction, testicular cancer, and tuberculosis or fungal epididymitis

        2.   For postpubertal boys and men <35 years, no follow up or test of cure is needed if symptoms resolve

        3.   In older men, repeat urine cultures are needed after completion of the therapy and further diagnostic tests can also be scheduled at this time

TESTICULAR TORSION

I.   Definition: Twisting of spermatic cord which results in compromised testicular blood flow

II.   Pathogenesis

    A.   Occurs when the free-floating testis rotates on the spermatic cord and occludes its blood supply

    B.   May occur spontaneously after activity or trauma

III.   Clinical Presentation

    A.   Commonly occurs during the newborn period and at puberty, but a significant number of patients with torsion are over the age of 21 years

    B.   Torsion: If not surgically treated, there will be ischemic injury and necrosis of the testis

        1.   Many patients have an anatomic defect known as "bell-clapper" deformity

        2.   Typical history is sudden onset of testicular pain which radiates to groin; but in some cases there is minimal swelling and little or no pain

3. May also have lower abdominal pain which leads to erroneous diagnosis of appendicitis or gastroenteritis
4. Nausea and vomiting occur in about half of the patients; usually there is no fever, urethral discharge or dysuria
5. Degree of injury is determined by the severity of the arterial compression and the interval between the onset and surgical intervention (for severe torsion, must intervene within 4-8 hours to salvage the testis)

IV. Diagnosis/Evaluation

    A. History: Testicular torsion is an urological emergency so rapidly gather a focused history
        1. Ask about onset and circumstances surrounding onset
        2. Ask about accompanying symptoms such as nausea, vomiting, fever, dysuria, urethral discharge
        3. Determine any occurrence of trauma or unusual physical activity
        4. To rule out epididymitis, question about recent change in sexual partners and symptoms of dysuria and urethral discharge

    B. Physical Examination: Perform a rapid but systematic exam
        1. Observe general appearance (patients with testicular torsion are in acute distress, have pain on ambulation, and prefer to lie quietly on the examination table)
        2. Inspect scrotal skin (often skin is erythematous, taut, and without normal rugations with torsion)
        3. Palpate testes (testis may be located high in the scrotum as a result of shortening of the cord by twisting)
        4. Palpate the epididymis which normally is located on the posterolateral surface of the testis and is smooth, discrete, and nontender (with testicular torsion the epididymis will not be in this typical position as a result of cord twisting and will be extremely tender)
        5. Palpate vas deferens from the testicle to the inguinal ring (normally vas deferens is smooth, discrete and nontender)
        6. Try to elicit the cremasteric reflex; positive reflex is testicular retraction when the upper, medial thigh is stroked (usually absent in torsion, but present in epididymitis)
        7. Perform a complete abdominal exam

    C. Differential Diagnosis
        1. Epididymitis is the most difficult condition to differentiate (see table in section on EPIDIDYMITIS, differentiating epididymitis from torsion)
        2. Torsion of the testicular appendage
            a. More common in pre-pubertal males
            b. Pain is usually less severe than with torsion of the entire testis; pain and swelling develop gradually
            c. "Blue dot" sign at superior aspect of testis is diagnostic of this problem
            d. Management is bedrest and scrotal elevation
            e. With appropriate management, symptoms resolve within a week
        3. Orchitis
        4. Incarcerated inguinal hernia
        5. Vasculitis
        6. Tumor
        7. Trauma
        8. Henoch-Schölein purpura is a systemic vasculitic syndrome characterized by nonthrombocytopenic purpura, arthralgia, renal disease, gastrointestinal pain and bleeding
        9. Idiopathic scrotal edema

    D. Diagnostic Tests: When clinical presentation is typical, surgical exploration is usually carried out without further testing. If uncertain, consider consulting a specialist and ordering the following:
        1. Urinalysis (will be normal in 90% of patients with testicular torsion, but will often be abnormal in epididymitis)
        2. Doppler ultrasound (absent testicular artery pulsations with torsion); the development of color Doppler imaging with pulsed Doppler has improved accuracy of this test

3. Nuclear testicular scanning allows evaluation of blood flow to the scrotal contents (decreased perfusion with torsion)

4. Scrotal ultrasonography can be ordered; does not distinguish torsion from epididymitis but is helpful in evaluating scrotal masses and trauma

V. Plan/Management:

A. Immediate consultation and surgical intervention; this is an urological emergency

B. Follow Up: Surgeon should arrange follow up to determine response to operation

VARICOCELE

I. Definition: Dilated plexus of scrotal veins situated above the testis in the scrotum

II. Pathogenesis: Due to valvular incompetence of the spermatic vein

A. Varicoceles on left side in adolescents are usually of unknown etiology; new left-sided varicocele in older men may be a renal tumor

B. Varicoceles on the right side may represent acute venous obstruction from a tumor or intra-abdominal pathology

C. In older men, new varicoceles may be secondary to renal tumors

III. Clinical Presentation

A. Usually found in older adolescents but can occur at a any age (onset in prepubertal males and in adult males is often associated with pathology)

B. Approximately, 15% of all adult males have a varicocele

C. Almost always varicoceles occur on left side; a unilateral right varicocele is rare; bilateral varicoceles are more common than previously thought

D. Testis resembles a bag of worms with a bluish discoloration which is visible through the scrotum (see Figure 13.1)

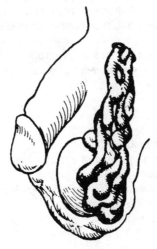

Figure 13.1. Varicocele.
Source: Judge, R.D., Zuidema, G.D., & Fitzgerald, F.T. (Eds.) (1989), <u>Clinical Diagnosis</u> (p. 381). Boston: Little, Brown and Company. Copyright 1989 by A.C. Judge, P.C. Judge, S.M. Judge, N.C. Judge. Reprinted by permission.

E. Varicocele is most prominent when the patient is standing; tends to collapse when the patient is sitting or supine

F. Patient is usually asymptomatic and testis is nontender, but may have mild pain or a feeling of heaviness in the scrotum

G. Varicoceles are associated with a time-dependent decline in testicular function; decreased sperm counts, infertility and testicular atrophy are associated in about 65%-75% of patients with varicoceles

H. Today, emphasis has shifted to early diagnosis, education and intervention in adolescence to prevent infertility in adulthood

IV. Diagnosis/Evaluation

A. History
1. Ask when patient first noticed varicocele
2. Determine the rate the scrotum is enlarging
3. Ask if the varicocele collapses upon sitting or standing
4. Inquire about testicular pain or discomfort
5. Question about problems with infertility

B. Physical Examination
1. Assess Tanner stage in adolescents to determine normal growth and development of testes
2. If varicocele is not visible, ask patient to stand and perform a Valsalva maneuver
3. Palpate testes, epididymis, and vas deferens in first standing then supine positions
4. Perform a rectal examination to assess prostate size since the prostate may shrink with testosterone deficiency that may occur with varicoceles

C. Differential Diagnosis
1. Hydrocele
2. Spermatocele
3. Testicular tumor
4. Epididymal cyst

D. Diagnostic Tests
1. In adolescents, order testicular ultrasound to assess testicular volume and significant testicular size variations between testes with and without varicocele
2. For right-sided varicoceles, suddenly appearing left-sided varicoceles, new onset varicoceles in adults consult specialist about ordering the following:
   a. Venography is the gold standard for diagnosing varicoceles in adults; also used to detect venous obstruction or renal carcinoma associated with varicoceles
   b. Doppler ultrasound, thermography, and scrotal scintigraphy are nonspecific for diagnosing varicoceles, but may be beneficial in some cases
3. Consult specialist about assessing reproductive function in adults with semen analysis, testis biopsy, and fine needle aspiration with flow cytometry

V. Plan/Management

A. Refer the following patients to a surgeon:
1. All patients with right-sided varicoceles
2. All adult males with new onset of varicoceles
3. The following adolescent males:
   a. When varicocele is voluminous, rapidly increasing in size, or does not disappear in sitting and supine positions
   b. When pain is present

c. When there is evidence of testicular atrophy defined as a two standard deviation in testicular size when compared with normal testicular growth curves

d. When there is greater than a 2 mL difference in testicular volume as noted on serial ultrasonography examination

B. If surgery is not recommended, explain that patient needs to monitor the growth and symptoms related to the varicocele

C. Follow Up: If surgery is not performed, explain to patient the need to return to clinic if he experiences increasing discomfort or if scrotum changes in size and shape

REFERENCES

Ahmed, Z., & Lee, J. (1997). Asymptomatic urinary abnormalities: Hematuria and proteinuria. Medical Clinics of North America, 81, 641-651.

Alexander, R.B., & Trissel, D. (1996). Chronic prostatitis: Results of an internet survey. Urology, 48, 568-574.

American Medical Directors Association. (1996). Urinary incontinence: Clinical practice guideline. Columbia, MD.

Anderson, J.E. (1997). Hematuria. In L. Dornbrand, A.J. Hoole, & R.H. Fletcher (Eds.). Manual of clinical problems in adult ambulatory care (3rd ed.). Philadelphia: Lippincott-Raven.

Bacheller, C.D., & Bernstein, J.M. (1997). Urinary tract infections. Medical Clinics of North America, 81, 719-729.

Barry, M.J., Fowler, F.J. Jr., Bin, L., Pitts, J.C. III, Harris, C.J., & Mulley, A.G. Jr. (1997). The natural history of patients with benign prostatic hyperplasia as diagnosed by North American urologist. Journal of Urology, 157, 10-14.

Barry, M.J., & Roehrborn, C.G. (1997). Benign prostatic hyperplasia. In L. Dornbrand, A.J. Hoole, & R.H. Fletcher (Eds.). Manual of clinical problems in adult ambulatory care (3rd ed.). Philadelphia: Lippincott-Raven

Beduschi, R., Beduschi, M.C., & Oesterling, J.E. (1998). Benign prostatic hyperplasia: Use of drug therapy in primary care. Geriatrics, 53, 24-40.

Benign Prostatic Hyperplasia Guideline Panel. (1994). Benign Prostatic Hyperplasia: Diagnosis and Treatment. AHCPR Pub. No. 94-0582. Rockville, MD: Agency for Health Care Policy and Research, Public Health Service, US Department of Health and Human Services.

Burnett, A.L. (1998). Erectile dysfunction: A practical approach for primary care. Geriatrics, 53 (2), 34-48.

Carson, C.C. III, Melman, A., Ruoff, G., & Saunders, C.S. (Spring,1998). Treatment of erectile dysfunction: Surveying the options. Supplement to Patient Care, 6-14.

Donovan, D.A., & Nicholas, P.K. (1997). Prostatitis: Diagnosis and treatment in primary care. Nurse Practitioner, 22 (4), 144-156.

Dull, P. (1998). Update on benign prostatic hyperplasia. Family Practice Recertification, 20 (2), 43-70.

Eardley, I. (1997). New oral therapies for the treatment of erectile dysfunction. British Journal of Urology, 81, 122-127.

Fang, L.S-T. (1995). Management of patient with chronic renal failure. In A.H. Goroll, L.A. May, & A.G. Mulley, Jr. (Eds.). Primary care medicine: Office evaluation and management of the adult patient (3rd ed.). Philadelphia: Lippincott.

Feld, L.G., Wza, W.R., Perez, L.M., & Joseph, D.B. (1997). Hematuria: An integrated medical and surgical approach. Pediatric Clinics of North America, 44, 1191-1211.

Fihn, S.D., et al. (1998). Use of spermicide-coated condoms and other risk factors for urinary tract infection caused by Staphylococcus saprophyticus. Archives of Internal Medicine, 158, 281-287.

Fourcroy, J.L. (1998). Urogynecology update: Incontinence. Hospital Practice, 33 (5), 63-81.

Gallo, M.L., Fallon, P.J., & Staskin, D.R. (1997). Urinary incontinence: Steps to evaluation, diagnosis, and treatment. Nurse Practitioner, 22 (2), 21-44.

Goldstein, I., Lue, T.F., Padma-Nathan, H., Rosen, R.C., Steers, W.D., & Wicker, P.A. (1998). Oral sildenafil in the treatment of erectile dysfunction. New England Journal of Medicine, 338, 1397-1404.

Guay, A.T., Levine, S.B., Montague, D.K., & Saunders, C.S. (March 15, 1998). New treatments for erectile dysfunction. <u>Patient Care,</u> 30-52.

Guthrie, R. (1997). Benign prostatic hyperplasia in elderly men: What are the special issues in treatment? <u>Postgraduate Medicine, 101,</u> 141-161.

Harrington, J.T. (1998). Chronic renal failure. In R.E. Rakel (Ed.), <u>1998 Conn's current therapy</u>. Philadelphia: Saunders.

Hebel, S.K. (Ed.). (1996). <u>Drugs Facts and Comparisons.</u> St. Louis: Facts and Comparisons, Inc.

Junnila, J., & Lassen, P. (1998). Testicular masses. <u>American Family Physician, 57,</u> 685-692.

Kass, E.J., & Lundak, B. (1997). The acute scrotum. <u>Pediatric Clinics of North America, 44,</u> 1251-1266.

Knapp, P.M. (1998). Identifying and treating urinary incontinence. <u>Postgraduate Medicine, 103,</u> 279-294.

Krieger, J.N. (1998). Epididymitis. In R.E. Rakel (Ed.), <u>1998 Conn's current therapy</u>. Philadelphia: Saunders.

Kurgan, A., Nunnelee, J.d., & Ailberman, M. (1994). The importance of the early detection of varicocele in adolescent males. <u>Nurse Practitioner, 19</u> (10), 36-37.

Kurowski, K. (1998). The woman with dysuria. <u>American Family Physician, 57,</u> 2155-2164.

Langermann, S., et al. (1997). Prevention of mucosal *Excherichia coli* infection by FimH-adhesion-based systemic vaccination. <u>Science, 276,</u> 607-614.

Lepor, H., Williford, W.O., Barry, M.J., Brawner, M.K., Dixon, C.M., Gormley, G., et al. (1996). α-blocker was more effective for benign prostatic hyperplasia. <u>New England Journal of Medicine, 335,</u> 533-539.

Lowe, F.C., & Ku, J.C. (1996). Phytotherapy in treatment of benign prostatic hyperplasia: A critical review. <u>Urology, 48,</u> 12-19.

Malhotra, D., & Tzamaloukas, A.H. (1997). Nondialysis management of chronic renal failure. <u>Medical Clinics of North America, 81,</u> 749-765.

Marberger, M.J. (1998). Long-term effects of finasteride in patients with benign prostatic hyperplasia: A double-blind, placebo-controlled, multicenter study. <u>Urology, 51,</u> 677-686.

Mattern, W.D. (1997). Chronic renal failure. In L. Dornbrand, A.J. Hoole, & C.G. Pickard. <u>Manual of clinical problems in adult ambulatory care</u> (3rd ed.). Boston: Little, Brown and Company.

McCarthy, J.J. (1997). Outpatient evaluation of hematuria: Locating the source of bleeding. <u>Postgraduate Medicine, 101,</u> 125-131.

McConnell, J.D. (1998). Benign prostatic hyperplasia. In R.E. Rakel (Ed.). <u>1998 Conn's current therapy</u>. Philadelphia: Saunders.

Montague, D.K., Barada, J.H., Belker, A.M., Levine, L.A., Nadig, P.W., Roehrborn, C.G., Sharlip, I.D., & Bennett, A.H. (1996). Clinical guidelines panel on erectile dysfunction. <u>Journal of Urology, 156,</u> 2007-2011.

Nickel, J.C. (1998). Prostatitis: Myths and realities. <u>Urology, 51,</u> 362-366.

Nygaard, I.E., & Johnson, J.M. (1996). Urinary tract infections in elderly women. <u>American Family Physician, 53,</u> 175-182.

Peters, S. (May, 1997). Don't ask, don't tell: Breaking the silence surrounding female urinary incontinence. <u>Advance for Nurse Practitioners,</u> 41-44.

Pittler, E.E. (1998). Yohimbe for erectile dysfunction: A systematic review and meta-analysis of randomized clinical trials. <u>Journal of Urology, 159,</u> 433-436.

Rahman, J., & Smith, M.C. (1998). Chronic renal insufficiency: A diagnostic and therapeutic approach. <u>Archives of Internal Medicine, 158,</u> 1743-1751.

Roberts, S.O., Lieber, M.M., Bostwick, D.G., & Jacobsen, S.J. (1997). A review of clinical and pathological prostatitis syndromes. <u>Urology, 49,</u> 809-821.

Robinson, D., Pearce, K.F., & Preisser, J.S. (1998). Relationship between patient reports of urinary incontinence symptoms and quality of life measures. <u>Obstetrics and Gynecology, 91,</u> 224-228.

Rosen, R.C., Riley, A., Wagner, G., Osterloh, I.H., Kirkpatrick, J., & Mishra, A. (1997). The International Index of Erectile Function (IIEF): A multidimensional scale for assessment of erectile dysfunction. <u>Urology, 49,</u> 822-830.

Schaeffer, A.J. (1998) . Prostatitis. In R.E. Rakel (Ed.), <u>1998 Conn's current therapy</u>. Philadelphia: W.B. Saunders.

Stamm, W.E. & Hooton (1993). Management of urinary tract infections in adults. <u>The New England Journal of Medicine</u>, <u>329</u>(18), 1328-1334.

Urinary Incontinence Guideline Panel. (1992). <u>Urinary Incontinence in Adults: Clinical Practice Guideline</u>. AHCPR Pub. No. 92-0038. Rockville, MD: Agency for Health Care Policy and Research, Public Health Service, US Department of Health and Human Services.

Urinary Incontinence in Adults Guideline Update Panel. (1996). <u>Urinary Incontinence in Adults: Acute and Chronic Management: Clinical Practice Guideline No. 2</u>. Rockville, MD: Agency for Health Care Policy and Research, Public Health Service, US Department of Health and Human Services.

US Department of Health and Human Services, Centers for Disease Control. (1998). 1998 guidelines for treatment of sexually transmitted diseases treatment guidelines. <u>Morbidity and Mortality Weekly Report, 47</u>(RR-1).

Whelan, C.A. (1998). Chronic renal failure--Non-dialysis care for the primary care provider. <u>American Journal for Nurse Practitioners, 2</u> (7), 21-31.

Wein, A.J. (1998). Pharmacologic options for the overactive bladder. <u>Urology, 51</u> (Suppl 2A), 43-47.

Weiss, B.D. (1998). Diagnostic evaluation of urinary incontinence in geriatric patients. <u>American Family Physician, 57,</u> 2675-2684.

Winkler, H.A., & Sand, P.K. (1998). Stress incontinence: Options for conservative treatment. <u>Women's Health in Primary Care, 1,</u> 279-294.

Wisinger, D.B. (1996). Urinary tract infection: Current management strategies. <u>Postgraduate Medicine, 100,</u> 229-239.

Gynecology

ABNORMAL CERVICAL CYTOLOGY

I.   Definition: All classifications of cervicovaginal cytology other than "within normal limits" using the revised Bethesda system

II.   Pathogenesis: An atypical Papanicolaou smear may be due to the following causes

    A.   Infection (fungal, bacterial, protozoal, or viral)

    B.   Reactive and reparative changes (inflammation and miscellaneous factors related to patient history, such as chemotherapy, radiation, use of IUD, and DES exposure)

    C.   Neoplastic (lower genital tract, upper genital tract, extragenital)

III.   Clinical Presentation

    A.   Incidence of cervical cancer is significantly higher in married and widowed women than in never married women

    B.   Although all sexually active women are at risk for cervical cancer, the disease is more common among women of low socioeconomic status, those with a history of multiple sex partners or early age at first intercourse, and smokers

    C.   Authorities agree that the cause of cervical dysplasia is a DNA mutation in an immature metaplastic cell
        1.   Dysplasia is caused by human papilloma virus (HPV) infection together with other carcinogenic cofactors
        2.   HPV types 16, 18, 31, 33, and 35 have a strong epidemiologic association with cervical dysplasia
        3.   HPV is found in 95% of cervical cancers

    D.   May be asymptomatic, or may have symptoms of fungal, bacterial, protozoan, or viral infection, if the atypia is due to an infectious cause

IV.   Diagnosis/Evaluation

    A.   The cytopathology report is considered a medical consultation

    B.   Every cytopathology report based on Bethesda system has statement on specimen adequacy in the first section of the report. The possible specimen categories are the following
        1.   <u>Satisfactory for evaluation</u>: Provides assurance that sample and preparation were adequate in that the smear had both endocervical and metaplastic ectocervical cells easily visible with ≤ 50% of cells obscured by inflammation, blood or debris (**Note**: The smear can be satisfactory but deficient in other ways, i.e, abnormal cells are present)
        2.   <u>Satisfactory for evaluation but limited by (reason)</u>: Smear may be limited by one or more of four factors which are listed here
            a.   **Lack of metaplastic or endocervical cells**--occurs when transformation zone is not sampled (most common reasons are excessive mucus, a nulliparous, pregnant, or atrophic cervix, or a cervix after an ablative/excisional procedure)
            b.   **Inflammation, blood, or debris** partially obscure >50% but less than 75% of cells on smear (inflammation can be caused by use of douching, tampons, cervical caps, or having sexual intercourse within 48 hours of exam; can also be caused by infection or cellular changes of the cervix that occur with cancer)
            c.   **Air drying** which causes an increased nuclear-cytoplasmic ratio mimicking cell dysplasia
            d.   **Lack of patient information** (name, LMP, history of ablative or excisional therapy)

3. <u>Unsatisfactory for evaluation:</u> Usually means the smear was improperly prepared or that inflammation was so extensive the examination was meaningless (≥75% of cells obscured)

4. **Note**: Two new Pap smear techniques--ThinPrep and MonoLayer--have been shown to increase the detection of abnormal cells by 65%

    a. A cervical broom or brush is used to obtain a cervical specimen that is placed in preservative-filled vial

    b. Specimen is filtered in lab to remove mucus, blood, and inflammatory cells making slides easier to read

    c. Techniques have a lower false negative rate but are more expensive than conventional Pap testing

C. The second section of the Bethesda system report contains three possible categories

    1. Within normal limits

    2. Benign cellular changes; see descriptive diagnoses

    3. Epithelial cell abnormalities; see descriptive diagnoses

D. The descriptive diagnoses section makes up the third part of the report

    1. Benign cellular changes reflect either reactive, reparative changes, or an underlying infection

        a. Reactive changes refer to reparative alterations from inflammation due to such conditions as atrophic vaginitis, mechanical or chemical irritation, or use of an IUD

        b. Infectious causes include common genital infections with pathogens such as *Trichomonas vaginalis*, herpes simplex, *Chlamydia trachomatis, Neisseria gonorrhoeae,* and *Candida* species, among others

    2. Epithelial cell abnormalities are either of squamous or glandular origin

        a. Squamous cell abnormalities are addressed first and these are classified into four categories from the **least to the most serious**

SQUAMOUS CELL ABNORMALITIES

Atypical squamous cells of undetermined significance (ASCUS)
- ❖ A description of cells that have nuclear atypia that are not normal yet are not consistent with low grade squamous intraepithelial lesion (LSIL)
- ❖ Diagnosis of ASCUS should be qualified by indicating whether it favors a reactive or neoplastic process

Low-grade squamous intraepithelial lesion (LSIL)
- ❖ Cellular changes of HPV previously termed koilocytosis, koilocytotic atypia, or condylomatous atypia are included in this category

High-grade squamous intraepithelial lesion (HSIL)
- ❖ Encompasses moderate and severe dysplasia as well as carcinoma in situ

Squamous cell carcinoma

---

        b. Glandular cell abnormalities are considered in the next category and are classified from the **least to the most serious**

GLANDULAR CELL ABNORMALITIES

Benign endometrial cells
- ❖ An abnormal finding in post-menopausal women, but insignificant in premenopausal women with normal ovulatory cycling

Atypical glandular cells of undetermined significance (AGUS)
- ❖ Includes a spectrum of findings ranging from minimally abnormal cells to adenocarcinoma in situ
- ❖ The diagnosis should include the origin of the atypical glandular cells, whether endometrial or endocervical

Adenocarcinoma in situ (AIS) and Adenocarcinoma

---

        c. Other, less common malignant neoplasms of the genital tract are then considered

    3. Finally, a hormonal evaluation (applies to vaginal smears only) is provided in the last part of the descriptive diagnoses section

        a. Hormonal pattern compatible with age and history

        b. Hormonal pattern incompatible with age and history (specify)

        c. Hormonal evaluation not possible due to (specify)

V.   Plan/Management

A.   Pap smear report of "Satisfactory for evaluation" and "Within normal limits": Counsel woman regarding findings and repeat the Pap smear in 1-3 years, depending on patient risk factors and history

B.   Pap smear report of "Specimen unsatisfactory for evaluation." Obtain a second specimen in 6-8 weeks, preferably when woman is at midcycle and has not had intercourse or used vaginal products for at least 24 hours; if poor specimen quality is due to atrophy in postmenopausal woman, consider prescribing a topical estrogen cream for 4-6 weeks, then repeat the test no earlier than one week after completing the medication

C.   Pap smear report of "Satisfactory but no endocervical cells." Repeat the test if the woman has any risk factors, if she has had no prior screening, or has a history of abnormal test in past

D.   Pap smear report of benign cellular changes: Consult descriptive diagnoses section to determine possible cause
       1.   If report of *Trichomonas vaginalis* or other specific infection
              a.   Review chart to determine if patient was treated at time Pap smear was obtained
              b.   If no treatment at that time, contact patient to return for evaluation by pelvic exam and appropriate diagnostic tests before treatment
       2.   If report of reactive changes with inflammation
              a.   Evaluate the patient for possible infection including gonorrhea and chlamydia
              b.   Repeat the Pap test in 3-6 months
              c.   Colposcopy is indicated if the inflammation persists and remains unexplained
       3.   If report of reactive changes associated with atrophy--prescribe a topical estrogen cream if the woman has symptomatic atrophic vaginitis (not necessary for the asymptomatic woman)
       4.   If report of reactive changes associated with an intrauterine device or radiation therapy-- continue with the routine screening schedule

E.   Pap smear report of atypical squamous cells of undetermined significance (ASCUS) should be managed as follows

---

INTERPRETATION OF ASCUS

If ASCUS is not qualified or if a reactive process is favored
- A repeat Pap test should be conducted every 4-6 months for 2 years; the pattern should be continued until 3 consecutive smears are negative
- A routine testing schedule should be returned to at that point
- If ASCUS is reported a second time, the patient should be referred for colposcopy

When ASCUS is associated with severe inflammation
- Infection must be ruled out, but treatment is not indicated without a specific diagnosis
- Pap testing should be repeated in 2-3 months
- Colposcopy is indicated if the repeat test is abnormal

When ASCUS is associated with vaginal atrophy (postmenopausal women not using HRT)
- Consider prescribing a topical estrogen cream, unless contraindicated
- Repeat the Pap smear in 2-3 months
- Some experts recommend that patients use the topical estrogen cream even if they are taking the hormone orally
- A colposcopy is indicated if the diagnosis remains equivocal

When ASCUS is qualified as favoring a neoplastic process
- For low-risk compliant patient, repeat Pap smears every 4-6 months for 2 years until three consecutive smears are negative; return to regular Pap smear testing routine at that point; if the repeated smears show abnormalities, colposcopy is indicated
- For high-risk poorly compliant patient, a colposcopy should be done without further Pap testing

---

F.   Pap smear report of low-grade squamous intraepithelial lesion (LSIL); Manage as above under WHEN ASCUS IS QUALIFIED AS FAVORING A NEOPLASTIC PROCESS

G.   Pap smear report of high-grade squamous intraepithelial lesion (HSIL); Endocervical curettage (ECG), colposcopy, and directed biopsy are required in patients with these high-grade lesions

518

H. Pap smear report of endometrial cells; endometrial cells found in a cytologically benign smear of a post-menopausal woman not on estrogen replacement therapy are an indication for an endometrial biopsy

I. Pap smear report of atypical glandular cells of undetermined significance (AGUS); the diagnosis should include origin--endometrial or endocervical--of the atypical glandular cells
1. Endometrial origin of the atypical cells requires an evaluation that includes endometrial biopsy, fractional dilation, and curettage, or hysteroscopy
2. Endocervical origin of the atypical cells is an indication for colposcopy and endocervical curettage (ECC)

J. Pap smear report of squamous cell carcinoma or adenocarcinoma requires a prompt referral to an expert in the management of gynecologic cancers

K. Pap smear report of other malignant neoplasms: Women with abnormalities in this section should be referred immediately for evaluation

L. Hormonal evaluation
1. Hormonal evaluation should be consistent with clinical picture of the patient
2. Evidence of an estrogenic effect in a 75 year old not on HRT is an example of abnormal findings in this area

M. Follow Up: Variable depending on cytopathology report (see appropriate sections above)

ABNORMAL VAGINAL BLEEDING

I. Definition: Vaginal bleeding not associated with normal menses. Important terms:

A. Menorrhagia/hypermenorrhea: Menstrual bleeding of greater than 80 mL or greater than 7 days in duration

B. Polymenorrhea: Menstrual interval < 21 days (regular interval)

C. Metrorrhagia: Irregular menstrual bleeding with frequent intervals

D. Menometrorrhagia: Irregular, heavy or prolonged menstrual bleeding

E. Oligomenorrhea: Bleeding that occurs in intervals greater than 5 weeks (35 days)

II. Pathogenesis

A. Dysfunctional uterine bleeding (DUB) results from persistent stimulation of endometrium by estrogen which is unopposed by periodic influence of progesterone; 70-80% of DUB is associated with anovulation
1. Unopposed estrogen causes endometrium to become thicker and more vascular (hyperplasia); without progesterone the structural support needed to sustain vascularity is absent which results in spontaneous superficial hemorrhages which occur randomly
2. This is a diagnosis of exclusion
3. DUB is the cause of approximately 85% of abnormal vaginal bleeding cases
4. Pathophysiology of DUB varies with age
   a. In adolescent years there is an immaturity of the hypothalamic-pituitary-gonadal axis
   b. In perimenopausal women, DUB is due to decreased sensitivity of the ovary to follicle stimulating hormone (FSH) and luteinizing hormone (LH) stimulation

B. Pregnancy related
    1. Ectopic pregnancy
    2. Gestational trophoblastic neoplasm (Hydatid mole)
    3. Threatened, incomplete, or missed abortion
    4. Placenta previa or low lying placenta

C. Trauma resulting from sexual abuse, tampon use, IUD use, or foreign body

D. Medications such as oral contraceptives, steroids, anticoagulants, neuroleptics, major tranquilizers

E. Organic gynecologic pathology such as benign polyps, myomas, endometrial hyperplasia, and malignancy (cervical, endocervical, ovarian, tubal)

F. Systemic diseases such as coagulation disorders, thyroid disorders, adrenal disorders, liver disease, and renal disease

G. Stress, exercise, and nutrition related such as excessive exercise and excessive weight loss

III. Clinical Presentation: Age of the patient, pattern of bleeding, and associated signs and symptoms provide clues to the possible etiology

A. In adolescents, the following are likely causes
    1. DUB is the most frequent cause of bleeding in this age group, accounting for about 75% of cases
        a. Some 50% of cycles are anovulatory for the first 1-2 years after menarche
        b. External forces can disrupt the often slow maturation of the hypothalamic-ovarian axis
            (1) Physical and mental stress can interfere with normal ovulation
            (2) Excessive exercise in ballet dancers, gymnasts and other athletes results in low body fat and can interrupt ovulation
            (3) Eating disorders such as anorexia and bulimia can disrupt ovulation even in women of normal or excess weight
    2. Infection is common
    3. Disorders of pregnancy, particularly ectopic pregnancies and abortions, are important factors causing bleeding
    4. Breakthrough bleeding from taking oral contraceptives is a common cause
    5. Among adolescent females the most frequent foreign body that is retained is a tampon; bleeding is usually accompanied by foul-smelling discharge

B. In women aged 20-35 years, the most common causes are accidents of pregnancy, infection, leiomyomas (uterine fibroids), and DUB
    1. Anovulatory DUB is less frequent cause of sustained menstrual irregularity during this age group as compared with adolescents and older women
    2. Most women will experience occasional anovulatory cycles that may be identified by delayed or increased flow

C. In perimenopausal women (35 years to menopause), likely causes in addition to DUB are endometrial hyperplasia, onset of menopause, anatomic lesions, cervical carcinoma, and endometrial carcinoma

D. In all postmenopausal women who have an intact uterus, concern is endometrial carcinoma
    1. Only 5% of all cases occur under age 40; incidence rises after age 45 with peak at age 70 years
    2. Today, it is twice as common as cervical cancer but the mortality is lower
    3. Risk factors include obesity, hypertension, diabetes, nulliparity, late menopause, polycystic ovary syndrome, estrogen replacement therapy, endometrial hyperplasia

E. Pattern of bleeding and associated signs and symptoms provide additional clues to possible causes
    1. DUB results in irregularity of menstrual interval, episodes of amenorrhea, and periods of heavy, prolonged bleeding
    2. Women with coagulation disorders may have signs of petechia, ecchymoses, or epistaxis
    3. Ectopic pregnancy has variable spotting due to hemorrhage, usually with cramping and possibly signs and symptoms of pregnancy
    4. Infection is usually associated with vaginal discharge, lower abdominal pain, and pain on intercourse
    5. Leiomyomas are a common cause of bleeding and result in uterine enlargement; abdominal exam may be positive for a large mass if the leiomyoma has grown larger than a 12 week pregnant uterus
    6. In cervical carcinoma, bleeding is frequently postcoital, intermenstrual, and described as slight spotting
    7. Endometrial carcinoma begins with intermenstrual discharge which is watery with small amounts of blood and then progresses to heavier bleeding

IV. Diagnosis/Evaluation

    A. History
        1. **Data relating to LMP**: Inquire about timing and duration of last normal menses and ask woman if she has kept a menstrual calendar
        2. **Timing and amount of abnormal bleeding**: Ask when bleeding begins, whether it is spotting or heavy, how long bleeding lasts, whether it is daily spotting, and how heavy the heavy days (**Note**: Daily spotting is suggestive of a polyp or infectious cause; heavy flow tapering to spotting, with no bleeding for several days, then returning to heavy flow again is characteristic of anovulatory bleeding)
        3. **Associated signs and symptoms**: Ask about presence of abdominal pain, vaginal discharge, pain on intercourse, pain with urination, defecation, or pelvic heaviness (**Note**: Pelvic pain/heaviness may indicate a persistent corpus luteum cyst, endometriosis, or myomas)
        4. **Contraceptive use and sexual practices/history**: Obtain this essential information
        5. **Drugs and medications**: Ask about medications, including oral contraceptives
        6. **Past medical history**: Inquire about past/present problems including endocrine, hematological, and gynecological problems (**Note**: Ask: "Are you seeing or have you recently seen a health care provider for any other problem?")
        7. **Gynecologic/obstetric history**: Obtain complete history in these areas
        8. **Behavior/lifestyle**: Ask about recent changes in weight, life, activity, exercise patterns

    B. Physical Examination
        1. Determine whether blood loss is significant by obtaining orthostatic B/P and pulse readings
        2. Inspect skin for bruising, petechia, or purpura
        3. Always do pelvic and speculum examinations
            a. Insure that bleeding is uterine and not from urethra or rectum
            b. Assess for foreign body in vault, examine cervical os for erosion, polyps, and mucopurulent discharge
            c. Evaluate the uterus for tenderness, size, and shape
            d. Carefully assess the adnexa
        4. Assess for signs of hypothyroidism such as skin thickening and abnormal deep tendon reflexes
        5. Assess thyroid and check for abdominal masses

    C. Differential Diagnosis: Rule out all conditions noted under Pathogenesis

    D. Diagnostic Tests
        1. Order urine or serum HCG (**Note**: May be the most important test!)
        2. CBC, and platelet count
        3. If anovulation is suspected, a prolactin, thyroid panel, TSH
        4. Obtain Pap smear with maturation index

5. Test for *N. gonorrhoae* and *C. trachomatis*
6. Coagulation studies are useful in adolescents and in women with bruising or history of bleeding diathesis
7. For women over age 35 years, consider ordering FSH, LH, FSH:LH, and doing a progesterone challenge test to determine menopausal status
8. For women over 40, or in any woman with a history suggestive of chronic anovulation, endometrial sampling should be performed to rule out hyperplasia and malignancy
9. For women younger than 40 with symptoms that are acute or of short duration, endometrial sampling is usually not necessary and should only be done if endometrial hyperplasia or neoplasia is suspected
10. Another diagnostic test for abnormal bleeding is endovaginal ultrasound which can be used to rule out ectopic pregnancy, to assess myomas and abnormal uterine size, and to measure endometrial thickness

V. Plan/Management

A. Refer patient to an expert if bleeding is severe (HCT <25) or if patient is unstable (orthostatic hypotension); also refer patients with suspected malignancy or serious systemic disease

B. Treat all known causes of vaginal bleeding such as the following
  1. Removal of foreign body from the vagina (most often impacted tampon)
     a. Under good visualization, and with the patient in the lithotomy position, grasp the tampon with a pair of sponge holding forceps
     b. Place a basin of water as close to the introitus as possible (to minimize malodor)
     c. Quickly immerse the tampon under water without releasing the forceps
     d. Flush the tampon and water down toilet
     e. **Note**: The unpleasant odor that envelopes the room is the most problematic; immersing the removed tampon into water the instant it is removed from the vagina reduces the malodor and the embarrassment to the patient
  2. Prescribe antibiotics for infections that are diagnosed
  3. Urethral prolapse is treated with sitz baths and application of topical estrogen cream and topical antibiotics
  4. For breakthrough bleeding from oral contraceptives
     a. Counsel that breakthrough bleeding decreases dramatically after first 3 months of pills
     b. Instruct to take pills at same time each day
     c. Last, change oral contraceptive to one with a higher progestational activity (usually effective regardless of when bleeding occurs in the cycle) such as Desogen, Ortho-Cept, or Demulen 1/35

C. If bleeding is light, patient has normal hemoglobin level (>12 g/dL) and DUB is suspected
  1. Ask patient to maintain menstrual calendar
  2. Reevaluate in 3-6 months
  3. Prescribe mefenamic acid (Ponstel) 500 mg orally TID for 3 days starting with menses to correct relative prostaglandin overproduction

D. If bleeding is moderate, hemoglobin is 10-12 g/dL, and DUB is suspected based on an absence of systemic disease or uterine disorder, a number of options are available and are outlined in the following table

TREATMENT FOR MODERATE DUB	
Goal of Treatment: Convert proliferative endometrium into secretory endometrium, thereby resulting in predictable uterine withdrawal bleeding	
Many different treatment regimens have been suggested; only 3 are considered here, but consult the literature for other options	
Select One of the Following Therapies	
Drug	**Dosage**
Medroxyprogesterone acetate (Provera)	5-10 mg QD for 12-14 days in the second half of the month
Any combination oral contraceptive with one not being preferred over another	One pill taken daily as directed and continued so long as the patient tolerates well and desires to continue (This regimen is recommended by Beckmann et al., 1998, pp. 379-380)
An oral contraceptive containing 50 mcg of estrogen such as Ovral	One pill QID x 5-7 days, then one pill QD for 21 days, followed by 7 pill-free days; repeat this regimen for several months (This particular regimen is recommended by Hatcher et al., 1998, pp. 435-436)

E.   If bleeding persists in women treated with hormonal therapies, endometrial sampling is indicated

F.   After successful hormonal therapy, a long-term plan should be established
   1.   For women with first episode of bleeding, a 3 month treatment with an oral contraceptive unless contraindicated is usually sufficient (**Note:** DUB may return after therapy is discontinued)
   2.   Patients with a second or third episode (and no etiology has been found) may need to be treated with the **addition** of NSAIDs to correct relative prostaglandin overproduction
      a.   Mefenamic acid (Ponstel) 500 mg initially, then 250 mg TID for 3 days starting with menses OR
      b.   Naproxen (Naprosyn) 500 mg BID for 3 days starting with menses

   3.   Follow-up with patients on a regular schedule depending on the clinical situation

AMENORRHEA

I.   Definition: Absence of menses at any age when menstrual function should be present

II.   Pathogenesis

   A.   The hypothalamic-pituitary-ovarian-uterine axis needs to function in a coordinated manner for menstruation to occur

   B.   If any part of the system functions incorrectly, withdrawal menses do not occur and amenorrhea is the symptom

III.   Clinical Presentation

   A.   Diagnostic Criteria: Primary Amenorrhea
      1.   No bleeding by age 14 in the absence of growth and development of secondary sexual characteristics
      2.   Failure to have menses by age 16, regardless of presence of normal growth and development with the appearance of secondary sexual characteristics

B. Diagnostic Criteria: Secondary Amenorrhea
1. Woman must have had at least one spontaneous menstrual period
2. Six months of amenorrhea (this is controversial, some say 3, others 12)

C. Common causes of primary amenorrhea along with usual presenting signs are the following
1. Gonadal dysgenesis -- there is a lack of mature (stages 4 or 5) breast/pubic hair development, but small amounts of development (stages 2 or 3) may be present secondary to only adrenal hormone secretion
2. Müllerion (uterovaginal) anomalies -- normal breast/pubic hair development occurs
3. Hypothalamic/pituitary disorders -- normal breast/pubic hair development does not occur
4. Constitutional delay secondary to an immature hypothalamic-pituitary axis -- short stature (under 5 feet at age 14) is found

D. Common causes of secondary amenorrhea
1. Pregnancy
2. Prolactin-secreting pituitary adenomas
3. Hypothalamic amenorrhea secondary to excessive stress, weight loss, and/or exercise (As many as half of all competitive female athletes may experience some menstrual abnormality, with luteal phase deficiency, anovulation, and amenorrhea the three most common)
4. Polycystic ovarian disease (PCOD)
5. Androgen excess, endocrine disorders such as thyroid disease and diabetes mellitus

E. There are numerous uncommon causes of amenorrhea including onset of systemic debilitating diseases such as Crohn's disease and lupus erythematosus

IV. Diagnosis/Evaluation

A. History: Primary Amenorrhea
1. Question about growth and development; occurrence of growth spurt (Ask: "Was there a period of 6 months - 1 year when you grew out of all your clothes, shoes?")
2. Ask questions about puberty (breast and pubic hair -- when development began and how far it has advanced)

B. Physical Examination: Primary Amenorrhea
1. Height, weight
2. Observe for common anomalies associated with gonadal dysgenesis
   a. Neck folds, setting of ears
   b. Chest configuration, whether 4th metacarpal is short, cubitus, valgus
3. Assess breast and pubic hair development using Tanner stages
4. Speculum exam for imperforate hymen, presence of vagina and uterus, and bimanual exam for adnexal masses
   a. Estrogen exposed vaginal mucosa is thick, with rugae
   b. Presence of cervix at end of canal is sufficient evidence that uterus is present
   c. Clear cervical mucus in os is good indication that estrogen is present
   d. Bimanual exam to confirm presence, size of uterus, and any masses

C. Differential Diagnosis: Primary amenorrhea is a symptom. There are numerous etiologies for this symptom

D. Diagnostic Tests: Primary Amenorrhea
1. Refer patient to specialist for management
2. Initial tests are usually HCG, TSH, prolactin, and progesterone challenge tests

E. History: Secondary Amenorrhea
1. Question patient regarding the following
   a. Age at menarche, cycle regularity, duration of menstrual flow (was it fairly constant month to month?) (**Note**: The presence of cycle regularity leads to a strong presumption of ovulation)

        b.   Presence of symptoms suggesting ovulation -- mittelschmerz, bloating, breast tenderness

        c.   When and how deviation from prior menstrual cyclicity occurred

        d.   Number and outcomes of pregnancies, postpartal course

        e.   Type of contraception and possibility of pregnancy

    2.   Obtain past medical history, medications currently taking

    3.   Question regarding growth of excess hair on face, chest, abdomen, upper back; ask about presence of acne

    4.   Ask about galactorrhea (breast milk). Persistent galactorrhea, even slight and unilateral, is significant

    5.   Question regarding weight changes, skin texture, energy level, bowel habits, and temperature tolerance

    6.   Take social history including exercise, eating habits and patterns, and stress at home, school, and work

    7.   If woman is competitive athlete, obtain information about intensity and duration of training (**Note**: A triad of disordered eating, amenorrhea, and osteoporosis occurs in the elite athlete)

  F.   Physical Examination: Secondary Amenorrhea

    1.   Vital signs, height and weight, and calculate BMI (see OBESITY section for how to calculate and interpret BMI)

    2.   Examine skin for signs of androgen excess--acne and hirsutism

    3.   Examine thyroid for size, presence of nodularity

    4.   Assess breast development for Tanner staging and presence of galactorrhea

    5.   Speculum exam for degree of vaginal rugation, type of cervical mucus (amount, stretchability, ferning pattern when dried on glass slide)

    6.   Bimanual exam for masses; for example, a unilateral ovarian enlargement can mean a steroid-producing tumor. Assess deep tendon reflexes as index of thyroid status

  G.   Differential Diagnosis: Secondary amenorrhea is a symptom. There are numerous etiologies for this symptom

  H.   Diagnostic Tests: Secondary Amenorrhea

    1.   Focused diagnostic tests are useful to isolate the underlying cause to the hypothalamic/pituitary, ovarian, or uterine/vaginal compartments, or to other organ systems

    2.   HCG, TSH, LH, FSH, prolactin, and progesterone challenge test are usually the initial tests

V.   Plan/Management

  A.   Primary Amenorrhea: Refer all patients with primary amenorrhea to specialist for further work-up

  B.   Secondary Amenorrhea: Consult with specialist regarding management based on history, physical exam and diagnostic test results

BARTHOLIN GLAND CYSTS AND ABSCESSES

I.   Definition: An occlusion and/or infection of the Bartholin gland or its ducts

II.   Pathogenesis:

  A.   Bartholin's glands are bilateral vulvovaginal structures located at about the 4 and 8 o'clock positions on the posteriolateral aspect of the vestibule (area enclosed by the labia at the mouth of the vagina) (see Figure 14.1)

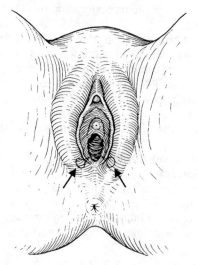

Figure 14.1. Bartholin's Glands.

B. These vestibular glands are nomally about the size of a pea and are made up of mucin-producing and excreting acini that drain into transitional and squamous epithelium-lined ducts about 2.5 cm long; the ducts exit into a fold between the hymen and labium

C. Obstruction of a Bartholin's duct occurs most commonly near the orifice
    1. The exact etiology is usually unknown although infection with inflammation probably plays a major role
    2. The duct becomes closed, while the mucus-secreting gland continues to produce fluid

D. An enlargement in the absence of inflammation is a cyst

E. With acute inflammation, an abscess develops
    1. Bartholin's duct abscesses may be caused from gonoccoccal or chlamydial infections
    2. However, other organisms such as *Staphylococcus aureus*, *Streptococcus fecalis*, and *Escherichia coli* also commonly cause the infection

III. Clinical Presentation

A. Dilatation of the Bartholin gland's duct due to obstruction is probably the most common finding in women complaining of vulvar masses and tends to be recurrent in some women

B. A normal Bartholin's gland and duct are nonpalpable, and any cystic swelling in the labia minora on the posteriolateral aspect of the vestibule usually represents a cyst or abscess

C. Cysts are generally 1 to 3 cm in size and are usually asymptomatic
    1. The patient may notice a bulge in the labia or mass may be found during routine clinical exam
    2. Cysts tend to grow slowly and noninfected cysts are nomally sterile (see Figure 14.2)

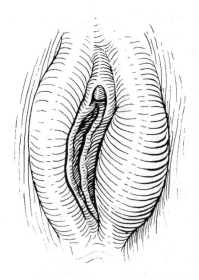

Figure 14.2. Bartholin's Gland Cyst.

D. With acute inflammation, an abscess develops with symptoms of swelling, tenderness, and erythema; patient may be unable to engage in sex or sports due to pain

IV. Diagnosis/Evaluation

    A. History
        1. Ask about onset, duration of cyst/abscess
        2. Ask about presence of associated symptoms such as pain, swelling, erythema and ask if presence of cyst/abscess has limited normal activities
        3. Determine if there are any symptoms present that might indicate presence of a sexually transmitted disease--discharge, irregular bleeding, dyspareunia
        4. Ask about trauma to the site
        5. Ask about history of recurrent cysts/abscesses

    B. Physical Examintion
        1. Inspect external genitalia for presence of lesions and masses, other abnormalities
        2. Carefully palpate the vaginal introitus with the thumb and forefinger for presence of swelling/masses, presence of fluctuance, areas of tenderness
        3. Palpate inguinal nodes for enlargement

    C. Differential Diagnosis
        1. Sebaceous cyst
        2. Vaginal inclusion cyst
        3. Fibromas
        4. Lipomas
        5. Hematoma

    D. Diagnostic Tests: None indicated unless abscess is recurrent; then culture and sensitivity testing of discharge from the abscess should be performed

V. Plan/Treatment

    A. Asymptomatic Bartholin's gland cysts in patients under age 40 may not require treatment
        1. Many small ductal cysts do not interfere with intercourse, or cause discomfort with walking, sitting, or other activities, and usually wax and wane in size. Treatment consists of daily sitz baths or warm compresses applied to area and spontaneous resolution of the cyst usually occurs
        2. Others eventually become symptomatic and require treatment

3. Referral to a specialist for drainage of the cyst and placement of a Word catheter in the cyst cavity is recommended
4. Word catheter is left in place for up to 4 weeks to allow drainage and formation of an epithelized outflow tract

B. Asymptomatic Bartholin's gland cysts in patients over 40 are usually excised because of concern about Bartholin's gland carcinoma (rare)

C. Most ductal abscesses will eventually "point" and spontaneously rupture resulting in immediate relief; the process will be hastened with frequent sitz baths
1. Because of the polymicrobial nature of most abscesses, broad-spectrum antibiotic coverage is recommended (erythromycin, 250 mg QID x 10 days)
2. Advise patient to continue with frequent sitz baths to provide relief and facilitate healing
3. Abscess may recur and definitive treatment with placement of a Word catheter may be necessary

D. Early abscesses (that have not ruptured) should be treated with sitz baths until the abscess points which makes incision and definitive treatment easier; broad spectrum antibiotics should also be prescribed
1. Refer the patient for incision, drainage, and placement of a Word catheter for up to 4 weeks to facilitate drainage and formation of an epithelized outflow tract
2. This procedure usually results in complete resolution of the condition

E. Follow Up: None indicated unless cyst/abscess fails to resolve

BREAST MASS

I. Definition: Benign and malignant lesions of the breast

II. Pathogenesis

A. Common benign lesions
1. Fibrocystic changes of the breast (FCB)
a. Abnormal restructuring in the layering of the parenchyma most likely related to estrogen/progestin imbalance resulting in excessive ductal stimulation and proliferation
b. Result of restructuring is atrophic epithelial segments and fibrous replacement
2. Fibroadenoma
a. Originates from the terminal duct -- lobular unit, and believed to be hormonally induced
b. Composed of fibrous and epithelial elements
3. Intraductal papilloma
a. Arises from dilated ductules in unfolding lobules
b. Found in both small and large ducts

B. Breast cancer
1. Arises from transformed epithelium that originates within ducts or lobules
2. For a period of time, these transformed cells are non-invasive; if undisturbed, eventually there is local, lymphatic and hematogenous spread

III. Clinical Presentation

A. The existence of a "dominant" area (lump, nodule, mass, or thickening) that is different from surrounding tissue or asymmetric compared to the opposite breast constitutes an abnormal finding

1. The basic question is whether a dominant area exists; issues of smoothness, hardness, distinctness from surrounding tissue are secondary
2. Causes of a specific dominant area must be determined by means other than physical examination

B. Benign lesions
   1. Fibrocystic changes of the breast (FBC)
      a. Most common of all benign breast conditions
      b. Occurs in about 50% of women with highest incidence among women aged 20-50 who are in reproductive, premenopausal years; symptoms cease with menopause (unless hormone replacement is begun)
      c. Risk factors include nulliparity, late age of natural menopause, middle class, and Caucasian race
      d. Condition is characterized by cyclic bilateral breast pain (mastalgia), which usually worsens premenstrually and resolves after onset of menses
      e. Multiple small cysts are usually palpable, particularly prior to menses as the internal fibroglandular tissue changes in consistency based on hormonal effects
   2. Fibroadenoma
      a. The second-most common form of benign breast disease occurring in about 10% of women, most often in 20-30 year age group, and decreasing in incidence with advancing age
      b. May be stimulated by pregnancy and regress with menopause
      c. Usually presents as single, smooth, round, mobile lumps which are usually painless (**Note**: Can feel firm or "rubbery")
      d. In about 15%-20% of patients, multiple, often bilateral fibroadenomas are involved
   3. Intraductal papilloma
      a. Tend to occur perimenopausally (median age of occurrence is 40)
      b. Usually presents as a spontaneous bloody or serous nipple discharge from a single duct
      c. Can cause a breast mass and nipple retraction, but often there is no associated palpable mass

C. Breast cancer
   1. Lifetime risk is 1 in 8 for US women (estimated lifetime risk of dying from breast cancer is 3.6%)
   2. Rare in women under 25; 48% of new breast cancer cases and 56% of breast cancer deaths occur in women age 65 and over
   3. Approximately 32% of all newly diagnosed cancers in women are cancers of the breast
   4. Risk factors include the following:
      a. Female gender, residence in North America or northern Europe and older age
      b. Family history of breast cancer in first degree relative, especially if bilateral and/or premenopausal in onset
      c. Menarche occurrence before age 11 or after age 14
      d. Onset of menopause after age 55 or more than 35 years duration of menses
   5. Usually presents as a painless, firm, fixed mass that does not change with menstruation; most common in upper, outer-quadrant though may occur in other areas
   6. Spontaneous nipple discharge that is most often clear may be associated with malignancy

D. Age is an important factor with most women <25 with masses having benign conditions and 75% of women >70 with palpable masses having cancer

IV. Diagnosis/Evaluation

A. History
   1. Question regarding presence/location of mass, characteristics of mass -- tenderness, mobility, size, single or multiple. Ask if any lymph nodes have seemed enlarged
   2. If presenting complaint is mastalgia, ask regarding frequency, severity, duration, location (localized, diffuse, or bilateral). Ask if the pain is cyclic occurring during the premenstrual phase or noncyclic. Determine if the pain is due to **trauma**

3. Inquire about changes of breast mass with menstruation (if not postmenopausal), presence of nipple discharge (spontaneous rather than elicited), type of discharge (bloody, serous, clear, milky), and laterality (one or both nipples)

4. Obtain detailed menstrual history including age at menarche, dates of last period, and age at menopause (if appropriate). Determine in which phase of menstrual cycle the patient is in at presentation (**Note:** Clinical breast exam is best performed a week or so after onset of menses when tissue is least congested)

5. Question about medication history, including current and past use of oral contraceptives and hormone replacement therapy

6. Obtain history of risk factors for breast cancer (see above), as well as information relating to previous breast masses, biopsies, and breast surgery

7. Determine and document in chart time since last clinical breast exam, when last mammogram was done and the results, and breast self-examination practices

B. Physical Examination
1. With patient sitting on table
   a. Inspect for symmetry, contour, and vascular pattern variation
   b. Inspect skin, noting discoloration, retraction, dimpling, edema
2. Have patient raise arms above head and place hands on hip
3. Palpate the axillary, supraclavicular, and infraclavicular nodes for adenopathy
4. With patient supine and arm extended and slightly bent on side being examined
   a. Inspect breast and skin as in the upright position
   b. Palpate the breast tissue, supraclavicular region, and chest wall following a vertical strip pattern
   c. Gently palpate the entire nipple-areolar complex; do not squeeze the nipple unless the patient has complained of nipple discharge
5. Teach BSE during exam
6. If a dominant area (i.e., lump, mass, nodule, or thickening different from surrounding tissue or asymmetric compared to the opposite breast) is found, the area should be assessed and then described
   a. Use tip of forefinger as a ruler
   b. Do simultaneous mirror image palpation bilaterally
   c. Description of dominant area should be noted on a drawing in the chart and labeled appropriately

C. Differential Diagnosis: Benign versus malignant tumor

D. Diagnostic Tests: When a dominant mass is encountered, patients under age 30 may be rescheduled after their next menstrual period for re-evaluation of the mass, to assess whether it has gotten smaller or gone away, before proceeding with diagnostic tests
1. Mammogram is the initial test ordered to evaluate a breast mass
2. Alternative: Fine needle aspiration (FNA) biopsy may be performed in office procedure when mass is easily palpable and cyst-like
3. Alternative: Ultrasound may also be used to differentiate a fluid-filled cyst from a solid tumor, but aspiration has the advantage of also treating the cyst; ultrasound may be more useful than mammogram in young women with dense breast tissue
4. Open biopsy is the definitive step in determining if a breast mass is malignant

V. Plan/Management

A. If mammographic abnormalities are found, refer patient for open biopsy

B. If fibrocystic breast changes are diagnosed via FNA, the aspiration itself may be therapeutic for benign cysts and may relieve localized pain. Patient may be managed as follows to control symptoms
1. Counsel patient that no cure exists for FBC but symptomatic therapy will control symptoms in most cases
2. Wear support bra to stabilize the breasts
3. Dietary modifications are controversial but reduction in caffeine intake and salt intake may help some patients

4.	If there are no contraindications, prescribe oral contraceptives that are low dose estrogen (20 mcg) and relatively high dose progesterone (1 mg) [product example is Loestrin 1/20]; patient usually has reduction in pain after a few months of therapy

5.	Low-dose danazol (Danocrine), a synthetic androgen, is the first-line treatment for severe mastalgia (works by blocking midcycle surges of LH and FSH; also reduces estrogen effects)

    a.	Dosing: 50-200 mg BID x 4-6 months (**Note**: Begin therapy during menses or perform appropriate tests to ensure patient is not pregnant)

    b.	Available as 50, 100, 200 mg caps

    c.	Several months of use may be needed before drug becomes effective

    d.	**Note**: Drug can cause alterations in the lipid profile and hepatic dysfunction

6.	Premenstrual use of diuretics, NSAIDs and vitamin E may be helpful in some patients

    a.	Hydrochlorothiazide 25-50 mg/day for 7-10 days before menses

    b.	Ibuprofen, 400 mg tabs, Q 4-6 hours for 2-3 days at time of maximal engorgement

7.	Vitamin E (150-600 IU/day) taken daily

8.	Patients whose breast pain does not resolve with above measures should be referred to a specialist for management

C.	If fibroadenoma is diagnosed via FNA or ultrasound, refer for surgical excision (**Note**: If cytologic assessment of the aspirate from FNA provides a clear diagnosis of fibroadenoma, the mass can be left in place and followed with monthly self-exam, annual clinical breast exam, and annual mammogram)

D.	If intraductal papilloma is diagnosed via excisional biopsy, the biopsy itself provides both diagnosis and treatment

E.	Follow Up: None indicated unless condition does not improve

CONTRACEPTION

I.	Definition: Prevention of pregnancy by reversible or irreversible methods used by either or both sexual partners

II.	Pathogenesis: Not applicable

III.	Clinical Presentation

A.	Requests for contraceptives and contraceptive counseling are among the most frequent reasons women visit a health care provider

B.	The proportion of never-married women currently in a sexual relationship has increased for all age categories over the past decade

C.	Pregnancy rates among teens are greater in the US than in any other developed country with a least 1 in 5 sexually active teens not using contraception

D.	Half of all pregnancies are unintended with 3.2 million unintended pregnancies in 1994, the last year for which data are available

E.	Female sterilization, oral contraceptives, male condoms, and male sterilization are the dominant contraceptive methods in the US today

IV.	Diagnosis/Evaluation

A.	History
1.	**Obtain a menstrual history** including age at menarche, duration, frequency of, interval between menstrual periods, the last menstrual period (LMP, which is dated from the first day of the last normal menses), any intermenstrual bleeding, pain with menses, and perimenstrual symptoms
2.	**Obtain an obstetric history**, including number of pregnancies and outcome of each
3.	**Obtain a gynecologic history** including breast history, previous gynecologic surgery, infectious diseases involving the reproductive tract, any history of infertility, use of douching/feminine hygiene products, and diethylstilbestrol (DES) exposure in utero
4.	**Obtain a sexual history** eliciting age at first intercourse; present sexual partner(s) and their gender; number of lifetime partners; types of sexual practices; level of satisfaction with sex lives
5.	**Obtain a contraceptive history** including contraceptive method currently used and reason for its choice; when begun, any problems, and satisfaction with method; inquire about previous methods used and why discontinued
6.	**Inquire about** past or present **sexual abuse** or assault
7.	**Obtain a complete medical and surgical history**, including information about cardiovascular disease, thromboembolic disease, liver problems, diabetes mellitus and blood transfusions
8.	**Inquire about substance use** including tobacco, alcohol, and drug use; ask what medications are currently being taken
9.	**Question about allergies** and any history of adverse drug reactions
10.	**Determine childhood diseases**, especially rubella, and immunization status
11.	**Obtain family history**, asking about stroke, CVD, cancer, DM in first degree relative

B.	Physical Examination
1.	**General Principles**: Have patient empty bladder, get completely undressed, and don the gown provided
2.	Obtain height, weight, temperature, pulse, respirations, and blood pressure
3.	Complete physical exam, including funduscopic exam, palpation of thyroid gland for irregularities, abdominal exam for organomegaly, examination of extremities for evidence of varicose veins, edema, arterial competency (peripheral pulses)
4.	Pelvic exam must include the following
a.	Inspection and examination of external genitalia
b.	Speculum examination of the internal structures
c.	Pap smear and specimens as appropriate
d.	Bimanual examination of the pelvic organs
e.	Rectovaginal exam of posterior aspect of pelvic organs (if indicated)
5.	Breast exam and instruction in breast self exam (BSE)

C.	Differential Diagnosis: Not applicable

D.	Diagnostic Tests
1.	Variable depending on history and physical
2.	Screening tests commonly ordered are the following
a.	CBC
b.	VDRL or RPR
c.	Urine dipstick
d.	Pregnancy test
e.	Pap smear
f.	DNA probe for gonorrhea and chlamydia
g.	Wet prep of vaginal secretions to evaluate for vaginitis

V.   Plan/Treatment

   A.   All patients should be counseled regarding the following and the counseling must be documented
         in the chart
         1.   Anatomy and physiology of reproduction
         2.   Contraceptive methods, including how they work, effectiveness, advantages, and
               disadvantages
         3.   The need to use condoms to prevent STDs, regardless of contraceptive method selected
         4.   Risks and benefits of all methods, as well as informed consent that is signed by patient
               and placed in chart when IUD, implants, injections, or oral contraceptives are chosen by
               patient
         5.   Techniques of breast self exam (BSE)

   B.   Assist patient to select one of the methods contained in the following overview of commonly used
         contraceptive methods, and provide counseling appropriate to the method selected

VI.   Brief Overview of Commonly Used Contraceptive Methods

   A.   **Spermicides** contain nonoxynol-9 (in the US) which disrupts the integrity of the sperm
         membrane. Spermicides are available as creams, gels, foams, film, tablets, and suppositories
         and should be placed deep in vagina near cervix prior to intercourse
         1.   Effectiveness: About 5-50% of women experience an unintended pregnancy during a year
               of typical use; there is no significant difference among various forms
         2.   Advantages: Inexpensive, easily available, convenient with infrequent intercourse, few
               side effects or user risk; provides some protection against some STDs
         3.   Disadvantages: May cause local irritation

   B.   **Male condoms** are more commonly used today to prevent transmission of STDs than for
         pregnancy prevention. They are thin sheaths made from latex or polyurethane. The condom acts
         as a physical barrier
         1.   Effectiveness: There is a 3% probability of pregnancy during a year of perfect use; causes
               of failure include slippage and breakage during intercourse and improper application
         2.   Advantages: Inexpensive, easy to use, easily available, reduce risk of STDs
         3.   Disadvantages: May decrease tactile sensation; condoms made of polyurethane are
               compatible with oil-based lubricants, but those made from latex are not
         4.   Application of condoms

         > Roll condom to base of erect penis
         >
         > Pinch tip of condom as it is unrolled and leave ½" of empty space at tip

   C.   **Female condoms (Reality)** have been in use since 1992 and are the first barrier contraceptive
         for women offering some protection against STDs. Composed of a thin polyurethane sheath that
         is 7.8 cm in diameter and 17 cm in length, the sheath has two polyurethane rings. The inner ring
         is at the closed end of the sheath that is placed inside the vagina and a larger ring remains
         outside the vagina providing some protection to the labia and the base of the penis. The inner
         ring provides stability for the condom which is prelubricated with a dry silicone-based lubricant.
         The condom can be inserted up to 8 hours prior to intercourse and is intended for one-time use
         1.   Effectiveness: About 5% of women experience an unintended pregnancy during a year of
               perfect use
         2.   Advantages: Controlled by woman and provides some STD protection
         3.   Disadvantages: Anatomy of women may make stable placement difficult

         > **Patient Education Relating to Use of Spermicides and Condoms**
         > ✔ The correct way to used spermicides and condoms including appropriate
         >   lubricants to use with condoms, and how to put on and remove both male
         >   and female condoms should be included
         > ✔ Follow Up: In 1 year for annual exam

D. **Diaphragms** are dome-shaped rubber caps with a flexible rim that fits over the cervix and blocks the passage of sperm; spermicides are applied to the inner aspect of the dome which is placed against the cervix

    1.   Effectiveness: Approximately 6% of women experience an unintended pregnancy during a year of perfect use

    2.   **Types**: Three types are commonly used

        a.   Flat spring rim: A thin rim with gentle spring strength, appropriate for use in women with normal vaginal size, contour, a shallow arch behind the symphysis pubis and normal vulvar tone

        b.   Arching spring rim: A sturdy rim with considerable strength, used in women with less than optimal vaginal support (indicated for women who have had a vaginal delivery which usually causes some amount of first degree cystocele) [**Note:** This type is the most commonly used]

        c.   Coil spring rim: A thin but sturdy rim useful in women with normal vaginal size, contour, and with an average or deep arch behind the symphysis pubis

    3.   **Goal** for fitting is to find the largest size that remains comfortable for the patient; most common problem in diaphragm fitting is selecting a size that is too small

        a.   Generally, a nulliparous woman will be fitted with sizes 65, 70, or 75

        b.   A multiparous woman, with sizes 75, 80, or 85

        c.   A grand multiparous woman, with size 85 or larger

    4.   **Procedure** for fitting with diaphragm

        a.   May use fitting rings or sets of various sizes of diaphragms (for the purpose of this explanation, a diaphragm will be used)

        b.   Begin with a size in the middle of the probable range or estimate diaphragm size by using technique described below

---

DIAPHRAGM FITTING

★ Insert your index and middle fingers into vagina until middle finger reaches vaginal posterior wall
★ With tip of your thumb, mark the place where your index finger touches the pubic bone.
★ Remove your fingers
★ Diaphragm is sized appropriately if it fits between mark on index finger and tip of middle finger

---

        c.   After selecting the size believed to be appropriate, introduce the diaphragm into the vagina (first, lubricate the rim of the diaphragm; then compress the sides with fingers and thumbs of one hand, and place in vagina as one would place a speculum--inserting downward and inward)

        d.   Check placement to make certain that the lower rim is in the posterior fornix, the circumference is against the lateral vaginal walls, and the upper rim is secured behind the symphysis pubis

        e.   Determine if the size is right by referring to the table below

---

IS THE DIAPHRAGM TOO SMALL, TOO LARGE, OR JUST RIGHT?

It's Too Small if
- it moves around in the vagina
- can't be stabilized behind the symphysis pubis
- it is loose
- comes out when woman coughs/bears down
- there is more than enough space to place your fingertips between rim and symphysis pubis

It's Too Large if
- rim buckles forward against the vaginal walls
- woman feels discomfort when the diaphragm is in place
- there is not enough space to place your fingertips between rim and symphysis pubis

It's Just Right if
- it fits snugly in the vagina without buckling forward
- it covers the cervix
- it fits both into posterior fornix and up behind symphysis pubis
- woman cannot feel the diaphragm and it does not cause discomfort
- there is just enough space to place your fingertips between rim and symphysis pubis

    f.   Teach the woman how to insert, place, check, and remove the diaphragm; give woman detailed instructions on how to use and care for diaphragm
5.   Advantages: May be inserted up to 6 hours prior to intercourse; reduced risk of STDs and a reduced risk of cervical cancer; works well with infrequent intercourse
6.   Disadvantages: UTIs are more common; some women are sensitive to contraceptive jelly; use has been associated with toxic shock syndrome, so should be avoided during menses and left in place no longer than 24 hours

E.   **Cervical caps** are soft rubber cups with a firm, round rim (Prentif Cavity Rim Cervical Cap) that fit snugly around the base of the cervex. Spermicide is placed inside the cap prior to insertion
1.   Effectiveness: About 9-26% of women experience an unintended pregnancy during a year of perfect use (nulliparous women are less likely than parous women to become pregnant)
2.   Advantages: Provides continuous contraception protection for 48 hours with no need to remove for additional spermicide
3.   Disadvantages: Must be removed after 48 hours because of possible risk of TSS; some women experience odor problems with use for more than a few hours. Device must be fitted by a health care provider and thus requires a visit and replacement every year

---

Patient Education Relating to Use of Diaphragm and Cervical Cap
★ Provide patient with insertion and removal instructions and how to care for devices
★ Include information on application of spermicidal jelly or cream when using the devices and when to remove
★ Follow up: In 1 year for annual exam

F.   **Intrauterine devices (IUDs)** are inserted into the uterus and their mechanisms of action is believed to be via preventing sperm from fertilizing ova
1.   Effectiveness: About 0.6 to 1.5% of women experience unintended pregnancy in first year of use with perfect use
2.   Types: Presently there are two intrauterine contraceptive devices marketed in the US: the Copper T-380A (ParaGard) and the intrauterine progesterone contraceptive system (Progestasert)
        a.   The ParaGard is a T-shaped polyethylene device whose stem is wrapped with copper wire, and whose cross-arms are partly covered by copper tubing; fertilization is prevented primarily through creation of an intrauterine environment that is spermicidal; it is approved for 10 years of use
        b.   The Progestasert is a plastic T-shaped device, whose stem contains a reservoir of 38 mg progesterone, along with barium sulfate; 65 mcg of progesterone per day is released for at least one year
        c.   IUDs are not abortafacients
3.   Contraindications to IUD use outlined in following table

---

CONTRAINDICATION TO IUD USE

Absolute Contraindications
- PID within the past 3 months, or current PID
- Known or suspected pregnancy

Strong Relative Contraindications
- History of ectopic pregnancy
- Abnormal vaginal bleeding whose cause remains unknown
- Risk factors for PID which includes multiple sexual partners
- Past history of infection with gonorrhea or chlamydia, or with mucopurulent cervicitis
- History of postpartum endometritis or
- infection following abortion in past 3 months
- Abnormal Pap smear which is unresolved

(continued)

CONTRAINDICATION TO IUD USE (CONTINUED)

- Poor access to health care
- Impaired ability to check for IUD string
- Known or suspected bleeding disorder
- Valvular heart disease
- Anatomic variations that make inserting difficult
- Severe dysmenorrhea, heavy menses, endometriosis, anemia
- History of fainting or vasovagal response
- Allergy to copper (ParaGard only)
- History of impaired fertility in patient desiring future pregnancy

---

4. Timing of insertion: Usually recommended during menses to avoid pregnancy
5. Advantages: High efficacy, which is sustained over 10 years for the ParaGard but only 1 year for the Progestasert; absence of systemic metabolic effects; method is not related to coitus; immediately reversible
6. Disadvantages: Risk of uterine perforation, increase in spontaneous abortion, ectopic pregnancy, uterine bleeding and pain, pelvic infection; need to return for annual replacement (Progestasert only)

Patient Education Relating to Use of IUDs

★ Instruct on how to check for strings, especially during first few months when expulsion is more likely
★ Instruct on signs of infection to be alert for (fever, chills, pelvic pain, severe cramping, unusual bleeding)
★ Instruct to contact health care provider immediately if period is missed
★ Provide a copy of the FDA-approved and manufacturer-supplied leaflet or pamphlet to each IUD user; consent forms can be written to include a statement such as "I have been given a copy of (title) and have been encouraged to read it carefully"
★ Follow up after woman's next menses (3-6 weeks after insertion) to make certain IUD is in place and that there are no signs of infection; further routine visits are not required. Schedule annual exam

---

G. **Combination oral contraceptives** prevent pregnancy by a number of effects of estrogen and progestin: they inhibit ovulation, presumably as a result of gonadotropin suppression induced by the estrogen and progestin effects on the hypothalamic/pituitary axis; they act directly on the cervical mucus, making it thicker which inhibits sperm penetration, and; they act directly on the endometrium, inhibiting its development into a state favorable for implantation
   1. Effectiveness: About 0.1% of women experience an unintended pregnancy within the first year of use with perfect use (combined pills); the figure is 0.5% with progestin-only pills
   2. Advantages: Easy to use convenient, rapidly reversible, use controlled by woman, many noncontraceptive benefits such as prevention of gynecologic malignancies (endocervical and ovarian), prevention of benign conditions such as fibrocystic breast changes
   3. Disadvantages: Dependent on user adherence to daily use, provides no protection against STDs, expensive, prescription needed, many possible side effects
   4. Absolute contraindications to the use of oral contraceptives are the following

---

ABSOLUTE CONTRAINDICATIONS TO USE OF ORAL CONTRACEPTIVES

- Thrombophlebitis, thromboembolic disorders
- Past history of deep vein thrombophlebitis or thromboembolic disorder
- Cerebral vascular or coronary artery disease
- Known or suspected carcinoma of the breast
- Known or suspected carcinoma of the endometrium and known or suspected estrogen-dependent neoplasia
- Undiagnosed abnormal genital bleeding
- Cholestatic jaundice of pregnancy or jaundice with prior pill use
- Hepatic adenomas, carcinomas, or benign liver tumors
- Known or suspected pregnancy
- Marked impaired liver function
- Benign or malignant liver tumor that developed during prior use of OCs or other estrogen-containing products
- Leiden factor V mutation
- Type II hyperlipidemia (hypercholesterolemia)

Adapted from Dickey, R.P. (1998). Managing contraceptive pill patients. Durant, OK: EMIS, Inc.

5. Strong relative contraindications are the following

STRONG RELATIVE CONTRAINDICATIONS TO USE OF ORAL CONTRACEPTIVES
• Severe headaches, particularly vascular or migraine headaches which begin after institution of oral contraceptives • Diastolic blood pressure of 90 mm Hg or greater or hypertension by any other criteria • Cardiac or renal dysfunction • Impaired glucose tolerance or history of gestational diabetes • Psychic depression • Varicose veins • Age ≥35 for smokers (considered absolute contraindication by some) • Sickle-cell or sickle cell-hemoglobin C disease • Cholestatic jaundice during pregnancy • Worsening of any chronic condition during pregnancy • Hepatitis or mononucleosis during past year • Breast feeding • Asthma • First degree family histories of nonrheumatic cardiovascular disease or diabetes before age 50 • Use of drugs know to interact with OCs • Ulcerative colitis

Adapted from Dickey, R.P. (1998). Managing contraceptive pill patients. Durant, OK: EMIS, Inc.

6. Most women (those without absolute contraindications and strong relative contraindications) can be prescribed any sub-50 mcg OC based on its cost, availability, or the woman's prior experience
   a. No single OC in the sub-50 mcg category is clearly superior to another
   b. One approach is to prescribe the lowest dose
   c. OCs such as Alesse provide one-third less ethinyl estradiol (EE) than is present in a 30 mcg OC such as Nordette
   d. Ovcon-35 has a total of 8.4 mg norethindrone per cycle compared with Tri-Norinyl which has 15 mg
   e. Tri-Levlen has a total of 1.925 mg of levonorgestrel per cycle which is over one-third less than in Nordette
   f. OCs containing more than 35 mcg of estrogen should rarely be used (clinical situations such as dysfunctional uterine bleeding [DUB] may be an indication for short-term use of higher estrogen dose in some women)
7. Women who are not candidates for estrogen-containing OCs should be considered for progestin-only pills such as Micronor or others listed in table of contraceptives categorized according to composition
8. Clinical considerations that might be a factor in OC choice are summarized in the following table

CHOICE OF ORAL CONTRACEPTIVE BASED ON PATIENT CHARACTERISTICS		
Characteristics	**Type of OC Indicated**	**Product Examples**
Risk for thrombosis which includes women 40-50 years of age, young women who are heavy smokers, women with diabetes, and those who are very overweight*	Lowest estrogen	Loestrin 1/20 Alesse
Women who complain of nausea, breast tenderness, who have vascular headaches and other estrogen-related side effects	Low estrogen	Loestrin 1/20 Alesse Estrostep
Women who have spotting or break through bleeding (BTB)	Intermediate estrogenic or progestogenic activity (can either alter progestin dose or increase the estrogen dose)	Lo-Ovral Estrostep (increases the amount of EE from 20 mcg to 35 mcg during cycle)
		(continued)

Characteristics	Type of OC Indicated	Product Examples
Women with androgenic effects such as acne, hirsuitism, oily skin, or weight gain	Low dose norethindrone or a new progestin OC**to decrease androgen effects	Ovcon 35 Desogen
Women in whom lipid changes are a concern	New progestin OCs tend to increase HDL cholesterol and decrease LDL cholesterol***	Ortho-Cyclen, Desogen, Ortho-Cept

* For complete listing of absolute contraindications as well as relative contraindications, always consult the product information inserts and the PDR

**New progestin refers to the fourth generation progestins--desogenstrel, norgestimate, and gestodene

***Oral contraceptives containing a new progestin (gestoden, desogestrel, or norgestimate) were associated with increased risk for DVT in women based on findings from several epidemiologic studies conducted in England and transnationally; however, these findings have been questioned due to poor research design, methodolgical weaknesses, and failure to replicate the data in subsequent studies. The FDA concluded that the additional risk of DVT due to use of oral contraceptives containing these new progestins is not great enough to justify switching to other products

Adapted from Hatcher et al. (1998). Contraceptive technology. New York: Ardent Media, Inc.

9.   The following table lists oral contraceptives categorized according to composition:

ORAL CONTRACEPTIVE CATEGORIZED BY COMPOSITION

Type	Preparation	Estrogen (mcg)	Progestin (mg)	Color of active tablets
COMBINATION ESTROPHASIC *Ethinyl estradiol/ norethindrone acetate*	Estrostep 21	(5 tabs)20 (7 tabs) 30 (9 tabs) 35	1 1 1	white (triangle) white (square) white (round)
	Estrostep Fe	(5 tabs) 20 (7 tabs) 30 (9 tabs) 35	1 1 1	white (triangle) white (square) white (round)
COMBINATION TRIPHASIC Ethinyl estradiol/ norethindrone	Ortho-Novum 7/7/7	(7 tabs) 35 (7 tabs) 35 (7 tabs) 35	0.5 0.75 1	white light peach peach
	Tri-Norinyl	(7 tabs) 35 (9 tabs) 35 (5 tabs) 35	0.5 1 0.5	blue yellow-green blue
Ethinyl estradiol/ norgestimate	Ortho Tri-cyclen	(7 tabs) 35 (7 tabs) 35 (7 tabs) 35	0.18 0.215 0.25	white light blue blue
Ethinyl estradiol/ levonorgestrel	Tri-Levlen	(6 tabs) 30 (5 tabs) 40 (10 tabs) 30	0.05 0.075 0.125	brown white light yellow
	Triphasil	(6 tabs) 30 (5 tabs) 40 (10 tabs) 30	0.05 0.075 0.125	brown white light yellow
COMBINATION BIPHASIC Ethinyl estradiol/ norethindrone	Ortho-Novum 10/11	(10 tabs) 35 (11 tabs) 35	0.5 1	white peach
	Jenest-28	(7 tabs) 35 (14 tabs) 35	0.5 1	white peach

(continued)

538

Type	Preparation	Estrogen (mcg)	Progestin (mg)	Color of active tablets
COMBINATION MONOPHASIC Ethinyl estradiol/ norethindrone	Loestrin 1/20	20	1	white
	Loestrin (Fe) 1/20	20	1	white
	Loestrin 1.5/30	30	1.5	green
	Loestrin (Fe) 1.5/30	30	1.5	green
	Brevicon	35	0.5	blue
	Modicon	35	0.5	white
	Norethin 1/35E	35	1	white
	Norinyl 1+35	35	1	yellow-green
	Ortho-Novum 1/35	35	1	peach
	Ovcon-35	35	0.4	peach
	Ovcon-50	50	1	yellow
Ethinyl estradiol/ levonorgestrel	Alesse	20	0.10	Pink
	Levlen	30	0.15	light orange
	Nordette	30	0.15	light orange
Ethinyl estradiol/ norgestiel	Lo/Ovral	30	0.3	white
	Ovral	50	0.5	white
Ethinyl/estradiol/ ethynodiol diacetate	Demulen 1/35	35	1	white
	Demulen 1/50	50	1	white
Mestranol/ norethindrone	Norethin 1/50 m	50	1	white
	Norinyl 1+ 50	50	1	white
	Ortho-Novum 1/50	50	1	yellow
Ethinyl estradiol/ desogestrel	Desogen	30	0.15	White
	Ortho-Cept	30	0.15	orange
Ethinyl estradiol/ norgestimate	Ortho-Cyclen	35	0.25	blue
PROGESTIN-ONLY Norethindrone	Micronor	-	0.35	lime
	Nor-QD	-	0.35	yellow
Norgestrel	Ovrette	-	0.075	yellow

Adapted from Murphy, J.L. (1998, May). Tables: Oral contraceptives. Monthly Prescribing Reference.

Patient Education Relating to Use of Oral Contraceptives

★ Instruct to use a backup method of birth control during first pack of pills
★ Provide instructions on when to start the pills based on information in the following table
★ Instruct patient to contact you if she does not have a menstrual period when expected while taking OCs
★ Teach the patient the OC danger sign and symptoms which signal that the OC should be discontinued immediately. Use the acronym ACHES (*A*bdominal pain, *C*hest pain, *H*eadaches, *E*ye problems, *S*evere leg pain) and also include teaching on unilateral numbness, weakness, or tingling, slurring of speech (possible stroke), hemoptysis (pulmonary embolism)
★ Provide a copy of the FDA-approved and manufacturer-supplied leaflet or pamphlet to each oral contraceptive OCs user; consent forms can be written to include a statement such as "I have been given a copy of (title) and have been encouraged to read it carefully"
★ When starting a woman on the OCs for the first time, give her a 3 month supply and have her return to the clinic for a BP check and for evaluation on how she is doing on the OCs; then give her enough OCs to last for the remainder of the year
★ Follow Up: In 1 year for annual exam

INSTRUCTIONS FOR STARTING ORAL CONTRACEPTIVES

- Advise woman to start the OCs on the first day of her menstrual cycle or on a the first Sunday after her period begins (if period begins Sunday, she should take the first pill on that day)
- Instruct patient to take 1 pill a day until pack is finished, then
- If on 28-day pack, begin a new pack immediately; skip no days
- If using 21-day pack, stop for 7 days, and then restart (Note: Caution patient to not wait until period starts, but to wait 7 days after completing pack, and then start next pack)
- Instruct to take at the same time each day and to associate with something that is done regularly at same time of day (going to bed, brushing teeth, etc.)
- Explain that a backup method such as condoms or foam should be used for first seven days during the first few cycles

Adapted from Dickey, R.P. (1998). Managing contraceptive pill patients. Durant, OK: EMIS, Inc.

INSTRUCTIONS ABOUT EARLY SIDE EFFECTS

- Advise that some side effects are common during the first few cycles of use, but that they should disappear after that time
- Side effects to expect include the following
  - ❖ Breakthrough bleeding (BTB) and spotting
  - ❖ Symptoms associated with early pregnancy, especially nausea
- Encourage patient to not make a decision about discontinuing the pill until after the 3rd cycle so that side effects will have had a chance to resolve

Adapted from Dickey, R.P. (1998). Managing contraceptive pill patients. Durant, OK: EMIS, Inc.

INSTRUCTIONS FOR DEALING WITH MISSED PILLS

First, explain to patients the difference between the 21-pill pack and the 28-pill pack (first 21 pills in 28-pill pack contain hormones and the last 7 contain no hormones)

Patients who are taking the 28-pill pack and miss any of the last 7 pills can discard the missed pill(s), take the remaining pills as scheduled to finish the pack
They should then start the next pack on usual schedule

Patients who are taking either the 21-pill or the 28-pill pack, and miss any of the 21 hormonal pills must do the following

Use back-up contraception even if one pill was missed, or even if a pill was taken as much as 12 hours late (if only 1 pill was missed or taken late, back-up contraception such as condoms should be used for 7 days or patient should abstain from sex for 7 days)

Advise Patient to Get Back on Schedule by Following These Guidelines

If patient is <24 hours late in taking a pill	Take the missed pill immediately and return to the daily pill-taking routine making sure to take the next pill at the regular time
If patient is 24 hours late in taking a pill	Take both the missed pill and today's pill at the same time
If patient is >24 hours late in taking one pill, and is late for or completely missed a second pill as well	Take the last pill that was missed immediately; take the next pill on time; throw out the other missed pills, and take the rest of the pills in pack right on schedule

If a pill was completely missed during the third week of pills (pills 15-21), advise the patient to do the following
- ✦ Finish the remainder of the hormonal pills in pack (take through pill 21 if using a 28-pill pack)
- ✦ Do not take a week off pills if using a 21-day pill pack OR do not take the last 7 pills (the nonhormonal pills) in the 28-pill pack
- ✦ Begin taking a new pack of pills as soon as the hormonal pills in the current pack have been taken
- ✦ Advise patient that she might not have a period until the end of the second pack of pills, but missing a period is not harmful
- ✦ In all cases, back-up contraception for at least 7 days must be used

Adapted from Hatcher et al. (1998). Contraceptive technology. New York: Ardent Media, Inc.

H.   **Norplant** is a long-acting subdermal contraceptive implant of the progestin levonorgestrel that suppresses ovulation in at least half the cycles; each set of implants contains 36 mg of progestin which is released at a slow, steady rate
   1.   Effectiveness: About 0.05% of women experience an unintended pregnancy within the first year of use with perfect use; rates are highest for women weighing 70 kg or more, but then is only 2.4% over 5 years

2. Advantages: Highly effective contraception; need little motivation on patient's part; rapid reversibility; avoids risks of estrogen
3. Disadvantages: Disruption of menstrual bleeding pattern and difficult removal
4. Indication: Sexually active women who
   a. Desire long-term contraception that is highly effective
   b. Have experienced estrogen-related side-effects with OCs
   c. Have difficulty taking OCs correctly
   d. Have completed childbearing but do not wish permanent sterilization
   e. Have a history of anemia with heavy menstrual bleeding
5. Contraindications are generally the same as with oral contraceptives; consult the package insert and PDR for more detail
6. Relative contraindications are generally the same as with oral contraceptives; consult the package insert and PDR for more detail
7. Overview of insertion
   a. Should be done during the first 7 days after the onset of menstruation; pregnancy should be ruled out
   b. Insertion is through a 3-5 mm incision in the skin located on the medial aspect of the upper inner arm
   c. Implants are placed beneath skin in fan distribution with ends nearly touching to facilitate removal
   d. Insertion is through a specially designed trocar sleeve in a largely painless procedure requiring 5-10 minutes
   e. A pressure bandage is applied post-insertion to reduce bruising
8. Generally, it is recommended that the implants be removed at the end of the fifth year

---

Patient Education Relating to Use of Norplant
- ★ Advise to use a backup form of contraception for first 7 days after the implant placement
- ★ Explain that Norplant will change pattern of menses with periods usually becoming less regular, and sometimes stopping altogether
- ★ Review "red flags" with patient--purulent discharge at implant site, expulsion of an implant, severe headaches, blurred vision, heavy vaginal bleeding, delayed menses after long interval of regular periods
- ★ If breast tenderness is a problem, she should contact provider (treatment with vitamin E 600 U/day may be helpful)
- ★ Encourage patient to call with questions

I. **Depo-Provera** is an injectable form of long-acting progestins with a mechanism of action similar to that of other progestin-only contraceptives; a good choice for women in whom estrogen-containing OCs are contraindicated, barrier methods are inadvisable because of compliance problems, and in women older than age 35 who smoke
   1. Effectiveness: About 0.3% of women experience an unintended pregnancy within the first year of use with perfect use
   2. Advantages: Easy to use, decreased menstrual flow and avoidance of the rare but serious complications attributable to estrogen use
   3. Disadvantages: Unpredictable vaginal bleeding, adverse changes in lipids
   4. How Administered: Usual dose is 150 mg, given IM every 12 weeks
      a. Initial dose should be administered by the 5th day of menses in nonpostpartum women
      b. In non-nursing postpartum women, initial dose should be given 5 days postpartum and at 6 weeks postpartum for breast feeding mothers (breast feeding must be well established)
      c. Approximately half of women using this method experience amenorrhea after a year of injections

J. **Emergency postcoital contraception** using emergency contraceptive pills (ECPs) has recently been approved by the FDA

1. ECPs are birth control pills containing ethinyl estradiol and norgestrel or levongestrel

2. These hormones are found in seven brands of combined oral contraceptives available in the US

3. The following table presents regimens for administering these drugs for emergency contraception

REGIMENS FOR ORAL EMERGENCY CONTRACEPTIVE USE IN THE UNITED STATES*			
Brand	Pills per dose	Ethynyl estradiol per dose (μg)	Levonorgestrel per dose (mg)[a]
Ovral	2 white pills[b]	100	0.50
Alesse	5 pink pills[b]	100	0.50
Nordette	4 light-orange pills[b]	120	0.60
Levlen	4 light-orange pills[b]	120	0.60
Lo/Ovral	4 white pills[b]	120	0.60
Triphasil	4 yellow pills[b]	120	0.50
Tri-Levlen	4 yellow pills[b]	120	0.50
Ovrette	20 yellow pills[c]	0	0.75

*Ovral, Alesse, Nordette, Levlen, Lo/Ovral, Triphasil, and Tri-Levlen have been declared safe and effective for use as emergency contraceptives by the FDA
[a]The progestin in Ovral, Lo/Ovral, and Ovrette is norgestrel, which contains two isomers, only one of which (levonorgestrel) is bioactive; the amount of norgestrel in each tablet is twice the amount of levonorgestrel
[b]The treatment schedule is one dose within 72 hours after unprotected intercourse, and another dose 12 hours later
[c]Treatment schedule using levonorgestrel only was tested in a clinical trial in which 0.75 mg was given within 48 hours after unprotected intercourse followed by 0.75 mg 12 hours later. The WHO has completed a study indicating that this same regimen is effective when initiated up to 72 hours after unprotected intercourse

Adapted from Hatcher, R.A. et al. (1998). Contraceptive technology. New York: Ardent Media.

4. Preven Emergency Contraceptive Kit was recently approved by the FDA

a. Kit is composed of 4 tabs containing both ethinyl estradiol 50 mcg and levonorgestrel 250 mcg

b. Dosing: 2 tabs within 72 hours of unprotected intercourse or a contraceptive failure and 2 tabs 12 hours later

c. **Note**: Kit also contains a urine pregnancy test

5. Effectiveness: Reduces the risk of pregnancy by about 75% (**Note**: Risk of becoming pregnant during unprotected intercourse during 2nd or 3rd week of cycle is about 8 of every 100 women; with ECPs, this is reduced to about 2 out of every 100 women, which represents a 75% reduction)

6. Side effects: Almost half of women who take ECPs have nausea and about a fourth have vomiting; if vomiting occurs within 2 hours after taking a dose, some authorities recommend repeating that dose

        a.   Antiemetics such as trimethobenzamide hydrochloride (Tigan) 250 mg caps or 200 mg suppositories may be administered 1 hour prior to the first dose, and then as needed every 6-8 hours x 24 hours

        b.   Recommend that the medication be taken with food to reduce nausea

   7.   Safety: Almost all women can safely use ECPs

        a.   The only absolute contraindication is confirmed pregnancy

        b.   Treatment may not be appropriate in women with active migraine or marked neurologic symptoms

        c.   In women with a history of stroke or blood clots in the lungs or legs, treatment with progestin-only pills may be preferable (consult table above)

K.   The Copper-T IUD has also been approved for emergency contraception and can be inserted up to five days after unprotected intercourse; reduce the risk of pregnancy following unprotected intercourse by more than 99%

DYSMENORRHEA

I.   Definition: Painful menstrual cramps

II.   Pathogenesis

   A.   Primary dysmenorrhea is painful uterine contractions associated with increased production and release of prostaglandins in the absence of pelvic pathology; a role may also be played by increased production of leukotrienes and vasopressin

   B.   Secondary dysmenorrhea is painful uterine contractions due to a clinically identifiable cause, and may be classified as follows:

       1.   External to the uterus (examples are endometriosis, tumors, adhesions, and nongynecologic causes)

       2.   Within the wall of the uterus (examples are adenomyosis, leiomyomas)

       3.   Within the cavity of the uterus (examples are polyps and infection)

III.   Clinical Presentation

   A.   Approximately 25% of women of childbearing age in the US have dysmenorrhea, with about 10% having levels of discomfort that cause absence from school or work

   B.   Incidence of primary dysmenorrhea is as follows

       1.   Greatest in women in teens and early 20s

       2.   Declines in women in their 30s and 40s

       3.   Uncommon during initial 3-6 menstrual periods when ovulation is not yet well established

   C.   Secondary dysmenorrhea increases in incidence as women grow older due to the increased prevalence of processes that cause the condition among older women

   D.   Pain of primary dysmenorrhea is characterized by the following

       1.   Occurs first day or two of menstruation

       2.   Located in suprapubic area and radiates to back, upper thighs

       3.   Associated with diarrhea, nausea, and vomiting

   E.   Women with secondary dysmenorrhea usually experience pain consistent with the underlying pathology such as the following

       1.   GI symptoms, UTI symptoms, and so on suggest nongynecologic causes

       2.   Dyspareunia and pelvic pain unrelated to menses (but also occurring with menses) suggest causes such as endometriosis, infection (PID), adenomyosis, and leiomyomas

IV. Diagnosis/Evaluation

    A. History
        1. Obtain a complete menstrual history and contraceptive history (including use of IUD)
        2. Question patient about location of pain, when it begins, if it radiates, if there are associated symptoms of nausea, vomiting, and diarrhea
        3. Inquire if pain occurs independently of menses in addition to occurring with menses. Ask if there is dyspareunia
        4. Ask if there are urinary tract symptoms, if there is any vaginal discharge
        5. Question patient about treatments tried and results

    B. Physical Examination
        1. Measure blood pressure (in 2 positions if blood loss is suspected), pulse rate, temperature
        2. Evaluate heart and lungs
        3. Perform abdominal exam, evaluating for bowel sounds, tenderness, masses, rigidity, guarding, rebound tenderness
        4. Do pelvic exam; inspect cervix for mucopurulent discharge draining from the endocervix. Gently scape cervix to test for friability
        5. Perform bimanual exam to check for adnexal tenderness, uterine tenderness, and cervical motion tenderness

    C. Differential Diagnosis
        1. For primary dysmenorrhea, the most important differential diagnosis to consider is that of secondary dysmenorrhea
        2. For secondary dysmenorrhea, must consider the following
            a. Intrauterine causes such as adenomyosis, myomas, polyps, IUDs, infection
            b. Extrauterine causes such as endometriosis, tumors, inflammation, adhesions, and nongynecologic causes

    D. Diagnostic Tests
        1. For primary dysmenorrhea, none indicated
        2. For secondary dysmenorrhea, H & P should guide test selection

V. Plan/Management

    A. For secondary dysmenorrhea, treatment of the underlying cause is indicated; if no obvious cause is uncovered, refer to expert for management

    B. For primary dysmenorrhea, drugs that suppress the production of prostaglandins are indicated; best accomplished by using nonsteroidal anti-inflammatory drugs (NSAIDs)

    C. NSAIDs inhibit prostaglandin synthesis and exhibit antiinflammatory and analgesic activity
        1. The most commonly used NSAIDs for dysmenorrhea come from two classes: propionic acids and fenamates
        2. Propionic Acids
            a. Ibuprofen (Motrin) 400 mg Q 4 H, OR
            b. Naproxen (Naprosyn) 500 mg initial dose, then 250 mg Q 6-8 H, OR
            c. Naproxen sodium (Anaprox) 550 mg initial dose, then 275 mg Q 6-8 H, OR
        3. Fenamates
            a. Mefenamic acid (Ponstel) 500 mg initial dose, then 250 mg Q 4-6 H, OR
            b. Meclofenamate (Meclomen) 100 mg initial dose, then 50-100 mg Q 6 H
        4. Drug that is selected for treatment should be tried over the course of 2-4 cycles before success or failure is judged
        5. If treatment failure occurs with one class, the second trial should utilize the other class
        6. Patients should be reminded to take drug at the onset of menstruation or symptoms, and continue taking for as long as symptoms would normally last if medication were not being taken

D. Oral contaceptives are also highly effective and may be used in addition to (reduce dose of NSAID) or instead of NSAIDs
   1. Oral contraceptives are first-line therapy for patients who also desire contraception
   2. Almost all patients with primary dysmenorrhea achieve good pain relief with use of OCs
   3. Low dose combination oral contraceptives should be prescribed if there are no contraindications

E. Nonpharmacologic management
   1. A regular aerobic exercise program may be helpful and should be recommended
   2. Use of acupuncture and acupressure on a weekly basis may also be helpful
   3. Use of a transcutaneous electrical nerve stimulation (TENS) unit is effective in some patients

F. Follow Up: In 6 months to evaluate treatment efficacy

PREMENSTRUAL SYNDROME

I. Definition: A cyclical symptom complex that occurs with greatest frequency and severity in the late luteal phase (5-11 days prior to onset of menses) and abates within 1-2 days of the onset of menses

II. Pathogenesis

   A. No single etiology has been identified and several mechanisms for pathogenesis have been described

   B. Mechanisms such as reductions in endorphin and serotonin levels, underproduction and excess production of prostaglandins, nutritional imbalance, endocrine and neuroendocrine alterations have been studied in relation to possible etiology of PMS, but findings have been inconclusive

III. Clinical Presentation

   A. Incidence of PMS is reported to be between 20-90% of women, with only about 20% having symptoms severe enough to limit daily functioning

   B. Disorder is more prevalent in women from 30-40 years of age, and is more frequent in women with history of postpartum depression or affective illness

   C. PMS presents as irritability, depression, crying spells, mood swings, sleep disturbance, appetite changes, and changes in libido; this presentation is similar to those seen in mood disorders and anxiety

   D. Patients with true PMS will have symptoms in the luteal phase only

   E. Diagnosis is made on the basis of history of a symptom-free follicular phase in contrast to emotional and physical disturbances that characterize the luteal phase

   F. Diagnostic critera for premenstrual dysphoric disorder (PMDD) are contained in the table on page 662, and are adapted from the fourth edition of the Diagnostic and Statistical Manual of Mental Disorders (1994); focus is on psychological symptoms rather than on physical symptoms

   G. Clinically, the two conditions--PMS and PMDD--overlap
      1. Many women with PMS meet the diagnostic criteria for PMDD
      2. PMDD is a much more narrowly defined disorder than PMS
      3. Presently, PMS and PMDD appear to be two points on a continuum, but further research is needed

545

<table>
<tr><td colspan="2">DIAGNOSTIC CRITERIA FOR PREMENSTRUAL DYSPHORIC DISORDER</td></tr>
</table>

- The woman must have **five or more** of the following 11 symptoms, including at least one of the first four for most of the time during the last week of the luteal phase in most menstrual cycles over the past 12 month period
  - Depressed mood, feelings of hopelessness, or self-deprecating thoughts
  - Marked anxiety or tension; feeling "keyed up"
  - Significant mood lability
  - Persistent anger or irritability
  - Decreased interest in usual activities
  - Difficulty concentrating
  - Lethargy, or marked lack of energy
  - Changes in appetite
  - Hypersonmia or insomnia
  - Feeling of being overwhelmed
  - Physical symptoms such as breast tenderness, headache, joint/muscle pain, bloating, or weight gain
- Symptoms must start or resolve within a few days of onset of menses and be absent in week after menstruation ceases
- Additionally, symptoms must markedly impair patient's ability to work/attend school, or conduct usual social activities
- The diagnosis must be confirmed by prospective daily ratings for at least two consecutive symptomatic menstrual cycles

Adapted from American Psychiatric Association. (1994). Diagnostic and statistical manual of mental disorders (4th ed.). Washington, DC: Author.

IV.   Diagnosis/Evaluation

    A.   History: (**Note**: Be cautious in accepting patient's self-diagnosis of PMS)
        1.   Ask about age at onset of symptomatology; when in cycle symptoms are experienced; most significant symptoms; degree of severity
        2.   Inquire about variations from cycle to cycle
        3.   Using the diagnostic criteria for PMDD, ask patient if the 11 symptoms listed are present during last week of luteal phase during menstrual cycles (**Note**: This is the best approach to the patient who reports significant impairment)
        4.   Inquire about previous history of depression; previous treatment for PMS and results
        5.   Determine if patient is experiencing dysmenorrhea (many women confuse PMS with dysmenorrhea), situational depression, or eating disorders
        6.   Obtain data regarding drug and alchol use
        7.   Use the SAFE Questions to screen for spousal abuse (see DOMESTIC VIOLENCE: PARTNER ABUSE section)

    B.   Physical Examination: No specific physical findings aid in diagnosis; physical and pelvic exams as part of a general health survey may be completed, however

    C.   Differential Diagnosis
        1.   Depression
        2.   Anxiety disorder
        3.   Relationship discord/domestic violence
        4.   Drug/alcohol abuse
        5.   Eating disorder
        6.   Dysmenorrhea

    D.   Diagnostic Tests: None indicated (**Note**: Make certain patient understands that laboratory testing is not helpful)

V.   Plan/Management

    A.   Prospective data collection by the patient for at least 2 menstrual cycles must be done to establish pattern of symptoms and establish diagnosis

    B.   Several commercially available checklists can be used by the patient to record occurrence and severity of symptoms on a daily basis throughout entire cycle. Available forms are the Menstrual Distress Questionnaire (Moos, 1969) and the Premenstrual Syndrome Symptomatology Questionnaire (Vargyas, 1986) [see reference list]

C. After 2 months of data collection related to occurrence and severity of symptoms, interpretation of data can be made
   1. The suspected diagnosis of PMS is confirmed if other disorders (see differential diagnosis) are ruled out, and patient's symptomatology is limited to luteal phase
   2. Patients who report a high degree of symptomatology throughout menstrual cycle should be referred for further evaluation, as PMS is unlikely

D. Treatment must be individualized based on symptoms

E. Conservative measures such as the following should be instituted first
   1. **Support and reassurance**: Patient should know that her problems are not uncommon
   2. **Stress reduction**: Many women benefit from formal instruction in stress management techniques such as relaxation exercises, biofeedback, and reflexology
   3. **Education**: Monitoring daily symptoms will help patient obtain a degree of control in life and will allow her to avoid making major decisions when symptoms are worse
   4. **Diet**: Advise to eat a well-balanced diet (see NUTRITION IN ADOLESCENCE AND ADULTHOOD); according to some sources, carboyhdrate-rich, low-protein foods, especially when eaten during the luteal phase may improve mood symptoms
   5. **Caffeine**: Sugggest that patient attempt a trial of caffeine elimiation to determine if this alleviates her symptoms (**Note**: Suggest that use be tapered to avoid caffeine-withdrawal headaches)
   6. **Exercise**: Personal preferences should be taken into account, but some type of regular daily activity should be undertaken (**Note**: Exercise is a great stress-reducer)
   7. **Vitamin Supplementation**: Studies to date suggest that vitamin B_6 supplementation may be helpful (<200 mg/day)
   8. **Herbal and other therapies**: Women should not be discouraged from trying therapies such as teas and herbs so long as ingredients are clearly identified, the products are safe, and the patient's symptoms are not severe; ask patient to bring in product for you to evaluate the ingredients

F. Pharmacologic therapies may also be used in conjunction with the conservative measures listed above
   1. NSAIDs can be prescribed for those patients with premenstrual and menstrual pain including headache, cramping, low back pain, breast tenderness. See section on DYSMENORRHEA for appropriate NSAIDs and dosages
   2. Selective serotonin reuptake inhibitors are often used as the drug of choice for treating PMS
      a. Fluoxetine (Prozac) 10-20 mg PO QD in AM OR
      b. Paroxetine (Paxil) 10 mg PO QD at bedtime
      c. Advise patient about common side effects, be aware of drug interactions and monitor response at 3 months
   3. Oral contraceptives work well for some women; this method is most appropriate in women needing contraception and who have also failed other treatments

G. Follow Up
   1. In 2 months to review diary
   2. Every 3-6 months until symptoms controlled

MENOPAUSE

I. Definition: Physiologic cessation of menses for 12 consecutive months as a result of decreased ovarian function; other important definitions include the following:

   A. Perimenopause: Years during which women report signs of transition; years before and after the actual experience of menopause or cessation of menses (35-60 years)

   B. Climacteric: 7-10 years of physiological change in the reproductive system that ends with the last menses

   C. Postmenopause: Period which occurs for 12 months after the last menses

   D. Premature menopause: Ovarian failure of unknown etiology before age 30-40

   E. Artificial menopause: Cessation of menses following surgery

   F. Delayed menopause: Cessation of menses after age 54

II. Pathogenesis

   A. Number of follicles in ovaries decrease and less estrogen is synthesized.

   B. There is decreased negative feedback on anterior pituitary with increased levels of follicle stimulating hormone (FSH) and luteinizing hormone (LH)

   C. When ovaries no longer produce estrogen, menses stops

III. Clinical Presentation

   A. Average age of onset is 51.4 years

   B. First sign is change in menses such as cycles become farther apart, menstrual flow is scanty, or there is heavy bleeding

   C. The hallmark symptom is the hot flash or hot flush

   D. Other neuroendocrine symptoms include night sweats, sleep disturbance, nausea, dizziness, fatigue, headaches, palpitations, paresthesia and formication (a sensation that small insects are creeping under the skin)

   E. Urogenital atrophy occurs
      1. Uterus and cervix become smaller
      2. Vulvar epithelium thins and may become irritated
      3. Labia majora and minora become flattened
      4. Vagina mucosa atrophies and becomes thin and pale with increased risk for trauma and infection (see section on ATROPHIC VAGINITIS)
      5. Urethra atrophies with increased risk of recurrent abacterial urethritis
      6. Supporting ligaments and tissue possibly become atrophied resulting in uterine prolapse, cystoceles, rectoceles

   F. Amount of collagen in skin decreases; skin is thinner and dryer

   G. Buccal mucosa atrophies with mouth dryness and increased dental caries

   H. Cardiovascular disease risk for women and men is equal after menopause

I. Controversy concerning whether psychological symptoms such as depression, irritability, and nervousness are related to menopause

J. Osteoporosis often develops in women not on hormone replacement and calcium supplementation (see section on OSTEOPOROSIS)

IV. Diagnosis/Evaluation

A. History
1. Determine severity, onset, and duration of symptoms
2. Obtain a complete menstrual history
3. Inquire about birth control methods
4. Determine medication history
5. Obtain a complete medical history
6. Ask about risk status for osteoporosis, coronary heart disease, breast cancer, and endometrial cancer

B. Physical Examination
1. Measure vital signs
2. Examine the mouth for gingivitis, caries, and lesions
3. Observe and palpate skin
4. Perform complete breast examination
5. Auscultate heart and palpate peripheral pulses
6. Auscultate lungs
7. Perform abdominal examination to rule out masses and hepatomegaly
8. Perform pelvic and speculum examinations; consider KOH and saline wet smear of vaginal secretions and determine pH
    a. Examine external genitalia, noting the following:
        (1) Candida vulvitis which is characterized by erythematous vulvar skin and satellite lesions (common in incontinent and diabetic women)
        (2) Lichen sclerosis (benign condition) which presents with a white lesion over a thin, pale vulva
        (3) Multicentric lesions of diverse appearance may represent intraepithelial neoplasia which may progress to invasive cancer
    b. Examine vagina noting patches of erythema and/or petechiae which may represent atrophic vaginitis (see section on ATROPHIC VAGINITIS)
    c. Examine cervix, noting size and shape
    d. Perform a bimanual examination; one third of masses which are detected in women >50 years are malignant
        (1) Typically the postmenopausal uterus is about half the size of a woman's fist; a size larger than this should lead to further evaluation
        (2) Consider a malignancy, endometrial hyperplasia, or a fibroid when the uterus size or shape is abnormal
        (3) Usually the ovaries are not palpable in women this age, so any adnexal mass should be considered malignant unless proven otherwise
    e. Perform a rectovaginal examination; colon cancer is the fourth most common cancer in women and can be detected about 50% of time with a rectal exam
9. May need to do complete musculoskeletal and neurological examinations if patient has symptoms and signs related to osteoporosis and paresthesias

C. Differential Diagnosis
1. Diabetes mellitus
2. Thyroid disease
3. Hyperparathyroidism
4. Any cause of amenorrhea (see section on AMENORRHEA)
5. Always consider pregnancy

D. Diagnostic Tests

    1. Determine menopausal status. The following are characteristics of menopause:

        a. FSH >30-40 mIU/ml; LH >30 mIU/ml; FSH:LH >1 (recent large study found that elevated FSH and LH are only predictive of menopausal status when other clinical manifestations of menopause are present)

        b. Vaginal smear and/or maturation index (parabasal and intermediate cells predominate when estrogen is low)

        c. Progesterone challenge: Administer 10 mg medroxyprogesterone acetate (Provera) for 13-day course

            (1) If positive response occurs and patient has withdrawal bleeding, estrogen is still being secreted and endometrial sampling should be performed to R/O endometrial lesion

            (2) Absence of withdrawal bleeding suggests menopause

    2. Obtain pap smear

    3. Order mammogram if one has not been done in past 12 months

    4. If considering hormone replacement therapy (HRT), order routine blood chemistries, lipid screen, and liver function tests

    5. Endometrial biopsies should be considered for the following women: before unopposed estrogen therapy is started, in women who are taking unopposed estrogen and have any bleeding, in women who have bleeding at unexpected times and are taking sequential combination therapy, in women on continuous estrogen-progestin therapy

    6. Consider dilation and curettage if biopsy is not possible or if endometrium is >4mm thick

    7. Some experts suggest a transvaginal ultrasound as the initial test to determine thickness of the endometrium and the need for an endometrial biopsy

    8. Dual energy x-ray absorptiometry (DEXA) can be ordered to determine bone mass and osteoporosis (see section on OSTEOPOROSIS)

V. Plan/Management

A. Consider estrogen replacement therapy (ERT) or hormone replacement therapy [(HRT) or estrogen/progesterone combination] for prevention of osteoporosis, cardiovascular disease, or symptom management; combination HRT rather than ERT is recommended for women with intact uteri

    1. Contraindications: Recent myocardial infarction, recent cardiovascular accident or transient ischemic attacks, acute liver disease, history of or active malignant breast cancer, endometrial cancer, recurrent or active thromboembolic disease, pregnancy, undiagnosed vaginal bleeding

    2. Relative contraindications: Ischemic heart disease, hypertension, diabetes mellitus, hyperlipidemia, pancreatitis, migraine headaches, epilepsy

    3. Discuss risks of hormone replacement therapy (HRT):

        a. Possibly breast cancer if women remains on estrogen for >15 years (this risk is probably nonexistent if using progestin supplement)

        b. Endometrial cancer (this risk is nonexistent if using progestin supplement)

        c. Gall bladder disease (this risk is nonexistent if using progestin supplement)

        d. Coagulation and thrombosis; women who are at high-risk for developing thromboembolisms such as when they are immobilized following trauma or surgery should consider discontinuing HRT temporarily

        e. Progestin supplement may negate some of cardiovascular benefits

    4. Discuss benefits of HRT

        a. Alleviation of symptoms such as hot flashes

        b. Alleviation of urogenital atrophy

        c. Osteoporosis prevention

        d. Postmenopausal Estrogen/Progestin Interventions (PEPI) Trial was a large 3-year study which found the following:

            (1) Estrogen increased high density lipid (HDL) cholesterol and decreased levels of low density lipid (LDL) cholesterol with no increased incidence of cancer

            (2) Combination of estrogen and progesterone reduced risk of endometrial hyperplasia and still had favorable effects on cholesterol although not as significant as when estrogen was used alone

      e.   Some studies have found a reduction in mortality (as high as a 40% reduction) when women are on HRT

      f.   Other possible benefits include reduction of strokes, reduced risk of Alzheimer's disease, and improved brain functioning

    5.   The American College of Physicians recommended the following in 1992:

      a.   All women should consider preventive hormone therapy

      b.   Women with coronary heart disease (CHD) or who are at increased risk for CHD should benefit from HRT

      c.   In women who are at risk for breast cancer, the risks of HRT may outweigh the benefits

B.   Oral regimes of HRT are usually the preferred route of administration

    1.   Estrogen should be taken continuously or daily; cyclic schedules were recommended in the past but continuous estrogen is now the standard of care for most women

      a.   The appropriate dose depends on the indication:

          (1)   For preventive use prescribe 0.625 mg of conjugated equine estrogens (Premarin) QD (see following table for other available oral estrogen products)

          (2)   For vasomotor symptoms, the dose should be adjusted based on effects; typically 1.25 mg QD of conjugated equine estrogen is needed

      b.   The most frequent side effects are bloating, nausea, and breast tenderness; these adverse effects usually resolve after a few months on therapy

ORAL ESTROGEN EQUIVALENCIES

Generic (Trade) Names	Dose Range	Dosage Recommendations for Preventive Therapy
Conjugated estrogens (Premarin)	0.3-2.5 mg	0.625 mg
Esterified estrogens (Estratab)	0.3-2.5 mg	0.625 mg
Micronized estrogen (Estrace)	0.5-2.0 mg	0.5-1 mg
Estropipate (Ogen)	0.625-5.0 mg	0.625 mg

    2.   Oral progestin should be given in combination with estrogen in women who have intact uteri; progestin is not needed in women who have had hysterectomies

      a.   Medroxyprogesterone acetate (Provera) is used most commonly in U.S.

      b.   Micronized progesterone (sometimes referred to as natural progesterone) has received increased interest because in the PEPI trial this form had a more positive effect on high-density lipoprotein (HDL) than medroxyprogesterone acetate; in 1998, natural progesterone is not FDA approved but can be obtained at specialty compounding pharmacies (see following table)

NATURAL PROGESTERONES

Route	Dose (mg)	Plasma concentration (ng/mL)*	Availability
Oral--micronized	100	3.0 - 6.0	Most US pharmacies
	200	30.3 ± 7.0	
Transdermal	45	3.0	Health food stores, Mail-order companies, Compounding pharmacies*
Vaginal cream	300	19.2	Compounding pharmacies*
Vaginal gel	90	3.9	Most US pharmacies
Vaginal suppository	100	9.5 - 19.0	Compounding pharmacies*
	400	17.0 - 34.5	
Rectal suppository	100	15.0 - 51.9	Compounding pharmacies*
Intramuscular	100	40.0 - 50.0	Most US pharmacies
Sublingual/buccal	10	5.0	Compounding pharmacies*

*Information about compounding pharmacies can be obtained from: The Internation Academy of Compounding Pharmacists (IACP), PO Box 1365, Sugar Land, TX 77487, 800/927-4227.

Adapted from Murray, J.L. (1998). Natural progesterone: What role in women's health care. Women's Health in Primary Care, 1, 671-687.

c. Progestin can be given either cyclically (sometimes called sequential use) or continuously
  (1) Cyclic progestin (Provera) is prescribed at a minimal dose of 5 mg to a maximum dose of 10 mg; drug is given for 10-12 days of the month, typically at the beginning of each month
  (2) Continuous progestin (Provera) is given in doses of 2.5 mg, 5 mg, or 10 mg (typically given in 2.5 mg dose) every day
  (3) Cyclic and continuous progestin have the same effect on the endometrium so the choice of regimen is left up to the woman
    (a) Cyclic progestin will result in monthly withdrawal bleeding
    (b) Continuous progestin may cause unpredictable bleeding or spotting
  (4) Progestin used alone or in combination with estrogen may have adverse effects that resemble premenstrual tension syndrome (breast tenderness, bloating, edema, cramping, anxiety and depression)

3. The following combination HRT products are available
  a. Premphase: Conjugated estrogens 0.625mg (14 tabs) first blister card; conjugated estrogens 0.625mg plus medroxyprogesterone acetate 5mg (14 tabs) second blister card
  b. Prempro: Conjugated estrogens 0.625mg plus medroxyprogesterone acetate 2.5mg tabs or conjugated estrogens 0.625mg plus medroxyprogesterone acetate 5mg tabs

C. Other routes of administration for HRT
1. Transdermal administration of estrogen is a useful alternative for certain women although the patch has less favorable effects on high density lipoproteins (HDL) than oral estrogens
  a. The patch is particularly beneficial in the following women:
    (1) Women who do not like to take pills or have adverse gastrointestinal effects from the pills
    (2) Women who smoke cigarettes, have gall bladder disease, fibrocystic breasts, history of thromboembolisms, high triglycerides, migraine headaches and women who develop hypertension on oral preparations
  b. Prescribe one of the following
    (1) Estraderm 0.05 mg/day, apply patch twice a week
    (2) Climara 0.05 mg/day, apply patch once a week
    (3) Vivelle 0.0375-0.1 mg/day, apply patch twice a week
    (4) Usually patch should be on skin for 3 weeks and then off for one week
    (5) Rotate application sites and avoid applying to breast and waistline
  c. Add progestational agent in women with intact uteri; Combi Patch (estradiol, norethindrone), a transdermal patch that combines estrogen and progestin; change twice weekly
2. Vaginal estrogen creams and rings are available to reduce symptoms of vaginal atrophy and genitourinary complaints (see section on ATROPHIC VAGINITIS)
3. Progesterone body creams (Gentle Changes and Pro-Gest PG) are available and mainly used to relieve menopausal symptoms
4. Vaginally administered progesterone is used in Europe and awaiting FDA approval in U.S. for preventive therapy, symptom management, and for protection of the endometrium

D. Management of hot flashes and other symptoms
1. For women with hot flashes, patient education is helpful
  a. Help identify precipitating factors such as hot drinks, caffeine, alcohol, stress, warm environment.
  b. Counsel to stop smoking
  c. Suggest dressing in layers of clothes
2. Estrogen replacement therapy (ERT) is often the first line of therapy
  a. Oral and transdermal forms are used to manage the vasomotor symptoms
  b. Vaginal cream or the estrogen ring may be used to treat atrophic vaginitis and urogenital atrophy (see section on ATROPHIC VAGINITIS)
  c. Usually need 3-5 years for symptom management

d. Prescribe estrogen in the lowest dose to control symptoms
   (1) Typically, 0.9-1.25 mg of conjugated estrogen (Premarin) is needed
   (2) Low dose estrogen patch (0.05 mg/day) may also be used

3. Although research is limited, the following alternative approaches may be beneficial; remember, however, that these therapies may have side effects and/or risks:
   a. Vitamin E doses between 100 IU to 1,200 IU (most experts recommend 400-800 IU)
   b. High-vegetable, low-meat, low-saturated fat diets, high in phytoestrogens may reduce vasomotor symptoms; the following are foods that contain phytoestrogens: soy beans (most potent source), soy milk, tofu, legumes, bean sprouts, red clover, sunflower seeds, rye, wheat, sesame seeds, linseed, flaxseed, berries
   c. Herbal preparations including ginseng, dong quai, and black cohash may also be beneficial
   d. Vitamin B complex also may be effective

4. The following nonestrogen drugs are not as effective as estrogen but may reduce symptoms
   a. Medroxyprogesterone acetate (Provera) 10-20 mg daily or progesterone body cream
   b. Megestrol acetate (Megace) 20 mg BID
   c. Depo-medroxyprogesterone acetate (Depo-Provera) 150 mg IM every 1-3 months
   d. Clonidine (Catapres) 0.1-0.2 mg BID (or 1 skin patch changed every 4 days)
   e. Methyldopa (Aldomet) 250-500 mg BID
   f. Phenobarbital, ergotamine tartrate, levorotatory alkaloids of belladonna (Bellergal-S) 1 tablet BID

5. Estrogen-androgen therapy may relieve menopausal symptoms and increase libido
   a. This therapy holds promise but is still considered investigational
   b. Women with osteopenia or osteoporosis of the spine and women with decreased libido are the best candidates for this therapy
   c. Androgen therapy is available as oral methyltestosterone [typically combined with estrogen in a single tablet (Estratest)] in a usual dose range of 1.25 to 5.0 mg daily

E. Patient Education
   1. For women taking HRT review danger signs of HRT: abnormal vaginal bleeding, pain in calf, chest pain, shortness of breath, coughing blood, severe headache, visual problems, breast lump, jaundice
   2. Advise patient regarding the need to exercise and increase calcium intake to prevent osteoporosis (see section on OSTEOPOROSIS)
   3. Instruct patient in breast self examination with annual breast exam by provider and annual mammogram.
   4. Instruct in Kegel exercises or other behavioral interventions to prevent or reduce the symptoms of incontinence (see section on INCONTINENCE)

F. Provide counseling about birth control
   1. Women over age 40 can continue to take oral contraceptives if they are a nonsmokers, have normal blood pressure, mammogram, lipid profile, and glucose screening, weigh no more than 30% above ideal body weight, negative family history of early cardiovascular or thromboembolic disease (i.e., no risk factor other than age)
      a. Type of OC recommended: 35μg estrogen or less and low potency progestin
      b. Examples: Ortho-Cyclen, Triphasil
      c. Controversy arises as to how long perimenopausal women should continue to take OC and when to begin HRT. Authorities recommend one of the following approaches:
         (1) Choose an age such as 49 or 50 and stop pills; if women resumes period use OC or some other barrier method -- do not start HRT
         (2) Measure FSH level on the last pill-free day; if it is elevated the patient is likely to be menopausal; however, if it is not elevated the patient may be menopausal because it may take longer for the suppressive effect of the pill to wear off
   2. Other available methods include male or female sterilization, barrier methods, intrauterine device (IUD); the fertility awareness method is problematic because of menstrual cycle irregularities

G. Health Maintenance Issues
1. Patients using HRT require pap smear with maturation index every year plus mammogram.
2. Consider annual endometrial biopsy. American College of Physicians (1992) recommends the following:
    a. Yearly endometrial biopsy and biopsy for any episode of bleeding for women taking unopposed estrogen
    b. No routine endometrial biopsy for women taking estrogen plus progestin; biopsy needed for bleeding which occurs at unexpected times

H. Follow Up
1. Return to health care provider 1-2 months after beginning drug therapy
2. Then, will need regular 3-6 months return visits to check side effects, BP, and response to therapy (may see nurse)
3. Annual visits needed for complete history and physical exam

ATROPHIC VAGINITIS

I. Definition: Thinning and fragility of vaginal and vulvar epithelium due to estrogen deficiency

II. Pathogenesis

A. Common disorder of postmenopausal women or women with premature ovarian failure

B. Due to estrogen deficiency the following occurs
1. The vagina becomes smaller, less compliant with decreased lubrication
2. The epithelium changes from having glycogen-rich superficial cells to parabasal and intermediate cells
3. Vagina becomes alkaline as the pH increases to as high as 7.0
4. All these changes provide an environment in which pathogenic bacteria can flourish

III. Clinical Presentation

A. Symptoms include thin, blood-tinged vaginal discharge, bleeding after intercourse, dysuria and dyspareunia

B. Signs include pale, dry nonrugated vagina with patches of erythema and/or petechiae

IV. Diagnosis/Evaluation

A. History
1. Determine onset and duration of symptoms
2. Ask patient to describe amount, color, and consistency of vaginal discharge
3. Explore sexual practices such as number of sexual partners or new sexual partners
4. Inquire about dysuria, urinary frequency and urgency, abdominal pain, flank pain, dyspareunia, vaginal and vulvar dryness and itching
5. Question about vasomotor symptoms that accompany menopause such as hot flashes, paresthesias, and dizziness
6. Explore self treatments
7. Obtain a medication history

B. Physical examination
1. Obtain vital signs
2. Perform a complete abdominal examination

3. Perform a speculum and pelvic examination (see section on MENOPAUSE for further description of gynecological exam in perimenopausal women)
4. Assess for flank tenderness

C. Differential diagnosis includes *Candida vulvitis*, bacterial vaginosis, trichomoniasis, gonorrhea or chlamydia, lichen sclerosis, intraepithelial neoplasia (see Physical Examination in section on MENOPAUSE)

D. Diagnostic Tests
1. Perform potassium hydroxide and saline vaginal wet prep examination to rule out other causes of vaginitis; Increased WBCs and decreased lactobacillus suggest atrophic vaginitis
2. In the past, a diagnostic smear of the vaginal wall maturation index was suggested but is no longer recommended

V. Plan/Management

A. Discuss benefits of regular sexual activity to decrease problems of atrophic vaginitis

B. Atrophic vaginitis may be treated with any form of estrogen
1. Initial therapy with intravaginal cream may be more effective than oral or transdermal estrogen because the cream delivers a higher dose of estrogen to the vaginal epithelium
   a. Prescribe topical vaginal estrogen cream, estradiol 0.01% (Estrace cream): 1/2 (2 gm) to 1 (4 gm) applicator HS for 1-2 weeks followed by every other night application for 1-2 weeks, then gradually taper frequency of administration and dosage, then discontinue until symptoms develop again
   b. Intermittent, long-term use of vaginal estrogen cream does not appear to increase the risk of endometrial cancer so intermittent progestin is not required
   c. Rather than intermittent use, some women prefer maintenance therapy with application of 1 gm 1-3 times per week (with this regimen, progestin is required if women have intact uteri)
2. Estradiol vaginal ring (Estring Vaginal Ring) is a good alternative to estrogen cream
   a. Estring is a flexible, soft elastomer ring that is inserted into the vagina and releases a low, continuous dose of estradiol
   b. Ring must be replaced every 90 days
   c. Estring does not measurably increase serum estradiol levels or endometrial growth; thus, intermittent progestin is not required
3. May use hormone replacement therapy (HRT) such as conjugated estrogen 0.625 mg PO QD (Premarin) plus medroxyprogesterone acetate 10 mg po QD (Provera) days 1-12 (progestin is needed if woman has an intact uterus)
4. Transdermal estrogen
   a. Estraderm patch: 0.05 mg/day patch twice a week applied to trunk; administer cyclically (3 weeks on and 1 week off) and progestin if woman has an intact uterus
   b. Combination patch: Combi Patch (estradiol, norethindrone), change twice a week

C. Alternative treatments may or may not be helpful
1. Recommend wearing cotton underwear to reduce chance of infections
2. Sitz baths provide symptomatic relief
3. Yogurt products have a high acidophilus count and help maintain vaginal pH as the vaginal flora become altered with menopause; try one of the following approaches:
   a. Yogurt douches
   b. Acidophilus tablets 460 mg/day can be taken orally or inserted into the vagina
4. Replens Vaginal Moisturizer maintains vaginal moisture for 2-3 days after a single vaginal application
5. Olive oil, vegetable oil, or Lubrin may be beneficial as vaginal lubricants; caution patients that petroleum-based products can break down latex condoms and foster infections

D.   Follow Up
1.   Estrogen administered by any route, even topical vaginal estrogen cream, is absorbed and can cause systemic effects
2.   Return to health care provider 1-2 months after beginning any type of estrogen drug therapy
3.   Then, schedule regular 3-6 months return visits to check side effects, B/P and response to therapy (may see nurse)
4.   Annual visits for complete history and physical exam

VULVOVAGINAL CANDIDIASIS

I.   Definition: Infection of the vulvar area and vagina by *Candida albicans* and other candida species

II.   Pathogenesis

A.   Little is known about factors that contribute to the overgrowth of normal flora in the vagina

B.   When the complex balance of microorganisms changes, however, potentially pathogenic endogenous microorganisms that are part of the normal flora such as *Candida albicans* proliferate to numbers that cause symptoms

C.   *C. albicans* causes 80% to 90% of vaginal fungal infections and other *Candida* species and *Torulopsis* sp., or other yeasts cause the remainder

III.   Clinical Presentation

A.   Approximately 25% of all vaginal infections are due to vulvovaginal candidiasis (VVC); this condition is not transmitted sexually but is often diagnosed in women being evauated for STDs

B.   An estimated 75% of women will have at least one episode of VVC, and approximately 40% will have two or more episodes; a small percentage, less that 5% experience recurrent VVC

C.   Primarily a disease of the childbearing years; the majority of premenarcheal and postmenopausal women who develop the disease have recently taken antibiotics, estrogen, or will be found to have diabetes

D.   Pregnancy is the most common predisposing factor

E.   Depressed cell-mediated immunity (such as with HIV+ status) also is risk factor

F.   Vulvar pruritus is the cardinal symptom and a white dischage may also be present; vulvar erythema is the most often observed sign, with edema and excoriation of the vulva also often observed; vaginal secretions have a normal pH ($\leq$4.5)

G.   Diagnosis can be made in a woman with typical signs and symptoms and when either a) wet preparation or Gram stain of vaginal discharge demonstrates yeasts or pseudohyphae or b) culture yields a positive result for a yeast species

IV.   Diagnosis/Evaluation

A.   History
1.   Question about vulvar itching, discharge, odor, dysuria, dyspareunia
2.   Ask about previous occurrences of yeast infections
3.   Ask about predisposing factors such as pregnancy, recent antibiotic or estrogen therapy, history of diabetes, HIV+ status
4.   Ask about douching and use of feminine hygiene products

B.   Physical Examination
      1.   Examine vulva for erythema, edema, and excoriation
      2.   Perform pelvic exam and examine vagina for erythema, white patches/plaques; note odor
            of secretions (should not be malodorous)

C.   Diagnostic Tests
      1.   Obtain sample of vaginal secretions from anterior or lateral vaginal walls on a dry swab
            and apply to pH paper. In candidiasis, pH of vaginal secretions is ≤4.5 (normal pH of
            vagina is 3.5-4.5)
      2.   Microscopic examination of slide containing vaginal secretions mixed with 10% potassium
            hydroxide (KOH) shows typical hyphae and budding yeast (see Figure 14.3)

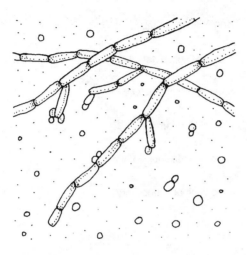

Figure 14.3. Hyphae and Yeast Buds.

D.   Differential Diagnosis
      1.   Other common causes of vaginitis -- bacterial vaginosis and trichomoniasis
      2.   Common causes of cervicitis -- chlamydia and gonorrhea which can sometimes cause a
            vaginal discharge

V. Plan/Management

A. Recommended regimens for the treatment of VVC are contained in the following table

RECOMMENDED REGIMENS FOR TREATMENT OF VULVOVAGINAL CANDIDIASIS		
Medication	Dose	Application
Intravaginal agents		
Butoconazole OR	2% cream	5 g intravaginally for 3 days*†
Clotrimazole OR	1% cream	5 g intravaginally for 7-14 days*†
Clotrimazole OR	100 mg vaginal tablet	for 7 days*
Clotrimazole OR	100 mg vaginal tablet	2 tablets for 3 days*
Clotrimazole OR	500 mg vaginal tablet,	1 tablet single application*
Miconazole OR	2% cream	5 g intravaginally for 7 days*†
Miconazole OR	200 mg vaginal suppository	1 suppository for 3 days*†
Miconazole OR	100 mg vaginal suppository	1 suppository for 7 days*†
Tioconazole OR	6.5% ointment	5 g intravaginally in a single application*†
Terconazole OR	0.4% cream	5 g intravaginally for 7 days*
Terconazole OR	0.8% cream	5 g intravaginally for 3 days*
Terconazole	80 mg suppository	1 suppository for 3 days*
Oral agent		
Fluconazole	150 mg oral tablet	1 tablet in single dose

*These creams and suppositories are oil-based and may weaken latex condoms and diaphragms. Refer to product labeling for further information

†Over-the-counter (OTC) preparations

Source: US Department of Health and Human Services, Centers for Disease Control and Prevention. (1998). 1998 guidelines for treatment of sexually transmitted diseases. Morbidity and Mortality Weekly Report, 47(RR-1), 76.

B. Treatment of pregnant women: Only topical azole therapies should be used for the treatment of pregnant women
   1. Most effective treatments that have been studied for pregnant women are clotrimazole, miconazole, butoconazole, and terconazole
   2. Many experts recommend 7 days of therapy during pregnancy

C. Treatment of sexual partners is not necessary unless candidal balanitis is present

D. Treatment considerations in patients with recurrent VVC (RVVC) [defined as **four** or more episodes of symptomatic VVC in a 12 month period]
   1. Pathogenesis of RVVC is poorly understood but risk factors include uncontrolled diabetes, immunosuppression, corticosteriod use, and repeated use of topical or systemic antibacterials (**Note**: The majority of women with RVVC have no apparent predisposing conditions)
   2. Use of either topical or oral azoles for a period of 10-14 days is recommended

3. After the 10-14 days of initial therapy, maintenance therapy should be initiated for at least 6 months with ketoconazole 100 mg orally once daily for ≤ 6 months

4. **Note:** All cases of recurrent VVC should be confirmed by culture before maintenance therapy is initiated

E. Follow Up: None indicated

REFERENCES

Ahlgrimm, M., Battistini, M., Ravnikar, V., Reed, S., Schiff, I., & Ringel, M. (April 30, 1998). Beyond hormones: Other treatments for menopausal symptoms. Patient Care, 28-52

American Psychiatric Association. (1994). Diagnostic and statistical manual of mental disorders (4th ed.). Washington, DC: Author.

Baker, S. (1998). Menstruation and related problems and concerns. In E.Q. Youngkin & M.S. Davis (Eds.), Women's health: A primary care clinical guide. Stamford,CN: Appleton & Lange.

Bayer, S.R., & DeCherney, A.H. (1993). Clinical manifestations and treatment of dysfunctional uterine bleeding. Journal of American Medical Association, 269, 1823-1828.

Beckman, C.R., Ling, F.W., Herbert, W.N., Laube, D.W., Smith, R.P., & Barzansky, B.M. (1998). Obstetrics and gynecology. Baltimore: Williams & Wilkins.

Caufield, K.A. (1998). Controlling fertility. In E.Q. Youngkin & M.S. Davis (Eds.), Women's health: A primary care clinical guide. Stamford,CN: Appleton & Lange.

Dickey, R.P. (1998). Managing contraceptive pill patients. Durant, OK: Emis Medical Publishers.

Endicott, J., Feemna, E.W. Kielich, A.M., & Sondeimer, S.J. (1996, April). PMS: New treatments that really work. Patient Care, 88-120.

Ettinger, B., Friedman, G. D., Bush, T., & Quesenberry, C. P. (1996). Reduced mortality associated with long-term postmenopausal estrogen therapy. Obstetrics & Gynecology, 87, 6-12.

Fiorica, J.V., Schorr, s.J., & Sickles, E.A. (1997, Apr). Benign breast disorders. Patient Care, 140-154.

Glasier, A. (1997). Emergency postcoital contraception. The New England Journal of Medicine, 337, 1058-1064.

Hammond, C. B. (1997). Management of menopause. American Family Physician, 55, 1667-1674.

Hammond, C.B. (1996). Menopause and hormone replacement therapy: An overview. Obstetrics & Gynecology, 87, 2S-14S.

Hatcher, R.A., Trussell, J., Stewart, F., Cates, W., Stewart, G., Guest, F., & Kowal, D. (1998). Contraceptive technology. New York: Adrent Media.

Hill, D.A., & Lense, J.S. (1998). Office management of Bartholin gland cysts and abscesses. American Family Physicain 57(7), 1611-1616.

Hindle, W.H., & Ling, F.W. (1992). Diseases of the breast. In T.G. Stovall, R.L. Summitt, Jr., C.R. Beckmann, & F.W. Ling (Eds.), Clinical manual of gynecology. New York: McGraw-Hill.

Moe, R.E. (1996). Clinical approach to breast disease. In M.A. Stenchever (Ed.), Office gynecology. St. Louis: Mosby.

Hindle, W.H. (1998, March). Palpable breast mass: The physical examination. Hospital Practice, 42-45.

Johnson, S.R. (1998). Menopause and hormone replacement therapy. Women's Health Issues, Part 2, 82, 297-320.

Moos, R.H. (1969). The development of a premenstrual distress questionnaire. Psychosomatic Medicine, 30, 850-855.

Morgan, K.W., & Deneris, A. (1997). Emergency contraception: Preventing unintended pregnancy. Nurse Practitioner, 22(11), 34-48.

Mou, S.M. (1995). Gynecologic infections. In V.L. Seltzer & W.H. Pearse (Eds.), Women's primary heath care. New York: McGraw-Hill.

Murphy, E.J. (1998, May). Oral contraceptives: Classification of oral contraceptives. <u>Monthly Prescribing Reference</u>, 209.

Murray, J.L. (1998). Natural progesterone: What role in women's health care. <u>Women's Health in Primary Care, 1</u>, 671-687.

Nand, S.L., Webster, M.A., Baber, R., & O'Connor, V. (1998). Bleeding pattern and endometrial changes during continuous combined hormone replacement therapy. <u>Obstetrics and Gynecology, 91</u>, 678-684.

Nelson, A.L. (1997). A practical approach to dysfunctional uterine bleeding. <u>Family Practice Recertification, 19</u>(8), 14-40.

Nesse, R.E. (1997). Menometrorrhagia and causes of abnormal premenopausal vaginal bleeding. In J.A. Rosenfeld (Ed.). <u>Women's health in primary care</u>. Baltimore: Williams & Wilkins.

Pickar, J.H., Thorneycroft, I., & Whitehead, M. (1998). Effects of hormone replacement therapy on the endometrium and lipid parameters: A review of randomized clinical trials, 1985 to 1995. <u>American Journal of Obstetrics and Gynecology, 178,</u> 1087-1097.

Sarrel, P.M. (1997) Hormone replacement therapy in the menopause. <u>International Journal of Fertility, 42</u>, 78-84.

Scharbo-Dehaan, M. (1996). Hormone replacement therapy. <u>Nurse Practitioner, Continuing Education Supplement Part 2,</u> 1-13.

Shaw, C.R. (1997). The Perimenopausal hot flash: Epidemiology, physiology, and treatment. <u>The Nurse Practitioner, 22,</u> 55-66.

Shy, K.K. (1996). Contraception. In M.A. Stenchever (Ed.), <u>Office gynecology</u>. St. Louis: Mosby.

Steege, J.F. (1996). Subjective disorders: Dysmenorrhea, chronic pelvic pain, and premenstrual syndrome. In M.A. Stenchever (Ed.). <u>Office gynecology</u>. St. Louis: Mosby.

Stellato, R.K., et al. (1998). Can follicle-stimulating hormone be used to define menopausal status? <u>Endocrine Practice, 4,</u> 137-141.

Tamimi, H.K. (1996). Management of the abnormal or atypical papanicolaou smear. In M.A. Stenchever (Ed.), <u>Office gynecology</u>. St. Louis: Mosby.

The Writing Group for the PEPI Trial. (1996). Effects of hormone replacement therapy on endometrial histology in postmenopausal women. <u>JAMA, 275,</u> 370-375.

Trussell, J., Ellerston, C., Stewart, F., Koenig, J., & Raymond, E.G. (1998). Emergency contraception. <u>Women's Health in Primary Care, 1</u>(1), 52-69.

US Preventive Services Task Force. (1996). <u>Guide to clinical preventive services</u>. Baltimore: Williams & Wilkins.

US Department of Health and Human Services, Centers for Disease Control. (1998). 1998 guidelines for treatment of sexually transmitted diseases. <u>Morbidity and Mortality Weekly Report, 47</u>(RR-1).

Uy, S., & McNicoll, K. (1998). Are you up-to-date on Pap smears? <u>Family Practice Recertification, 20</u>(1), 53-84.

Vargyas, J.M., & Ling, F.W. (1992). Premenstrual syndrome. In T.G. Stovall, R.L. Summitt, Jr., C.R. Beckmann, & F.W. Ling (Eds.), <u>Clinical manual of gynecology</u>. New York: McGraw-Hill.

Vargyas, J.M. (1986). Premenstrual syndrome. In D.R. Mishell, & V. Davajan (Eds.), <u>Infertility, contraception, and reproductive endocrinology</u>. Cambridge, MA: Blackwell Scientific Publications.

Webb, T.S. (1996, Jan.). Common menstrual disorders: Primary care management. <u>Advance for Nurse Practitioners,</u> 20-23.

CHAPTER 15

Sexually Transmitted Disease

BACTERIAL VAGINOSIS

I.   Definition: Clinical syndrome resulting from replacement of the normal H_2O_2-producing *Lactobacillus sp.* in the vagina with high concentrations of anaerobic bacteria (e.g., *Prevotella* sp. and *Mobiluncus* sp.), *Garderella vaginalis*, and *Mycoplasma hominis*

II.   Pathogenesis

      A.   Causes of the microbial alteration are not fully understood

      B.   Bacterial vaginosis (BV) is associated with having multiple sex partners, but it remains unclear whether BV results from acquisition of a sexually transmitted pathogen

      C.   Women who have never been sexually active are rarely affected

III. Clinical Presentation

      A.   BV is the most prevalent cause of vaginal discharge and malodor in women

      B.   Approximately half of the women whose illness meet the clinical criteria for BV are asymptomatic

      C.   BV may be diagnosed by use of clinical or Gram stain criteria

      D.   Clinical criteria require three of the following signs or symptoms
            1.   A grayish-white, homogenous, malodorous discharge that may be scant or profuse, which adheres to the vaginal walls
            2.   The presence of clue cells on microscopic exam
            3.   pH of vaginal fluid >4.5
            4.   A fishy odor of vaginal discharge before or after addition of 10% KOH (whiff test)

      E.   When Gram stain is used, determining the relative concentration of the bacterial morphotypes characteristic of the altered flora of BV is an acceptable laboratory method for diagnosing BV

      F.   Because organisms do not invade vaginal wall, gross vulvitis and vaginitis do not occur; thus, few women experience irritative symptoms such as pruritus and burning

IV.   Diagnosis/Evaluation

      A.   History
            1.   Question about onset of symptoms, description of discharge (whether malodorous and appearance and amount)
            2.   Ask if other signs and symptoms are present
            3.   Ask if woman uses frequent douching, feminine hygiene products to control odor
            4.   Obtain complete menstrual history and history of contraceptive use including condom use

      B.   Physical Examination
            1.   Examine introitus for homogenous discharge
            2.   Do speculum exam and look for homogenous discharge coating vaginal walls; note odor for characteristic foul, fishy odor
            3.   Inspect cervix (should be normal) and complete bimanual exam

      C.   Differential Diagnosis
            1.   Other common cause of vaginitis -- trichomoniasis and vulvovaginal candidiasis
            2.   Common causes of cervicitis -- chlamydia and gonorrhea

D. Diagnostic Tests
1. Obtain sample of vaginal secretions from anterior or lateral wall on a dry swab and apply to pH paper. In bacterial vaginosis, pH of vaginal secretions is >4.5 (normal pH of vagina is 3.5-4.5)
2. Microscopic examination of slide containing vaginal secretions mixed with saline shows clue cells. Secretions have a fishy odor before or after being mixed with a drop of 10% KOH (positive whiff test)
3. Figure 15.1 depicts a clue cell, an epithelial cell to which many bacteria are attached

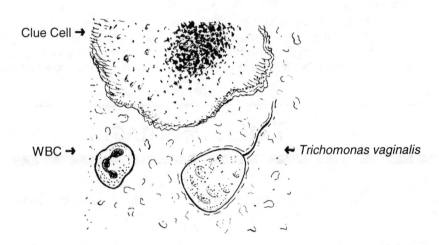

Clue Cell →

WBC →

← *Trichomonas vaginalis*

Figure 15.1. Clue Cell, WBC, & *Trichomonas vaginalis*

V. Plan/Management

A. The principal goal of therapy is to relieve signs and symptoms

B. All women with symptomatic disease require treatment, regardless of pregnancy status
1. BV during pregnancy is associated with adverse outcomes
2. Treatment of pregnant women who have BV and who are at high risk for preterm delivery might reduce risk for prematurity
3. High-risk pregnant women who do not have symptoms of BV may be evaluated for treatment
   a. Presently, treatment for high-risk pregnant women who have asymptomatic BV remains controversial
   b. A large clinical trial is underway to assess benefits and risks of treatment for asymptomatic high-risk pregnant women
4. Consideration should be given to treatment of women who have symptomatic or asymptomatic BV before invasive or surgical procedures such as endometrial biopsy, hysterectomy, cesarean section, and abortion are performed

C. Treatment of choice for nonpregnant women
1. Metronidazole (Flagyl) 500 mg orally BID x 7 days, OR
2. Metronidazole gel 0.75%, one full applicator (5 g) intravaginally BID x 5 days, OR
3. Clindamycin cream, 2%, one full applicator (5 g) intravaginally at bedtime x 7 days

D. Alternative regimens for nonpregnant women
1. Metronidazole (Flagyl) 2 g orally in a single dose, OR
2. Clindamycin 300 mg orally BID x 7 days

E. Treatment during pregnancy
1. High-risk pregnant women may be screened and treated for BV at the earliest part of the second trimester of pregnancy

2. Low-risk pregnant women who have symptomatic BV should be treated to relieve symptoms
   a. Recommended regimen is metronidazole 250 mg orally TID x 7 days
   b. Alternative regimens: Metronidazole 2 g orally in a single dose OR clindamycin 300 mg orally BID x 7 days
3. Use of clindamycin vaginal cream during pregnancy is not recommended

F. Routine treatment of sex partners in **not** recommended

G. Follow Up
   1. None indicated except in high-risk pregnant women who should receive follow-up 1 month after completion of therapy to evaluate efficacy of treatment
   2. Recurrence of BV is common but no long-term maintenance regimen is recommended
   3. Use alternative treatment regimens for treatment of recurrent disease

TRICHOMONIASIS

I. Definition: Infection of the vagina by *Trichomonas vaginalis*. May also involve Skene's ducts and lower urinary tract in women, and the lower genitourinary tract in men

II. Pathogenesis

   A. *Trichomonas vaginalis*, a unicellular flagellated protozoan, causes this primarily sexually transmitted disease

   B. Incubation period is 4-20 days with the average being 1 week

III. Clinical Presentation

   A. Trichomoniasis comprises about 10% of all vaginal infections and is observed primarily in women with normal estrogen levels

   B. Infection is frequently asymptomatic. If symptomatic, symptoms are usually worse immediately after menstruation and during pregnancy

   C. Cardinal symptom is a diffuse, malodorous, yellow-green discharge

   D. Diffuse edema and redness is usually apparent in vulvar and vaginal tissue; the cervix may be inflamed and friable. Rarely, punctate lesions on the cervix give a "strawberry" appearance

   E. Flagellated protozoa are seen in wet prep of vaginal secretions. Vaginal secretions have a pH of >4.5

   F. Urethritis and prostatitis may be seen in the male; almost 80% of men harboring the organism are asymptomatic

IV. Diagnosis/Evaluation

   A. History
      1. Question about presence of discharge, its odor, color and if dysuria, dyspareunia are present
      2. Obtain menstrual history and ask if menstruation makes symptoms worse
      3. In males, question about dysuria
      4. Obtain history of previous STDs; ask about condom use

B. Physical Examination
   1. Examine external genitalia for discharge pooling at introitus or posterior fourchette
   2. Do pelvic exam to determine if vagina has erythema, edema; note type, color, and amount of discharge; examine cervix for erythema, friability, discharge

C. Differential Diagnosis
   1. Other common causes of vaginitis -- bacterial vaginosis and vulvovaginal candidiasis.
   2. Common causes of cervicitis -- chlamydia and gonorrhea

D. Diagnostic Tests
   1. Obtain sample of vaginal secretions from anterior or lateral wall on a dry swab and apply to pH paper. In trichomoniasis, pH of vaginal secretions is >4.5 (normal pH of the vagina is 3.5-4.5)
   2. Microscopic examination of slide containing vaginal secretions mixed with saline solution shows organisms with whip-like flagellae that are motile and slightly larger than WBCs (see Figure 15.1 of trichomonad, WBC, and clue cell)
   3. In men, collect the first 5-30 mL of an early morning specimen of urine. Examine under microscope for trichomonads

V. Plan/Management

   A. Treatment of choice is metronidazole (Flagyl) 2 g orally in a single dose

   B. Alternative: Metronidazole (Flagyl) 500 mg twice daily for 7 days

   C. FDA has recently approved Flagyl 375 mg BID x 7 days

   D. Management of treatment failure
      1. If treatment failure occurs with either regimen, retreat with metronidazole (Flagyl) 500 mg twice daily for 7 days
      2. If treatment failure occurs frequently, patient should be treated with a 2 g dose of metronidazole QD x 3-5 days

   E. Sex partners should be treated and patients should be instructed to avoid sex until they have been cured (after therapy has been completed and patient and partner are asymptomatic)

   F. Treatment during pregnancy: Patients should be treated with 2 g of metronidazole in a single dose

   G. Follow Up: None indicated for men and women who become asymptomatic after treatment (or who are initially asymptomatic)

CHLAMYDIAL INFECTION

I. Definition: A sexually transmitted disease caused by *Chlamydia trachomatis*

II. Pathogenesis

   A. *C. trachomatis,* a bacterial agent with at least 15 serologic variants (serovars) divided between the following two biologic variants: oculogenital (serovars A-K) and LVG (serovars L1-L3); genital infections are caused by serovars B and D-K

   B. Infects the genital tract of women most commonly at the transition zone of the endocervix and infects the urethra in men

   C. Incubation period is variable but is usually at least 1 week

565

III. Clinical Presentation

A. One of the two most frequent causes of cervicitis in women and urethritis in men; *Neisseria gonorrhoeae* is the other

B. Over 4 million new cases of chlamydial infection occur annually; presently the most common bacterial STD in the US

C. Screening sexually active adolescent females for chlamydial infection is recommended as a routine screening test because of the high prevalence of this infection among females in this age group

D. In women, several important sequelae can result from infection including PID, ectopic pregnancy, and infertility

E. In women, chlamydial infection can cause mucopurulent cervicitis, urethritis, salpingitis, and proctitis

F. In men, chlamydial infection can cause nongonococcal urethritis (NGU) and acute epididymitis (see NGU and EPIDIDYMITIS)

G. Women may complain of vaginal discharge, dysuria, abnormal vaginal bleeding, and pelvic pain

H. Men may complain of discharge of mucopurulent or purulent material from the urethra and burning during urination

I. Asymptomatic infection is common among both men and women

IV. Diagnosis/Evaluation

A. History
1. In women, ask about presence of vaginal discharge, dysuria, abnormal bleeding, pelvic pain, and dyspareunia
2. In women, obtain menstrual history and contraceptive history
3. In men, ask about presence of mucopurulent/purulent discharge from urethra, presence of burning on urination
4. Inquire about sexual history including age at first intercourse, number of partners in past year, types of sexual practices, use of condoms
5. Ask about past history of STDs including types, frequency, and treatment

B. Physical Examination
1. In women, perform speculum exam to inspect cervix for mucopurulent discharge from the endocervix. Gently scrape cervix to test for friability
2. Bimanual exam to check for adnexal tenderness, uterine tenderness, and cervical motion tenderness
3. In men, examine the urethra for mucopurulent/purulent discharge
4. In women, obtain specimen of vaginal secretions for wet-prep or Gram stain

C. Differential Diagnosis
1. PID in women
2. Gonorrhea

D. Diagnostic Tests
1. Chlamydia culture is most definitive test but is expensive and takes 2-6 days to obtain results
2. Currently available tests for detection without cell culture include
   a. Direct fluorescent antibody (DFA) staining for elementary bodies in clinical specimens using monoclonal antibody
   b. Enzyme immunoassay (EIA)

   c. DNA probe

   d. Nucleic acid amplification (PCR and LCR) [in men, perform test on first-void urine]

  3. Always test for *N. gonorrhoeae* and also perform microscopic analysis of vaginal secretions (wet-prep or Gram stain)

V. Plan/Treatment

 A. Treatment of choice is azithromycin (Zithromax) 1 g orally in a single dose OR doxycycline 100 mg orally BID x 7 days

 B. Alternative regimens: Erythromycin base 500 mg orally QID x 7 day; OR erythromycin ethylsuccinate 800 mg orally QID x 7 days OR ofloxacin 300 mg orally BID x 7 days

 C. Selecting a treatment
  1. Doxycycline has the advantage of low cost and a long history of safety and efficacy
  2. Azithromycin has the advantage of single-dose administration and may be more cost effective in patients in whom compliance is an issue (single-dose, directly observed therapy in the clinical setting is possible)
  3. Ofloxacin is similar in efficacy to doxycycline and azithromycin, but it is more expensive than doxycycline and offers no advantage in dosing
  4. Erythromycin is less efficacious than either azithromycin and doxycycline and gastrointestinal side effects are common and reduce patient compliance
  5. Pregnant women should **not** be treated with doxycycline or ofloxacin

 D. Treatment of sex partners: Patients should be instructed to refer their sex partners for evaluation and treatment
  1. Sex partners should be evaluated and treated if they had sexual contact with the patient during the 60 days preceding onset of symptoms in the patient or diagnosis of chlamydia
  2. The most recent sex partner should be treated even if the time of the last sexual contact was >60 days before symptom onset or diagnosis
  3. Patients should be instructed to abstain from sexual intercourse until they and their sex partners have completed treatment (i.e., 7 days after a single-dose regimen or after completion of a 7-day regimen)

 E. Treatment during pregnancy: Erythromycin base 500 mg orally QID x 7 days OR amoxicillin 500 mg orally TID for 7 days

 F. Alternative regimens for pregnant women
  1. Erythromycin base 250 mg orally QID x 14 days OR
  2. Azithromycin 1 g orally in a single dose

 G. Follow Up: None indicated when treated with doxycycline, azithromycin, or ofloxacin; retesting may be considered 3 weeks after completion of treatment with erythromycin

GONORRHEA

I. Definition: A sexually transmitted disease caused by *Neisseria gonorrhoeae,* a Gram-negative diplococcus that prefers columnar and pseudo-stratified epithelium

II. Pathogenesis

 A. *N. gonorrhoeae* organisms are Gram-negative diplococci present in exudate and secretions of infected mucous surfaces

 B. Transmission results from intimate contact, such as sexual acts and parturition

C. Incubation period is usually 2-7 days

D. Gonococcal infections occur only in humans

III. Clinical Presentation

A. An estimated one million new infections with *N. gonorrhoeae* occur in the US each year

B. Rate of infection is highest in sexually active young adults

C. Transmission risk from an infected male to a woman is 70% after one exposure; from infected woman to male is as low as 20% with one exposure but rises to 60-90% with four exposures

D. At least 20% of neonates of infected women delivered vaginally acquire the disease

E. Most infections among men produce symptoms that cause the person to seek treatment before serious sequelae develop

F. Many infections among women, on the other hand, do not produce symptoms until complications have occurred

G. In women, common sites of infection are the urethra, endocervix, upper genital tract, pharynx, and rectum
   1. Presenting symptoms include increased vaginal discharge, abnormal uterine bleeding, and dysuria
   2. Twenty to forty percent of pelvic inflammatory disease (PID) is caused by gonorrhea
   3. Disseminated disease occurs most often when gonorrhea is acquired during menses or pregnancy; common features of disseminated disease include tenosynovitis, skin lesions, fever, and polyarthralgias
   4. A primary measure for controlling gonorrhea is the screening of high-risk women

H. In men, common sites of infection are the urethra, epididymis, prostate, rectum, and pharynx; disseminated disease may also occur

IV. Diagnosis/Evaluation

A. History
   1. Inquire about onset and duration of symptoms
   2. In women, ask about presence of vaginal discharge, dysuria, abnormal bleeding, abdominal/pelvic pain, and dyspareunia
   3. In women, obtain menstrual history and contraceptive history
   4. In men, ask about dysuria, urethral discharge, rectal pain or discharge
   5. Inquire about sexual history including age at first intercourse, number of partners in past year, types of sexual practices, and use of condoms
   6. Ask about past history of STDs, including types, frequency, treatments

B. Physical Examination
   1. Take temperature to determine if febrile
   2. In women, perform pelvic exam; inspect Bartholin's and Skene's glands for tenderness and enlargement and the urethra for discharge; inspect cervix for mucopurulent discharge; gently scrape cervix to test for friability
   3. In women, perform a bimanual exam to check for adnexal tenderness and masses, for uterine tenderness, and cervical motion tenderness
   4. In men, examine for urethral discharge; if anal sex practiced, perform rectal exam for tenderness and discharge

C. Differential Diagnosis
   1. Pelvic inflammatory disease in women
   2. Chlamydia

D. Diagnostic Tests
   1. Microscopic examinations of Gram-stained smears (for Gram-negative intracellular diplococci) of exudate from the endocervix in females and the urethra in males are helpful in the initial evaluation
   2. Cervical or urethral culture for *N. gonorrhoeae* using modified Thayer-Martin media
   3. In men, nucleic acid amplification tests on first-void urine
   4. DNA probe can also be used for both men and women to diagnose gonorrhea and chlamydia

V. Plan/Treatment

A. Treatment of adults with uncomplicated gonococcal infections of the cervix, urethra, and rectum (**Note**: Routine dual therapy for gonococcal and chlamydial infections is necessary)

> Ceftriaxone (Rocephin) 125 mg IM in a single dose
> OR
> Cefixime 400 mg orally in a single dose
> OR
> Ciprofloxacin 500 mg orally in a single dose
> OR
> Ofloxacin 400 mg orally in a single dose
> **PLUS**
> A regimen effective against possible coinfection with C. trachomatis--azithromycin
> 1 g orally in a single dose OR doxycycline 100 mg orally BID x 7 days

B. Alternative Regimens: Spectinomycin 2 g IM in a single dose OR ceftizoxime 500 mg IM in a single dose

C. Many other antimicrobials are active against *N. gonorrhoeae*. See <u>1998 Guidelines for Treatment of Sexually Transmitted Diseases</u> available from US Department of Health and Human Services, Centers for Disease Control and Prevention (CDC), Atlanta, GA 30333 for additional drugs that can be used

D. Pregnant women should be treated with a recommended or alternative cephalosporin as listed above. Either erythromycin or amoxicillin should also be used for presumptive or diagnosed chlamydia infection (see CHLAMYDIAL INFECTIONS section above for treatment of pregnant women) [**Note: Pregnant women should not be treated with quinolones or tetracyclines**]

E. Patients should be instructed to refer sex partners for evaluation and treatment
   1. All sex partners of patients who have *N. Gonorhoeae* should be evaluated and treated for both *N. Gonorrhoeae* and *C. Trachomatis* infections if their last sexual contact with the patient was within 60 days before onset of symptoms or diagnosis of infection in the patient
   2. If the patient's most recent sexual encounter was >60 days before onset of symptoms or diagnosis, the patient's most recent sex partner should be treated

F. Patients should be instructed to avoid sexual intercourse until therapy is completed and symptoms are no longer present

G. Persons with disseminated gonococcal infection (bacteremia) should be hospitalized for initial parenteral antibiotic therapy

H. Follow Up
   1. Patients with uncomplicated gonorrhea and who are treated with any of the recommended regimens need not return for a test of cure
   2. Patients with persistent symptoms after treatment need to be re-evaluated for antimicrobial susceptibility
   3. Persistence of symptoms usually results from reinfection rather than treatment failure

MUCOPURULENT CERVICITIS

I.   Definition: A sexually transmitted syndrome in which there is purulent or mucopurulent endocervical exudate visible in the endocervical canal or in an endocervical swab specimen

II. Pathogenesis

   A.   Mucopurulent cervicitis (MPC) can be caused by *Chlamydia trachomatis* and *Neisseria gonorrhoeae*, but in **most cases** neither organism can be isolated
   B.   Other non-microbiologic determinants (e.g., inflammation in an ectropion) could be involved

III. Clinical Presentation

   A.   MPC is often asymptomatic, but some women have an abnormal vaginal discharge and vaginal bleeding (e.g., after sexual intercourse)

   B.   MPC can persist despite repeated courses of antimicrobial therapy

   C.   Some experts consider an increased number of polymorphonuclear leukocytes on Gram stain of endocervical secretions as being helpful in the diagnosis of MPC; however, this criterion has not been standardized and is not available in some settings

   D.   Important to keep in mind that most women who have *C. trachomatis* or *N. gonorrhoeae* do not have MPC

IV. Diagnosis/Evaluation

   A.   History
        1.   Inquire about the onset and duration of symptoms, if present
        2.   Ask about presence of vaginal discharge, dysuria, abnormal bleeding particularly after sexual intercourse
        3.   Obtain menstrual history and contraceptive history
        4.   Inquire about sexual history including age at first intercourse, present partner(s), types of sexual practices, and use of condoms
        5.   Inquire about past history of STDs, including types, frequency, treatments

   B.   Physical Examination
        1.   Determine if febrile
        2.   Perform speculum exam to inspect cervix and sample secretions for purulent or mucopurulent discharge; gently scrape cervix to determine friability
        3.   Perform bimanual exam, checking for adnexal tenderness, masses

   C.   Differential Diagnosis
        1.   Urinary tract infection
        2.   Chlamydia
        3.   Gonorrhea
        4.   Trichomonal vaginitis

   D.   Diagnostic Tests
        1.   Gram stain of endocervical secretions looking for PMNs and intracellular Gram-negative diplococci
        2.   DNA probe to test for *C. trachomatis* and *N. gonhrrhoeae*
        3.   Wet mount exam for trichomonas
        4.   Urine for culture and sensitivity (if symptomatic)

V.   Plan/Management

   A.   Results of tests for *C. trachomatis* and *N. gonorrhoeae* should determine the need for treatment

   B.   Empiric treatment should be considered for patients in whom gonorrhea and/or chlamydia is SUSPECTED if the patient might be difficult to locate for treatment (see GONORRHEA and CHLAMYDIA sections for treatment recommendations)

   C.   Sex partners of women with MPC should be notified, examined, and treated for the STD identified or suspected in the index case

   D.   Follow Up
      1.   Should be as recommended for the infections for which the woman is being treated
      2.   If symptoms persist, woman should be instructed to return for reevaluation and to abstain from sexual intercourse even if the course of prescribed therapy has been completed

NONGONOCOCCOL URETHRITIS (NGU)

I.   Definition: Inflammation of the urethra not caused by gonococcal infection and characterized by a mucoid or purulent urethral discharge

II.   Pathogenesis

   A.   *Chlamydia trachomatis* is the most frequent cause of NGU (23%-55% of cases)

   B.   Etiology of most cases of nonchlaymdial NGU is unknown; *Ureaplasma urealyticum*, and possibly *Mycoplasma genitalium* are implicated in about one third of cases

   C.   *Trichomonas vaginalis* and HSV sometimes cause NGU

   D.   Complications of NGU among men infected with *C. Trachomatis* include epididymitis and Reiter's syndrome

III.   Clinical Presentation

   A.   Most common STD syndrome in males living in industrialized countries

   B.   NGU is substantially more common than gonococcal urethritis in most areas of US

   C.   Many men are entirely asymptomatic

   D.   In symptomatic males, primary complaints are urethral discharge (yellow, white, or cloudy), dysuria, or urethral itching

   E.   Urethritis can be documented by the presence of **any** of the following signs:
      1.   Mucopurulent or purulent discharge
      2.   Gram stain of urethral secretions demonstrating ≥ 5 WBCs per oil immersion field
      3.   Positive leukocyte esterase test on first-void urine, or microscopic examination of first-void urine demonstrating ≥ 10 WBCs per high power field

IV.   Diagnosis/Evaluation

   A.   History
      1.   Ask about onset, duration of symptoms
      2.   Inquire about presence and color of discharge, presence of dysuria, and urethral itching

3. Inquire about sexual history including age at first intercourse, number of partners in the past year, types of sexual practices, use of condoms
4. Inquire about past history of STDs, including types, frequency, and treatments

B. Physical Examination: Examine urethra for mucopurulent discharge

C. Differential Diagnosis: Gonorrhea

D. Diagnostic Tests
1. Gram-stain urethral smear (>5 WBCs per oil immersion field PLUS no intracellular Gram-negative diplococci are expected findings)
2. Positive leukocyte esterase test on first void urine, or microscopic examination of first-void urine demonstrating ≥10 WBCs per high power field
3. Test for *N. gonorrhoeae* and *C. trachomatis* using DNA probe

V. Plan/Treatment

A. If none of the criteria for confirming urethritis are met (see III. E. above), treatment should be deferred until the test results for *N. gonorrhoeae* and *C. trachomatis* tests are obtained
1. If the results are positive for either infection, the appropriate treatment should be given and sex partners referred for evaluation and treatment
2. Empiric treatment of symptoms without documentation of urethritis is recommended only for patients at high risk for infection who are unlikely to return for follow-up (such patients should be treated for both gonorrhea and chlamydia) [see GONORRHEA and CHLAMYDIA for treatment recommendations]

B. Management of sex partners: Should be evaluated and treated appropriately based on evaluation (see exposure intervals to base treatment on under section on CHLAMYDIA)

C. Recurrent NGU may be due to a lack of compliance, or more often, reinfection by untreated sex partner
1. Men with persistent or recurrent urethritis should be re-treated with the initial regimen if they failed to comply with the treatment regimen or if they were re-exposed to an untreated sex partner
2. Otherwise, a wet mount exam and culture of an intraurethral swab specimen for *T. vaginalis* should be performed;
3. If negative, the man should be retreated with an alternative regimen extended to 14 days (e.g., erythromycin base 500 mg orally 4 times a day for 14 days)
4. Refer for evaluation by an expert if objective signs of urethritis continue after adequate treatment

D. Follow Up: None required unless patient remains symptomatic

PELVIC INFLAMMATORY DISEASE (PID)

I. Definition: A spectrum of inflammatory disorders of the upper female genital tract, including any combination of endometritis, salpingitis, tubo-ovarian abscess, and pelvic abscess, and pelvic peritonitis

II. Pathogenesis

A. Sexually transmitted organisms, especially *Neisseria gonorrhoeae* and *Chlamydia trachomatis*, are implicated in most cases

B. Microorganisms that can be part of the vaginal flora (e.g., anaerobes, *G. vaginalis*, *H. influenzae*, enteric Gram-negative rods, and *Streptococcus agalactiae*) also can cause PID

C. In addition, *M. hominis* and *U. urealyticum* might be etiologic agents of PID

III. Clinical Presentation

    A. Incidence of PID is highest among sexually active adolescents

    B. Variables that **increase** risk of PID include adolescence, multiple sex partners, previous episode of STD, use of an intrauterine device, and douching

    C. Variables that **decrease** risk include use of oral contraceptives, barrier contraceptives, and spermicide use

    D. Most typical presentation is continuous bilateral lower abdominal or pelvic pain that may be accompanied by fever, nausea, and vomiting

    E. In many patients the infection is asymptomatic (silent PID) or symptoms are vague and mild with abnormal vaginal bleeding, dyspareunia, or change in vaginal discharge as the only signs and symptoms (atypical PID)

    F. PID symptoms most often begin within one week of onset of menses

    G. The diagnosis of PID usually is based on clinical findings; no single historical, physical, or laboratory finding is both sensitive and specific for the diagnosis

    H. The following recommendations for diagnosing PID are made by the CDC to help health-care providers recognize when PID should be suspected and when there is a need to obtain additional information to increase diagnostic certainty

DIAGNOSTIC CRITERIA FOR PID
Minimum Criteria

Empiric treatment of PID should be instituted in sexually active young women and others at risk for STDs if all the following **minimum criteria** are present and no other cause(s) for the illness can be identified
 	
  ❖ Lower abdominal tenderness
  ❖ Adnexal tenderness, and
  ❖ Cervical motion tenderness

Additional Criteria

For women with severe clinical signs, more elaborate diagnostic evaluation is warranted because incorrect diagnosis and management may cause unnecessary morbidity. These additional criteria may be used to increase the specificity of the minimum criteria listed above
 	
Listed below are the **additional criteria** that support a diagnosis of PID
 	
  ❖ Oral temperature >101°F (>38.3°C)
  ❖ Abnormal cervical or vaginal discharge
  ❖ Elevated erythrocyte sedimentation rate
  ❖ Elevated C-reactive protein
  ❖ Laboratory documentation of cervical infection with *N. gonorrhoeae* or *C. trachomatis*

Definitive Criteria

The **definitive criteria** for diagnosing PID include the following
 	
  ❖ Histopathologic evidence of endometritis on endometrial biopsy
  ❖ Transvaginal sonography or other imaging techniques showing thickened fluid-filled tubes with or without free pelvic fluid or tubo-ovarian complex, and
  ❖ Laparoscopic abnormalities consistent with PID

Source: Centers for Disease Control and Prevention. (1998). 1998 guidelines for treatment of sexually transmitted diseases. MMWR, 47(No.RR-1), 80.

IV.   Diagnosis/Evaluation

    A.   History
        1.   Ask about presence of lower abdominal/pelvic pain, including onset, duration, location, and character or pain
        2.   Ask the patient if she has had fever
        3.   Inquire about presence of vaginal discharge, postcoital bleeding, spotting between menstrual periods, fever, and gastrointestinal symptoms
        4.   Obtain sexual history including age at first intercourse, number of partners in past year, types of sexual practices, and contraceptive history (ask if IUD is used)
        5.   Inquire about past history of STDs, including type, frequency, treatments; ask about HIV+ status.
        6.   Obtain complete menstrual history including pattern of recent menstrual cycles and a description of the last menses (Ask: "Did onset of pain coincide with LMP?")

    B.   Physical Examination
        1.   Determine if febrile
        2.   Examine abdomen for tenderness, masses, signs of peritonitis
        3.   On speculum exam, inspect cervix for inflammation; insert a cotton swab into cervix to sample mucus and examine its gross appearance. (A thick transparent discharge similar to styling gel is normal; secretions that appear yellow on a cotton-tipped swab are not normal)
        4.   Perform bimanual exam to check for adnexal masses, uterine tenderness, and for cervical motion tenderness (pain that occurs when cervix is moved from side to side)

    C.   Differential Diagnosis
        1.   Appendicitis
        2.   Ectopic pregnancy
        3.   Tubo-ovarian abscess
        4.   Ovarian cyst
        5.   Pyelonephritis

    D.   Diagnostic Tests
        1.   Pregnancy Test
        2.   Endocervical and rectal cultures for *N. gonorrhoeae* and an endocervical test for *C. trachomatis* should be obtained before treatment
        3.   CBC with differential and sedimentation rate
        4.   Wet prep or Gram stain of endocervical secretions
            a.   If number of epithelial cells > than number of WBCs per high-powered field, then patient almost certainly does not have PID
            b.   If number of WBCs > epithelial cells per high powered field, patient may have PID
        5.   VDRL or RPR

V.   Plan/Management

    A.   Inpatient therapy for every case of PID is unrealistic. The CDC has made recommendations for when to select inpatient therapy and these recommendations are contained in the following table

SITUATIONS WHEN HOSPITALIZATION OF PATIENTS WITH ACUTE PID IS INDICATED
✓ Diagnosis is uncertain, and surgical emergencies such as appendicitis and ectopic pregnancy cannot be excluded
✓ Patient has a tubo-ovarian abscess
✓ Patient is pregnant
✓ Patient has severe illness, nausea and vomiting, or high fever
✓ Patient is immunodeficient
✓ Patient fails to respond clinically to oral antimicrobial therapy
✓ Patients is unable to follow or tolerate an outpatient oral regimen

B. Outpatient therapy for PID is described in the table below

RECOMMENDED REGIMENS FOR AMBULATORY TREATMENT OF ACUTE PID
Regimen A
Ofloxacin 400 mg orally BID for 14 days
PLUS
Metronidazole 500 mg orally BID for 14 days
Regimen B
Cefoxitin 2 g IM plus Probenecid 1 g orally in a single dose concurrently, **OR** ceftriaxone 250 mg IM in a single dose, **OR** other parenteral equivalent third-generation cephalosporin
PLUS
Doxycycline 100 mg orally BID for 14 days

C. Management of sex partners:
1. Sex partners of patients with PID should be examined and treated if they had sexual contact with patient during the 60 day period preceding onset of symptoms in patient
2. Evaluation and treatment of sex partners of women with PID is imperative because of the risk of reinfection
3. Sex partners should be treated empirically with regimens effective against both *C. trachomatis* and *N. gonorrhoeae* regardless of the apparent etiology of PID

D. Counsel woman about importance of using condoms to prevent STDs and also importance of partner treatment

E. Follow Up
1. Patients treated on an ambulatory basis need to be monitored closely and reevaluated in 72 hours for clinical improvement (**Note**: Clinical improvement is defined as defervescence; reduction in direct or rebound abdominal tenderness; reduction in uterine, adnexal, and cervical motion tenderness within 3 days after initiation of therapy)
2. Patients who do not demonstrate improvement within this time require additional diagnostic test, surgical intervention, or both
3. Some experts recommend rescreening for *C. trachomatis* and *N. gonorrhoeae* 4-6 weeks after therapy is completed

SYPHILIS

I. Definition: A systemic sexually transmitted disease involving multiple organ systems and caused by *Treponema pallidum*, a spirochete

II. Pathogenesis

A. *T. pallidum* is a thin, delicate organism with humans as the sole host

B. Organism penetrates intact skin or mucous membrane during sexual contact, multiplies, and rapidly spreads to regional lymph nodes

C. Spirochetes enter the blood stream within hours and are transported to other tissues

D. Congenital syphilis results from transplacental passage of the organism

E. Incubation period for acquired primary syphilis is about 3 weeks, but ranges from 10-90 days after exposure

III. Clinical Presentation

    A. Since the end of the nationwide syphilis epidemic between 1986 and 1990, the syphilis rate has never been lower in the US, having declined by 84% between 1990 and 1997

        1. The syphilis rate has declined 95% in the Northeast, 91% in the West, 80% in the South, and 73% in the Midwest

        2. Despite declines in the South, that region has the highest syphilis rate in the nation

    B. To guide therapeutic decisions and disease intervention strategies, acquired syphilis has been divided into the following clinical stages: Primary, secondary, latent, and tertiary

    C. Primary syphilis: Characterized by appearance of ulcer or chancre at site of inoculation, usually on genitals 3-4 weeks after exposure

        1. Genital lesions are usually indurated and painless

        2. Extragenital lesions (e.g., lips, breast) are often painful

        3. Regional lymphadenopathy usually present

        4. Chancre persists for 1-5 weeks and heals spontaneously

    D. Secondary syphilis: Occurs about 6-8 weeks later and is characterized by flu-like symptoms -- headache, generalized arthralgia, malaise, fever, and lymphadenopathy, followed by a generalized rash

        1. Rash is macular, papular, annular, or follicular; often involves the palms and soles

        2. Rash persists for 2-6 weeks then spontaneously heals

        3. Mucous patches often occur in mouth, throat, on cervix; flat, papular lesions (condylomata lata) occur in intertriginous areas

        4. About 25% of infected persons have at least one cutaneous relapse

        5. Secondary syphilis is the most contagious state of the disease

        6. Even without treatment, signs of first 2 stages resolve spontaneously, and persons enter the next state: the latent state

    E. Latent syphilis: Arbitrarily divided into early and late latent stages

        1. Infection of <1 year is defined as early latent (infectious)

        2. Infections of >1 year is late latent or syphilis of unknown duration (non-infectious)

        3. Difficult to make this distinction in practice, because exact date of infection is usually difficult to establish

        4. Latent syphilis begins with the healing of the lesions in the secondary stage and may last a few years or a lifetime

        5. About 1/3 of persons with latent syphilis are little inconvenienced by the disease

        6. After a variable period of latency, about 1/3 of untreated cases go on to develop tertiary syphilis, and about 28% of these will die because of the disease

    F. Tertiary syphilis: May take the form of gummatous, cardiovascular (both rare forms), or neurosyphilis

    G. Congenital syphilis involves multiple organ systems with the stage of syphilis in the mother determining the effects on the fetus

        1. Early congenital syphilis occurs from birth to age 2 and is characterized by mucocutaneous lesions, rhinitis, and other symptoms

        2. Congenital syphilis can be asymptomatic, especially in the first weeks of life

        3. Late congenital syphilis is characterized by bone and joint disorders, cranial neuropathies, and interstitial keratitis which causes blindness if untreated

IV. Diagnosis/Evaluation

    A. History

        1. Question about onset, duration of symptoms

        2. Ask about presence or history of chancre (when it appeared, where located, if symptomatic, when healed)

        3. Ask about presence (or history of) rash, mucous patches, condylomata lata

        4. Ask about sexual behavior, use of condoms

5. Ask if sex partner has had similar symptoms
6. Ask about past history of STDs, including types, frequency, duration, treatment
7. Ask about HIV status
8. Obtain past medical history, medication history, drug and alcohol use, allergies

B. Physical Examination
1. Examine genital area and other skin surfaces (breast, buttocks) for characteristic chancre (primary syphilis)
2. Look for mucocutaneous lesions of secondary syphilis

C. Differential Diagnosis
1. Primary syphilis: Syphilis can mimic all lesions that appear to be genital ulcers: genital herpes, chancroid, lymphogranuloma venereum, scabies, balanitis should all be suspect
2. Secondary syphilis: Syphilis can mimic many skin disorders: all undiagnosed mucous or cutaneous eruptions should be suspect

D. Diagnostic Tests
1. Darkfield microscopy and direct fluorescent antibody tests of lesion exudate or tissue are the definitive methods for diagnosing early syphilis
2. A presumptive diagnosis is possible with the use of two types of serologic tests for syphilis
   a. Nontreponeal-specific tests: rapid plasma reagin (RPR) test and Venereal Disease Research Laboratory (VDRL) test
   b. Treponemal-specific tests: Fluorescent Treponemal antibody absorbed (FTA-ABS) and microhemagglutination assay for antibody to *T. Pallidum* (MHA-TP)
3. VDRL and RPR are used for initial screening and titers; fall in titer correlates with response to therapy; RPR is test most often used today, but the tests are comparable
4. For sequential serologic tests, the same test (VDRL or RPR) should be used
5. Treponemal tests are used to confirm diagnosis of syphilis in persons with positive VDRL or RPR
   a. Usually remains positive for life regardless of treatment or disease activity
   b. Reported as positive or negative

V. Plan/Treatment

A. Treatment is based on clinical and serologic staging of the disease and is summarized in the following table

RECOMMENDED TREATMENT OF SYPHILIS IN ADULTS	
Stage	**Treatment**
Primary, secondary, and early latent disease	Benzathine penicillin G 2.4 million units IM in a single dose. For patients allergic to penicillin: doxycycline 100 mg orally BID x 14 days, or tetracycline 500 mg orally QID x 14 days
Late latent syphilis or syphilis of unknown duration	Benzathine penicillin G 7.2 million units total, given as three doses of 2.4 million units IM each at 1-week intervals. For patients allergic to penicillin: doxycycline 100 mg orally BID for 4 weeks, or tetracycline 500 mg orally QID x 4 weeks
Tertiary disease, excluding neurosyphilis	As for late latent disease, with appropriate management of complications
Neurosyphilis	Aqueous crystalline penicillin G, 18-24 million units/day given as 3-4 million units IV every 4 hours for 10-14 days, or procaine penicillin 2-4 million units IM a day PLUS Probenecid 500 mg orally QID both for 10-14 days
Exposure: Sexual contacts of persons with infectious syphilis	Refer to MANAGEMENT OF SEX PARTNERS table below

B.   Management of sex partners should be guided by the following recommendations

MANAGEMENT OF SEX PARTNERS
Patients exposed sexually to a patient who has syphilis in any stage should be evaluated both clinically and serologically as follows:
Persons exposed within the 90 days preceding the diagnosis of primary, secondary, or early latent syphilis in a sex partner might be infected even if seronegative--**Treat presumptively**
Persons exposed >90 days before the diagnosis of primary, secondary, or early latent syphilis in a sex partner and in whom serologic test results are not available immediately and the opportunity for follow-up is uncertain--**Treat presumptively**
For purposes of **partner notification and presumptive treatment of exposed sex partners**, patients with syphilis of unknown duration with high nontreponemal serologic test titers (defined as ≥1:32) may be considered as having early syphilis
Note: Serologic titers should not be used to differentiate early from late latent syphilis for the purpose of determining treatment for the index case

C.   Congenital syphilis
  1.   Infants born to seroreactive mothers should be evaluated with a quantitative nontreponemal serologic test (RPR or VDRL)
      a.   Test should be performed on infant serum
      b.   Umbilical cord blood may be contaminated with maternal blood and might yield a false-positive result
      c.   A treponemal test of a newborn's serum is not necessary
  2.   Evaluation of infant includes the following
      a.   Complete physical exam of neonate for evidence of congenital syphilis
      b.   Examination of the placenta or umbilical cord using specific fluorescent antitreponemal antibody staining
      c.   Darkfield microscopic examination or direct fluorescent antibody staining of any suspicious lesions or body fluids (example, nasal discharge)
  3.   Consult expert regarding therapy decisions and treatment guidelines for all infants born to seroreactive mothers

D.   Syphilis in HIV infected persons
  1.   Diagnostic considerations
      a.   Both treponemal and non-treponemal serologic tests for syphilis can be interpreted in usual manner for most patients who are coinfected with *T. pallidum* and HIV
      b.   When clinical findings suggest syphilis, but serologic tests are nonreactive or unclear, alternate tests such as biopsy of lesion, darkfield examination or direct fluorescent antibody staining of lesion material may be helpful
  2.   Treatment
      a.   Treatment the same as for HIV-negative patients is recommended
      b.   HIV-infected patients who have either late latent syphilis or syphilis of unknown duration should have a CSF examination before treatment

E.   Follow Up
  1.   Patients with primary and secondary syphilis should be examined clinically and serologically at 6 months and 12 months; more frequent evaluation may be prudent if follow-up is uncertain
  2.   If nontreponemal antibody titers (either VDRL or RPR) have not declined fourfold within 6 months after therapy for primary or secondary syphilis, person is at risk or treatment failure
  3.   Optimal management of such patients is unclear, but the following steps should be taken
      a.   First, reevaluate for HIV infection (if positive for HIV, see V.D. above)
      b.   Then, provide more frequent follow-up (every 3 months instead of 6)
      c.   If additional follow-up cannot be ensured, re-treatment is recommended
      d.   Note: Some experts recommend CSF examination in such situations
      e.   Retreatment (according to most experts): 3 weekly injections of benazthine penicillin G 2.4 million units IM [unless CSF examination indicates neurosyphilis is present]

4. Patients with latent syphilis should be followed up with non-treponemal serologic testing at 6, 12, and 24 months; patient should be evaluated for neurosyphilis and retreated appropriately if
   a. Titers increase fourfold
   b. An initially high titer (≥ 1:32) fails to decline at least fourfold within 12-24 months
   c. Signs or symptoms attributable to syphilis develop in the patient

F. HIV infected persons should have more frequent follow up, including serologic testing at 3, 6, 9, 12, and 24 months after therapy

GENITAL HERPES SIMPLEX VIRUS INFECTION

I. Definition: Infections with herpes simplex viruses, large DNA viruses. Two major types have genomic and antigenic differences--Type 1 (HSV-1) usually involves the face and skin above the waist, but an increasing number of genital herpes cases are attributable to HSV-1; Type 2 (HSV-2) usually involves the genitalia and skin below the waist in sexually active adolescents and adults (see SKIN PROBLEMS IN ADULTS for Herpes Simplex infections of the skin and mucous membranes)

II. Pathogenesis

A. HSV-1 and HSV-2 are epidermotropic viruses with infection occurring within keratinocytes

B. Transmission is only by direct contact with active lesions, or by virus-containing fluid such as saliva or cervical secretions in persons with no evidence of active disease

C. Inoculation of the virus into skin or mucosal surfaces produces infection, with an incubation period of 2-14 days

D. About 48 hours after entering the host, the virus transverses afferent nerves to find host ganglion
   1. The trigeminal ganglia are the target of the oral virus -- primarily HSV-1
   2. The sacral ganglia are the target of the genital virus -- most often HSV-2

E. Upon reactivation, the virus retraces its route, causing recurrence in the cutaneous area affected by the same nerve root, but not necessarily in the original site

F. Generally HSV-1 is associated with infection of the lips, face, buccal mucosa, and throat; HSV-2, with the genitalia

G. In spite of the distinctive sites of herpetic lesions with each serotype, there is overlap in site of infection in approximately 25% of individuals who are infected
   1. Type 1 strains can be recovered from the genital tract
   2. Type 2 strains probably can be recovered from the pharynx as a result of oral-genital activity
   3. Whereas type 1 HSV genital infections in children also can result from autoinoculation of virus from the mouth, sexual abuse must always be considered in prepubertal children with genital herpes

III. Clinical Presentation

A. Based on serologic studies, approximately 45 million persons in the US have been diagnosed with genital HSV-2

B. Most HSV-2 infected persons have not received a diagnosis of genital herpes
   1. Infections in these persons are either mild or unrecognized with the virus shed intermittently in the genital tract

2.   Many cases are transmitted by persons unaware that they are infected or asymptomatic when transmission occurs

C.   A small minority of first-episode genital herpes cases are manifest by severe disease that requires hospitalization

D.   The usual sequence of disease in which signs/symptoms occur is painful papules followed by vesicles, ulceration, crusting, and healing

E.   First clinical episode of genital herpes
1.   Symptoms of primary infection that is symptomatic often consists of hyperesthesia, burning, itching, dysuria, pain, and tenderness in the genital area
2.   Fever and lymphadenopathy are frequently present
3.   More systemic manifestations are present than with recurrent episodes
4.   Viral shedding is prolonged (average 12 days) and healing of lesions takes 21 days on average
5.   Persons with genital infection with HSV-1 (about 20-30% of patients with first episode herpes) have a much lower risk of symptomatic recurrent outbreaks

F.   Recurrent episodes of HSV infection
1.   Most patients (about 50%) with symptomatic first episode HSV-2 infection will have recurrent episodes within 6 months after the first clinical episode
2.   Frequently have prodrome with recurrence
3.   Lesions often localized in recurrent episodes
4.   Length of viral shedding reduced compared to primary episode (average 7 days)
5.   Healing of lesions is also faster (5 days on average)

IV.   Diagnosis/Evaluation

A.   History
1.   Question regarding location, onset, duration, and appearance of lesions; ask if pain, burning, or paresthesia present prior to eruption
2.   Ask about associated symptoms of fever, myalgia, malaise
3.   Ask regarding previous occurrence of similar lesions, symptoms
4.   Inquire about exposures to infected persons and use of condoms

B.   Physical Examination
1.   Examine genital area for characteristic location, distribution, appearance of lesions
2.   Check for enlarged lymph nodes in inguinal area

C.   Differential Diagnosis
1.   Syphilis
2.   Chancroid
3.   Folliculitis
4.   Molluscum contagiosum

D.   Diagnostic Tests
1.   Viral culture is the most sensitive and commonly available test for confirming the diagnosis of genital herpes
        a.   Unroof vesicle and scrape the material with Dacron-tipped swab
        b.   Place swab in viral transport media
        c.   Virus grows rapidly and cultures may be positive within 2-3 days (can take longer)
        d.   Additional advantage of culture is that it permits viral typing which is useful prognostic information for patients with primary episodes (**Note**: Patients with genital infection with HSV-1 have a much lower risk of symptomatic recurrent outbreaks)
2.   Direct fluorescent antibody test is an alternative when viral culture is not possible
        a.   Yield rapid results at a relatively low cost
        b.   Most antigen tests do not differentiate HSV-1 from HSV-2
3.   The Tzanck test is not recommended by the CDC for diagnosing HSV infection

V.   Plan/Management

   A.   Management of first clinical episode of genital herpes is outlined in the following table

---

RECOMMENDED REGIMENS: FIRST CLINICAL EPISODE

Select one of the following regimens

Acyclovir 400 mg orally TID x 7-10 days   Famciclovir 250 mg orally TID x 7-10 days
Acyclovir 200 mg orally 5 times/day x 7-10 days   Valacyclovir 1 g orally BID x 7-10 days

Note: Treatment may be extended if healing is incomplete after 10 days of therapy

---

COUNSELING FOR MANAGEMENT OF PATIENTS WITH GENITAL HERPES

Natural history of the disease with emphasis on recurrent episodes, asymptomatic viral shedding, and sexual transmission
        Sexual transmission can occur during asymptomatic periods
        Asymptomatic viral shedding occurs more frequently in persons with genital HSV-2 than
            HSV-1 and also occurs more frequently in those with infection <12 months

After first episode,
        Episodic antiviral therapy during recurrent episodes might shorten duration
        Suppressive antiviral therapy can modulate or prevent recurrences

There is a risk for neonatal infection in pregnant women

Importance of use of condoms during all sexual exposures

Need to abstain from all sexual activity when lesions or prodromal symptoms are present

---

   B.   Management of recurrent episodes of HSV infection is outlined in the following table

---

RECOMMENDED REGIMENS FOR EPISODIC RECURRENT INFECTION

Select one of the following regimens

Acyclovir 400 mg orally TID x 5 days   Famciclovir 125 mg orally BID x 5 days
Acyclovir 200 mg orally 5 x/day x 5 days   Valacyclovir 500 mg orally BID x 5 days
Acyclovir 800 mg orally BID x 5 days

Options for treatment of recurrent episodes should be discussed with all patients
Treatment is most efficacious when begun during the prodrome or within 1 day after onset of lesions

If treatment for recurrence is chosen, patient should be provided with antiviral therapy, or a prescription for the medication, so that treatment can be initiated at the first sign of prodrome or genital lesions

---

RECOMMENDED REGIMENS FOR DAILY SUPPRESSIVE THERAPY

Select one of the following regimens

Acyclovir 400 mg orally BID   Valacyclovir 500 mg orally QD*
Famciclovir 250 mg orally BID   Valacyclovir 1,000 mg orally QD

Daily suppressive therapy reduces the frequency of genital herpes recurrences by ≥75% among patients who have frequent recurrences (defined as 6 or more recurrences per year)

Suppressive therapy with acyclovir reduces but does not eliminate asymptomatic viral shedding

Suppressive therapy has not been associated with emergence of acyclovir resistance among immunocompetent patients

After 12 months of continuous suppressive therapy, discontinuation should be discussed with patient

Famciclovir and valacyclovir should **not be used for over 12 months**

Safety and efficacy have been documented among patients using daily acyclovir for as long as 6 years

*May be less effective than other dosing regimens of valacyclovir in patients with ≥10 outbreaks per year

C. Management of sex partners
   1. Can usually benefit from evaluation and counseling
   2. Symptomatic sex partners should be evaluated and treated

D. Lesions caused by HSV are common among HIV-infected patients and may be severe
   1. Whereas the dosage of antiviral drugs for HIV-infected persons is controversial, clinical experience suggests the need for increased doses of antiviral drugs
   2. For initial and recurrent episodes, acyclovir 400 mg PO 3-5x/day, continued until clinical resolution is obtained is recommended
   3. For suppressive therapy, famciclovir 500 mg PO BID has been shown to be effective in decreasing the recurrence rate
   4. For severe cases, patients should be referred for expert care

E. Consult a specialist for management of pregnant women with HSV infection (**Note**: The safety of acyclovir and valacyclovir therapy in pregnant women has not been established)

F. Follow Up: None indicated

HUMAN PAPILLOMAVIRUS INFECTION (GENITAL WARTS)

I. Definition: A sexually transmitted disease caused by certain types of the human papillomavirus (HPV) that produces epithelial tumors of the skin and mucous membranes

II. Pathogenesis

   A. Of the more than 60 HPV types identified in humans, more than 20 infect the lower genital tract

   B. The virus enters the body via an epithelial defect and infects the stratified squamous epithelium of the lower genital tract

   C. Visible genital warts usually are caused by HPV types 6 or 11

   D. Other HPV types in the anogenital region--types 16, 18, and 31--have been strongly associated with cervical dysplasia

III. Clinical Presentation

   A. Most HPV infections are asymptomatic, subclinical, or unrecognized

   B. Genital warts are generally benign growths that cause minor or no symptoms aside from their cosmetic appearance

   C. HPV infections are very common and account for an increasing proportion of primary care gynecologic visits

   D. Clinical HPV infections develop following an incubation period of unknown length but is estimated to range from 3 months to several years

   E. Present as small flesh-colored warty lesions

F.   In males, warts may be found on shaft of penis, penile meatus, scrotum, and perianal areas

G.   In females, warts are seen on labia and perianal areas with asymptomatic nonverrucous infections occurring in the vagina and on the cervix

H.   Most anogenital infections are asymptomatic but can sometimes cause itching, burning, local pain, or bleeding

I.   Individual warts may become confluent and appear as a single, large fleshy lesion

J.   Growth of warts may be stimulated by pregnancy, oral contraceptive use, immunosuppression, and local trauma

IV.   Diagnosis/Evaluation

A.   History
   1.   Question about location, onset, duration, and presence of any associated symptoms
   2.   Inquire about exposures to sexually transmitted diseases (unprotected intercourse)
   3.   Ask if partner has similar lesions
   4.   Inquire about past history of HPV
   5.   Question regarding pregnancy, use of oral contraceptives, and immune status

B.   Physical Examination
   1.   Examine external genitalia and rectal areas for characteristic lesions
   2.   To assist in visualization of warts, apply 3-5% acetic acid to the vulva (women), penis (men) and perianal areas to reveal acetowhitening
   3.   Perform Pap smear in women to detect cervical dysplasia

C.   Differential Diagnosis
   1.   Herpes simplex
   2.   Syphilis

D.   Diagnostic Tests: Most anogenital warts are diagnosed by clinical inspection

V.   Plan/Management

A.   Primary goal of treating visible warts is the removal of symptomatic warts
   1.   Treatment can induce wart-free periods in most patients
   2.   Currently available treatments do not affect the natural history of HPV infection
   3.   Most genital warts are asymptomatic and many warts resolve on their own, when left untreated
   4.   There is no evidence that treatment of visible warts affects development of cervical cancer in women

OVERVIEW OF TREATMENT

Treatment of genital warts should be guided by
> Preference of the patients after they have been informed of the options
> Available resources
> Experience of health care provider

Most patients have 1-10 warts with a total wart area of 0.5-1.0 cm^2
Most warts are responsive to most treatment modalities

Factors that influence selection of treatment

Wart size and number	Patient preference
Anatomic site of wart	Convenience and cost of treatment
Wart morphology	Provider experience

Treatment protocol is important because many patients require a course of therapy rather than a single treatment!
> Treatment modality should be changed if
>> Patient has not improved substantially after 3 provider-administered treatments, OR
>> Warts have not cleared after 6 treatments

Avoid overtreatment!

To increase efficiency and efficacy, providers should be knowledgeable about
> At least one patient-applied treatment
> At least one provider-administered treatment

Note: Most experts believe that combining modalities does not increase efficacy but may increase complications; therefore, it is best to not combine therapies (use two or more modalities on same wart at same time)

Because of the limitations of currently available treatments, some providers employ combination therapy

EXTERNAL GENITAL WARTS: RECOMMENDED TREATMENT

Patient-Applied (Note: for patient-applied treatments, patient must be able to identify and reach warts!)

Podofilox 0.5% solution or gel
Dosing: Apply BID x 3 days, followed by 4 days of no therapy
Repeat cycle as necessary for a total of 4 cycles
Instruction to patient:
Apply solution with cotton swab, gel with finger to visible genital warts
Total wart area treated should be ≤10 cm^2, and total volume of podofilox should be ≤0.5 mL per day
Most patients experience mild/moderate pain or local irritation after treatment
If possible, provider should apply initial treatment to demonstrate proper application technique and identify
> which warts should be treated

Not for use in pregnancy

Imiquimod 5% cream
Dosing: Apply QD at bedtime, 3 times/week for as long as 16 weeks
Instructions to patient:
Apply cream with a finger at bedtime and wash off with mild soap/water after 6-10 hours
Many patients may be clear of warts by 8-10 weeks
Not for use in pregnancy

Provider-Administered

Select **one** of the following
> Cryotherapy with liquid nitrogen or cryoprobe
> Repeat applications Q 1-2 weeks
> Pain after application followed by necrosis and sometimes blistering are common

Note: Major limitation of this modality is that proper use requires substantial training; most warts are overtreated or undertreated by providers who have not been trained resulting in poor efficacy or increased complications

Podophyllin resin 10%-25% in compound tincture of benzoin
Apply small amount to each wart and allow to air dry
Limit application to ≤0.5 mL of podophyllin or ≤10 cm^2 of warts per session
Instruct patient to thoroughly wash preparation off 1-4 hours after application
Repeat weekly if necessary
Not for use in pregnancy

Trichloroacetic acid (TCA) or bichloroacetic acid (BCA) 80%-90%
Apply small amount to warts only
Allow to dry--a white "frosting" develops
Powder with talc or sodium bicarbonate to remove untreated acid (if excess amount was applied)
Repeat weekly if necessary

B. For treatment of cervical and vaginal warts, referral to an expert is recommended

C. For treatment of urethral meatus warts, referral to an expert is recommended

D. For treatment of anal warts, use of cryotherapy with liquid nitrogen or TCA or BCA 80%-90%; apply as directed above under EXTERNAL GENITAL WARTS: RECOMMENDED TREATMENT

E. Management of warts on rectal mucosa should be referred to an expert

F. Subclinical genital HPV infection (without exophytic warts)
1. Subclinical genital HPV infection occurs more frequently than visible warts in both men and women
2. Infection is usually diagnosed via Pap smear, colposcopy, or biopsy of vulva in women, and via biopsy of penis in men. In both men and women, the use of acetic acid soaks and examination of genital skin with light and magnification may be helpful
3. Screening for subclinical genital HPV infection using DNA or RNA tests or acetic acid is not recommended
4. In the absence of coexistent dysplasia, treatment is not recommended for subclinical genital HPV infection diagnosed via Pap smear, colposcopy, biopsy, acetic acid soaking of genital skin/mucous membranes, or DNA/RNA methodologies

G. Management of pregnant women: Refer to specialist

H. Management of sexual partners
1. Examination of partners not necessary because most partners of infected patients probably are already infected subclinically with HPV
2. Partner should be cautioned that patient remains infectious even though warts are gone
3. Use of condoms reduces, but does not eliminate risk of transmission

I. Recommendations relating to cervical cancer screening for women who attend STD clinics or have a history of STDs
1. If woman has not had a Pap smear during previous 12 months, a Pap smear should be obtained as part of the routine pelvic examination
2. Provide woman with printed information about Pap smears and a report containing a statement that a Pap smear was obtained during her clinic visit
3. A copy of the Pap smear result should be provided to the patient for her records
4. **Note:** Women who have a history of STD are at increased risk for cervical cancer
5. Counsel woman about need for an annual Pap smear, and provide her with names of local clinics/providers where Pap smears can be obtained on an annual basis

J. Follow Up
1. After visible warts have cleared (which may require several visits for provider-administered treatments), a follow-up evaluation is not necessary
2. Patient should be advised to watch for recurrences, which occur most often during first 3 months after treatment
3. Women should be reminded of the need for regular cytologic screening (Pap smear) as recommended for women without genital warts [annual screening]

REFERENCES

American Medical Association. (1997). Genital herpes: A clinician's guide to diagnosis and treatment, part I. Chicago: Author.

American Medical Association. (1997). Genital herpes: A clinician's guide to diagnosis and treatment, part II. Chicago: Author.

Baker, D.A. (1997). Diagnosis and treatment of viral STDs in women. International Journal of Fertility, 42 (2), 107-114.

Centers for Disease Control and Prevention. (1998). 1998 guidelines for treatment of sexually transmitted. Morbidity and Mortality Weekly Report, 47(No. RR-1)

Cox, J.T. (1998). HPV testing: Is it useful in triage of minor pap abnormalities? Journal of Family Practice, 46 (2), 121-132.

Dull, P., & Miller, K.E. (1997). STDs in women: An update. Family Practice Recertification, 19 (6), 13-30.

Eschenbach, D.A. (1996). Diagnosis and treatment of vaginitis. In M.A. Stenchever (Ed.). Office gynecology. St. Louis: Mosby.

Faro, S., Apuzzio, J., Bohannon, N., & Elliott, K. (1997). Treatment considertions in vulvovaginal candidiasis. The Female Patient, 22, 21-36.

Hook, E.W., & Marra, C.M. (1992). Acquired syphilis in adults. New England Journal of Medicine, 326(16), 1060-1067.

Mayeaus, E.J., & Spigener, S.S. (1997, Nov). Epidemiology of human papillomarirus infections. Hospital Practice, 39-41.

Mayeaus, E.J., & Spigener, S.S. (1997, Dec). Treatment of human papillomarirus infections. Hospital Practice, 87-90.

Moran, G. (1997, Jan). Diagnosing STDs: Ulcerating diseases. Emergency Medicine, 59-72.

Moran, G. (1997, Feb). Diagnosing and treating STDs: Lesionless disorders. Emergency Medicine, 20-31.

Slade, C.S. (1998, Mar). HPV and cervical cancer: Breaking the deadly link. Advance for Nurse Practitioners, 39-55.

Rosen, T., & Ablon, G. (1997, Aug). Cutaneous herpesvirus infections update. Consultant, 2021-2042.

Verdon, M.E. (1997). Issues in the management of human papillomavirus genital disease. American Family Physician, 55 (5), 1813-1817.

Vincent, M.T., & Adeyele, E. (1998). Are you comfortable taking the sexual history? Family Practice Recertification, 20 (1), 87-101.

Wolner-Hanssen, P. (1996). Acute pelvic inflammatory disease. In M.A. Stenchever (Ed.), Office gynecology. St. Louis: Mosby.

CHAPTER 16

Human Immunodeficiency Virus Infection and Acquired Immunodeficiency Syndrome

Human Immunodeficiency Virus (HIV) Infection and Acquired Immunodeficiency Syndrome (AIDS) in Adults

Health-Care Worker Exposures to Blood and Other Body Fluids That May Contain Human Immunodeficiency Virus (HIV)

HUMAN IMMUNODEFICIENCY VIRUS (HIV) INFECTION AND ACQUIRED IMMUNODEFICIENCY SYNDROME (AIDS) IN ADULTS

I. Definitions:

    A.   HIV infection: Infection with human retrovirus, Human Immunodeficiency Virus (HIV)

    B.   AIDS: Disease characterized by opportunistic infections (see following table for case definition of AIDS)

CONDITIONS INCLUDED IN THE 1993 AIDS SURVEILLANCE CASE DEFINITION

- HIV+ persons with CD4 cells counts <200/μL or a CD4 percent <14%*
- Candidiasis of bronchi, trachea, or lungs
- Candidiasis, esophageal
- Cervical cancer, invasive*
- Coccidioidomycosis, disseminated or extrapulmonary
- Cryptococcosis, extrapulmonary
- Cryptosporidiosis, chronic intestinal (>1 mo duration)
- Cytomegalovirus disease (other than liver, spleen, or nodes)
- Encephalopathy, HIV-related
- Herpes simplex: Chronic ulcer(s) (>1 mo duration); or bronchitis, pneumonitis, or esophagitis
- Histoplasmosis, disseminated or extrapulmonary
- Isosporiasis, chronic intestinal (>1 mo duration)
- Kaposi's sarcoma
- Lymphoma, Burkitt's (or equivalent term)
- Lymphoma, immunoblastic (or equivalent term)
- Lymphoma, primary, of brain
- *Mycobacterium avium* complex or *M. kansasii*, disseminated or extrapulmonary
- *Mycobacterium tuberculosis*, any site (pulmonary* or extrapulmonary)
- *Mycobacterium*, other species or unidentified species, disseminated or extrapulmonary
- *Pneumocystis carinii* pneumonia
- Pneumonia, recurrent*
- Progressive multifocal leukoencephalopathy
- *Salmonella* septicemia, recurrent
- Toxoplasmosis of brain
- Wasting syndrome due to HIV

*Added January 1993

Source: Center for Communicable Diseases. 1992. 1993 revised classification system for HIV infection and expanded surveillance case definition of AIDS among adolescents and adults. MMWR, 41 (RR-17).

II. Pathogenesis

    A.   HIV invades the body and may enter any cell, but it has a propensity to infect and kill cells of the immune system, particularly the CD4+ T-cells (T-lymphocytes)

    B.   HIV actively replicates which leads to immune system damage and results in susceptibility to opportunistic infections (OIs), cancer, neurologic diseases, wasting, and death

C. Transmission occurs by direct contact of a person's blood or body secretions with the blood or body secretions of a person infected with HIV virus
  1. Body fluids considered to be infectious include blood, tissues, cerebrospinal fluid, synovial fluid, peritoneal fluid, pleural fluid, pericardial fluid, amniotic fluid, semen and vaginal secretions
  2. Body fluids that are **not** considered infectious include feces, nasal secretions, sputum, sweat, tears, urine, vomitus and saliva (unless contaminated with blood)
  3. Certain activities are associated with high risk of infection such as unprotected anal, oral, or vaginal sex with multiple partners; unprotected sex with an HIV positive person; IV drug abuse; blood transfusions outside the U.S. or during 1977-1985; unprotected sex with a person who has recent or past history of sexually transmitted diseases
  4. Highest percentage of HIV transmissions occurs during sex acts where body fluids are exchanged
  5. IV drug use is the second most frequent route of transmission

III. Clinical Presentation

A. Epidemiology
  1. The first AIDS cases were reported in 1981
  2. Seroprevalence of HIV in U.S. is 0.3%
  3. Highly active antiretroviral therapy (HAART) has revolutionized HIV care
    a. In late 1995 and early 1996, introduction of 3TC, non-nucleoside reverse transcriptase inhibitors and protease inhibitors brought a new wave of hope that there would be chronic nonprogressors
      (1) To date, however, there are no cures
      (2) Studies show that these new drugs (i.e., protease inhibitors) have potent activity in most recipients for up to 1-2 years, but there are few studies to confirm long-term benefits
    b. During transition period from late 1995 through 1997, there has been a 60-80% decline in AIDS-defining complications, a 60-80% decrease in the number of hospitalizations, and a 44% decrease in mortality rate
  4. White men who had sex with men had the largest proportional decline in AIDS incidence
  5. Incidence of AIDS has proportionately increased among black men, Hispanic men, and black women with heterosexual exposures
  6. In U.S., there is growing incidence of AIDS in persons older than 50 years; older persons are often diagnosed late in the course of their disease and progress more rapidly
  7. HIV infection is no longer the leading cause of death in individuals between the ages of 25 and 44 in U.S.

B. Viral load and CD4+ T-cell counts help to assess the prognosis of HIV-infected patients
  1. Viral load measures the level of circulating plasma HIV-RNA
    a. Viral load is the most powerful predictor of progression to AIDS and death
    b. The greater the number of virus, the more active the infection and the worse the prognosis
  2. CD4+ T-cell counts are obtained to assess the general level of immunity or the extent of HIV-induced immune damage already suffered; the lower the CD4+ T-count the greater the risk for opportunistic infections
  3. A decrease in viral load of one log is associated with an average increase in CD4+ T-cells of about 85/mm^3

C. The natural history of HIV infection encompasses a wide spectrum of disease
  1. There is great variability in the progression of the disease among individuals
  2. Infection with HIV is always harmful; true long-term survival free of major immune damage is uncommon

D. The acute retroviral syndrome develops after HIV exposure and a 1-3 week incubation period
   1. Symptoms resemble those of infectious mononucleosis or influenza and are usually self-limited
      a. Fever, fatigue, lymphadenopathy, pharyngitis, and arthralgias are typical
      b. Rash, diarrhea, nausea, vomiting, hepatosplenomegaly, thrush, weight loss, and neurological are less common problems
   2. Syndrome is accompanied with rapid HIV replication or high viral load
   3. Recovery is usually in 1-3 weeks
   4. There is a sharp decrease in viral replication after recovery; however, replication is probably continuing in various tissues such as the lymphatic tissue and the central nervous system even though it can no longer be detected by blood tests

E. Early HIV disease: period between seroconversion to 4 months following HIV transmission
   1. Approximately at 4 months, the plasma levels of HIV RNA reach a set point that shows a very gradual increase averaging 7% a year over several years in the absence of antigenic stimuli such as intercurrent illness or immunizations or antiretroviral therapy
   2. This set point predicts the subsequent rate of progression
      a. High concentrations (>100,000 copies/mL) are associated with median survival of 4.4 years
      b. Low concentrations (<5,000 copies/mL) are associated with median survival exceeding 10 years
   3. Symptoms occurring early in the course of disease include the following:
      a. Lymphadenopathy and dermatologic abnormalities (seborrheic dermatitis, psoriasis, eosinophilic folliculitis)
      b. Oral lesions such as aphthous ulcers, herpes simplex labialis, and oral hairy leukoplakia usually occur later but may present
   4. As the disease progresses, patients have more frequent skin disorders, oral lesions, and infections as well as the following symptoms: recurrent diarrhea, intermittent fevers, night sweats, chills, unexplained weight loss, myalgias, arthralgia, headache and fatigue

F. Symptomatic HIV disease: complications are due to direct effects of the virus or to immunosuppression which occurs after a significant quantity of CD4+ T-cells has been destroyed
   1. Direct effect of HIV: persistent generalized lymphadenopathy, HIV-associated dementia, lymphocytic interstitial pneumonia, HIV-associated nephropathy, and progressive immunosuppression; other possible consequences are anemia, neutropenia, thrombocytopenia, cardiomyopathy, myopathy, peripheral neuropathy, chronic meningitis, polymyositis, and Guillain-Barré syndrome
   2. Immunosuppression results in opportunistic infections and tumors, primarily from compromised cell-mediated immunity (see tables in V.E.1.2.3.4 for further clinical presentation of opportunistic infections)
   3. Only about 2% or less of HIV-infected patients can maintain CD4+ T-cell counts in the normal range for lengthy periods of time (>12 years) without antiretroviral therapy
   4. In untreated patients, CD4+ T-cells average a 40-60/mm^3 decrease per year
   5. Opportunistic infections, particularly pneumocystic pneumonia, may occur when CD4+ T-cell counts fall below 200/mm^3
   6. Risk for opportunistic infections increases dramatically as CD4+ T-cell counts drop below 50/mm^3 (see tables in V.E.1.2.3.4 for further clinical presentation of opportunistic infections)

IV. Diagnosis/Evaluation

A. History
   1. Determine risk factors for HIV; because a recent study found that many primary health care providers are missing opportunities to identify and test persons at high risk for HIV infection, the following questions may be helpful (see following table)

30-SECOND ROUTINE ASSESSMENT TO IDENTIFY PATIENTS AT RISK FOR HIV INFECTION

* Did you receive transfusion of blood products outside the U.S. or between 1977 and 1985?
* Have you ever, even once, used any kind of injected drugs?
* For men: Have you ever, even once, had sex with a man, a prostitute, or with someone who has used injected drugs?
* For women: Have you any reason to suspect that you have had sex with a bisexual man or one who has used injected drugs?
* Do you have any reason to suspect you might be at risk for AIDS or HIV infection?
* Do you want to be tested for HIV infection?

2. History at initial visit after the diagnosis is confirmed; at this initial visit the patient's health status may range from asymptomatic to advanced immunodeficiency; this first encounter sets the stage for a partnership with the patient that may last for years
   a. Explore the duration of HIV positivity as well as when and how the patient was infected
   b. Document when the patient was first diagnosed with HIV infection
   c. Inquire about testing (when and where was it done?; what led to testing?)
   d. Ask about results of prior diagnostic tests
   e. Inquire about prior treatments and responses to treatment
   f. Obtain past risk history (see preceding table) including a detailed sexual history such as number of partners within last year, use of condoms, and history of other sexually transmitted diseases
   g. Determine immunization status (pneumovax, flu vaccine, tetanus, hepatitis B, varicella)
   h. Document significant past medical history (opportunistic infections, hospitalizations, chicken pox, and other chronic diseases, particularly tuberculosis, hepatitis, shingles)
   i. In women, obtain a gynecological history including current menstrual pattern, date of last pelvic exam and pap smear, history of abnormal pap smear, and history of vaginal bleeding
   j. Inquire about travel to Ohio and Mississippi River Valleys (risk of histoplasmosis) and to Southwestern desert (risk of coccidioidomycosis)
   k. Assess patient's and family's knowledge about HIV
   l. Obtain a detailed social and mental health history to determine psychosocial assets and needs
   m. Screen for domestic violence (see section on DOMESTIC VIOLENCE for recommended questions)
   n. Perform an HIV-related review of systems (ROS) directed toward uncovering symptoms of infection (fevers, night sweats, weight change, lymphadenopathy, skin changes, new headaches, memory problems, mouth lesions, difficulty swallowing, cough/chest pain, diarrhea, nausea, vomiting, vaginitis, peripheral neuropathy)
3. History on subsequent visits
   a. Document most recent CD4+ T-cell count and HIV viral load
   b. Document medications used for treating HIV infection
      (1) Inquire about adverse effects from medications
      (2) Always ask about adherence; a simple, direct question such as "How many doses have you missed in the past 24 hours?" may be nonthreatening
   c. Inquire about new or worsening symptoms
   d. Perform an HIV-related ROS (see IV.A.2.n.)

B. Physical Examination
   1. Vital signs (fever is a sign of opportunistic infections and neoplasms)
   2. Measure weight (important in detecting "wasting syndrome" and determining the type of dietary intervention that is needed)
   3. Observe general appearance, noting signs of distress and depression
   4. Examine skin for lesions, ecchymosis, and signs of dehydration
   5. Perform ophthalmological exam including a fundoscopic exam for retinopathy
   6. Examine mouth, noting thrush, hairy oral leukoplakia, herpes simplex, peridontal problems, ulcerations

7. Palpate for lymphadenopathy as generalized lymphadenopathy is frequently present; localized lymphadenopathy may indicate carcinoma
8. Perform pulmonary and cardiac exam for pneumonia and cardiomyopathy
9. Perform examination of abdomen, noting organomegaly
10. Examine anal area for detection of sexually transmitted diseases, ulcerations, and fissures
11. Perform pelvic and speculum exam on women for cervical dysplasia, vaginal candidiasis, and sexually transmitted diseases; perform a complete genitourinary examination on men
12. Perform complete neurologic exam, including testing of cranial nerves, cerebellar function, reflexes, sensory function, and mental status for dementia and neuropathy
13. Perform a psychiatric examination

C. Diagnostic tests
1. Methods to **determine the diagnosis of HIV**
   a. Typically, the diagnosis is made with antibody testing using enzyme-linked immunoabsorbent assay (ELISA) and a Western blot (both tests must be positive to confirm the diagnosis)
      (1) ELISA is the initial test; it is sensitive but not highly specific (may have false positives)
      (2) Either a Western blot (WB) or an immunofluorescence assay (IFA) is used for confirmation of positive ELISA tests; WB and IFA are specific but labor intensive
      (3) Testing should be preceded by pretest counseling
      (4) Test results are usually available in 1-3 weeks and should be given in person with posttest counseling
   b. Other tests for detection of antibodies
      (1) FDA approved HIV ELISA and Western Blot urine tests are available but they are less accurate and cause more false positive results than serum tests
      (2) Orasure HIV-1 can detect antibodies from a sample of oral mucosal transudate
      (3) Home Access is an anonymous, finger-stick blood test for antibodies which can be done by an individual at home and purchased over-the-counter
   c. Rapid tests
      (1) Three FDA approved rapid tests are SUDS, Recombigen latex agglutination assay, Genie HIV-1
      (2) Results are available within 10 minutes
      (3) Advantageous in settings in which there are occupational exposures to health care workers and where reliable follow-up is unlikely such as in emergency rooms and STD clinics
   d. Persons with positive antibody tests are considered HIV seropositive; however, a negative antibody test does not guarantee that an individual is seronegative
      (1) A window period exists: it may take 1-3 months after HIV exposure for antibodies to form in sufficient amounts to be detectable by antibody tests
      (2) Because of this window period, it is recommended that persons with initial negative antibody tests and low risks have retesting at 6 months and high risk persons have repeat testing at 6 months and 1 year
2. **Antigen tests** are expensive, but can directly detect the virus
   a. Nucleic acid testing can detect the presence of HIV and is used for patients suspected of having acute retroviral syndrome which occurs before antibody tests become positive
   b. HIV blood culture is labor intensive and reliability is low
   c. p24 antigen can identify the presence of the HIV protein, but cannot quantify the amount of HIV
   d. RNA polymerase chain reaction (PCR) and branched DNA (bDNA) assay can measure the amount of HIV RNA in the plasma of infected persons

3. **Tests to monitor disease progress**
   a. RNA PCR or bDNA assay (viral load) is the most important test to order when making decisions to initiate and change antiretroviral drug therapy; order at the following times:
      (1) At time of diagnosis and then every 3-4 months in untreated patients
      (2) Immediately prior to and again at 4-8 weeks after initiating or changing antiretroviral drug therapy (ideally viral loads should be ordered on two occasions before beginning or altering drugs)
      (3) Once patient is stable, order every 3-4 months
      (4) Do not measure viral load during or within 4 weeks after successful treatment of any intercurrent infection, resolution or symptomatic illness, or immunization because of the immune activation of virus associated with these events
      (5) "Third generation" assays or ultra sensitive RNA PCR will detect HIV RNA at a threshold of 20-50 copies/mL
   b. Measurement of CD4+ T-cell counts, CD8 and CD4/CD8 ratio are the primary tests for monitoring immune function
      (1) Determine stage of HIV infection, prognosis of disease, and need for prophylaxis of opportunistic infections; these tests play a secondary role in helping providers determine when to initiate and change drug therapy (viral loads are the essential test in decisions concerning drug therapy)
      (2) Changes >50% (0.3 log) are considered significant
      (3) Order at time of diagnosis and generally every 3-6 months thereafter

4. **Tests to screen for concomitant diseases, immunity status and as a base-line before drugs are administered;** ordered at first visit after diagnosis is confirmed
   a. Mantoux method using the purified protein derivative (PPD) to screen for tuberculosis (anergy testing is no longer recommended); positive PPD for person with HIV is >5 mm of induration
   b. Rapid plasma reagin (RPR) or the Venereal Disease Laboratories (VDRL) to screen for syphilis which occurs in approximately 20% of patients with HIV infection; for patients with high-risk of developing STDs order annually
   c. Pap smear for women to screen for cervical dysplasia; perform every 6-12 months
   d. Typically the following additional tests are recommended:
      (1) Chemistry panel including liver function tests and renal profile: useful as a baseline since patient may be receiving drugs with potential hepatic or renal toxicity
      (2) Hepatitis B serology (HbsAg) to determine hepatitis immunity and need for vaccination as well as to detect hepatitis B infection which is common in HIV infected patients
      (3) Hepatitis C serology to detect infection, particularly important in patients who are/were IV drug users and those with liver function abnormalities
      (4) Toxoplasmosis serology (anti-toxoplasma antibody or IgG titer)
         (a) Patient is at risk for reactivation toxoplasmosis when CD4+ T-cells drop below 100/mm^3
         (b) Consider repeating in seronegative patients when their CD4+ T-cell is <100/mm^3
      (5) Cytomegalovirus (CMV) IgG; CMV retinitis is a common complication and develops in seropositive patients when CD4+ T-cell drops below 50-75/mm^3
      (6) Glucose-6-phosphate dehydrogenase deficiency (G-6-PD): If test is positive, patient has a deficiency and should not be prescribed dapsone and possibly should not be given a sulfonamide
      (7) Varicella IgG to determine need for post-exposure prophylaxis with varicella zoster immune globulin
      (8) CBC with differential and platelet count; anemia, leukopenia, or thrombocytopenia are common in HIV infection and can also result from drug therapy
      (9) Chest x-ray to screen for latent TB and as a baseline

5. **New monitoring tests** that are being developed
   a. Resistance testing is available but not currently recommended for routine clinical practice
   b. CD4+ cell subset determinations to enumerate memory and naive cells are used in clinical trials to help define the degree of immune reconstitution
   c. Therapeutic drug level monitoring is available but is not recommended at this time

V. Plan/Management (care should be supervised by infectious disease specialist); because treatment of HIV infection changes rapidly consult following websites for updated information: CDC Clearinghouse (http://www.cdc.org) and the HIV Information Network (http://www.hivatis.org)

A. Provide **patient education and counseling** at each visit; adjust amount and complexity of teaching and counseling based on patient's degree of stress, prior knowledge, readiness to learn, and cognitive abilities
   1. Provide information about transmission and how to prevent spread of infection such as not sharing razors or toothbrushes, carefully cleaning up blood spills, disposing of used feminine sanitary products
   2. Discuss ways to handle notification of partners and others; the local health department can assist with anonymous partner notification/elicitation
   3. Discuss lifestyle choices and safe sex practices such as latex barriers including condoms and female vaginal pouches
      a. Even patients with undetectable viral loads should be considered infectious and should practice safe sex
      b. HIV infected males should wear condoms even when engaging in sexual activity with other HIV infected individuals to prevent transmission of drug-resistant strains of HIV and other sexually transmitted diseases
   4. Discuss healthy diet; referral to nutritionist is beneficial
      a. Recommend eating a variety of foods from different food groups
      b. Encourage nutrient density or making every bite of food count; avoid foods with little protein, vitamins, and minerals
      c. Choose foods that are close to their natural states as possible; use whole wheat instead of white bread or brown rice instead of white
      d. Use olive and canola oils instead of margarine and vegetable oils which are rich in polyunsaturated fatty acids and may suppress the immune system
      e. One or two daily multivitamin/mineral supplement(s) is(are) recommended
   5. Encourage smoking cessation and decreasing or eliminating other types of substance abuse (alcohol, recreational drugs)
   6. Teach about food safety
      a. Foods should be well done and thoroughly cooked; avoid raw/rare meat, fish and poultry, raw eggs, or unpasteurized dairy products
      b. Wash hands after contact with raw meat
      c. Wash fruits and vegetables before eating
      d. Consider using filtered or bottled water
   7. Recommend that patient wash hands after gardening or other contact with soil; avoid changing cat liter box due to risk of toxoplasmosis; avoid rough play with kittens due to risk of cat scratch disease
   8. Reinforce the importance of good oral hygiene
   9. Discuss susceptibility to contagious disease and how to protect self
   10. Discuss ways to improve sleep habits and receive sufficient rest
   11. Explore stress levels, and recommend stress reduction interventions such as exercise, relaxation techniques, and guided imagery; massage therapy and referral to a psychologist may be beneficial
   12. Provide information on available community services
   13. Listen to fears and concerns and provide social support
   14. Provide information on prognosis and future therapy plans
   15. Discuss what to do if an emergency arises and which symptoms require immediate attention
   16. Help empower patients to become actively involved in their care through support groups, learning about the disease and treatments, and developing a partnership with the health care provider
   17. For patients in the late stage of disease offer information on advance directives; discuss living wills, health care surrogates; consider referral for home care or hospice care

B. **Immunization** recommendations
1. Administer annual influenza vaccine to all patients with CD4+ T-cell counts >100/mm^3 who are on effective antiretrovirals
2. Administer pneumococcal (Pneumovax) vaccine, 05 mL IM X 1
3. *Haemophilus influenzae* type B vaccine is no longer recommended as most infections in HIV-infected persons involve nontypable strains
4. Consider Hepatitis B vaccine (series of 3) in all susceptible persons (anti-HB$_c$-negative), especially if patient is continuing to share needles or having unsafe sex
5. Tetanus-diphtheria, mumps, rubella, measles identical to patients without HIV
6. If polio vaccine is needed, use enhanced inactivated polio vaccine (eIPV)
7. Do **not** use any of the following vaccines: Live polio, varicella zoster, BCG, or any live or attenuated vaccine except measles, mumps, and rubella

C. **Health maintenance referrals**
1. Schedule twice-yearly dental examinations
2. Periodic ophthalmology examinations are recommended; screening for CMV retinitis by a trained ophthalmologist or optometrist is recommended every 4-6 months once the patient's CD4+ T-cell count falls below 75/mm^3

D. Medications should be given to **prevent opportunistic infections** when a person's CD4+ T-cell counts fall to certain levels or after exposure to certain pathogens (see following table)

PREVENTION OF OPPORTUNISTIC DISEASE IN HIV-INFECTED ADULTS AND ADOLESCENTS

Pathogen	Indication	Preventive regimens	
		First Choice	Alternatives
I. Strongly recommended as standard of care			
Pneumocystis carinii	CD4+ count <200/μL or prior PCP or oropharyngeal candidiasis or unexplained fever ≥2 weeks	Trimethoprim-sulfamethoxazole (TMP-SMZ), 1 DS PO QD; TMP-SMZ, 1 SS PO Q.D.	TMP-SMV, DS PO three times a week; dapsone, 50 mg PO BID or 100 mg PO QD or aerosolized pentamidine, 300 mg every month via Respirgard II™ nebulizer
Mycobacterium tuberculosis	PPD reaction ≥5 mm or prior positive PPD result without treatment or contact with case of active tuberculosis	Isoniazid, 300 mg PO plus pyridoxine, 50 mg PO QD x 12 mo or isoniazid, 900 mg PO plus pyridoxine, 50 mg PO twice a week x 12 mo	Rifampin, 600 mg PO QD x 12 mo
Toxoplasma gondii	IgG antibody to *Toxoplasma* and CD4+ count <100/μL	TMP-SMZ, 1 DS PO QD	TMP-SMZ, 1 SS PO QD; dapsone, 50 mg PO QD plus pyrimethamine, 50 mg PO QW plus leucovorin, 25 mg PO QW
Mycobacterium avium complex	CD4+ count <50μL	Clarithromycin, 500 mg PO BID or azithromycin, 1,200 mg PO QW	Rifabutin, 300 mg PO QD
Varicella zoster virus (VZV)	Significant exposure to chickenpox or shingles for patients who have no history of either condition or, if available, negative antibody to VZV	Varicella zoster immune globulin (VZIG), 5 vials (1.25 mL each) IM administered ≤96 h after exposure, ideally within 48 h	Acyclovir, 800 mg PO 5 times/d for 3 weeks
II. Not recommended for most patients; indicated for use only in unusual circumstances			
Candida species	CD4+ count <50/μL	Fluconazole, 100-200 mg PO QD	
Cryptococcus neoformans	CD4+ count <50/μL	Fluconazole, 100-200 mg PO QD	Itraconazole, 200 mg PO QD
Cytomegalovirus (CMV)	CD4+ count <50/μL and CMV antibody positivity	Oral ganciclovir, 1 g po TID	None

Adapted from U.S. Department of Health and Human Services. (1997). 1997 USPHS/IDSA guidelines for the prevention of opportunistic infections in persons infected with human immunodeficiency virus. MMWR, 46(RR-12), 1-46

E. It is important to recognize the signs and symptoms of **opportunistic diseases** and to diagnose and treat appropriately and then provide prophylaxis to prevent recurrences (see V.F. for prevention of recurrences)

  1. See following table for diagnosis and treatment of bacterial infections

ASSESSMENT, DIAGNOSIS, AND TREATMENT OF COMMON BACTERIAL OPPORTUNISTIC INFECTIONS			
Transmission	**Clinical Characteristics**	**Diagnosis**	**Treatment**
Mycobacterium Avium Intracellulare (MAI) or M. Avium Complex Infections			
Widely dispersed in environment and found in most water supplies	Diarrhea, abdominal pain, organomegaly, high fevers, weight loss, fatigue, enlarged nodes, elevated alkaline phosphatase	Cultures of blood, stool, or bone marrow; Lymph node and liver biopsy	Clarithromycin 500 mg BID **plus** ethambutol 15-25 mg/kg/day ± rifabutin 300 mg/day or ciprofloxacin 500-750 mg BID; Alternatively, substitute azithromycin 500 mg QD for clarithromycin
Mycobacterium Tuberculosis			
Spread through droplet nuclei coughed up by persons with untreated TB	Productive, prolonged cough; fever, chills, night sweats, fatigue, weight loss, hemoptysis, lymphadenopathy	PPD skin test, chest x-ray, sputum smear and culture	**PPD but no active disease:** Isoniazid (INH)* 300 mg QD x 12 months **Active disease: 12 months treatment;** INH*, Rifampin, Pyrazinamide, & Ethambutol for 8 weeks; then INH & Rifampin
Syphilis			
Caused by *Treponema pallidium*; Sexually transmitted disease	Primary: chancre Secondary: Rash on palms and soles Tertiary: No outward signs Neurosyphilis: CNS problems	RPR or VDRL and then FTA-ABS and a lumbar puncture	If VDRL is ≥1:32 **and** CSF VDRL is negative: 2.4 million units Bicillin q week x 3 weeks; If VDRL is ≥1:32 and CSF VDRL is positive: 3.5 million units Penicillin G IV q 4 hrs. x 10 days followed by 2.4 million units of Bicillin q week x 3 weeks

*If on INH, give pyridoxine 50 mg/day

  2. See following table for diagnosis and treatment of fungal infections

ASSESSMENT, DIAGNOSIS, AND TREATMENT OF COMMON FUNGAL OPPORTUNISTIC INFECTIONS			
Transmission	**Clinical Characteristics**	**Diagnosis**	**Treatment**
Candidiasis			
Caused by *candida albicans* when CD4+ T-cells drop below 500/mm³	Oral: White plaques anywhere in oral cavity, burning sensation, absence of taste, pain when swallowing	Swab lesion: KOH prep	Clotrimazole 10 mg troches; dissolve in saliva, 1 troche 5 times daily for 14 days; Fluconazole 100 mg PO QD for 7-14 days
	Vaginal: Thick white vaginal discharge; itching, burning, redness in vaginal area	Swab vagina: KOH prep	Terconazole vaginal suppositories: 1 suppository HS X 3 nights; Fluconazole 150 mg tab. PO single dose
Cryptococcal Meningitis			
Yeast-like fungus found widely in environment, especially in soil contaminated with bird excrement	Fever, headache, fatigue, nausea, memory loss, confusion, problems with coordination	Cryptococcal serum antigen; Lumbar puncture: India ink, cryptococcal antigen, culture	Amphotericin B 0.7 mg/kg/day IV X 10-14 days or Fluconazole 400 mg/day for 8-10 weeks; Lifelong suppressive therapy with 200 mg/day

3. See following table for diagnosis and treatment of protozoal infections:

ASSESSMENT, DIAGNOSIS, AND TREATMENT OF COMMON PROTOZOAL OPPORTUNISTIC INFECTIONS

Transmission	Clinical Characteristics	Diagnosis	Treatment
Pneumocystis Carinii Pneumonia (PCP)			
Believed to infect most humans during childhood, and then remains dormant	Dry, non-productive cough; shortness of breath, fever, fatigue, weight loss	Chest X-ray; Induced sputum; Broncho-alveolar lavage	Mild-Moderate Disease TMP/SMX* PO 15 mg/kg, TMP equivalent in 4 divided doses times PO of IV 21 days (usually 2 DS tabs TID); TMP 5 mg/kg PO q 6 hours plus Dapsone 100 mg/day times 21 days for sulfa allergy Severe Disease:TMP/SMX 15 mg/kg TMP equivalent/day in 4 divided doses for 21 days with prednisone
Toxoplasmic Encephalitis			
30% U.S. adults infected with parasite which remains dormant until immune system is damaged	Fever, headache, neurological problems such as seizures, changes in mental status, coma	CT scan or MRI of brain for ring enhancing lesions; Positive toxoplasma IgG in serum	Pyrimethamine 100-200 mg QD PO then 50-75 mg QD with sulfadiazine 4-8 g PO QD plus folinic acid 10-20 mg PO QD for 6 weeks
Cryptosporidiosis			
Transmitted to humans via contact with feces, contaminated water or food	Chronic watery diarrhea, abdominal cramps, nausea, fever, weight loss, headache	Modified acid fast stain of stool; endoscopy with biopsy or bowel biopsy	Treatment is difficult - refer to specialist; sometimes Paromomycin 500 mg PO QID with food X 14-28 days then 500 mg BID may be effective

*Trimethoprim/sulfamethoxazole

4. See following table for diagnosis and treatment of viral infections:

ASSESSMENT, DIAGNOSIS, AND TREATMENT OF COMMON VIRAL OPPORTUNISTIC INFECTIONS

Transmission	Clinical Characteristics	Diagnosis	Treatment
Cytomegalovirus Retinitis			
High percentage of US adults are infected with virus which remains dormant until immune system is damaged	Cytomegalovirus may infect GI tract, brain, and other organs but common site is the eye with blurred vision, floaters, flashing lights, loss of peripheral vision, area of vision that is missing	Diagnosis made with indirect fundoscopy by a trained ophthalmologist	Need chronic IV therapy or ocular implant plus oral therapy with ganciclovir or foscarnet (refer to specialist)
Oral Hairy Leukoplakia			
Caused by Epstein-Barr virus	White, non-removable lesion with a corrugated surface on lateral margins of tongue	Clinical presentation	None usually needed; may treat with acyclovir 400 mg PO QID
Progressive Multifocal Leukoencephalopathy (PML)			
Caused by J. C. virus; most people are infected by 2 years of age, but virus remains latent in brain until immune system is sufficiently damaged	Insidious onset with rapid progression; confusion, lack of energy, loss of balance, memory and speech problems, blurred or double vision, hallucinations, seizures, paralysis and eventual death	CT scan or MRI which may reveal focal brain lesions which do not enhance or cause surrounding edema	Refer to specialist; no universally accepted treatment
Herpes Simplex, Herpes Zoster, and Molluscum Contagiosum (see Chapter 7, SKIN PROBLEMS)			

5. See following table for diagnosis and treatment of cancers:

ASSESSMENT, DIAGNOSIS, AND TREATMENT OF CANCERS ASSOCIATED WITH HIV INFECTION

Transmission	Clinical Characteristics	Diagnosis	Treatment
Kaposi's Sarcoma			
May be sexually transmitted and is caused by herpes virus, HHV-8	Red, brown or pink blotches on skin which change to hard, raised purplish-red lesions; can be on internal organs as well as common places of arms, legs, and chest	Visual examination or skin biopsy	Referral to specialist, sometimes left untreated or can remove with alpha interferon, radiation, chemotherapy
Lymphomas			
Cancers of lymphoid cells; B-cell non-Hodgkin's lymphoma is most common	Spreads quickly, occurs in brain and outside of the lymph nodes	Depending on site; biopsy or CT/MRI	Refer to specialist

F. Patients who have a history of opportunistic diseases should be administered chemoprophylaxis to prevent recurrence (see following table)

PROPHYLAXIS FOR RECURRENCE OF OPPORTUNISTIC DISEASE (AFTER CHEMOTHERAPY FOR ACUTE DISEASE) IN HIV-INFECTED ADULTS AND ADOLESCENTS

Pathogen	Indication	Preventive regimens	
		First choice	Alternatives
I. Recommended for life as standard of care			
Pneumocystis carinii	Prior *P. carinii* pneumonia	Trimethoprim-sulfamethoxazole (TMP-SMZ), 1 DS PO QD TMP-SMZ 1 SS PO QD	TMP-SMZ DS PO three times a week; dapsone, 50 mg PO BID or 100 mg PO QD; aerosolized pentamidine, 300 mg QM via Respirgard II™ nebulizer
Toxoplasma gondii	Prior toxoplasmic encephalitis	Sulfadiazine 500-1000 mg PO QID plus pyrimethamine 25-75 mg PO QD plus leucovorin 10 mg PO QD	Clindamycin, 300-450 mg PO Q 6-8 h plus pyrimethamine, 25-75 mg PO QD plus leucovorin, 10-25 mg PO QD-QID
Mycobacterium avium complex	Documented disseminated disease	Clarithromycin, 500 mg PO BID plus one or more of the following: ethambutol, 15 mg/kg PO QD; rifabutin, 300 mg PO QD	Azithromycin, 500 mg PO QD plus one or more of the following: ethambutol, 15 mg/kg PO QD; rifabutin, 300 mg PO QD
Cytomegalovirus	Prior end-organ disease	Ganciclovir, 5-6 mg/kg IV 5-7 days/wk or 1,000 mg PO TID or foscarnet, 90-120 mg/kg IV QD; or cidofovir 5 mg/kg every other week; or (for retinitis) ganciclovir sustaned-release implant every 6-9 months	
Cryptococcus neoformans	Documented disease	Fluconazole, 200 mg PO QD	Amphotericin B, 0.6-1.0 mg/kg IV QW-TIW; itraconazole, 200 mg PO QD
II. Recommended only if subsequent episodes are frequent or severe			
Herpes simplex virus	Frequent/severe recurrences	Acyclovir, 200 mg PO TID or 400 mg PO BID	
Candida (oral, vaginal, or esophageal)	Frequent/severe recurrences	Fluconazole, 100-200 mg PO QD	Ketoconazole, 200 mg PO QD; itraconazole, 200 mg PO QD

Adapted from Center for Disease Control. (1997). 1997 USPHS/IDSA guidelines for the prevention of opportunistic infections in persons infected with Human Immunodeficiency Virus. MMWR, 46, 1-46.

G.   Summary of the **principles of antiretroviral drug therapy** of HIV infection (see following table)

PRINCIPLES OF THERAPY
1. Because rates of disease progression vary among patients, treatment decisions must be individualized by level of risk indicated by viral loads and CD4+ T-cell levels
2. Maximum achievable suppression of HIV replication is the goal of drug therapy
3. Simultaneous initiation of combinations of effective anti-HIV drugs that the patient has not previously received and that are not cross-resistant with antiretroviral agents that the patient has previously received is the most effective method to achieve durable suppression of HIV replication
4. Drug monotherapy is **NOT** a recommended option as it presents risk for development of drug resistance and potential development of cross-resistance to related drugs
5. Each antiretroviral drug should be used according to optimum schedules and dosages
6. Any change in antiretroviral therapy increases future therapeutic constraints
7. Women need optimal antiretroviral therapy regardless of pregnancy status
8. Patient adherence is extremely important as intermittent use leads to resistance; emphasize that patient should not stop any medications without consulting health care provider

Adapted from NIH Panel To Define Principles of Therapy of HIV Infection. (1998). Report of the NIH Panel To Define Principles of Therapy of HIV Infection. Annals of Internal Medicine, 128, 1057-1078

H.   **Initiating antiretroviral therapy** (see V.H 2. & 4. for discussion of combination therapies; see K.L. & M. for discussion of specific drug classifications and agents)
   1.   Criteria of when to offer antiretroviral therapy to patients
      a.   In asymptomatic patients begin therapy when CD4+ T-cell counts are <500/mm^3 or plasma HIV RNA levels are > 5,000-10,000 copies/mL (bDNA) or >10,000-20,000 copies/mL (RT-PCR)
         (1)   Some experts recommend treating all patients who have a detectable viral loads, particularly if the patient has a concomitant pattern of declining CD4+ T-cells
         (2)   Treatment decisions for asymptomatic patients should also be based on patient's willingness to begin a complicated regimen, likelihood of adherence, and benefits/risks of early initiation (see following table)
      b.   Symptomatic patients should be treated regardless of laboratory values

BENEFITS AND RISKS OF EARLY INITIATION OF ANTIRETROVIRAL THERAPY		
Potential Benefits:	Control of viral replication and mutation Prevention of progression of immunodeficiency Delayed progression to AIDS	Decreased risk for selection of resistant virus Decreased risk for drug toxicity
Potential Risks:	Reduction in quality of life from adverse drug effects Inconvenience of drug administration Earlier development of drug resistance Limitation of future choices of antiretroviral agents Unknown long-term toxicity of drugs Unknown duration of effectiveness of current antiretroviral agents	

Adapted from NIH Panel to Define Principles of Therapy of HIV Infection. (1998). Guidelines for the use of antiretroviral agents in HIV-infected adults and adolescents. Annals of Internal Medicine, 128, 1079-1100

   2.   Initiating therapy with a naive patient (patient who has never been on antiretroviral medications):
      a.   Begin with 2 nucleoside reverse transcriptase inhibitors (NRTIs) and 1 protease inhibitor (PI)
      b.   Alternative regime: Ritonavir and saquinavir (soft-gel capsule) plus one or two NRTI(s) or nevirapine as a substitute for PI
      c.   When initiating therapy, start all drugs simultaneously and at a full dose with following exceptions: Dose escalation needed with ritonavir, nevirapine, and in some cases ritonavir plus saquinavir

3. Patients on monotherapy and dual therapy regimes should be offered triple combination therapy; even if these patients have no detectable virus in the plasma, triple combination therapy is more effective in preventing virologic failure than regimens with one or two drugs

4. See following table for acceptable antiretroviral combinations

ANTIRETROVIRAL COMBINATIONS
Acceptable combinations include the following:
Zidovudine (AZT) and lamivudine (3TC) plus a protease inhibitor (PI)
Lamivudine (3TC) and stavudine (d4T) plus PI
Zidovudine (AZT) and didanosine (ddl) plus PI
Didanosine (ddl) and stavudine (d4T) plus PI
Zidovudine (AZT) and zalcitabine (ddC) plus PI
Saquinavir-SGC (Fortovase) and ritonavir (Norvir) plus a NRTI
Alternative therapy which is less likely to provide sustained virus suppression
1 non-nucleoside reverse transcriptase inhibitor (NNRTI) plus 2 NRTI (listed above)
The following are generally not recommended:
Saquinavir-HGC (Invirase) with any combination
Two NRTIs
Unacceptable combinations of NRTI used in triple therapy include the following:
Didanosine (ddl) and zalcitabine (ddC)
Stavudine (d4T) and zidovudine (AZT)
Zalcitabine (ddC) and stavudine (d4T)
Lamivudine (3TC) and didanosine (ddl)

5. If possible, nevirapine should not be combined with a PI, because dose of PI must be increased if combined with nevirapine

6. If only one NRTI is used in a triple combination use zidovudine, stavudine, or didanosine; never use lamivudine as high-level resistance develops within 2-4 weeks in partially suppressive regimens

7. PI-sparing regimens: Because of fears of treatment failures leading to cross-resistance to all PIs and serious side effects, some experts recommend that patients with modest degrees of immunocompromise and no treatment experience should defer exposure to PIs and instead should be prescribed combinations of NRTIs and a NNRTI

I. Interruption of antiretroviral therapy: stop all antiretroviral agents simultaneously

J. Considerations for **changing an antiretroviral regimen**
1. If change is due to drug toxicity, substitute one or more alternative drugs of same potency from the same class of agents as causing suspected toxicity
2. Criteria to use when deciding whether or not to change regimens (see following table)

CRITERIA THAT SHOULD PROMPT CONSIDERATION OF CHANGING THERAPY
1. < a 0.5- to 0.75-log reduction in plasma HIV RNA by 4 weeks after initiation of therapy or < a 1-log reduction by 8 weeks
2. Failure to suppress plasma HIV RNA to undetectable levels within 4-6 months after initiation of therapy*
3. Repeated detection of virus in plasma after initial suppression of undetectable levels which suggests development of resistance
4. Any reproducible significant increase (defined as threefold or greater) from nadir of plasma HIV RNA levels not attributable to intercurrent infection, vaccination, or test methods
5. Patients on monotherapy and dual therapy regimens should be considered for triple combination therapy, regardless of viral load
6. Persistently declining CD4+ T-cell counts (measured on two separate occasions)
7. Clinical deterioration**

*Before changing therapies, consider the degree of initial decrease in plasma HIV RNA and the overall trend in decreasing viremia (patients with high initial viral loads may have slower rates of declining plasma HIV RNA)

**Professional judgement is needed; a new opportunistic infection may not suggest failure of drug therapy if there has been a sufficient decline in viremia

Adapted from NIH Panel to Define Principles of Therapy of HIV Infection. (1998). Guidelines for the use of antiretroviral agents in HIV-infected adults and adolescents. Annals of Internal Medicine, 128, 1079-1100.

3. With drug failure, best approach is to change to all new drugs, not previously taken
4. Limited information is available on restarting a drug that the patient has previously received; avoid if possible
5. Because of the likelihood of high-level cross resistance avoid the following:
   a. Changing from ritonavir to indinavir or vice versa
   b. Changing from nevirapine to delavirdine or vice versa
6. See the following table for possible regimens for patients in whom antiretroviral therapy has failed

TREATMENT OPTIONS WHEN CHANGING ANTIRETROVIRAL REGIMENS	
Prior Regimen	**New Regimen (Not listed in priority order)**
2 NRTIs +	2 new NRTIs +
Nelfinavir	RTV; or IDV; or SQV + RTV; or NNRTI# + RTV; or NNRTI + IDV*
Ritonavir	SQV + RTV*; NFV + NNRTI; or NFV + SQV
Indinavir	SQV + RTV; NFV + NNRTI; or NFV + SQV
Saquinavir	RTV + SQV; or NNRTI + IDV
2 NRTIs + NNRTI	2 new NRTIs + a protease inhibitor
2 NRTIs	2 new NRTIs + a protease inhibitor 2 new NRTIs + RTV + SQV 1 new NRTI + 1 NNRTI + a protease inhibitor 2 protease inhibitors + NNRTI
1 NRTI	2 new NRTIs + a protease inhibitor 2 new NRTIs + NNRTI 1 new NRTI + 1 NNRTI + a protease inhibitor

#Of the two available NNRTIs, clinical trials support a preference for nevirapine over delavirdine based on results of viral load assays. These two agents have opposite effects on the CYP450 pathway and this must be considered in combining these drugs with other agents
*There are some clinical tests with viral burden data to support this recommendation

Adapted from NIH Panel to Define Principles of Therapy of HIV Infection. (1998). Guidelines for the use of antiretroviral agents in HIV-infected adults and adolescents. Annals of Internal Medicine, 128, 1079-1100.

K. Nucleoside reverse transcriptase inhibitors (NRTIs)
1. Mechanism of action: Blocks the conversion of virus RNA into viral DNA through inhibition of reverse transcriptase; inhibits viral spread to uninfected cells rather than eradicating the virus
2. Factors to consider when selecting a NRTI: advantages and disadvantages

SELECTION OF NUCLEOSIDE REVERSE TRANSCRIPTASE INHIBITORS		
Drug	**Advantages**	**Disadvantages**
Zidovudine (Retrovir, AZT, ZDV, Azidothymidine)	✓ Superior CNS penetration compared to other NRTIs ✓ Twice daily dosing ✓ Can be combined with lamivudine in one tablet (Combivir)	✓ Numerous nuisance adverse effects ✓ Major objective adverse effect: bone marrow suppression with anemia and/or granulocytopenia ✓ May not be given with stavudine
Didanosine (ddI, dideoxyinosine, Videx)	✓ Efficacious ✓ Twice daily dosing	✓ Must be taken on empty stomach ✓ Only available in chewable tablets, powder or liquid ✓ Decreases absorption of other drugs when taken simultaneously ✓ Adverse effect of pancreatitis which can be fatal
Zalcitabine (ddC, dideoxycytidine, Hivid)	✓ None	✓ Efficacy is less than other NRTIs ✓ TID dosing ✓ Adverse effect of peripheral neuropathy is common (continued)

SELECTION OF NUCLEOSIDE REVERSE TRANSCRIPTASE INHIBITORS (CONTINUED)

Drug	Advantages	Disadvantages
Stavudine (d4T, Zerit)	✓ Twice daily dosing	✓ Adverse effect of peripheral neuropathy is common ✓ May <u>not</u> be given with zidovudine
Lamivudine (3TC, Epivir)	✓ Twice daily dosing ✓ Few adverse effects ✓ Can be combined with zidovudine in one tablet (Combivir) ✓ Has activity against Hepatitis B	✓ Resistence develops rapidly if not given with another antiretroviral

NUCLEOSIDE REVERSE TRANSCRIPTASE INHIBITORS

Dosing	Adverse Effects	Contraindications/ Precautions	Comments
Zidovudine: 600 mg/day in 2-3 divided doses; Available 100 mg and 300 mg caps **or** with lamivudine as **Combivir** 1 tab BID	✓ Major: bone marrow suppression with anemia and/or neutropenia ✓ Common subjective: nausea, headaches, insomnia, fatigue, malaise, vomiting, GI pain ✓ Less common: myopathy and muscle pain ✓ Long term: nail pigmentation	✓ Consider dose adjustment in patients with liver dysfunction	✓ Do **not** use with ganciclovir or other marrow-suppressing drugs ✓ Do **not** use with stavudine ✓ Discontinue if hemoglobin falls below 7.5 g/dL ✓ Monitor CBC 2-4 weeks after initiating and then periodically
Didanosine: <60 kg: 125 mg q 12 hours; ≥60 kg: 200 mg q 12 hours; Available 25, 50, 100, 150 mg chewable tablets and 100,167, 250 mg packets of buffered powder; must take on empty stomach	✓ Pancreatitis (potentially fatal) ✓ Peripheral neuropathy ✓ Diarrhea and GI problems	✓ Consider dose adjustment in patients with renal and liver dysfunction; do not prescribe to alcoholics, patients with history of pancreatitis, and those with poor seizure control	✓ Do not give within two hours following drugs requiring an acid environment: ketoconazole, dapsone, tetracyclines, quinolones, cimetidine, indinavir, delavirdine ✓ Monitor amylase levels and assess for abdominal pain, nausea, and vomiting ✓ Contains 8.6 mEq of magnesium hydroxide ✓ Must chew tabs
Zalcitabine: <45 kg: 0.375 mg q 8 hours; ≥45 kg 0.75 mg q 8 hours; Available 0.375, 0.75 tabs	✓ Peripheral neuropathy ✓ Aphthous ulcers ✓ Pancreatitis (less frequently than with didanosine)	✓ Extreme caution when given to patients with Hepatitis B; consider dose adjustment in patients with renal disease	✓ Used infrequently today because it is less efficacious than other NRTIs
Stavudine: <60 kg: 30 mg BID; ≥60 kg 40 BID; Available 15, 20, 30, 40 caps	✓ Peripheral neuropathy	✓ Consider dose adjustment in patients with renal and liver dysfunction	✓ Use cautiously with other drugs that cause peripheral neuropathy
Lamivudine: 150 mg BID; Available 150 mg tabs **or** with zidovudine as **Combivir** 1 tab BID	✓ Minimal toxicity but may have headache, nausea, diarrhea, abdominal pain, insomnia	✓ Consider dose adjustment in patients with renal dysfunction	✓ Increased drug absorption when given with trimethoprim/sulfamethoxazole ✓ Delays or reverses resistance of zidovudine ✓ Best to always administer concurrently with a protease inhibitor ✓ Not recommended with ddC and ddl

L. Protease inhibitors (PI)
   1. Mechanism of action: Inhibit HIV replication in cells that are chronically infected with HIV; competitively inhibit the HIV protease enzyme, a necessary enzyme for formation of the protein capsule surrounding the viral RNA in mature virions

2. Factors to consider when selecting a PI
   a. Saquinavir (Invirase) hard-gel formulation has decreased bioavailability; use Fortovase, soft-gel formulation
   b. Saquinavir and nelfinavir have less cross-resistance than other PIs
   c. Ritonavir is the most potent PI but has many drug interactions and adverse effects
   d. Indinavir is the least expensive PI, but is difficult for patient to take because it must be taken on an empty stomach and patient must drink >48 ounces of fluids
3. Toxicities of PIs sometimes limit their use
   a. Elevated glucose, serum triglycerides, and cholesterol are often reported
      (1) Monitor these levels every 3 months
      (2) Teach patients to maintain a healthy diet by reducing intake of saturated fatty acids, cholesterol and simple sugars
      (3) Consider prescribing gemfibrozil (Lopid) 1.2 g/day in 2 divided doses 30 minutes before morning and evening meals if trigylceride levels are >1000
   b. Changes in body habitus: peripheral lipodystrophy (fat wasting of face and limbs with central obesity), posterior cervical fat pads ("buffalo hump"), and breast enlargement in women
4. Patient adherence is a major consideration; to enhance adherence
   a. Use combination medications if possible such as combivir
   b. Simplify medication regimen
   c. Individualize therapy and seek patients' input on their preferences for drug regimens
5. See following tables for selecting PIs, drug interactions and other drugs requiring dose modifications

CHARACTERISTICS OF PROTEASE INHIBITORS

Characteristic	Indinavir (Crixivan)§	Ritonavir (Norvir)*	Saquinavir-SGC* (Fortovase)	Nelfinavir (Viracept)§
Form	200-,400-mg caplets	600 mg/7.5 mL po solution	200-mg soft gel caps	250-mg tablets 50-mg/g oral powder
Dosing recommendations	800 mg q8h Take 1 h before or 2 h after meals; may take with skim milk or low-fat meal Reduce dose to 600 mg q 8 hours with ketoconazole or itraconazole	600 mg q 12h*† Take with food if possible	1,200 mg TID* Take with large meal	750 mg TID Take with food (meal or light snack)
Patient Teaching	Drink >48 ounces of fluid to reduce risk of nephrolithiasis Grapefruit juice decreases levels Separate by 2 hrs. from ddI Can use with oral contraceptives	Liquid contains alcohol; caution about driving and working with machinery; avoid in patients with alcohol abuse problems Reduces effectiveness of oral contraceptives Tobacco decreases levels	Not bioequivalent to Invirase or hard gel formulation Grapefruit juice increases levels	Do not take with carbonated beverages due to high phosphorus content Reduces effectiveness of oral contraceptives
Adverse effects	Nephrolithiasis GI intolerance, nausea Laboratory: increased indirect bilirubinemia (inconsequential) Miscellaneous: headache, asthenia, blurred vision, dizziness, rash, metallic taste, thrombocytopenia Hyperglycemia ↑Cholesterol ↑Triglycerides	GI intolerance, nausea, vomiting, diarrhea Paresthesias– circumoral and extremities Hepatitis Asthenia Taste perversion Laboratory: ↑ triglycerides, ↑ aminotransferase, ↑ creatine phosphokinase and uric acid, ↑glucose	GI intolerance, nausea, diarrhea, abdominal pain, and dyspepsia Headache Elevated aminotrans-ferace enzymes Hypergylcemia	Diarrhea Hyperglycemia

*Combination of ritonavir 400 mg BID and saquinavir-SGC 400 mg BID
†Dose escalation of ritonavir: days 1-2, 300 mg BID; days 3-5, 400 BID; days 6-13, 500 mg BID; day 14, 600 mg BID.
§Twice-daily regimens of indinavir 1200 mg BID (three 400 mg caps BID) and nelfinavir 1000 mg. in am (four 250 mg tabs) and 1250 mg in pm (five 250 mg tabs) in combination with zidovudine and lamivudine is not recommended in 1998

Adapted from NIH Panel to Define Principles of Therapy of HIV Infection. (1998). Guidelines for the use of antiretroviral agents in HIV-infected adults and adolescents. Annals of Internal Medicine, 128, 1079-1100.

DRUG INTERACTIONS: PROTEASE INHIBITORS

Indinavir (Crixivan)	Ritonavir (Norvir)	Saquinavir-SGC (Fortovase)	Nelfinavir (Viracept)
Inhibits cytochrome p450 (less than ritonavir) Do not use with rifampin Contraindicated for concurrent use: terfenadine, astemizole, cisapride, triazolam, midazolam, and ergot alkaloids Indinavir increased by ketoconazole*, delavirdine, and nelfinivir Indinavir reduced by rifampin, rifabutin, grapefruit juice, and nevirapine Didanosine reduces indinavir absorption unless taken >2 h apart	Inhibits cytochrome p450 (potent inhibitor) Ritonavir increases levels of multiple drugs that are not recommended for concurrent uses§ Didanosine may reduce absorption of both drugs; should be taken ≥2 h apart Ritonavir decreases ethinyl estradiol, theophylline, sulfamethoxazole, and zidovudine Ritonavir increases clarithromycin and desipramine	Inhibits cytochrome p450 Saquinavir increased by ritonavir, ketoconazole, grapefruit juice, nelfinavir, and delavirdine Saquinavir reduced by rifampin, rifabutin, and possibly phenobarbital, phenytoin, dexamethasone, carbamazepine, and nevirapine Contraindicated for concurrent use: rifampin, rifabutin, terfenadine, astemizole, cisapride, ergot alkaloids, triazolam, and midazolam	Inhibits cytochome p450 (less than ritonavir) Nelfinavir reduced by rifampin and rifabutin Contraindicated for concurrent use: triazolam, midazolam, ergot alkaloids, terfenadine, astemizole, and cisapride Nelfinavir decreases ethinyl estradiol and norethindrone Nelfinavir increases rifabutin, saquinavir, and indinavir Not recommended for concurrent use: rifampin

§Drugs contraindicated for concurrent use with ritonavir: amiodarone (Cordarone), astemizole (Hismanal), bepridil (Vascar), bupropion (Wellbutin), cisapride (Propulsid), clorazepate (Tranxene), clozapine (Clozaril), diazepam (Valium), encainide (Enkaid), estazolam (ProSom), flecainide (Tambocor), flurazepam (Dalmane), meperidine (Demerol), midazolam (Versed), piroxicam (Feldene), propoxyphene (Darvon), propafenone (Rythmol), quinidine, rifabutin, terfenadine (Seldane), triazolam (Halcion), zolpidem (Ambien), and ergot alkaloids
*Decrease indinavir to 600 mg every 8 hours

Adapted from NIH Panel to Define Principles of Therapy of HIV Infection. (1998). Guidelines for the use of antiretroviral agents in HIV-infected adults and adolescents. Annals of Internal Medicine, 128, 1079-1100.

DRUG INTERACTIONS BETWEEN PROTEASE INHIBITORS AND OTHER DRUGS REQUIRING DOSE MODIFICATIONS

Drug	Indinavir	Ritonavir	Saquinavir*	Nelfinavir
Fluconazole Ketoconazole and Itraconazole	No dose change Decrease dose to 600 mg q8h	No dose change Increases ketoconazole >3-fold; dose adjustment required	No data Increases saquinavir levels 3-fold; no dose change†	No dose change No dose change
Rifabutin	Reduce rifabutin to half dose: 150 mg qd	Consider alternative drug or reduce rifabutin dose to one quarter	Not recommended with either Invirase or Fortovase	Reduce rifabutin to half dose: 150 mg qd
Rifampin	Contraindicated	Unknown‡	Not recommended with either Invirase or Fortovase	Contraindicated
Oral contraceptives	Modest increase in Ortho-Novum levels; no dose change	Ethinyl estradiol levels decreased; use alternative or additional contraceptive method	No data	Ethinyl estradiol and norethindrone levels decreased; use alternative or additional contraceptive method
Miscellaneous	Grapefruit juice reduces indinavir levels by 26%	Desipramine levels increased by 145%: reduce dose Theophylline levels decreased; increase dose	Grapefruit juice increases saquinavir levels†	

*Several drug interaction studies have been completed with saquinavir given as Invirase or Fortovase. Results from studies conducted with Invirase may not be applicable to Fortovase.
†With Invirase.
‡Rifampin reduces ritonavir levels by 35%. Increased ritonavir dose or use of ritonavir in combination therapy is strongly recommended. The effect of ritonavir on rifampin is unknown. Concurrent use may increase liver toxicity. Therefore, patients on ritonavir and rifampin should be monitored closely.

Adapted from NIH Panel to Define Principles of Therapy of HIV Infection. (1998). Guidelines for the use of antiretroviral agents in HIV-infected adults and adolescents. Annals of Internal Medicine, 128, 1079-1100.

M. Non-nucleoside reverse transcriptase inhibitors (NNRTI)
  1. Mechanism of action: Act on a nonsubstrate binding site of the enzyme which alters the shape of the active site
  2. Drugs in this class should be used only in regimens designed to be maximally suppressive because of the potential for high-level resistance
  3. See following table for characteristics of NNRTIs

NON-NUCLEOSIDE REVERSE TRANSCRIPTASE INHIBITORS		
Variable	**Nevirapine (Viramune)**	**Delavirdine (Rescriptor)**	**Efavirenz (Sustiva)***
Form Dosing recommendations	200-mg tablets 200 mg po QD x 14 days, then 200 mg po BID	100-mg tablets 400 mg po TID (four 100-mg tabs in ≥3 oz of water to produce slurry) Decrease dose to 600 mg TID with indinavir	200-mg tablets 600 mg HS
Drug interactions	Induces cytochrome p450 enzymes The following drugs have suspected interactions that require careful monitoring if coadministered with nevirapine: rifampin, rifabutin, oral contraceptives, protease inhibitors, triazolam, and midazolam	Inhibits cytochrome p450 enzymes Not recommended for concurrent use: terfenadine, astemizole, alprazolam, midazolam, cisapride, rifabutin, rifampin, triazolam, ergot derivatives, amphetamines, nifedipine, and anticonvulsants (phenytoin, carbamazepine, phenobarbitol) Delavirdine increases levels of clarithromycin, dapsone, quinidine, warfarin, indinavir, and saquinavir Antacids or didanosine: separate delavirdine administration by ≥1 hr	Metabolized by cytochrome P450 Induces metabolism of indinavir (increase indinavir dose to 1000 mg every 8 hours)
Adverse events	Rash Increased aminotransferase levels Hepatitis Reduces effectiveness of oral contraceptives	Rash Headaches	Central nervous system symptoms (dizziness, light-headedness, nightmares, drowsiness, insomnia, impaired concentration) Rash Birth defects (use with caution in women of reproductive age)

*May be given with indinavir, zidovudine, lamivudine
Adapted from NIH Panel to Define Principles of Therapy of HIV Infection. (1998). Guidelines for the use of antiretroviral agents in HIV-infected adults and adolescents. Annals of Internal Medicine, 128, 1079-1100.

N. Investigational therapies
  1. Several investigational drugs are in the advanced stages of clinical evaluation:
    a. Abacavir (1592, Ziagen) is a potent NRTI with good bioavailability that penetrates the cerebrospinal fluid
      (1) Dosage is 300 mg every 12 hours; may be combined with any PI and with zidovudine and lamivudine (no known clinically significant drug interactions with other antiretroviral agents)
      (2) Usually well tolerated but may have mild nausea, headache, malaise, abdominal pain, diarrhea, and rash
      (3) Serious hypersensitivity reaction with flu-like symptoms, fever, nausea, vomiting, malaise and rash mandates stopping the drug **permanently**
    b. Amprenavir (141W94) is a new PI
      (1) Dosage is 800 mg TID or 1200 mg BID
      (2) Available in 150 mg tablets
      (3) Can be taken with or without food
      (4) May be given with other PIs or NRTIs; metabolized by cytochrome P450 so drug interactions with other PIs may prove to be important
      (5) Does not have high-level cross-resistance to other PIs which suggests it may be good first-line option
      (6) Usually well tolerated, but may have gastrointestinal symptoms and rash

      c.   Adefovir dipivoxil (bis-POM, Preveon) is in a different category than any of other currently approved antiretrovirals; it is a nucleotide analogue

          (1)   It has activity against herpes simplex virus; may have activity against hepatitis B and CMV

          (2)   Does not appear to be as potent as the other new agents, but it has limited cross-resistance to other currently available antiretroviral agents

          (3)   Once daily dosing; 60-120 mg QD

          (4)   No drug interactions with other antiretroviral agents

          (5)   Usually well tolerated but may have mild nausea, vomiting, malaise, and diarrhea

          (6)   Most common adverse effects are abnormal levels of creatinine and proteinuria (monitor renal function routinely)

          (7)   It can cause lowered L-carnitine levels, so L-carnitine should be administered with adefovir

2.   Hydroxyurea (Hydrea) in combination with other antiretrovirals therapies is being investigated

    a.   Best to prescribe hydroxyurea with didanosine (ddI) plus a protease inhibitor and a NRTI (stavudine is often recommended)

    b.   Dosages are 1.0 gram daily in single dose; 500 mg BID; or 300 mg TID

3.   HIV vaccine is in the exploratory stage

O.   **Treatment regimen for primary HIV infection (acute retroviral syndrome)**

1.   Prescribe a combination of two NRTIs and one potent PI (see V.H.4)

2.   Testing for plasma HIV RNA levels and CD4+ T-cells counts should be performed on initiation of therapy, after 4 weeks, and every 3-4 months thereafter

3.   The optimal duration and composition of therapy is unknown; some experts recommend that treatment should be indefinite whereas others treat for 1 year and then re-evaluate the patient with HIV RNA measurements and CD4+ T-cell counts

P.   **Symptom management**

1.   Wasting syndrome defined as otherwise unexplained loss of 10% of body weight

    a.   Causative factors include;

        (1)   Decreased food intake due to mouth or esophageal ulcers, anorexia (often related to depression), early satiety, or nausea

        (2)   Decreased absorption from loss of enzymes causing lactose intolerance; to avoid this problem teach patient to avoid all milk products by reading labels

        (3)   Increased metabolic demand from infection and fever

        (4)   Malabsorption due to infections and bacterial overgrowth

    b.   Order following diagnostic tests to rule-out infection and treat as needed: stool culture, blood culture, cryptococcal serum antigen and other tests based on patient's clinical presentation

    c.   Recommend daily multivitamin

    d.   Consider prescribing one of the following appetite stimulants

        (1)   Megestrol acetate (Megace) 40 mg/ml susp.; 800 mg/day; adverse effects include impotence, decreased libido, hypertension

        (2)   Dronabinol (Marinol)

            (a)   2.5 mg BID before lunch and supper, may gradually increase to maximum of 20 mg/day

            (b)   Adverse effects include abuse potential, euphoria, psychomimetic reactions, altered mental status

    e.   Recommend nutritional supplements (10 cans per day are needed for total daily caloric needs)

        (1)   If patient needs to gain weight and can tolerate milk use Carnation Instant Breakfast or SportsShake

        (2)   If the patient needs to gain weight but cannot tolerate milk give Ensure, Sustacal, Scandishake

        (3)   If patient has constant diarrhea give a low or special fat supplement such as Lipisorb or a supplement with special dietary fiber such as Ensure with Fiber

        (4)   For patients with severe diarrhea an elemental diet (with easily absorbed nutrients) is needed such as Criticare HN or Peptamen

        (5)   Advera and Hi-Cal VM are specifically formulated for persons with HIV/AIDS

        (6)   Elemental formulas: Vivonex TEN

    f.   Consider other beneficial therapies such as serostim (growth hormone) 6 mg SC QD X 12 weeks, recombinant growth hormone, thalidomide 100 mg PO/day, anabolic steroids (oxandrolone 20 mg/day PO)

2. Testosterone failure may cause a decrease in energy levels and muscle mass

    a.   To diagnose, order serum testosterone level

    b.   Treatment is testosterone injections 200 mg IM every 2 weeks or testosterone patch (Testoderm TTS), apply 5 mg patch every 22-24 hours to arm, back or upper buttocks (application site rotation is not necessary)

3. Diarrhea

    a.   Order following diagnostic tests to rule-out parasites or infection: Stool for ova and parasites, bacterial stool culture, *C-difficile* toxin, acid-fast bacterial smear of stool can sometimes detect *Myobacterium avium* and cryptosporidiosis

    b.   If infection is ruled-out, prescribe one of following

        (1)   Imodium (Loperamide) 2 mg. caps, two in am and one after each BM up to maximum of 8 caps

        (2)   Alternative: Lomotil (diphenoxylate) 2.5 mg; 2 tabs or 10 ml four times a day

    c.   Patient education

        (1)   Increase fluids

        (2)   Follow a low lactose, low fat, high fiber diet

        (3)   Use LactAid instead of milk

        (4)   Avoid caffeine, fried foods, carbonated beverages, cabbage, broccoli

4. Nausea and vomiting

    a.   Rule out infections

    b.   Symptomatically treat with metroclopramide (Reglan) 10 mg PO QID, or prochlorperazine (Compazine) 5-10 mg QID, or ondansetron (Zofran) 4-10 mg QID

5. Pain is a common symptom (see section on PAIN)

6. Fever

    a.   Common causes are *Mycobacterium avium complex*, tuberculosis, lymphoma, cytomegalovirus infection, secondary syphilis

    b.   Following diagnostic tests should be obtained: blood culture for acid-fast bacteria, cryptococcal serum antigen, CBC; consider PPD, RPR, chest x-ray

    c.   Symptomatic treatment (see section on FEVERS)

7. Anemia may develop due to drugs such as zidovudine or may result from the HIV infection

    a.   Order the following diagnostic tests

        (1)   Iron profile, reticulocyte count, erythropoietin levels, B_{12}, folate

        (2)   If patient has normal WBCs but decreased RBCs consider infection with parvovirus

    b.   If patient is on zidovudine, consider switching to another NRTI

    c.   For severe anemia (<7.5 hemoglobin), prescribe erythropoietin (Epogen, Procrit)

        (1)   Need to determine endogenous levels of erythropoietin; if >500 units of endogenous erythropoietin, patient won't respond to this drug

        (2)   Measure ferritin levels, patient must have adequate iron stores to respond to drug

        (3)   Administer 100-250 U/kg, 3 subcutaneous injections every week

    d.   Neutropenia may be due to drugs (zidovudine, ganciclovir) or HIV infection: give G-CSF, filgrastim (Neupogen) 5-10 micrograms/kg 2-4 times a week; available 300 micrograms/ml

8. Mouth ulcers are common, particularly if patient is on zalcitabine (See sections on APHTHOUS ULCERS, HERPES SIMPLEX, CANDIDIASIS)

9. Dermatological problems

    a.   Eosinophilic folliculitis or red, itchy bumps: prescribe astemizole (Hismanal) 10 mg QD and one of following:

        (1)   Camphor 0.5/Menthol 0.5 lotion (sarna)

        (2)   Topical steroids

    b.   See treatment of other dermatological conditions in SKIN chapter

10. Peripheral neuropathy: treat with one of following:
    a. Nortriptyline (Pamelor) 10 mg HS; increase dose by 10 mg q 5 days to maximum of 50 mg HS or 10-20 mg TID
    b. Ibuprofen 600-800 mg TID
    c. Capsaicin-containing ointments (Zostrix) for topical application
11. Mental health problems are common (see sections on DEPRESSION, INSOMNIA, and ANXIETY)

Q. Ethical issues
    1. Disclosure of HIV status to sexual partners
       a. Recent study found that 40% of HIV infected patients failed to tell their sexual partners that they were HIV positive; 43% of those who did not disclose failed to used condoms all the time
       b. Persons sometimes fail to disclose due to fear of abuse and abandonment
       c. Assist patients to safely and readily disclose; state health departments can help with confidential partner notification
    2. Needle exchange programs have been developed to reduce the spread of HIV infection; research results have been inconclusive
    3. The need for post-sexual exposure prophylaxis programs is being debated; programs typically offer the following:
       a. Assess sexually exposed persons risk of HIV infection
       b. Provide HIV testing and STD evaluation (see section on HEALTH-CARE WORKER EXPOSURE)
       c. If risks are evident, prescribe postexposure prophylaxis regimen (PEP) within 72 hours after sexual exposure; delaying treatment more than 24 to 36 hours dramatically decreases the likelihood of effectiveness (see Plan/Management V.D. in section on HEALTH-CARE WORKER EXPOSURE for appropriate medication prophylaxis)

R. Follow Up; adjust followup to clinical condition of patient
    1. Patients who are asymptomatic and not on antiretroviral therapy should be seen every 3-6 months
    2. Patients who begin antiretroviral therapy or begin a new antiretroviral regimen should be reevaluated in one month
    3. Patients who are stable and on antiretroviral therapy should be seen every 1-3 months depending on their clinical situation

HEALTH-CARE WORKER EXPOSURES TO BLOOD AND OTHER BODY FLUIDS THAT MAY CONTAIN HUMAN IMMUNODEFICIENCY VIRUS (HIV)

I. Definitions:

   A. Health care worker (HCW) is any individual (employee, student, contractor, attending clinician, public-safety worker, or volunteer) whose activities involve contact with patients or with blood or other body fluids from patients in a health care or laboratory setting

   B. An exposure that may place the HCW at risk for HIV infection includes the following incidents involving blood, tissue or other body fluids such as semen, vaginal secretions or other fluids contaminated with visible blood; cerebrospinal, synovial, pleural, peritoneal, pericardial and amniotic fluids have an undetermined risk
      1. Percutaneous injury such as a needlestick or cut with a sharp object
      2. Contact of mucous membrane or nonintact skin such as when the exposed skin or mucous membrane is chapped, abraded or has dermatitis
      3. Contact with intact skin when the duration of contact is prolonged (> several minutes), or involves an extensive area
      4. Any direct contact with concentrated HIV in a research laboratory or production facility

II. Pathogenesis: (see section on HIV/AIDS in Adults)

III. Clinical Presentation

   A. Through September 1997, 52 U.S. HCWs have reported documented occupationally acquired HIV infection (negative HIV-antibody tests at the time of exposure and subsequent conversion); another 114 health care workers have possible occupationally acquired HIV infection (lack documented seroconversion as a result of occupational exposure)

   B. Nurses are the most commonly exposed professional group

   C. The risk of HIV seroconversion depends on several factors
      1. Risk after a needlestick when the source patient is HIV positive ranges from 0.36 to 0.42%
         a. There is increased risk for transmission when the needle involved in the injury was placed directly into the source patient's vein or artery, was large gauge, and was hollow bore
         b. Needlesticks with great depth of penetration and which involved increased amounts of injected blood pose greater risks
         c. There is increased risk when the source patient has a high viral load
         d. Host defenses may also play a role in the risk profile
      2. Risk of mucocutaneous transmission is less than 0.1%

   D. Approximately 81% of HCWs with documented seroconversions had symptoms suggesting acute retroviral syndrome or primary infection

   E. Time course of HIV seroconversion in HCWs is similar to that of other individuals who acquire HIV through other modes of transmission

IV.   Diagnosis/Evaluation

   A.   History
          1.   Evaluate exposure
                 a.   Determine type of fluid that was involved in exposure
                 b.   Carefully explore and document exact type of exposure such as needlestick, skin contact, mucous membrane contact
                 c.   If it was a needlestick, document gauge of needle, whether it was hollow bore, depth of needlestick, and whether needle had visible blood
                 d.   If it was a skin or mucous membrane exposure, ask about abrasions, chafing, lesions, dermatitis
                        (1)   Determine duration of exposure
                        (2)   Determine type and amount of fluids that had contact with HCW
          2.   Evaluate exposure source person
                 a.   Explore prior HIV testing results and CD4+ T-cell levels
                 b.   History of possible HIV exposures such as IV drug use, sexual contact with a known HIV infected partner, unprotected sexual contact with multiple partners, etc.
                 c.   Ask exposure source about clinical symptoms that may suggest acute syndrome or undiagnosed HIV infection
                 d.   If exposure source is HIV positive, obtain information on current HIV RNA levels, CD4+ T-cells, and current and previous antiretroviral therapies
          3.   For purposes of considering postexposure prophylaxis, ask HCW about current use of medications and underlying medical conditions

   B.   Physical Examination
          1.   Thoroughly assess site of wound
          2.   Explore mental status and anxiety level of HCW

   C.   Differential Diagnosis: None

   D.   Diagnostic Tests
          1.   Testing considerations of source person
                 a.   If the HIV serostatus of the source person in not known, source person should be told of the incident and if consent is obtained, HIV-antibody testing should be performed
                 b.   If consent cannot be obtained, testing of the source patient should follow local and state laws
                 c.   If the source person is HIV negative no further testing is needed
          2.   Clinical evaluation and baseline testing of exposed HCWs
                 a.   Baseline testing or testing to establish serostatus at time of exposure with HIV antibody testing should be performed if the source person is HIV infected or has recently engaged in high risk behaviors
                 b.   Follow up HIV antibody testing of HCW should be considered at 6 weeks, 12 weeks and 6 months if the source person is HIV infected or has high risk for HIV infection
                 c.   Pregnancy testing should be offered to all nonpregnant women of childbearing age if pregnancy status is unknown

V.   Plan/Management

   A.   Occupational exposure should be documented in HCWs confidential medical record

   B.   Wound and skin sites should be washed with soap and water

   C.   Before treatment, assessment of infection risk should be determined

   D.   Postexposure prophylaxis (PEP)
          1.   Discuss risks and benefits of PEP
          2.   Selection of type of PEP regimen should involve consideration of the comparative risk of the exposure (see following table)

POSTEXPOSURE PROPHYLAXIS REGIMEN		
Regimen Category	Application	Drug Regimen
Basic	Occupational HIV exposures for which there is a recognized transmission risk	4 weeks (28 days) of both zidovudine 600 mg every day in divided doses (i.e., 300 mg twice a day, 200 mg three times a day, or 100 mg every 4 hours) and lamivudine 150 mg twice a day
Expanded	Occupational HIV exposures that pose an increased risk for transmission (e.g., larger volume of blood and/or higher virus titer in blood)	Basic regimen plus either indinavir 800 mg every 8 hours or nelfinavir 750 mg three times a day

Source:Center for Disease Control. (1998). Public Health Service guidelines for the management of health-care worker exposure to HIV and recommendations for postexposure prophylaxis. MMWR, 45 (22), 468-472

3. PEP should be started as soon as possible
4. PEP should be administered for 4 weeks if tolerated
5. If serostatus of source person in unknown or if exposure source is unknown, use of PEP should be decided on an individual or case-by-case basis

E. Counseling
1. Advise HCW to use the following measures to prevent secondary transmission during the period after occupational exposure: use sexual abstinence or condoms, refrain from donating blood, plasma, organs, tissue or semen, refrain from breastfeeding if applicable
2. Counsel on importance of completing the prescribed drug regimen

F. Follow Up
1. HCWs with exposure need follow up counseling, postexposure testing and medical evaluation regardless of whether they receive PEP; HIV antibody testing should be performed at 6 weeks, 12 weeks, and 6 months
2. Monitoring of PEP toxicity is important
   a. CBC, renal and hepatic chemical functioning tests should be performed at baseline and again 2 weeks after starting PEP
   b. Glucose levels should be obtained for HCWs taking protease inhibitors
   c. If HCW is receiving indinavir, monitor for crystalluria, hematuria, hemolytic anemia, hepatitis

REFERENCES

Association of Nurses in AIDS Care. (1996). In K.M. Casey, F. Cohen, & A.M. Hughes. (Eds.). ANAC's core curriculum for HIV/AIDS nursing. Nursecom: Philadelphia.

Bartlett, J.G. (1999). The John's Hopkins Hospital 1998-1999 guide to medical care of patients with HIV infection (8th ed.). Baltimore: Williams & Wilkins.

Burman, W.J., Reves, R.R. & Cohn, D.L. (1998). The case for conservative management of early HIV disease. JAMA, 280, 93-95.

Carpenter, C.C.J., Fischl, M.A., Hammer, S.M., Hirsch, M.S., Jacobsen, D.M., Katzenstein, D.A., Montaner, J.S.G., Richman, D.D., Saag, M.S., Schooley, R.T., Thompson, M.A., Vella, S., Yeni, P.G. & Volberding, P.A. (1998). Antiretroviral therapy for HIV infection in 1998. JAMA, 280, 78-86.

Center for Communicable Diseases. (1992). 1993 revised classification system for HIV infection and expanded surveillance case definition of AIDS among adolescents and adults. MMWR, 41 (RR-17).

Center for Disease Control. (1997). 1997 USPHS/IDSA guidelines for the prevention of opportunistic infections in persons infected with Human Immunodeficiency Virus. MMWR, 46, 1-46.

Center for Disease Control. (1998). Public Health Service guidelines for the management of health-care worker exposure to HIV and recommendations for postexposure prophylaxis. MMWR, 45 (22), 468-472.

Cotton, D. (1998). Post-sexual exposure prophylaxis: A roundtable discussion. AIDS Clilnical Care, 10 (2), 9-12.

Dube, M.P., & Sattler, F.R. (1998). Metabolic complications of antiretroviral therapies. AIDS Clinical Care, 10 (6), 41-44.

Flexner, C. (1998). HIV-protease inhibitors. The New England Journal of Medicine, 338, 1281-1292.

Gulick, R.M. (1998). HIV treatment strategies: Planning for the long term. JAMA,, 279, 957-958.

Hirsch, M.S., Conway, B., D'Aquila, R.T., Johnson, V.A., Brun-Vézinet, F., Clotet, B., Demeter, L.M., Hammer, S.M., Jacobsen, D.M., Kuritzkes, D.R., Loveday, C., Mellors, J.W., Vella, S., & Richman, D.D. (1998). Antiretroviral drug resistance testing in adults with HIV infection. JAMA, 279, 1984-1991.

Klaus, B.D., & Grodesky, M. J. (1998). Drug interactions and protease inhibitor therapy in the treatment of HIV/AIDS. The Nurse Practitioner, 23 (2), 102-106.

Klaus, B.D., & Grodesky, M.J. (1998). News from the 5th Conference on Retroviruses and Opportunistic Infections. The Nurse Practitioner, 23, 117-127.

Maenza, J., Flexner, C. (1998). Combination antiretroviral therapy for HIV infection. The American Family Physician, 57, 2789-2798.

Martin, J.E., & Pindaro, C. (1998). Clinician's antiretroviral medications guide. Journal of the Association of Nurses in AIDS Care, 9, 84-85.

Myers, R.A. Jr. (1998). Outpatient management of HIV-infected adults: The varied challenges for primary care. Postgraduate Medicine, 103, 219-225.

NIH Panel To Define Principles of Therapy of HIV Infection. (1998). Report of the NIH Panel To Define Principles of Therapy of HIV Infection. Annals of Internal Medicine, 128, 1057-1078.

NIH Panel to Define Principles of Therapy of HIV Infection. (1998). Guidelines for the use of antiretroviral agents in HIV-infected adults and adolescents. Annals of Internal Medicine, 128, 1079-1100.

Parra, E.O. (1997). Standardized forms to use in the management of HIV infection. The American Family Physician, 55, 2166-2172.

Perlmutter, B.L. & Harris, B.R. (1997). New recommendations for prophylaxis after HIV exposure. The American Family Physician, 55, 507-512.

Shands, J.W., Jr., & Bentrup, K.L. (Eds.). (1998). HIV/AIDS primary care guide: For health care professionals providing HIV/AIDS care. Gainesville, Fl: University of Florida.

Stegbauer, C. C. (1997). Human Immunodeficiency Virus: Early steps in management. Nurse Practitioner, 23, 94-100

Stein, M.D. (1998). Sexual ethics: Disclosure of HIV-positive status to partners. Archives of Internal Medicine, 158, 253-257.

Stephenson, J. (1998). AIDS vaccine moves into phase 3 trials. JAMA, 280, 7-8.

Walker, B.D., & Basgoz, N. (1998). Treat HIV-1 infection like other infections--Treat it. JAMA, 280, 91-92.

Musculoskeletal Problems

ANKLE SPRAIN

I.   Definition: Injury to the ligaments of the ankle

II. Pathogenesis:

    A.   Due to sudden stress on one or more of the supporting ligaments of the ankle

    B.   Often occurs from stepping off a curb or into a hole

    C.   If injury is sports-related, it is often due to jumping or falling on outstretched ankle; basketball, football, and cross-country running are the sports in which sprains occur most frequently

    D.   Inversion injuries which involve the anterior talofibular or the calcaneofibular ligaments occur most frequently

    E.   Eversion injuries which usually involve the deltoid ligament are the second most common type

III. Clinical Presentation

    A.   Approximately 85% of all ankle injuries in adults are due to sprains

    B.   Classification of sprains
        1.   First-degree sprain occurs when the ligament is minimally torn and the joint is stable with minimal pain and swelling
        2.   Second-degree sprain is a more severe injury with the ligament appreciably torn but the joint remains stable; tends to have more swelling and ecchymosis than Grade I injury; usually patient has difficulty bearing weight
        3.   Third-degree sprain is a complete tear of the ligament with an unstable joint; usually there is marked swelling, ecchymosis, pain, and difficulty bearing weight

    C.   Immediate pain is noticed and swelling over the injured ligament often occurs within 1 hour of the injury

    D.   Persons with previous ankle injuries have increased risk of reinjuring the same ankle

    E.   Characteristics of severe ankle injuries
        1.   Eversion injury
        2.   Immediate diffuse swelling which may indicate bleeding
        3.   Inability to bear weight immediately
        4.   Sensation of a "pop", "snap", locking of joint, or kick into the heel
        5.   On physical exam, patient often has a positive drawer sign and a positive squeeze test

IV. Diagnosis/Evaluation

    A.   History
        1.   Ask patient to precisely describe how the injury occurred
        2.   Ask patient to describe the foot position at the time of injury
        3.   Determine whether the patient was able to bear weight after injury
        4.   Determine whether the patient had a sensation of a "pop," a "snap," or had any locking of the joint which may indicate a partial- or full-tendon rupture
        5.   Question when and where the swelling and ecchymosis were first noticed
        6.   Ascertain whether there is any associated pain in the leg, knee or foot
        7.   Inquire about previous musculoskeletal injuries
        8.   Inquire about self-treatment

B.   Physical Examination
1.   Always compare injured side with unaffected side; examine most painful area last
2.   Observe ankle, concentrating on the lateral and medial aspects of the foot and ankle, for swelling, ecchymosis, and deformity
3.   Check neurovascular status of foot
4.   Palpation should be systematic (see Figure 17.1 of anatomical structures)
   a.   Start with bony structures: shaft of fibula, distal fibula over lateral malleolus, medial malleolus, base of the fifth metatarsal, all the tarsals, metatarsals, and phalanges
   b.   Next palpate the ligamentous structures
      (1)   Palpate the anterior tibiofibular ligament
      (2)   Palpate the anterior talofibular ligament
      (3)   Palpate the calcaneofibular ligament
      (4)   Palpate the medial compartment to determine deltoid ligament damage
   c.   Palpate tendons including the Achilles, the peroneal tendons, and the anterior tibial tendon

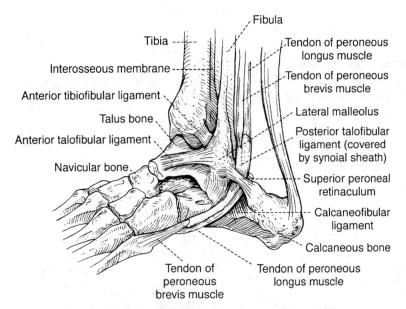

Figure 17.1. Anatomical Structures of the Ankle.

5.   Perform active range of motion and assess the limits of unassisted movement
6.   Perform passive range of motion and assess the limits of manipulation by the examiner without effort of the patient
7.   Perform resisted range of motion to determine muscular strength by measuring the patient's active movement against resistance
8.   Perform three special tests:
   a.   Anterior drawer test is used to assess the anterior talofibular and other ligaments of the lateral side of the ankle (see Figure 17.2)

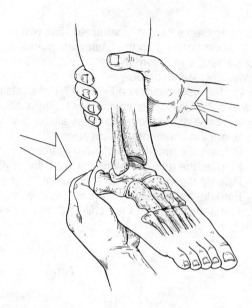

Figure 17.2. Anterior Drawer Sign.

Examiner grasps distal tibia with one hand and heel with other hand; Patient's foot is held firmly while backward force is applied to tibia; Positive test is graded 1+ for slight movement, 2+ for moderate movement, and 3+ for marked movement

      b.   Talar tilt test is used to assess stability of the calcaneofibular ligament (see Figure 17.3)

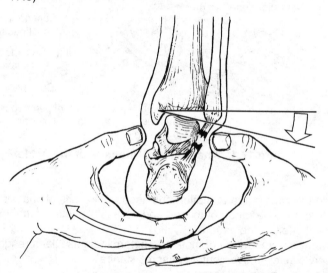

Figure 17.3. Talar Tilt Test.

Grasping the distal tibia and heel with other hand, apply gentle inversion force to affected ankle; ligaments are probably damaged if the talar tilt around the ankle is 5-10° greater around injured than around uninjured ankle

      c.   Squeeze test is not often performed but should be done if medial or severe lateral injury has taken place
          (1)   Examiner's hands are placed 6 inches inferior to the knee with thumbs on the fibula and fingers on the medial tibia
          (2)   Leg is squeezed as if to bring fibula and tibia together
          (3)   Pain with this test denotes syndesmotic injury which is a severe injury with a long rehabilitation time
    9.   Assess joints above and below injury

C. Differential Diagnosis
1. Strains: Injuries to the tendons and muscles; usually have gradual onset of pain due to overuse rather than trauma
2. Tenosynovitis usually occurs from a direct blow or overuse with repetitive overloads or faulty technique; Achilles tendonitis is an example and presents with pain on palpation of tendon and pain which is worse with active stretching and plantar flexion against resistance; tenderness is worse with hill running; treatment is rest, ice, and pain control
3. Tendon ruptures such as Achilles
   a. While exercising, patient has a sudden onset of shooting pain in calf, followed by weakness in leg and inability to stand or walk on toes
   b. Signs include absence of normal plantar reflex and a positive Thompson test (with patient prone, flex the affected leg 90° at knee and squeeze calf; if foot doesn't move, the tendon is ruptured)
   c. Refer to orthopedist
4. Fractures often occur in persons who engage in high velocity, high impact sports
   a. Four basic injury mechanisms for fractures: lateral displacement of talus (most common), medial displacement of talus, axial compression of talus, and repetitive microtrauma
   b. Refer to orthopedist
5. Gout, arthritis, or infection may present with a painful ankle, but examination findings and history are inconsistent with trauma

D. Diagnostic Tests
1. When to order x-rays is controversial; some authorities suggest x-rays should be routinely ordered to rule out bony involvement whereas the recently-developed Ottawa rules recommend the following:
   a. Order ankle series if there is pain near the malleoli and either inability to bear weight both immediately and in the emergency department or bone tenderness at the posterior edge or tip of either malleolus
   b. Order foot x-ray series if there is pain in the midfoot and either inability to bear weight both immediately and in emergency department or bone tenderness at the navicular or the base of the fifth metatarsal
2. Consider ordering of stress films when the ankle cannot be easily manipulated to test for stability or when the patient has chronically unstable ankles

V. Plan/Management

A. Refer patient to orthopedist with Grade III sprain; consider orthopedist referral for eversion injury

B. Patient education for the first 48 hours: follow RICE therapy (**R**est, **I**ce, **C**ompression, **E**levation)
1. Immediately after injury, stop all weight-bearing
2. Apply ice to injury as many times as possible a day for 20 minutes
3. Compression can be accomplished by using an ace wrap to hold ice in place and after ice application to prevent swelling (when wrapping ankle, make sure to include heel)
4. Elevate ankle above the level of heart
5. A posterior splint and crutches may also be needed

C. Patient education after first 48 hours if patient's pain and swelling are resolving normally
1. Use hot and cold contrast baths
   a. Submerge ankle in hot water (115°F) for 4 minutes then in cold water (50°F) for 1 minute
   b. Alternate between hot and cold water 4 times, ending with cold water
   c. Repeat procedure 4 times each day
2. Begin exercising
   a. Toe alphabet in which entire foot and ankle traces letters of alphabet in air
   b. Isometrics in which side of injured foot/ankle is placed against an immovable object and pressed

      c.   Toe raising in which patient raises up and down on toes while holding onto object to maintain balance

D.   Patient education 2 weeks post-injury for individuals who have no further problems:
    1.   Resistive exercises with surgical or bicycle tubing (see Figure 17.4)
    2.   Remind patient that once an injury has occurred, the joint will never be as strong which will increase likelihood of reinjury unless strengthening exercises are continued

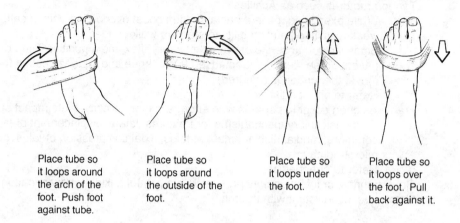

Place tube so it loops around the arch of the foot. Push foot against tube.

Place tube so it loops around the outside of the foot.

Place tube so it loops under the foot.

Place tube so it loops over the foot. Pull back against it.

Figure 17.4. Resistence Exercises.

E.   May order an air stirrup orthosis (e.g., Swede-O, Air Cast) to support ankle

F.   For pain, prescribe acetaminophen (Tylenol) 325 mg or 5-15 mg/kg/dose every 4 hours prn or ibuprofen (Motrin) 400 mg every 4-6 hours prn

G.   Prevention should include high-top lace-up shoes or a combination of proper shoes with a lace-up brace underneath (e.g., Swede-O)

H.   Follow Up
    1.   Examine ankle in 7-10 days or sooner if pain and swelling do not decrease
    2.   If there is little improvement or the condition has worsened in 2-3 weeks, consider referral to orthopedist or the ordering of additional films or bone scans

ELBOW PAIN

I.   Definition: Chronic or recurrent pain or discomfort of the elbow caused by selected common problems

II.   Pathogenesis

A.   Lateral epicondylitis or "tennis elbow"
    1.   Inflammation of the common tendinous origin of the extensor muscles of the forearm on the humeral lateral epicondyle
    2.   Exact mechanism of injury is uncertain but activities that combine excessive pronation and supination of the forearm with an extended wrist are probably responsible

B.   Medial epicondylitis or "golfer's elbow"
    1.   Inflammation of the common forearm flexor origin at the humeral medial epicondyle
    2.   Occurs in persons performing repetitive pronation activities

III.   Clinical Presentation

   A.   Lateral epicondylitis is one of the most common syndromes affecting the upper extremities
        1.   Commonly occurs in patients who frequently play tennis, badminton, or bowl
        2.   Also occurs in persons who engage in occupations that require using a wrench or screwdriver repetitively
        3.   The commonality among these activities is use of a strong grasp during wrist extension
        4.   Onset of symptoms is usually gradual with the patient complaining of tenderness on the lateral aspect of the elbow; swelling may occasionally be present

   B.   Medial epicondylitis is similar in presentation to "tennis elbow" described above but occurs less commonly
        1.   Occurs in golfers, but more commonly associated with certain manual activities such as the frequent carrying of objects with elbows flexed
        2.   Clinical presentation is similar to that of lateral epicondylitis except that the pain is located in the area of the medial, rather than the lateral, epicondyle
        3.   Inflammation can involve the ulnar nerve and compression of the nerve may cause numbness in the little and ring fingers on the affected side

IV.   Diagnosis/Evaluation

   A.   History
        1.   Inquire about onset, duration, and location of pain
        2.   Determine if associated symptoms of swelling, numbness and tingling of hand/fingers, or loss of strength in arm or hand are present
        3.   Inquire about participation in activities, either occupational or recreational that require the following
             a.   Strong grasp during wrist extension (if lateral epicondylitis is suspected)
             b.   Repetitive pronation of the arm or the carrying of heavy objects with elbows flexed (if medial epicondylitis is suspected)
        4.   Inquire about what makes the pain better or worse
        5.   Determine what treatments (either by the patient or another provider) have been tried and their result
        6.   Ask about past medical history and medication history

   B.   Physical Examination
        1.   If lateral epicondylitis is suspected, examine the elbow to determine the following
             a.   Assess for tenderness over the lateral epicondyle or over the radiohumeral joint
             b.   Assess range of motion (flexion and extension should be normal though extension may cause minimal pain)
             c.   Evaluate motor function of the hand by asking patient to abduct the thumb, index, and little fingers against resistance
             d.   Evaluate sensation at the dorsal web space between thumb and index finger (radial nerve), the tip of the long finger (median nerve), and the tip of the little finger (ulnar nerve)
             e.   Have the patient perform supination (palms up) and pronation (palms down) against resistance
             f.   To reproduce the patient's symptoms, perform the maneuver in Figure 17.5. Sharply localized tenderness in area of palpation or just distal is diagnostic of tennis elbow

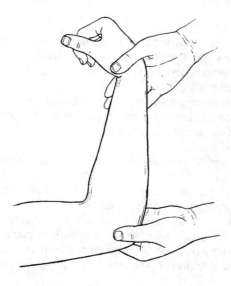

Figure 17.5. Palpation of the Lateral Epicondyle with the Thumb.

2.   If medial epicondylitis is suspected, examine the elbow to determine the following
    a.   Assess for point tenderness over the medial epicondyle
    b.   Assess range of motion (flexion and extension should be normal though extension may cause minimal pain)
    c.   Evaluate motor function of the hand by asking patient to abduct the thumb, index, and little fingers against resistance
    d.   Evaluate sensation at the dorsal web space between thumb and index finger (radial nerve), the tip of the long finger (median nerve), and the tip of the little finger (ulnar nerve)
    e.   To reproduce the patient's symptoms, perform the maneuver in the Figure 17.6. Tenderness on palpation occurs in golfer's elbow, tears of the ulnar collateral ligament, and injuries to the medial epicondyle

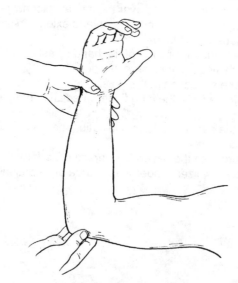

Figure 17.6. Palpation of the medial epicondyle.

C. Differential Diagnosis

D. Diagnostic Tests
   1. None indicated with history and physical examination that are consistent with the suspected diagnosis
   2. If atypical findings on history or physical examination, x-rays should be ordered

V. Plan/Management

   A. Lateral epicondylitis
      1. Focus is on reduction of the inflammation, strengthening the involved muscle, and avoidance of further injury
      2. Rest (immobilization in a sling for several days), ice, and use of rapidly acting NSAIDs (such as naproxen or piroxicam) are helpful in reducing the inflammation
      3. Referral to physical therapy can reduce symptoms and strengthen the involved muscle groups in the forearm and wrist through an appropriate exercise program, possibly preventing recurrences
      4. Avoidance of the activity that caused the problem for several weeks or months is necessary
      5. Use of an elbow strap (available at sporting goods stores) in the area of the muscle mass of the proximal portion of the forearm can be helpful, but is usually of limited value
      6. Patients who fail to respond to conservative therapy should be referred to a specialist for management

   B. Medial epicondylitis
      1. Treatment is the same as described under V.A. above
      2. If ulnar nerve involvement is suspected based on history and physical examination, prompt orthopedic referral is indicated

   C. Follow up: In one month to determine treatment effectiveness and to assess whether referral to a specialist is warranted

EXTREMITY PAIN, LOWER

I. Definition: Acute or chronic discomfort or pain in a limb

II. Pathogenesis

   A. Shin splints: inflammation of the sites of origin of the muscles originating from the shaft of the tibia; often due to overactivity

   B. Tibial and fibular stress fractures are due to repetitive forces being applied to the lower leg during strenuous activity; a malaligned lower leg may precipitate a stress fracture

   C. Osgood-Schlatter disease
      1. Degeneration of the tibial tubercle at the insertion site of the quadriceps ligament
      2. Associated with overuse and rapid growth, particularly during adolescence
      3. Result of repetitive, micro stress fractures

   D. Patellofemoral pain syndrome (PFPS) is due to one or both of the following:
      1. Mild malalignment of the extensor mechanism of the knee
      2. Repetitive microtrauma from overuse

E. Chondromalacia patellae is due to degeneration of the cartilage on the articular surface of the patella; overuse and malalignment of the lower leg predispose individuals to this condition

F. Patellar subluxation is associated with trauma and results in a lateral displacement of the patella

G. Iliotibial band syndrome is caused by overuse and excessive friction between the iliotibial band and the lateral femoral condyle; related to change in footwear, increase in running schedule, or prolonged downhill running

H. Legg-Calvé-Perthes disease results from compromise of the vascular supply to the femoral capital epiphysis which may be idiopathic or due to one of following:
1. Slipped capital femoral epiphysis
2. Trauma
3. Steroid use
4. Sickle cell crisis
5. Congenital dislocation of the hip

I. Slipped capital femoral epiphysis is a disorder of the growth and development of the upper femur due to a sudden or gradual dislocation of the head of the femur from its neck and shaft at the upper epiphyseal plate level; may be associated with endocrinopathies and heredity

J. Bursitis may be caused by acute trauma, contusion over bursae, overuse, or acute or chronic intra-articular inflammation (Baker's cyst)

K. Other important causes of lower extremity pain include osteomyelitis, neoplasms, fractures, sprains, sickle cell anemia, septic arthritis, thyroid disorders, and conditions with psychosocial origins

III. Clinical Presentation

A. Shin splints
1. Most often develop in persons who undergo exercise and are not properly conditioned, do not warm up properly, run on hard or uneven surfaces, wear improper shoes, and/or have anatomical abnormalities
2. Achy pain over the medial tibia that increases with exercise and improves with rest
3. Tenderness over the medial tibia

B. Tibial and fibular stress fractures
1. More common in adults than children; occur in athletes
2. Pain at the start of running activity; pain reproduced by jumping on affected leg
3. Diffuse tenderness over medial aspect of tibia or lateral aspect of fibula

C. Osgood-Schlatter disease
1. Most common in late childhood and adolescence
2. Painful swelling and point tenderness of the anterior aspect of the tibial tubercle; resisting knee extension worsens pain
3. Bilateral involvement occurs in 30% of cases
4. Occurs with strenuous activity, particularly involving the quadriceps muscles
5. May have permanent prominence of the tibial tubercle
6. Reoccurrence rate is 60%

D. Patellofemoral pain syndrome (PFPS)
1. Most common complaint in sports medicine clinics, particularly for the running athlete
2. Females are affected more than males, probably due to females having increased width of the gynecoid pelvis which results in an exaggerated Q angle (see IV.B.6)
3. Patients often complain of dull, achy knee pain of insidious onset which may have associated clicking or popping of knee on movement; pain is often poorly localized and bilateral
4. Pain is exacerbated with extended sitting, and activity involving knee flexion such as running and climbing and descending stairs

5. No history of swelling
6. Tenderness is elicited by compression of patella in the femoral groove
7. May have pain with movement of the patella laterally
8. Often associated with malalignment such as femoral anteversion, external tibial torsion, ankle valgus and excessive foot pronation
9. May lead to chondromalacia patellae and patellofemoral degenerative arthritis in adulthood

E. Chondromalacia patellae
   1. Occurs mainly in adults, infrequent incidence in adolescents
   2. Diffuse pain especially with climbing stairs or getting up from a squatting position
   3. Usually has a greater degree of malalignment than occurs with PFPS

F. Patellar subluxation
   1. Initial episode usually involves trauma
      a. Usually patient has severe knee pain and effusion
      b. Typically, patient can recall that knee "gave way"
   2. On pivoting and running, patients often complain of "locking" or "popping" of knee

G. Iliotibial band syndrome: typically involves mild pain over lateral side of knee

H. Legg-Calvé-Perthes Disease
   1. Most common in males, aged 4-8 years
   2. Limp may be presenting complaint
   3. Pain often is minimal, intermittent, and referred to medial aspect of knee
   4. Limitation of internal rotation and abduction of the femur is often present
   5. May have unequal iliac crest height and lower limb length discrepancy

I. Slipped capital femoral epiphysis
   1. Commonly affects sedentary, obese male adolescents
   2. Limp and varying degrees of ache and pain in the groin or referred pain in the knee are the common symptoms
   3. May have sudden dislocation of the head of the femur resulting in severe pain with associated inability to bear weight or gradual dislocation resulting in increasing dull pain
   4. Abduction, internal rotation, and flexion of the hip are the movements most limited
   5. Most cases are stable with a good prognosis if diagnosed early
   6. Unstable cases have a poorer prognosis because of high risk of avascular necrosis

J. Bursitis: Typically has swelling and pain over respective bursae (prepatellar, infrapatellar, and anserine bursae); may be associated with a Baker's cyst

IV. Diagnosis/Evaluation

A. History
   1. Inquire about mode of onset, duration, frequency and location of pain
   2. Question about discomfort in areas above and below the stated location of pain
   3. Ask patient to describe pain
   4. Ask about joint pain, especially without a history of trauma, as joint pain is often related to rheumatologic diseases and needs to be ruled out
   5. Query patient about recent trauma involving the lower leg
      a. Determine how injury occurred
      b. Ask patient to specifically describe the position and movement of his/her leg during the trauma
   6. Inquire about a history of a limp, stiffness, grinding, or any audible popping or snapping sound
   7. Inquire about exercise without pretraining, change in intensity or duration of exercise, recent viral infections, previous musculoskeletal problems, or repetitive activity
   8. Ask about medication use, particularly steroid use, and recent immunizations such as rubella

9. Inquire about family history of musculoskeletal problems, autoimmune disease, sickle cell disease, and recent exposure to infectious disease
10. Inquire about self-treatments and what aggravates and relieves pain
11. Perform a review of systems to rule-out systemic disease

B. Physical Examination
1. Assess vital signs as increased temperature may point to a systemic disease
2. Observe gait
3. Observe for misalignment of bones such as femoral anteversion and external tibial torsion
4. Observe for signs of trauma, development of muscles, deformities, swelling, and erythema
5. May need to measure limb length
6. Determine quadriceps angle (Q angle) if PFPS and chondromalacia patellae are suspected (see Figure 17.7)

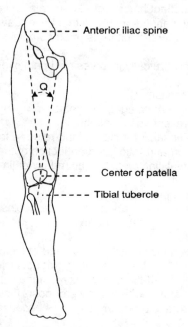

Figure 17.7. Measurement of Q-Angle or the Patellofemoral Angle.

Q angle is measured as the angle between a line drawn from the center of the patella to the anterior superior iliac spine and a line drawn from the center of the patella to the tibial tubercle. Average Q angle is 10-13° in males and 15-18° in females. Any angle less than or greater than average angles may be associated with PFPS.

7. Palpate limb and joints for tenderness, swelling and warmth
8. Perform range of motion of affected joints, noting any limitation in movement, crepitus, and tenderness
9. Assess peripheral vascular status by palpating pulses and determining capillary refill time distal to site of pain
10. Assess sensation of affected extremity
11. Assess muscle strength (distal weakness is often due to a neurological problem and proximal weakness is often due to a muscular problem)
12. Evaluate joint stability
13. Assess hamstring flexibility by having patient lie on back with hips flexed to 90° and then extend leg; failure to extend knee completely indicates hamstring tightness and may be a contributing factor in the extremity pain
14. Compare opposite limb for swelling, muscle wasting, color, mobility, strength, pulses, and sensation
15. A complete physical examination is often needed to rule out rheumatologic diseases

C. Differential Diagnosis:
1. Septic arthritis often involves abrupt onset of fever, malaise, pain and a tense, hot joint effusion
2. Inflammatory arthritis presents with warm, swollen, tender joints
3. Osteomyelitis commonly has extremity pain along with systemic signs of infectious disease such as fever and a septic appearance

D. Diagnostic Tests
1. If there is suspicion of systemic or infectious disease, or if pain has a longer duration than expected, is not relieved by common therapies, or is more intense than usually expected, the following tests may be helpful
   a. CBC
   b. Erythrocyte sedimentation rate
   c. Sickle cell preparation or hemoglobin electrophoresis
2. Consider rheumatologic studies for chronic pain
3. X-rays are usually ordered for the following:
   a. Pain due to trauma
   b. Suspected pathologic fractures, tumors or metabolic defects
   c. Pain lasting longer than 4-6 weeks
   d. Any history of swelling
4. Bone scan is often ordered if stress fractures or osteomyelitis is suspected
5. Diagnostic tests are usually ordered for suspected common causes of extremity pain:
   a. Shin splints: Order X-ray or bone scan if uncertain about diagnosis
   b. For suspected tibial and fibular stress fractures, x-rays (AP, lateral, and both oblique views of leg) are usually ordered; x-rays may be negative in early stages; technetium-99m bone scans and MRI are most helpful
   c. Osgood-Schlatter disease: None usually needed; may order x-ray to rule out other conditions or if diagnosis is uncertain
   d. PFPS: Order X-rays if pain lasts longer than 4-6 weeks
   e. Chondromalacia patellae: Order knee x-rays which include a tangential or sunrise view to look for lateral subluxation of the patella
   f. Patellar subluxation: Order knee x-rays; need a tangential or sunrise view
   g. Iliotibial band syndrome: none usually needed
   h. Legg-Calvé-Perthes disease: Order x-rays (anteroposterior and frog-leg lateral pelvis) or bone scan
   i. Slipped capital femoral epiphysis: Order x-rays
   j. Bursitis: Arthrography is ordered to definitively diagnose a Baker's cyst; otherwise none are needed

V. Plan/Management

A. Shin Splints
1. Rest: Unless the pain is severe, the athlete does not need to completely stop exercising but needs to reduce intensity and duration of exercise
2. Ice should be applied to reduce swelling and inflammation
3. Anti-inflammatory medication such as naproxen (Naprosyn) 250-500 mg every 6-8 hours
4. May need to treat concomitant hyperpronation of foot with flexible orthotics or sturdy, well-fitting footwear
5. Instruct patient to run on soft, flat surfaces

B. Tibial and fibular stress fractures
1. Initial treatment is rest, ice, and antiinflammatory medication
2. Often fractures heal without casting or surgery
3. Rest until there is no longer point tenderness on palpation or pain with running (usually takes 6-8 weeks to resolve)
4. Can bike, swim or do other activities that do not produce pain

C. Osgood-Schlatter disease: Rest, ice, quadriceps strengthening exercises, hamstring stretching exercises, and limited use of antiinflammatory medication

D.   PFPS
    1.   Modify activities to avoid full flexion of the knee and stress on the patellofemoral joint
    2.   Begin stretching and strengthening program for quadriceps muscles (perform three sets of 10 repetitions each day during the acute phase)
        a.   Quadriceps setting: Patient lies supine with affected knee fully extended, dorsiflexes foot, then tightens the thigh muscles or pushes the thigh into the floor
        b.   Straight leg raise: Patient sits on floor, leans back on elbows with one leg fully extended and the other leg flexed to 90 degrees; the extended leg is raised until it is parallel with the thigh of the flexed leg and held in this position for 5 seconds
        c.   Terminal-arc extension: Patient lies on floor with knees in about 20 degrees of flexion over a rolled towel of about 6 inches in diameter; patient then extends knee fully and holds for 5 seconds
        d.   After the acute phase, progressive resistance with ankle weights should be initiated
        e.   Encourage flexibility exercises as well
    3.   Consider flexible orthotics for malalignment of lower extremities
    4.   For exacerbations, use ice and antiinflammatory medication
    5.   Teach that pain tends to be chronic with exacerbations and remissions, but pain can be controlled; swimming or walking are better sports to participate in than running, basketball, and volleyball

E.   Chondromalacia patellae: Plan is similar to treatment for PFPS (see above)

F.   Recurrent patellar subluxation: Refer to orthopedist

G.   Iliotibial band syndrome: Rest for approximately 1-2 weeks (may take as long as 6 weeks), ice, limited use of NSAIDS, and gradual resumption of full activities with rehabilitation (quadriceps strengthening exercises); consider one-eighth-inch lateral heel wedge

H.   Legg-Calvé-Perthes disease: Refer to orthopedic surgeon

I.   Slipped Capital Femoral Epiphysis: Refer to orthopedic surgeon

J.   Bursitis
    1.   Rest (couple days to weeks), ice for 24 hours, and limited use of NSAIDS
    2.   Aspirate tense, inflamed bursa and inject corticosteroid solution
    3.   Aspirate Baker's cyst to relieve pressure and pain

K.   Follow up for extremity pain is variable depending on patient's problem

FIBROMYALGIA

I.   Definition: Complex syndrome involving fatigue and widespread, nonarticular musculoskeletal pain

II.   Pathogenesis

A.   Etiology is unknown

B.   The following mechanisms have been hypothesized to trigger fibromyalgia (FMS): metabolic processes, immunological abnormalities, sleep disturbances, stress and trauma from accidents or surgery and infection due to Epstein Barr virus, cytomegalovirus, human herpesvirus 6, enteroviruses, *B. burgdorferi*

III. Clinical presentation

   A. Age of onset is typically between 20-40 years; prevalence increases with age but can occur in childhood

   B. Females are affected 8-10 times more than men

   C. Most common symptoms are diffuse musculoskeletal pain, sleep disturbance, and persistent fatigue

   D. Other symptoms include swelling of hands and feet, morning stiffness, headaches, paresthesias, sensitivity to cold and/or hot, dypsnea, chest pain, night sweats, visual problems, dizziness, painful menses, gastrointestinal complaints, memory impairment, anxiety and depression

   E. Patients may have associated conditions such as mitral valve prolapse, episodic hypoglycemia, Raynaud's disease, and irritable bowel syndrome

   F. Symptoms can be severe and patients may become functionally disabled

   G. Because patients have chronic, multiple, vague complaints and no outward signs, they are often misdiagnosed as hypochondriacs and relationships with family and friends may deteriorate

   H. Patients often have disturbance of stage 4 of sleep; disturbance of this stage for 2-3 consecutive nights can produce physical symptoms of FMS even in normal controls

   I. Tender points (localized areas of muscle tenderness that result in pain when pressure is applied) are essential to the diagnosis; trigger points (pain is elicited at initial site of palpation as well as in a linear or circumferential pattern surrounding the site or at a distant site) are also common

   J. The American College of Rheumatology (ACR) established clinical criteria for diagnosing FMS (see table on ACR Criteria and Figure 17.8 on Tender Point Sites)

THE AMERICAN COLLEGE OF RHEUMATOLOGY 1990 CRITERIA FOR CLASSIFICATION OF FIBROMYALGIA

*1. History of widespread pain

Definition. Pain is considered widespread when all of the following are present: pain in the left side of the body, pain in the right side of the body, pain above the waist, and pain below the waist. In addition, axial skeletal pain (cervical spine or anterior chest or thoracic spine or low back) must be present. In this definition, shoulder and buttock pain is considered as pain for each involved side. "Low back" pain is considered lower segment pain.

2. Pain in 11 of 18 tender point sites on digital palpation.

Definition. Pain, on digital palpation must be present in at least 11 of the following 18 tender point sites:
   Occiput: Bilateral, at the suboccipital muscle insertions
   Low cervical: Bilateral, at the anterior aspects of the intertransverse spaces at C5-C7
   Trapezius: Bilateral, at the midpoint of the upper border
   Supraspinatus: Bilateral, at origins, above the scapula spine near the medial border
   Second rib: Bilateral, at the second costochondral junctions, just lateral to the junctions on upper surfaces
   Lateral epicondyle: Bilateral, 2 cm distal to the epicondyles
   Gluteal: Bilateral, in upper outer quadrants of buttocks in anterior fold of muscle
   Greater trochanter: Bilateral, posterior to the trochanteric prominence
   Knee: Bilateral, at the medial fat pad proximal to the joint line

For a tender point to be considered "positive" the subject must state that the palpation was painful.

*For classification purposes, patients must satisfy both criteria. Widespread pain must have been present for at least 3 months.

Source: Wolfe, F., et al. (1990). The American College of Rheumatology 1990 criteria for the classification of fibromyalgia. Arthritis and Rheumatism, 33(2), 160-173.

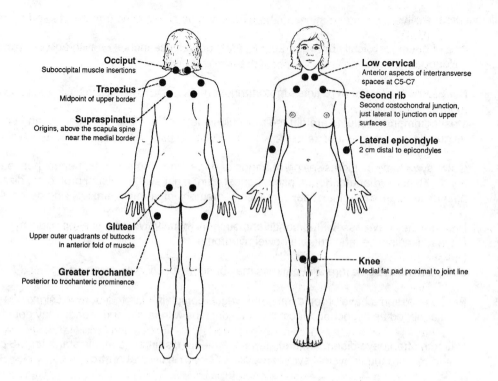

Figure 17.8. Tender Points Identified by American College of Rheumatology.

The figure labels include:

Occiput
Suboccipital muscle insertions

Trapezius
Midpoint of upper border

Supraspinatus
Origins, above the scapula spine near the medial border

Gluteal
Upper outer quadrants of buttocks in anterior fold of muscle

Greater trochanter
Posterior to trochanteric prominence

Low cervical
Anterior aspects of intertransverse spaces at C5-C7

Second rib
Second costochondral junction, just lateral to junction on upper surfaces

Lateral epicondyle
2 cm distal to epicondyles

Knee
Medial fat pad proximal to joint line

IV.   Diagnosis/Evaluation

    A.   History
        1.   Question about associated symptoms such as headaches, diarrhea, lack of concentration
        2.   Ask about factors that may precipitate symptoms
        3.   Explore how the disease has impacted on patient's family, interpersonal relationships, work, school, and activities of daily living

    B.   Physical Examination
        1.   Measure vital signs
        2.   Observe general appearance
        3.   Assess neck for thyromegaly
        4.   Perform bilateral digital palpation using a force of about 4 kg/cm$_2$ which is approximately equal to pressing finger on bathroom scale until it registers 10 pounds, or until the nail bed just begins to blanch; to meet criteria of a positive tender point, patient must label the palpation as "painful," not just tender
        5.   Perform a complete musculoskeletal, particularly assess each joint
        6.   Assess mental status and perform a mental health assessment

    C.   Differential Diagnosis
        1.   Patients with chronic fatigue syndrome have vague, systemic symptoms but do not usually complain of pain as is characteristic of FMS
        2.   Rheumatoid arthritis in contrast to FMS presents with warm, erythematous joints in addition to pain
        3.   Patients with FMS may have a mildly elevated ANA but other criteria of systemic lupus erythematosus (SLE) are not present (see section on RHEUMATOID ARTHRITIS for criteria for SLE)
        4.   Somatization and depression often accompany FMS but are not the primary diagnoses; patients with psychological problems do not have characteristic tender points
        5.   Myofascial pain syndrome presents with referred trigger points and occurs more frequently in men than women which is not characteristic of FMS

6. Polymyalgia rheumatica can be diagnosed by an elevated erythrocyte sedimentation rate (ESR)
7. Severe hypothyroidism can mimic FMS but usually patient has signs such as lid lag, dry skin, and an elevated thyroid stimulating hormone

D. Diagnostic Tests: no tests are available to detect FMS, consider the following tests to exclude other possible diagnoses
1. Complete blood count
2. Erythrocyte sedimentation rate (order in all persons >50 years who present with symptoms)
3. Measurement of muscle enzymes
4. Thyroid stimulating hormone
5. Rheumatoid factor

V. Plan/Management: a multifaceted approach with an interdisciplinary team is ideal

A. Patient Education
1. Provide reassurance that patient has a distinct, recognizable disease and that symptoms are real but can be managed
2. Help patient shift from a sense of helplessness and frustration to a sense of self-efficacy and hope
   a. Self-management courses to control symptoms and promote health are effective
   b. Social support interventions may be beneficial
   c. Cognitive behavioral therapy such as helping patients to prioritize their time and activities to include meaningful work, activities of daily living as well as leisure is helpful

B. Exercise: A program which includes pain reduction techniques of stretching, proper posture, body mechanics with careful and gentle exercise such as walking, bicycling, and swimming is helpful
1. Strenuous or excessive exercise should be avoided
2. Referral to a physical therapist can be beneficial

C. Pharmacological treatment
1. Medications to help the patient receive a restful sleep may be helpful
   a. Amitriptyline (Elavil) is commonly used and in the FMS patient this drug increases non-REM stage 4 sleep by increasing serotonin levels; prescribe amitriptyline 10 mg at HS and can increase to 50 mg over a few weeks
   b. Zolpidem (Ambien) 10 mg HS is an alternative drug to treat sleep problems; limit to 2-3 nights per week
   c. To help combat the concomitant fatigue and depression, a serotonin reuptake inhibitor like fluoxetine (Prozac) 20 mg can be given in the morning; a combination of amitriptyline and prozac was found to be more effective than either drug alone in a recent study
2. To treat muscle spasms, cyclobenzaprine (Flexeril) 10 mg TID can be prescribed; do not use more than three weeks
3. Tramadol (Ultram) 50-100 mg every 4-6 hours and topical anesthetics such as capsaicin (Zostrix) may be effective in relieving pain; because of chronic nature of FMS avoid narcotic agents; there are contradictory research findings concerning the benefits of nonsteroidal anti-inflammatory drugs

D. Massage therapy, acupuncture, local infiltration of trigger points with 1% solution of lidocaine, stress management, relaxation techniques, transcutaneous electrical nerve stimulation, visualization and meditation are additional effective therapies

E. Followup is variable and depends on the severity of symptoms as well as coping abilities and resources of the patients and their support systems

GOUT

I.   Diagnosis: Inflammatory disease of peripheral joints caused by monosodium urate crystal deposition

II.   Pathogenesis: Alteration in purine metabolism, the end product of which is uric acid

    A.   Primary gout is due to inborn error in production or excretion of uric acid (90% have an underexcretion problem)

    B.   Risk for developing primary gout is directly proportional to degree and duration of hyperuricemia

    C.   Secondary gout is due to a variety of acquired diseases such as myeloproliferative disease, lymphoproliferative disease, hemolytic anemia, glycogen storage disease, psoriasis, renal insufficiency, sarcoidosis

    D.   Secondary gout is associated with obesity, starvation, lead intoxication and ingestion of drugs (salicylates, diuretics, pyrazinamide, ethambutol, nicotinic acid, alcohol)

III.   Clinical Presentation

    A.   Men over age of 30 years are most affected; disease is rare in women until after menopause

    B.   Symptoms occur after many years of sustained hyperuricemia

    C.   Acute phase
        1.   Sudden onset of joint inflammation and excruciating pain; one joint, often the metatarsophalangeal joint of great toe (referred to as podagra) is involved, but other common sites are instep of foot, ankle, knee, wrist, or elbow
        2.   First attack often begins at night or early morning and pain peaks in 24-36 hours; even without treatment symptoms subside in few days to weeks
        3.   Signs include warm, tender, erythematous joint and possible fever

    D.   Intercritical period: between attacks patient is asymptomatic without abnormal physical findings

    E.   Chronic gout
        1.   Asymptomatic intervals become shorter and more joints are involved as disease progresses
        2.   Over time persistent symptoms such as morning stiffness, synovial tissue thickening, and joint deformity occur
        3.   Tophi, chalky deposits of sodium urate, can develop at sites of irritation such as Achilles tendon, joints of hand, pinnae of ears; tophi seldom become visible until 10 years after the onset of gout
        4.   Extra-articular manifestations include low grade fever, chronic gouty nephropathy, nephrolithiasis, and acute uric acid nephropathy

IV.   Diagnosis/Evaluation

    A.   History
        1.   Question about possible precipitating causes such as aspirin intake, diuretic and alcohol use, recent changes in dietary intake
        2.   Ask about family history of gout
        3.   Carefully determine number, duration and characteristics of previous attacks
        4.   For patients with chronic grout, explore associated symptoms such as fever, back pain, nausea

B. Physical Examination
    1. Measure vital signs noting elevated temperature and blood pressure
    2. Observe and palpate painful joints
    3. Observe for tophi and chronic joint deformity

C. Differential Diagnosis
    1. Pseudogout due to presence of calcium pyrophosphate dihydrate (CPPD) in the joints
        a. Affects the elderly
        b. Has three phases (acute, asymptomatic, and chronic) similar to gout but rarely has tophuslike collections
        c. Typical affected joints are the knees, wrists, MCP joints, elbows and shoulders
        d. Symptomatic treatment with NSAIDs and colchicine is recommended during the acute phase
        e. In chronic arthritis, NSAIDs are recommended; no medication is known to prevent CPPD crystal formation
    2. Cellulitis
    3. Septic arthritis
    4. Rheumatoid arthritis
    5. Bursitis related to a bunion
    6. Evaluate for gout associated with hypertension, hyperlipidemia, renal disease, obesity, and alcohol overuse

D. Diagnostic tests
    1. Aspirate joint fluid for smear and culture (to rule out infection) and to identify urate crystals
    2. Order serum uric acid levels
        a. A level >7.0 mg/dL supports the diagnosis of gout but is not specific; patients with chronic use of low-dose aspirin, renal insufficiency, and diuretic use may have elevated uric acid
        b. Serum uric acid levels also can be used to assess the risk for urate stones and the need for aggressive therapy
    3. Consider 24-hour urine to measure uric acid excretion which is normally between 600-900 mg on a regular diet; levels >900 mg suggest overproduction of urate
    4. During attack, sedimentation rate and white blood cell count may be elevated
    5. To help rule out rheumatoid arthritis may order rheumatoid factor titer
    6. X-rays may be ordered to rule out other conditions, but are not helpful in differentiating gout from other diseases except in advanced cases when affected joints show punched out lesions in subchondral bone

V. Plan/Management

A. General principles of pharmacological management
    1. Initiate medications early in disease course to enhance likelihood of response
    2. Drugs that affect serum urate levels should never be changed during an acute attack
    3. Acute attacks usually resolve within 48 hours if properly managed; seek other diagnoses if symptoms are not improved in this time frame

B. Acute phase
    1. Joint immobilization and decreased weight-bearing
    2. Analgesics
        a. Non-steroidal anti-inflammatory drugs (NSAIDs) are considered the first line drug; start drugs at high dose and then gradually reduce; consider one of the following:
            (1) Indomethacin (Indocin) 50 mg every 8 hours for 6-8 doses, then reduce to 25 mg every 8 hours until attack resolved (usually give high dose for 2-3 days and then taper dose over next 3-5 days)
            (2) Naproxen (Naprosyn), initially 750 mg followed by 250 mg every 8 hours

  b. Colchicine is used less frequently today due to potential adverse effects
    (1) Dosage depends on the severity of symptoms and individual characteristics of patient: traditionally 0.5 mg tablet was given every hour until total dose of 7.0 mg or 14 doses was reached, symptoms abated, or patient had diarrhea, abdominal cramping, nausea and vomiting; today, colchicine is usually titrated based on pain, but the maximum dosage should not be exceeded
    (2) For patients with severe gout who are unable to use NSAIDS or oral colchicine, intravenous colchicine is available
    (3) Extreme caution is necessary for patients with even mild renal impairment
  c. Low-dose oral corticosteroids (30 mg of prednisone given daily for 2-3 days then tapered over 5-7 days) and intra-articular injections of steroids may also be beneficial

C. Intercritical Phase: **daily prophylaxis** with NSAID or colchicine is often all that is needed to prevent development of frequent attacks and chronic gout
 1. Prescribe indomethacin 25 mg BID
 2. Alternatively, prescribe colchicine 0.5-0.6 mg BID
 3. Patients may also take 1 or 2 tablets of colchicine when they sense an impeding attack

D. Chronic gout
 1. Treatment with a urate lowering agent or hypouricemic treatment (allopurinol or probenecid) is indicated in the following patients:
  a. Frequent (more than 3 attacks/year) and disabling attacks
  b. Tophaceous deposits in soft tissues
  c. Destructive gouty joint disease as seen by erosions on x-rays
  d. Recurrent urolithiasis; most recent stone within last 2 years
  e. Severe hyperuricemia (>13 mg/dL in males; >10 mg/dL in females; >15 mg/dL in patients with renal failure)
  f. Severe uric acid overproduction (urinary uric acid excretion >1100 mg/day)
  g. Gout with renal damage, urate nephropathy
  h. Patients with high tumor burden of leukemia-lymphoma about to receive cytotoxic treatment
 2. If patients meets above criteria, begin urate lowering agent regimen that follows:
  a. Continue low doses of colchicine or NSAIDS for 2-12 months as prophylaxis to avoid fluctuation of uric acid levels which may precipitate an acute attack
  b. Do not start urate-lowering agent until at least one month after acute attack
  c. Order blood urea nitrogen (BUN), serum lipid levels, and CBC before drug therapy
  d. To decrease synthesis of uric acid, if patient is secreting too much uric acid (>900 mg/day in 24-hour urine) or in patients with nephrolithiasis, creatinine clearance less than 50 mL/minute or tophaceous deposits prescribe allopurinol (Zyloprim). Give allopurinol 100 mg for 1 week, then raise by 100 mg at weekly intervals until maintenance dose of 300 mg/day is attained; however, a few patients may need doses as high as 800 mg/day
    (1) Goal is to keep uric acid <6.5 mg/dL
    (2) Allopurinol hypersensitivity reaction consists of fever, rash, decreased renal function, liver damage, and leukocytosis
    (3) Patients with renal insufficiency should have reduced dose
  e. Alternatively, use probenecid (Benemid) (start low at 250 mg BID for 1 week then increase to 500 mg BID) <u>to increase renal excretion of uric acid</u>
    (1) Always encourage high fluid intake (>3L/day)
    (2) Patients at risk for stones should be given trisodium citrate 5 gm TID for urine alkalinization
  f. A uricosuric combination tablet of probenecid 500 mg and colchicine 0.5 mg given BID is available

E. Patient Education
   1. Gradual weight reduction
   2. Reduce alcohol consumption and reduce purine intake (anchovies, gravies, liver)
   3. Avoid salicylates
   4. Increase fluid intake to 3 L/day
   5. Patients with chronic gout on hypouricemic treatment, must be advised that control of disease is a lifelong commitment

F. Asymptomatic Hyperuricemia
   1. Search for causes
   2. Generally asymptomatic hyperuricemia is not treated but followed closely

G. Follow Up
   1. Patient with acute gout should be contacted or seen in 24 hours and return in 4 weeks to discuss maintenance therapy
   2. Followup for patients with chronic gout should be individualized, however, yearly uric acid levels are recommended

JOINT PAIN

I. Definition: Discomfort or tenderness in one or more joints

II. Pathogenesis: see clinical presentation for common causes

III. Clinical presentation of common forms of joint pain

   A. Pain involving multiple joints
      1. Rheumatoid arthritis (RA): Chronic inflammatory polyarthritis with symmetric joint involvement and rheumatoid factor positivity (see section on RHEUMATOID ARTHRITIS)
      2. Osteoarthritis: Joint pain and stiffness, usually lasting less than 30 minutes with lack of systemic symptoms (see section on OSTEOARTHRITIS)
      3. Gout: First attack usually involves only 1 joint, often metatarsophalangeal joint of great toe, which is painful, warm and red; subsequent attacks may involve one or several joints (see section on GOUT)
      4. Systemic lupus erythematosus (SLE): American Rheumatism Association Classification (1982) (see following table)

CLASSIFICATION OF SYSTEMIC LUPUS ERYTHEMATOSUS
• Malar rash: fixed, erythematous, flat, or raised rash over malar eminences
• Discoid rash: erythematous raised patches with scaling
• Photosensitivity
• Oral ulcers
• Arthritis involving 2 or more peripheral joints
• Serositis involving either pleuritis or pericarditis
• Renal disorder involving persistent proteinuria or cellular casts
• Neurologic disorder involving seizures or psychosis
• Hematologic disorders of hemolytic anemia, leukopenia, lymphopenia, or thrombocytopenia
• Immunologic disorder such as positive lupus erythematosus cell preparation or anti-DNA antibody to native DNA in abnormal titer or Anti-Sm or false positive serologic test for syphilis for at least 6 months
• Abnormal titer of antinuclear antibody

* A person is said to have SLE if 4 or more of 11 criteria are present

Adapted from Tan, E.M., Cohen, A.S., Fries, J.F., et al. (1982). The 1982 revised criteria for the classification of systemic lupus erythematosus. Arthritis Rheumatology, 25, 1275-1277.

5. Polymyalgia rheumatica usually presents in patients over age 50 with shoulder pain, hip-girdle stiffness and increased erythrocyte sedimentation rate
6. Fibromyalgia is a poorly understood syndrome involving widespread musculoskeletal pain and accompanied by fatigue, nonrestorative sleep, reduced functional ability and sometimes accompanied with headaches, irritable bowel syndrome, paresthesias, restless leg syndrome, and cold sensitivity (see section on FIBROMYALGIA)
7. Reiter's syndrome involves classic triad of arthritis, urethritis, and conjunctivitis
8. Psoriatic arthritis often presents with asymmetric joint involvement and characteristic nail and skin lesions
9. Gonococcal arthritis presents as migratory polyarthritis, tendinitis and often has vesicular-pustular skin lesions
10. Lyme arthritis usually has classic history of tick bite and rash with arthritis in knees (see section on LYME DISEASE)
11. Rheumatic heart disease presents in a migratory pattern of joint involvement with evidence of antecedent streptococcal infection
12. Inflammatory bowel disease such as ulcerative colitis and Crohn's disease are associated with gastrointestinal complaints
13. Ankylosing spondylitis presents with back pain and stiffness
14. Infections such as influenza, rubella, mumps, chickenpox, infectious mononucleosis, hepatitis, Rocky Mountain-spotted fever, and rat-bite fever can also involve joints
15. Sickle cell disease causes pain, swelling, tenderness, and effusion in large joints

B. Pain involving single joint
1. Infection
   a. Septic arthritis due to disseminated gonorrhea or gram positive bacteria, especially *Staphylococcus aureus,* is a serious condition, presenting with fever, chills, skin lesion, joint pain, and swelling
   b. Gram-negative bacterial infections and infections due to anaerobes are increasingly frequent causes of monarthritis due to the rising number of persons who are parenteral drug users and immunosuppressed persons
   c. Tuberculous arthritis with subsequent periarticular bone lesions and synovial involvement may occur even if pulmonary tuberculosis is not present
   d. Monarthritis can herald the onset of HIV infection
2. One joint may be involved in crystal-induced arthritis such as gout and pseudogout which results from crystals of calcium pyrophosphate inducing joint inflammation and seems to be associated with hyperparathyroidism and hemochromatosis in the older patient
3. Trauma and foreign-body reactions may present with sudden pain and swelling in one joint
4. Osteomyelitis involves localized swelling, limitation of joint mobility, erythema and tenderness over involved area, fever, and and/or an associated ulcer or skin lesion with possibly a sinus tract draining infected fluid; risk factors include history of bacteremia, peripheral vascular disease, diabetes mellitus, trauma, or surgery in the affected area

C. Other diseases such as rheumatoid arthritis, osteoarthritis, systemic lupus erythematosus, arthritis of inflammatory bowel disease, Lyme disease, psoriatic arthritis, Behcet's disease, Reiter's syndrome, and hemarthrosis (bleeding into a joint commonly due to a clotting abnormality) can result in pain in single or multiple joints

IV. Diagnosis/Evaluation

A. History
1. Ascertain pain characteristics, location, what aggravates pain, and what functional loss has occurred
2. Ask about distribution of involved joints (symmetric involvement of metacarpophalangeal joints (MCP) and wrists suggests rheumatoid arthritis (RA), whereas involvement of distal interphalangeal joints (DIP) suggests osteoarthritis (OA)
3. Determine severity of pain by asking if it awakens patient at night or hinders activities of daily living
4. Explore history of previous attacks; past episodes lend support for a crystalline or other noninfectious cause

5. Inquire about previous trauma to joint or surrounding tissues
6. Question about tick bites, fever, sexual risk factors, intravenous drug use, alcohol abuse, and travel in foreign countries -- all of which suggest an infectious cause
7. Inquire about rash, diarrhea, urethritis, or uveitis which supports a diagnosis of arthritides
8. Explore systemic symptoms such as fatigue, fever, sleep problems which suggest rheumatoid arthritis, SLE, fibromyalgia
9. Ask about history of gastrointestinal problems and determine whether there is a history of an ulcer, because this will affect choice of analgesic medication
10. A complete family history is important
11. Often a complete review of systems is needed to determine other involved organs

B. Physical Examination
   1. Measure temperature and other vital signs (fever suggests infection such as septic arthritis)
   2. Observe gait and general appearance
   3. Examine joints for presence of tenderness, erythema, warmth, effusion, bony enlargement, and mechanical abnormalities
      a. Assessment must distinguish an arthritis, which involves the articular space, from conditions involving the periarticular area, such as bursitis, cellulitis, or tendinitis; painful limitation of motion probably indicates joint involvement
      b. Helpful to compare paired joints
      c. Remember to inspect, palpate, perform range of motion activities, and perform additional tests such as Tinel's sign [percuss over median nerve on palmar side or volar surface of wrist; shooting pain in the long or index finger is a positive sign] (see Figure 17.22)
   4. Assess for muscle atrophy
   5. Detailed physical examination is often needed to detect extra-articular manifestations
      a. Observe eyes, nose, and mouth for dryness as occurs with sicca syndrome which suggests Sjögren's syndrome that often accompanies rheumatoid arthritis
      b. Palpate elbows, Achilles tendons, and pinnae for nodules and tophi (rheumatoid arthritis and gout, respectively)
      c. Observe nails for pitting (psoriatic arthritis)
      d. Observe skin for malar and discoid lesions of SLE and exanthem of gonococcal arthritis
      e. Examine eyes for conjunctivitis of Reiter's syndrome
      f. Inspect mouth for ulcers in Behcet's syndrome, Reiter's syndrome, and SLE
      g. Auscultate heart and lungs noting pleural rubs and heart murmurs from RA and SLE
      h. Urethral or cervical discharge suggests gonococcal arthritis

C. Differential Diagnosis: Rule out all conditions listed in section III.

D. Diagnostic tests are useful in differentiating the specific type of arthritis present.
   1. Synovial fluid analysis is done to differentiate inflammatory from non-inflammatory joint disease and to determine whether a joint is infected
   2. Erythrocyte sedimentation rate (ESR) can be useful as a screen for inflammatory disease
   3. Rheumatoid factor may be helpful in confirming the diagnosis of RA, but is also often positive when the patient has other conditions
   4. Antinuclear antibody (ANA) is sensitive but not specific in diagnosing SLE
   5. Uric acids levels are often elevated in gout
   6. X-rays are often ordered to obtain baseline data rather than to help determine diagnosis; best utilized in bone and joint evaluation
   7. Magnetic resonance imaging can sometimes localize an infectious or inflammatory process in a joint, tissue, or bone; best utilized in soft tissue evaluation
   8. Tests for HIV antibodies should be ordered when risk factors for this disease are present
   9. Blood cultures are needed when sepsis is suspected
   10. Bone biopsy or culture are needed when osteomyelitis is suspected

V.   Plan/Management

A.   Determine severity of disease and the need for hospitalization; rapid onset on pain, heat, swelling, and erythema of joint should be evaluated immediately for septic arthritis or osteomyelitis

B.   Treat known causes. For example, ceftriaxone (Rocephin) should be used to treat gonococcal arthritis

C.   Symptomatic therapy often includes rest of involved joint, hot and/or cold therapy and pain relief with aspirin (not gout) or NSAIDs

D.   Follow up is variable

KNEE INJURY, ACUTE

I.   Definition: Injury to the knee from acute trauma

II.   Pathogenesis

A.   Strains and sprains of the collateral and cruciate ligaments are caused by forces that create abduction of the leg at the knee, hyperextension of the knee, or a direct blow to the knee
1.   Strains involve stretching of the muscles or tendons
2.   Grade I sprains involve stretching fibers without significant structural damage
3.   Grade II sprains involve partial disruption of fibers with increased laxity
4.   Grade III sprains involve complete tearing of ligamentous tissues

B.   Tears of the medial and lateral meniscus are common and typically involve a simple twisting motion or a rotary force applied to a flexed knee joint; often caused by a noncontact injury

C.   Patellar subluxation or dislocation usually occurs with knee near extension and the tibia externally rotated or may result from a direct blow to knee; may accompany an anterior cruciate ligament (ACL) injury

D.   Fractures of the patellar result from falls or direct blows to the knee

E.   Hemarthrosis, or blood collecting in joint, is a serious injury and results from extensive trauma

F.   Excessive pronation of the foot or misalignment of an extremity can cause inappropriate stress on structures of the knee and result in injury

III.   Clinical Presentation

A.   Ligament injuries
1.   Most frequently injured ligament is the medial collateral ligament
2.   Patients have variable amounts of pain, stiffness, tenderness and swelling depending on severity of ligament damage
3.   Anterior cruciate ligament injury may involve an audible pop and "giving way" sensation (patient typically falls to ground and is unable to arise without assistance); involves a positive Lachman's test; large effusion develops within first few hours
4.   Posterior cruciate ligament injury has a positive posterior drawer test; observation of knee may reveal hyperflexion
5.   Collateral ligament injury involves local swelling, laxity, tenderness over the ligament and may or may not be painful; effusion is usually minimal

B. Meniscus injury
1. Medial meniscus injuries are more common than lateral meniscus injuries
2. Patient often recalls a twisting flexion injury of the knee following by pain and difficulty flexing the knee and bearing weight
3. May have clicking, locking, catching, or giving way of knee
4. Knee joint effusion and tenderness over the joint line are often noted

C. Patellar subluxation or dislocation occurs more frequently in women and involves medial tenderness and effusion; often the dislocation reduces when the leg is completely extended

D. Fractures are difficult to differentiate from other injuries; may result in severe pain, inability to bear weight, swelling, limited range of motion, and unequal leg length
1. Crepitus is palpable with patellar fractures
2. Neurovascular compromise may occur with femoral condylar fractures
3. Pain with compression of the side of joint may occur with tibial plateau fractures

IV. Diagnosis/Evaluation

A. History
1. Ask patient to precisely describe circumstances surrounding injury and mechanism of the injury; particularly ask if injury involved hyperextension of the knee, a direct blow to knee, or a twisting injury
2. Inquire about location of pain, tenderness, and swelling in knee as well as hip, thigh, shin, ankle and foot
3. Inquire about sensations of locking, clicking, catching, giving way or buckling of the knee
4. Ask patient to point to site of greatest pain
5. Ask how quickly after the injury the swelling developed; swelling in the joint within 24 hours suggests hemarthrosis
6. Ask about previous musculoskeletal injuries; important to determine if this is an acute problem or a preexisting condition which has been aggravated
7. Inquire about systemic symptoms such as fever, chills, night sweats
8. Determine patient's occupation and job requirements
9. Determine whether patient is involved in leisure or competitive athletics which will affect decisions about management
10. Inquire about self treatments

B. Physical Examination
1. Always compare injured side with unaffected side during observation, palpation, range of motion, and special tests
2. Observe gait and stance, noting lower extremity alignment
3. Observe knee while standing for deformity, discoloration, and swelling
4. With patient seated and knee flexed at 90°, look for bulge of fluid on either side of patellar ligament
5. Palpate in a proximal to distal direction with patient sitting and supine (see Figure 17.9 for anatomical structures)
   a. Begin with thigh, palpating quadriceps, hamstrings, and articular surfaces of the femoral condyles; consider measuring thigh girth to detect disuse atrophy
   b. Palpate patella and all around the joint line (tenderness at joint line suggests meniscal tear, whereas tenderness slightly above or below suggests ligament damage)
   c. Palpate muscles around patella and collateral ligaments
   d. Palpate tibial plateau and tibial tuberosity

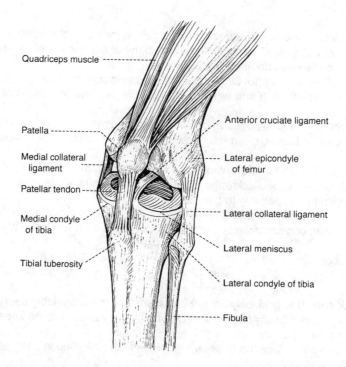

Figure 17.9. Anatomical Structures of the Knee.

6.   Assess for effusion or fluid in knee joint (see Figure 17.10)

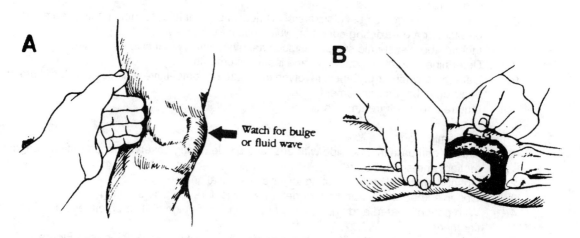

Figure 17.10. Testing for Fluid in the Knee Joint.

A. The bulge sign. B. The patellar tap will suggest fluid in the knee as the patella clicks against the femur. With greater amounts of knee fluid, the patella will be ballottable.

Source: Judge, R.D., Zuidema, G.D., & Fitzgerald, F.T. (Eds.), 1989. Clinical Diagnosis (p. 445). Boston: Little, Brown and Company. Copyright 1989 by A.C. Judge, P.C. Judge, S.M. Judge, N.C. Judge. Reprinted by permission.

7.   Perform range of motion of knee
8.   Assess mobility of patella by flexing knee 30° and applying medial and lateral pressure to determine amount of subluxation that is possible
9.   Determine the quadriceps or Q angle (see Figure 17.7 in section on EXTREMITY PAIN)
  a.   This angle is formed by lines drawn from center of patella to the tibial tubercle and from the center of patella to anterior superior spine
  b.   When angle exceeds 15° it is abnormal and may be associated with patellar subluxation and dislocation

10. Determine ligament stability (see Figure 17.11)
   a. Apply valgus (medial) or varus (lateral) stress when knee is at full extension and then at 30° flexion to assess stability of medial and lateral collateral ligaments
      (1) In first-degree sprains, end point is solid
      (2) In second-degree sprains, laxity is evident at 30° flexion but not at full extension
      (3) In third-degree sprains, there are no solid end points at either 30° flexion or full extension

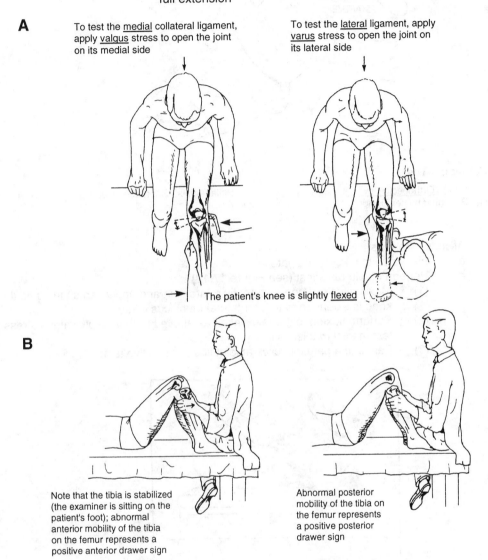

A

To test the medial collateral ligament, apply valgus stress to open the joint on its medial side

To test the lateral ligament, apply varus stress to open the joint on its lateral side

→ The patient's knee is slightly flexed

B

Note that the tibia is stabilized (the examiner is sitting on the patient's foot); abnormal anterior mobility of the tibia on the femur represents a positive anterior drawer sign

Abnormal posterior mobility of the tibia on the femur represents a positive posterior drawer sign

Figure 17.11. Collateral Ligament Testing.

A: Collateral ligament testing. B: The "drawer" sign for cruciate ligament testing.

Source: Reilly, B.M. (1991). Practical Strategies in Outpatient Medicine (p. 1193). Philadelphia: Saunders. Copyright 1991 by Saunders. Reprinted by permission.

   b. Assess stability of cruciate ligaments with the drawer test by applying anterior (see aforementioned illustration) and posterior forces to the proximal tibia when the knee is flexed and the foot is stabilized
   c. Lachman's test can also test cruciate ligaments and is performed with knee flexed to 30°; anterior drawer force is applied to the proximal tibia with one hand while the other hand stabilizes the femur (see Figure 17.12)

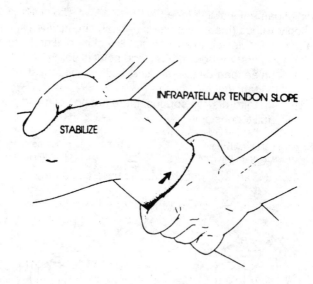

Figure 17.12. Lachman's Test.

Source: Magee, D.J. (1987). Orthopedic Physical Assessment (p. 284). Philadelphia: Saunders. Copyright 1987 by Uniform Copyright Convention. Reprinted by permission.

11.   Assess meniscus
    a.   Flex knee to 90° and palpate joint line
    b.   Perform McMurray's test (see Figure 17.13)
        (1)   Maximally flex knee, externally rotate tibia and apply varus stress as the knee is extended to test for lateral meniscus injury
        (2)   Perform flexion, external rotation as above but then apply valgus stress to test medial meniscus injury
        (3)   Pain and a palpable click at joint line are positive tests

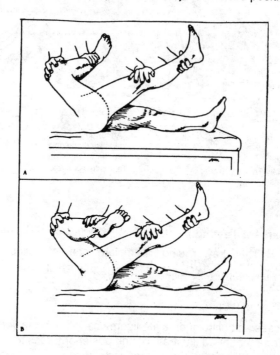

Figure 17.13. McMurray Maneuver.

A. Extension in internal rotation. A palpable or audible snap suggests a lesion in the lateral meniscus.
B. Extension in external rotation. A palpable or audible snap suggests a lesion in the medial meniscus.

Source: Judge, R.D., Zuidema, G.D., & Fitzgerald, F.T. (Eds.). (1989). Clinical Diagnosis (p. 448). Boston: Little, Brown and Company. Copyright 1989 by A.C. Judge, P.C. Judge, S.M. Judge, N.C. Judge. Reprinted by permission.

12. Assess hip and back whenever a history of knee pain is combined with normal findings on the knee exam

C. Differential Diagnosis: important to differentiate acute injuries from overuse injuries, inflammatory processes, infection, and neoplasms
   1. Overuse injuries have insidious onset and usually result from repetitive stress (see section on EXTREMITY PAIN, LOWER)
       a. Chondromalacia patellae
       b. Osgood-Schlatter disease
       c. Patellar tendinitis
       d. Stress fractures
   2. Inflammatory processes, infections, and neoplasms are typically associated with systemic symptoms
   3. Hip problems should be considered; referred pain from the hip occurs, especially in older patients who are at risk for metastatic disease, osteoarthritis, and fractures

D. Diagnostic Tests
   1. Consider ordering x-rays of the knee including anteroposterior, lateral and sunrise patella views; the Ottawa Knee Rule is helpful in deciding when to use radiography (see following table)

OTTAWA KNEE RULE

Order knee x-ray series for patients with the following findings:

1) Age 55 years or older
   Or
2) Isolated tenderness of patella*
   Or
3) Tenderness at head of fibula
   Or
4) Inability to flex to 90°
   Or
5) Inability to bear weight immediately or walk more than four steps immediately after injury

---

*No bone tenderness of knee other than patella

Adapted from Stiell, I.G., Wells, G.A., Hoag, R.H., et al. (1997). Implementation of the Ottawa Knee Rule for the use of radiography in acute knee injuries. JAMA, 278, 2075-2079.

   2. Aspirate a large effusion and order cell count, gram stain, and culture
   3. Injuries which do not heal after 2 weeks of conservative treatment may require magnetic resonance imaging or in the case of a meniscus injury, an arthrogram which is less accurate
   4. An arteriogram is ordered for suspected knee dislocations

V. Plan/Management

A. The following are indications for immediate orthopedic referral; patient's knee should be immobilized in a splint or rigid knee immobilizer
   1. Neurovascular compromise
   2. Suspected fracture or dislocated tibia or femur
   3. Suspected growth plate injury
   4. Torn ligaments (Grade II and III sprains)
   5. Locked knee which is unable to be manipulated into place
   6. Large meniscus tear or hemarthrosis
   7. Suspected infection or tumor

B. For other, less extensive knee injuries teach patient the following:
1. Rest depending on extent of injury; minor injuries may need only 1-2 days of rest, whereas more extensive injuries may need 8-10 weeks
2. Apply ice (never directly to skin) 20 to 30 minutes with at least 10 minute breaks in application as often as possible during first 48 hours after injury
3. After first 48 hours, hot and cold applications can be used (see section on ANKLE INJURY)
4. Elevate extremity
5. Consider prescribing NSAIDs such as ibuprofen (Motrin) 200-800 mg TID every 6 to 8 hours; some clinicians believe that NSAIDs hamper early healing and should be used conservatively
6. Teach crutch walking and the need to avoid weight-bearing until acute inflammation subsides
7. For injuries with pronounced symptoms, immobilize knee in brace for a minimal period of time
8. Exercise is important
   a. For minor injuries, exercise can be permitted within 1-2 days, but patient should be cautioned to gradually increase activity
   b. For more extensive injuries, activity should initially consist of isometric quadriceps tensing exercises
   c. Begin isotonic quadriceps exercises and range of motion exercises after acute inflammation subsides
9. Incision and drainage of large and fluctuant hematomas may be needed

C. Surgery is needed for more extensive knee injuries; a promising new method of repairing damaged knees is extraction of autologous chondrocytes from patient's cartilage which are grown in vitro and then reimplanted

D. Follow Up
1. For extensive injuries, schedule return visit in 24 hours
2. For less extensive injuries, return visits should be scheduled in two weeks or sooner if problems occur
3. Consult specialist for patients with ligament and meniscus injuries which have had only minimal improvement after 2 weeks of conservative treatment; patients with meniscus injuries may need magnetic resonance imaging and/or an arthrogram before orthopedic visit
4. At the return visit, all patients should be taught ways to prevent further injuries to their knees particularly by proper exercising and conditioning and possibly the use of prophylactic braces

LOW BACK PROBLEMS, ACUTE

I. Definition: Activity intolerance due to lower back or back-related leg symptoms of less than 3 months duration

II. Pathogenesis

A. Lumbosacral strain
1. Etiology is often unclear but results from stretching or tearing of muscles, tendons, ligaments or fascia of back secondary to trauma or chronic mechanical stress
2. Predisposing factors include chronic occupational strain, obesity, exaggerated lumbar lordosis, abnormal forward tipped-pelvis, weak paraspinal and/or abdominal muscles, leg length discrepancy, chronic poor posture, inadequate/inappropriate conditioning and sub-optimal lifting habits

B.	Herniated intervertebral disc
1.	Intervertebral discs are composed of collagenous annulus fibrosis and gelatinous nucleus pulposus
2.	Herniation occurs with tears in annulus fibrosis which allows contents of nucleus pulposus to protrude
3.	When nerve roots are compressed by these contents, pain and other neurological signs and symptoms develop

C.	Spinal stenosis results from soft tissue and bony encroachment of the spinal canal and nerve roots

D.	Spondylolysis is a break of the pars interarticularis; found in 5% of people over age 7

E.	Spondylolisthesis is a slip of the vertebrae (after spondylolysis) which allows one vertebrae body to slide forward on its neighbor; most common cause of back pain in persons <26 years, especially athletes

III.	Clinical Presentation of common syndromes of acute low back problems; 90% of patients with acute low back problems will recover spontaneously in 4 weeks

A.	Lumbosacral strain
1.	Occurs frequently between 20-40 years of age
2.	Typically, patient experiences minimal discomfort during or immediately after injury or activity with stiffness and pain occurring 12-36 hours later as soft tissue swells
3.	Pain is located in back, buttocks or in one or both thighs
4.	Pain is aggravated by standing and flexion; is relieved with rest and reclining

B.	Herniated intervertebral disc
1.	Occurs most frequently in young and middle-aged adults; In older persons the nucleus pulposus becomes more fibrotic and dehydrated resulting in a lower incidence of disk herniation compared with the incidence of degenerative disk disease
2.	Characterized by radicular pain which is described as shooting, sharp, electric-type pain, associated with foot and leg pain and worsened with valsalva maneuvers
3.	Paresthesia or numbness may occur in sensory distribution of nerve root.
4.	Deep tendon reflexes are absent or depressed in distribution of nerve root.
5.	Muscular weakness and atrophy may result.
6.	Most common disc ruptures affect L-5 or S-1, nerve roots.
7.	Cauda equina involvement (compression of the lower portion of the nerve roots inferior to spinal cord proper) may occur secondary to central disc herniation and presents as insidiously worsening rectal and/or perineal pain with decreased perineal sensation, loss of sphincter control, and disturbances in bowel and bladder functions
8.	Signs and symptoms depend on level of herniation (see Figure 17.14 on Common Disc Syndromes)

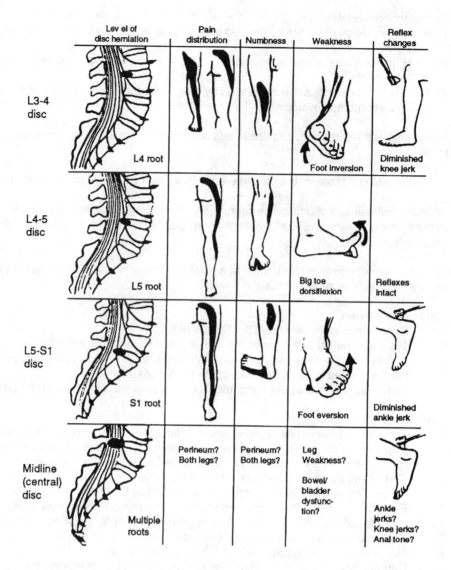

Level of disc herniation	Pain distribution	Numbness	Weakness	Reflex changes
L3-4 disc L4 root			Foot inversion	Diminished knee jerk
L4-5 disc L5 root			Big toe dorsiflexion	Reflexes intact
L5-S1 disc S1 root			Foot eversion	Diminished ankle jerk
Midline (central) disc Multiple roots	Perineum? Both legs?	Perineum? Both legs?	Leg Weakness? Bowel/ bladder dysfunction?	Ankle jerks? Knee jerks? Anal tone?

Figure 17.14. Common Disc Syndromes: Neurologic Findings.

Source: Reilly, B.M. (1991). Practical Strategies in Outpatient Medicine (p. 915). Philadelphia: Saunders. Copyright 1991 by Saunders. Reprinted by permission.

C. Spinal stenosis
  1. Occurs in middle-aged and older adults
  2. Gradual onset of bilateral neurogenic claudication (leg pain and/or leg paresthesias and weakness) when walking; neurogenic claudication may present as cramping in the buttocks with ambulation
    a. Differentiate neurogenic claudication from vascular claudification in which symptoms of vascular insufficiency can be relieved by stopping activity or standing
    b. Neurogenic claudication is usually relieved when patient flexes lumbar spine or sits
  3. In severe cases, may have bowel and bladder disturbances

D. Spondylosis and spondylolisthesis
  1. Often occurs from a stress fracture of the posterior vertebral elements or from hyperextension sports such as gymnastics, diving, or weight lifting
  2. Family history for spondylolysis is often positive
  3. Neurologic examination is usually normal, but patients may have tight hamstrings, and hyperextension (back bending) often reproduces pain at L5 or just below the iliac crests
  4. If spondylolysis is suspected x-rays are ordered; if x-rays are negative and suspicion is still high, a bone scan is ordered

E. Rare causes of low back pain include tumors, tuberculosis, and discitis (bacterial infection which causes narrowing of the disc space)

IV. Diagnosis/Evaluation

A. History
   1. Ask patient to point with one finger where he/she feels pain and then to describe pain and/or radiation of pain
   2. Determine onset because acute onset without trauma may signal serious conditions such as dissecting aortic aneurysm
   3. Differentiate whether pain is mechanical and worsens after bending or lifting or is nonmechanical, occurring at rest, and related to extraspinal disorders such as pelvic or intra-abdominal conditions
   4. Inquire about pattern of symptoms; ask whether symptoms are constant or intermittent
   5. Explore occurrence of systemic symptoms, such as weight loss, and fever, which could signal malignant disease
   6. Obtain careful past medical history, noting previous trauma, TB, cancer, immunosuppression, urinary infection, osteoporosis, previous back problems and surgery
   7. Ask about possible associated symptoms such as dysuria, bowel or bladder incontinence, muscle weakness, paresthesia, and loss of sensations
   8. Inquire about steroid and other drug use
   9. Determine patient's limitations in activities
   10. Use of pain drawings or visual analog scales may augment history

B. Physical Examination
   1. Observe gait and general appearance
      a. Patients with herniated discs usually are uncomfortable sitting and gait is cautious and awkward
      b. Limping or coordination problems suggest a possible neurological problem
      c. Severe guarding of lumbar motion may indicate spinal infection, tumor, or fracture
   2. Observe spine for alignment and abnormalities; observe skin overlying spine for signs of trauma or infection
   3. Perform range of motion.
      a. Increased pain with extension often indicates osteoarthritis.
      b. Increased pain with flexion most often indicates strain or injured or herniated disc
   4. Palpate spine and paraspinal structures noting point tenderness and paravertebral muscle spasm
      a. If fell on tailbone, need to do rectal exam checking for stability of coccyx
      b. Palpate ischial tuberosity and greater trochanter to rule out bursitis
   5. Perform traction maneuvers
      a. Straight leg raise (SLR): Elevate each leg passively with flexion at hip and extension of knee; positive SLR is radicular pain when leg is raised between 30-60°
      b. Crossed leg raise is very diagnostic for disc injury; positive when patient complains of radicular pain in the leg that is not raised
      c. Yeoman maneuver: Unilateral hyperextension in prone position (checking for lumbosacral mechanical disorders)
      d. Patrick's test in which heel is placed on opposite knee and lateral force is exerted on knee (check for hip or sacroiliac disease)
   6. Check for malingering
      a. Observe for overreaction
      b. Apply slight pressure to top of head (should not produce pain)
      c. Perform distracted straight leg raise
      d. Observe for nonanatomical motor or sensory regional disturbances
   7. Perform complete neurological examination
      a. Determine pain and sensation distribution; pain and diminished or absent sensation should follow nerve root distribution (see Figure 7.1 Dermatomes in HERPES ZOSTER in SKIN chapter)

b.   Do complete motor strength assessment, including dorsiflexion of great toe (only abnormality of the common L4-5 disc protrusion may be great toe weakness)
    (1)   Ask patient to toe walk which tests calf muscles and mostly S1 nerve root
    (2)   Ask patient to heel walk which tests ankle and toe dorsiflexor muscles, L5 and some L4 nerve roots
    (3)   Ask patient to perform a single squat and rise which tests quadriceps muscles, mostly L4 nerve root

c.   Circumferential measurements of calf and thigh bilaterally can detect muscle atrophy; differences of greater than 2 cm in measurements of the two limbs often indicate an abnormality

d.   Deep tendon reflex testing
    (1)   Ankle jerk tests mostly the S1 nerve root
    (2)   Knee jerk tests mostly the L4 nerve root
    (3)   Up-going toes in response to stroking the plantar footpad (Babinski or plantar response) may indicate motor-neuron abnormalities such a myelopathy or demyelinating disease

8.   Check sensation of perineum to rule out cauda equina syndrome (compression of the lower portion of the nerve roots inferior to the spinal cord proper).

9.   Examine abdomen (masses or bruits)

10.   Assessment of the legs and feet is necessary to differentiate spinal stenosis from vascular insufficiency

a.   Inspect legs and feet for loss of hair and color changes that may accompany vascular insufficiency

b.   Palpate legs and feet for temperature and tenderness

c.   Palpate femoral, popliteal, and pedal pulses

11.   Consider pelvic and rectal examinations

12.   Palpate peripheral pulses

C.   Differential Diagnosis

1.   Important to rule out red flags for potentially serious conditions (see following table)

RED FLAGS FOR POTENTIALLY SERIOUS CONDITIONS		
Possible Fracture	**Possible Tumor or Infection**	**Possible Cauda Equina Syndrome**
Major trauma such as vehicle accident or fall from a high place	Age >50 and <20 years	Saddle anesthesia
Minor trauma or even strenuous lifting (in older or potentially osteoporotic patient)	History of cancer	Recent onset of bladder dysfunction such as urinary retention, increased frequency, or overflow incontinence
	Constitutional symptoms such as fever, chills, or unexplained weight loss	Severe or progressive neurologic deficit in legs
	Risk factors for infection: recent bacterial infection, IV drug abuse, or immunosuppression	Unexpected laxity of anal sphincter
		Perianal/perineal sensory loss
	Pain that worsens when supine; severe nighttime pain	Major motor weakness such as knee extension weakness or foot drop

Adapted from Bigos, S., Bowyer, O., Braen, G., et al. (1994). <u>Acute low back problems in adults. Clinical practice guideline No. 14.</u> AHCPR Publication No. 95-0642. Rockville, MD: Agency for Health Care Policy and Research, Public Health Service, U.S. Department of Health and Human Services.

2.   Pseudosciatica with a normal neurologic exam includes simple mechanical back pain, disorders of hip, thigh, pelvis, rectum, and vascular claudication

3.   True radicular pain (sciatica or shooting, sharp pain down to the lower leg and foot) includes herniated intervertebral disc, spondylolisthesis, compression fracture, degenerative spondylosis, herpes zoster, and neoplasm

4.   Extreme, tearing pain with syncope and diaphoresis may indicate an aneurysm

5.   Fever or meningeal symptoms may suggest vertebral osteomyelitis

6. Other less common ominous causes: metabolic bone disease, inflammatory disease, spinal cord disease, unstable spine, pyelonephritis
7. Other diseases may or may not be accompanied with back pain: peripheral neuropathy, depression, hysteria, cystitis, prostatitis, endometriosis, osteoarthritis, bursitis, osteoporosis

D. Diagnostic Tests
1. For patients with low back pain less than 4 weeks and in the absence of signs and symptoms of dangerous conditions (see preceding table on RED FLAGS FOR POTENTIALLY SERIOUS CONDITIONS), no tests are needed
   a. If spinal fracture is a possibility, order plain x-ray of lumbosacral spine; if fracture still suspected after 10 days or there are multiple sites of pain, consider bone scan or consultation
   b. If cancer and/or infection is suspected, order CBC, erythrocyte sedimentation rate, urinalysis; if after these tests, there is still suspicion consider consultation or order bone scan, x-ray or other lab test
2. For patients whose back pain does not improve over 4 weeks:
   a. If symptoms are primarily in the low back consider ordering CBC, ESR, x-rays, or bone scan depending on symptomatology and risk factors
   b. If spinal stenosis is suspected, spinal x-ray (not diagnostic, but may demonstrate degenerative changes), MRI, or CT should be considered
   c. If sciatica symptoms are present >4 weeks, consult surgeon about choice of imaging study (MRI, CT) to define nerve root compression **or** order electromyography (EMG) if the level of nerve root dysfunction is not obvious from the physical examination; sensory evoked potentials may be added if spinal stenosis or spinal cord myelopathy is suspected

V. Plan/Management

A. Immediately consult specialist and arrange for emergency care and studies for patients with cauda equina or rapidly progressing neurologic deficit

B. Pharmacological therapy for acute back pain without ominous signs
1. Safest, effective medication is acetaminophen which may be used safely in combination with non-steroidal anti-inflammatory drugs (NSAIDs) or physical therapeutics
2. NSAIDs including aspirin are also effective but can cause gastrointestinal problems, renal or allergic problems
   a. Phenylbutazone is not recommended due to risks of bone marrow suppression
   b. Do not use combination of NSAIDs
   c. Naproxen (Naprosyn) 500 mg initially followed by 250 mg every 6-8 hours or Ibuprofen (Motrin) 400 mg every 4-6 hours
3. Muscle relaxants are a treatment option but are no more effective than NSAIDS in relieving low back symptoms and have adverse effects including drowsiness; cautiously consider prescribing cyclobenzaprine HCl (Flexeril) 10 mg QD to TID, or methocarbamol (Robaxin) initially 1.5 gm (2 tabs, 750 mg each) QID, then 750-1000 mg QID
4. Opioids should be avoided if possible, and if selected, used only for a short time
5. The following therapies are not recommended: oral steroids, colchicine, and antidepressants

C. Physical methods
1. Consider referral for manipulation (manual loading of the spine using short or long leverage methods)
   a. Safe and effective for patients in the first month of low back pain if they do NOT have radiculopathy
   b. Stop manipulation if there is no symptomatic or functional improvement after 4 weeks with this therapy

2. Self application of heat and cold therapy may provide temporary symptom relief
   a. Cold therapy for 20-30 minutes several times a day for first 24 hours.
   b. Topical heat 20-30 minutes several times a day after first day
3. The following have not been found effective: traction, massage, diathermy, ultrasound, biofeedback, transcutaneous electrical nerve stimulation, acupuncture, shoe lifts, back corsets, back belts

D. Activity
1. For most patients, no bed rest is needed; prolonged bed rest may have debilitating consequences
2. For patients with severe limitations, 2-4 days of bed rest may be beneficial
3. Teach patient to minimize stress to the back
   a. Avoid jerky, hurried movements when lifting
   b. Lift with legs by straddling the load; bend knees to pick up load; keep back straight (do not bend back)
   c. Keep objects close to the body at navel level when lifting
   d. Avoid twisting, bending, reaching while lifting
   e. Avoid prolonged sitting
   f. Change positions often while sitting
   g. A soft support at small of back, armrests to support some body weight, a slight recline in chair back may make sitting more comfortable
   h. Firm mattress/bed board, lying supine with hips and knees flexed on pillows is beneficial when sleeping
4. Low-stress, aerobic exercise (walking, riding bike, swimming, and eventually jogging) can be gradually and incrementally started within the first 2 weeks of symptoms; conditioning exercises for trunk muscles are not recommended during the first few weeks of symptoms

E. Surgery
1. Surgery should only be considered within the first 3 months of symptoms if the patient has serious spinal pathology or nerve root dysfunction from a herniated lumbar disc
2. Even patients with clinical findings of nerve root dysfunction due to disc herniation recover activity tolerance within one month; no research has found that delaying surgery for one month worsens outcomes
3. Surgical consultation should be considered if patients have any of the following:
   a. Severe and disabling sciatica
   b. Symptoms of sciatica persist without improvement for >4 weeks or with extreme progression
   c. Strong physiologic evidence of dysfunction of a specific nerve root with intervertebral disc herniation is confirmed at the corresponding level and side by imaging studies

F. Management of spinal stenosis
1. Symptomatic treatment as discussed above should be used for first three months
2. Consider surgery which is usually a complete laminectomy for posterior decompensation for patients who cannot manage activities of daily living or who have new signs of bowel or bladder dysfunction

G. Management of spondylolysis
1. Begin with rest, analgesics and hamstring stretching exercises
2. Back muscle strengthening exercises are recommended when the pain has subsided
3. Immobilization with back braces may be needed to achieve healing of fractures or to relieve irritation if patient is not responding to analgesics and exercises
4. Surgical fusion is rarely required

H. Management of spondylolisthesis: surgical consultation after an adequate trial of conservative, symptomatic therapy

I. Prevention of further back problems
   1. Discuss that low back pain, like other chronic conditions, will get worse unless preventive measures are taken.
   2. Exercises to condition specific trunk muscles can be added a few weeks after acute symptoms; encourage patient to do exercises such as partial sit-ups or extension exercises such as lying prone and lifting legs off floor or upper torso off floor for at least 5 minutes a day
   3. Instruct patient in proper lifting, sleeping position, and body mechanics (see V.D.3)

J. Follow Up
   1. For patients with severe pain which does not improve in 24 hours, reevaluate
   2. If patient is in moderate pain reevaluate in 7-10 days
   3. In 4-6 weeks, schedule office visit for further evaluation and further patient education

OSTEOARTHRITIS

I. Definition: Degenerative disease of the cartilage of joints

II. Pathogenesis

   A. Progressive structural breakdown of articular cartilage that lines joint surfaces occurs

   B. Dense, smooth-surfaced bone forms at the base of cartilage lesion and marginal osteophytes develop

   C. Variable synovial inflammation results

   D. Factors associated with development of osteoarthritis (OA): joint trauma, aging, obesity, occupational overuse, weak muscles around joints, congenital musculoskeletal disorders, metabolic disorders (i.e., Wilson's disease), endocrine disorders (i.e., diabetes mellitus), and crystalline deposit disease

   E. Contrary to common belief, active exercise without trauma is not associated with the development of secondary OA and may actually prevent development of the condition by strengthening muscles surrounding joints

   F. Estrogen excess is a possible contributory factor

III. Clinical Presentation

   A. OA is the most common form of chronic arthritis and affects one-fourth of adult population; by age 40, 90% of all persons have some joint problems; however, few people have major symptoms until 60 years or older

   B. Often presents with insidious, gradual onset of joint pain, tenderness and limitation of movement

   C. Morning stiffness or stiffness after prolonged immobility usually lasts less than 30 minutes

   D. Crepitus and occasional joint effusions are characteristic signs

   E. Joint deformity such as subluxation and formation of bony cysts may occur; Heberdens nodes in distal interphalangeal (DIP) joints appear in later stage

F. Joints most affected are the following: DIP, proximal interphalangeal (PIP), first metacarpophalangeal, knees, hip, cervical spine, and lumbar spine
1. OA of hip is the most disabling and painful
2. Knees are the most common symptomatic joints

G. Although there is no criteria for the general diagnosis of OA, criteria have been established for OA of the hip and knee (see table that follows)

CRITERIA FOR OSTEOARTHRITIS OF THE HIP AND KNEE
Hip
Hip pain **and** radiographic femoral or acetabular osteophytes
Or
Hip pain **and** radiographic joint space narrowing **and** erythrocyte sedimentation rate <20 mm/hour
Knee
Knee pain **and** radiographic osteophytes
Or
Knee pain **and** age ≥40 years **and** morning stiffness ≤30 minutes in duration **and** crepitus on motion

Adapted from Hochberg, M.C., Altman, R.D., Brandt, K.D., Clark, B.M., Dieppe, P.A., Griffin, M.R., Moskowitz, R.W. & Schnitzer, T.J. (1995). Guidelines for the medical management of osteoporosis, Part I: Osteoarthritis of the hip, Part II: Osteoarthritis of the knee. Arthritis and Rheumatism, 38, 1535-1541.

IV. Diagnosis/Evaluation

A. History
1. Question about location of joint pain which is usually asymmetric and poorly localized
2. Inquire about joint stiffness which usually lasts less than 30 minutes
3. Ask about systemic symptoms which are usually absent
4. Inquire about occupational activities related to overuse
5. Explore factors such as trauma and extremity malalignment which predispose persons to more serious degenerative changes
6. Obtain a complete past medical history, focusing on endocrine, musculoskeletal, and metabolic diseases
7. Determine the degree to which joint problems are affecting activities of daily living

B. Physical Examination
1. Observe gait; patients with OA of hip may have a "lurching" gait or favor the affected joint
2. Inspect affected joints for deformities, swelling, and color
3. Assess joint range of motion
4. Palpate for crepitus, warmth, edema, and tenderness
5. Observe muscles for atrophy, particularly inspect the quadriceps muscles
6. Evaluate muscle strength
7. Assess joint stability

C. Differential Diagnosis
1. Bone disease such as osteopenia, osteoporosis, malignancy
2. Periarticular soft tissue abnormalities such as tendinitis, bursitis
3. Neuromuscular disease such as neuropathy, Parkinson's Disease
4. Vascular disease such as vasculitis
5. Rheumatoid disease such as rheumatoid arthritis and gout

D. Diagnostic Tests
1. Consider ordering CBC, erythrocyte sedimentation rate (ESR), chemistry profile, urinalysis, serum calcium, serum phosphorus, uric acid, alkaline phosphatase (all normal with OA)
2. Rheumatoid factor may or may not be present
3. X-rays are often ordered as baseline to determine progression of disease; typically there is narrowed joint space, sclerosis of subchondral bone, bony cysts, and osteophytes

V.   Plan/Management: Goals are to control pain, maintain function, maximize independence and minimize complications

A.   Patient education is an essential part of plan
1.   Lessen weight-bearing by purchasing elevated toilet seats and high chairs
2.   Encourage weight reduction in overweight patients
3.   Self-help classes have been reported to decrease pain, decrease health care visits, and improve quality of life
4.   Community support groups and patient information are available through the Arthritis Foundation

B.   An exercise program is important
1.   Recommend eliminating or reducing the following aggravating factors: strenuous activity, stair climbing, prolonged sitting, jogging
2.   Low impact and low torsional loading (twisting motion) exercises are best; swimming or water exercise decreases stress on joints and allows flexibility
3.   Alternate exercise activities to decrease the amount of repetition and burden on joints
4.   For OA of the knee, quadriceps strengthening exercises may reduce pain and improve function (see table below for exercise technique)

TECHNIQUE FOR QUADRICEPS STRENGTHENING EXERCISES

❖   Lie on back with one knee bent and the other leg straight with ankle dorsiflexed to 90°

❖   Tighten quadriceps muscle of straight leg and lift straight leg 25-50 cm off the ground

❖   Hold position for 10 seconds

❖   Lower leg and relax muscle

❖   Repeat exercise at least 10 times, alternating legs

C.   Control of pain is important; a step-wise approach is recommended
1.   Local treatments of moisture, hot and cold therapy, and ultrasound may be beneficial
2.   Pain can usually be controlled with analgesics that do not have anti-inflammatory properties; drug of choice is acetaminophen 325 mg tabs (Tylenol), 2 tabs every 4-8 hours, up to 4,000 mg/day
3.   Nonsteroidal antiinflammatory drugs (NSAIDs) may be substituted if patients do not respond to acetaminophen
      a.   NSAIDs with shorter half lives and smaller dosages should be used with elderly patients
      b.   Begin with a low-dose NSAID [Ibuprofen (Motrin) 400 mg TID] and if that is not effective increase to a full dose NSAID such as one of the following
            (1)   Diclofenac sodium (Voltaren-XR), 100 mg tab QD
            (2)   Oxaprozin (Daypro) 1.2g once daily; Available in 600 mg caplets
      c.   Use regularly for 2-3 weeks before switching to another class of NSAIDs
      d.   Concurrent cytoprotective therapy is needed for individuals at risk for developing peptic ulcers: Give misoprostol (Cytotec), 200 microgram tabs, one tab 4 times daily with meals and HS; or prescribe Arthrotec 50 mg TID which consists of both diclofenac (50mg) and misoprostol (200 mcg)
4.   Capsaicin 0.025% cream (Zostrix) is sometimes beneficial. Apply thin layer over painful joints 3-4 times daily; can use concurrently with other pain medications; wash hands after applying
5.   Intra-articular injection with corticosteroids may be effective for patients with OA in the knee who have signs of inflammation, effusion or substantial pain
      a.   Before injection, joints should be aspirated and fluid evaluated for infection (cell count, gram stain, culture) and gout (crystals)
      b.   Because of possible damage from repeated injections, time interval for injections should be greater than every 3 months for large joints and greater than 4-6 months for small joints

6. Alternatively, sodium hyaluronate (Hyalgan) injection may provide pain relief, improve mobility, but not slow disease progression
   a. Treatment is a form of hyaluronic acid which is the viscous substance in the synovial fluid that lubricates and protects the joints
   b. Course of treatment consists of 5 injections into knee over 4 weeks
   c. Inform patient that it takes a few weeks to notice improvement, but relief usually lasts at least 6 months
   d. Expensive therapy

D. Adjunctive therapies
   1. Knee irrigation with saline solution can relieve pain and improve joint functioning
   2. Arthroscopic lavage with or without debridement may be helpful

E. Surgical procedures such as total joint arthroplasty or osteotomy are options for patients who do not respond to other therapies

F. Experimental treatments may be effective approaches in the future and include the following: cytokine modulation, iontophoresis, tissue transplants, chemically modified tetracyclines, Vitamin D, and Vitamin C

G. Follow Up
   1. May need to regularly monitor (i.e., every 3-6 months) CBC, electrolytes, LFTs, BUN, creatinine, and stool guaiac if on NSAIDs
   2. Return to clinic if there is a flare up of symptoms or symptoms are not improved in 4-6 weeks after beginning any new therapy

OSTEOPOROSIS

I. Definition: Bone density more than 2.5 deviations below the normal bone mass of women who are less than 35 years of age

II. Pathogenesis

A. Generalized and progressive disorder of bone metabolism characterized by loss of bone mass to a point where the skeleton is compromised.

B. In osteoporotic patients, bone resorption is increased whereas bone formation is normal

C. Primary osteoporosis
   1. Type I results from postmenopausal endocrine changes and occurs between ages 51-75 years
   2. Type II occurs in persons >70 years and probably results from age-related reduction in vitamin D synthesis

D. Secondary osteoporosis
   1. Endocrine: glucocorticoid excess, hyperthyroidism, hyperparathyroidism, hypogonadism, hyperprolactinism, diabetes mellitus
   2. Drug induced: corticosteroids, anticonvulsants, ethanol, tobacco, barbiturates, heparin, thyroid hormones, and possibly loop diuretics
   3. Other: chronic renal failure, liver disease, chronic obstructive pulmonary disease (COPD), rheumatoid arthritis, malignancy, Cushing's Syndrome

E. Risk factors include female sex, advanced age, menopause, bilateral oophorectomy, heredity, family origin in British Isles, Northern Europe, China or Japan, low initial bone mass, low body weight (<58 kg), physical inactivity, personal history of low-trauma fracture, low calcium and vitamin D intake

F. Possible risk factors include excessive intake of coffee, alcohol, salt and protein; smoking; irregular menstrual periods

III. Clinical Presentation

A. Approximately 90% of cases are postmenopausal women

B. Patients are often asymptomatic; considerable bone loss (over 35%) can occur before complaints are present or abnormalities are detected on x-rays

C. Fractures of the vertebrae, hip, or forearm may occur spontaneously or with minor trauma
   1. Vertebral fractures are most common, but fractures of the hip cause the most morbidity and mortality
   2. Approximately 80% of hip fractures are related to osteoporotic changes; almost half of patients with hip fractures die within 12 months of presentation

D. By age 60, 1 in 4 white females will have a spinal compression fracture related to bone loss
   1. Back pain is usually present
   2. Signs include spinal deformity (kyphosis, scoliosis) and loss of height
   3. Arm span is longer than body height

E. Approximately 1/3 of patients with senile osteoporosis who are older than 70 years are men
   1. A man's lifetime risk of hip fracture is greater than his risk of prostate cancer
   2. In men, osteoporosis is often a secondary disease due to endocrine disorders, hypogonadism, corticosteroid therapy, smoking, or excessive alcohol intake

IV. Diagnosis/Evaluation

A. History
   1. Ascertain onset, duration, location, and characteristics of pain
   2. Question about previous fractures, falls, and history of chronic back pain
   3. Ask whether patient has noticed loss of height
   4. Determine level of physical activity
   5. Ask about smoking history
   6. Determine medication history, particularly use of corticosteroids
   7. Inquire about diet; explore calcium, caffeine, and alcohol intake
   8. Explore whether patient is postmenopausal, has had a surgical menopause, or is amenorrheic
   9. Obtain complete medical history, focusing on endocrine problems
   10. Explore family history of spinal fractures and osteoporosis

B. Physical Examination
   1. Measure height and compare against patient's previous measurements
   2. Observe back for dorsal kyphosis and cervical lordosis from multiple compression fractures
   3. Palpate any painful area
   4. Assess for physical abnormalities that may interfere with mobility

C. Differential Diagnosis: Rule out conditions noted under pathogenesis

D. Diagnostic Tests: Consider ordering the following:
   1. CBC, erythrocyte sedimentation rate (ESR) and serum protein electrophoresis to R/O multiple myeloma and leukemia
   2. Thyroid stimulating hormone (TSH), parathyroid function tests, glucose level, estrogen level to R/O endocrine disease
   3. Alkaline phosphatase (serum and 24-hr urine) to R/O osteomalacia
   4. Primary osteoporotic patient will have normal serum levels of calcium, phosphate, vitamin D, parathyroid hormone and alkaline phosphatase (although alkaline phosphatase may be elevated in context of a healing fracture)

5. Bone markers are helpful; markers include urinary N-telopeptide or pyridinium cross links for bone resorption and serum osteocalcin for bone formation
   a. Markers help differentiate low from high rates of bone turnover; patients with high turnover may respond better to antiresorptive therapy
   b. Markers can help monitor response to therapy; if initial levels are high, repeat tests in 3-6 months; levels should decrease or normalize with therapy
6. Technetium-99m bone scan, computed tomography, and magnetic resonance imaging are recommended for detecting vertebral fractures
7. Bone mineral density tests should be ordered to determine bone mass loss and patient's response to therapy
   a. Dual energy, X-ray absorptiometry (DEXA) can be done rapidly and is the most reliable and safest diagnostic technique
      (1) Recommended initially for diagnosis and then every 2 years to evaluate effectiveness of treatments
      (2) Measuring the density of the proximal femur is most helpful for predicting fractures
      (3) Measuring density of the lumbar spine is most helpful for monitoring response to therapy
   b. Single photon absorptiometry, dual photon absorptiometry, and quantitative computed tomographic are not as effective as DEXA scanning
   c. Quantitative ultrasound measurement is an alternative to DEXA scanning, but more research is needed to determine its specific role; advantages are that it is portable, inexpensive, and patients are not exposed to ionizing radiation
   d. Plain x-rays are not reliable; detection of osteoporosis is not possible until 40-50% of skeletal mass is lost

V. Plan/Management

   A. Prevention; estimates indicate that 50% of osteoporotic hip fractures and 90% of vertebral fractures can be prevented; adequate calcium and Vitamin D intake and practice of other health-promoting behaviors are needed regardless of which preventive drug therapy is used
      1. Sufficient intake of calcium is an important area of counseling; remember, however, that adequate calcium intake alone is not sufficient for preventing osteoporosis in most women
         a. A high intake of calcium in childhood and throughout life increases mineral density and may decrease the risk of developing osteoporosis (see following table for recommended calcium intake)

RECOMMENDED CALCIUM INTAKE	
Age	Recommended Intake
Children and Adolescents 9-18 years	1,800 mg/day
Adults 19-50 years	1,000 mg/day
Adults older than 51 years	1,200-1,500 mg/day (higher dose if not on estrogen)

Source: National Academy of Sciences, Institute of Medicine, 1997 (as seen in Nurse Practitioner. (1997), 22(11), 104).

         b. See following table for good sources of calcium

FOODS WHICH ARE GOOD SOURCES OF CALCIUM			
Food Source	Approximate Calcium Content	Food Source	Approximate Calcium Content
Milk (skim, 1%, 2%, whole)	300 mg/cup	Cheddar cheese	200 mg/ounce
Ice cream	160 mg/cup	Swiss cheese	270 mg/ounce
Canned salmon with bones	60 mg/cup	Broccoli, turnip greens, collard greens	150-250 mg/cup
Cottage cheese	125 mg/cup	Orange juice, fortified	300 mg/cup

Adapted from Berarducci, A., & Lengacher, C.A. (1998). Osteoporosis in perimenopausal women. The American Journal for Nurse Practitioners, 2 (9), 9-14.

  c. Calcium supplement may be needed; supplementation need only add to dietary intake which means that most postmenopausal women need a supplementation of 400-600 mg per day; Suggest one of the following:

   (1) Calcium citrate is better absorbed than calcium carbonate; suggest Citracal 200 mg tabs, 1-2 tabs BID

   (2) Alternatively can recommend calcium carbonate, (Os-Cal) 500 mg, 1 tab, 1-3 times/day or Tums 500 mg, 1 tab, 2-3 times/day, both should be taken with meals, but remember that high fiber food may reduce absorption

 2. To enhance calcium absorption, recommend 800 IU of Vitamin D daily for people >51 years of age, particularly important in postmenopausal women who are house-bound, institutionalized, or who get little Vitamin D from sunlight or fortified dairy products

 3. Magnesium should be slightly increased for all adults 31 years of age and older

 4. Hormone replacement therapy (HRT) slows bone loss

  a. For postmenopausal women, hormone replacement is the gold standard for prevention if there are no contraindications and patient can tolerate

  b. Consider hormone replacement therapy (HRT) with estrogen and progesterone (use progesterone in women with intact uteri)

   (1) Prescribe conjugated equine estrogens (Premarin) 0.625 mg PO QD or transdermal estrogen (Estraderm) 0.5 mg/day (apply patch twice a week); lower doses of oral estrogen such as Premarin 0.3 mg PO QD if combined with 1,500 mg of calcium may prevent loss in women who cannot tolerate 0.625 mg of Premarin (see section on MENOPAUSE for more information on HRT)

   (2) In women with intact uteri, also prescribe medroxyprogesterone (Provera) 5 mg PO for 10-12 days of the month or 2.5-5 mg PO QD

  c. Estrogen appears to be most effective when started at the onset of menopause, but beginning HRT after the age of 60 is almost as effective; may need lifetime HRT

 5. Raloxifene HCl (Evista) is a selective estrogen receptor modulator that is approved for prevention

  a. Mechanism of action is similar to estrogen, but it is less effective in increasing bone density and lowering blood lipid levels; raloxifene appears to have no effect on triglycerides whereas HRT increases

  b. Prescribe one 60-mg tab orally without regard to food

  c. Most common adverse effect is hot flash; rare adverse effect is increase in venous thromboembolic events

  d. Discontinue drug 72 hours before and during prolonged immobilization

 6. Alendronate sodium (Fosamax) in a 5-mg dose is also approved for prevention (see V.B.2.d. for patient teaching when taking this drug)

 7. Recommend daily exercise particularly weight-bearing activity such as walking

 8. Avoidance of cigarette smoking, excessive alcohol intake, and caffeine may reduce risk of osteoporosis and should be discussed

 9. Educational interventions to prevent falls should be implemented: patients should rise slowly from sitting or lying, look around room before walking, wear flat, rubber-soled shoes, use proper lifting techniques, install hand grips and safety mats in tubs, remove throw rugs, keep halls and stairways well lit and free of clutter; hip padding may provide protection against hip fractures

B. Treatment; adequate calcium and Vitamin D intake is needed regardless of which drug is used; however, there is no data that combination of the following drugs are more effective than monotherapy:

 1. Estrogen is drug of choice

  a. Inhibits osteoclast activity, possibly binds to osteoblasts; main effect is reduction in the rate of bone absorption; classified as an resorption-inhibiting drug

  b. Prescribe oral estrogen with progesterone in women with intact uterus or prescribe estrogen only in women without uterus plus calcium supplementation; transdermal estrogen should not be used to treat osteoporosis because its effects on bones are not apparent until 12 or more months of therapy (see section V.A.4.b. for dosing of HRT)

2. Alendronate (Fosamax), a bisphosphonate, is the most effective treatment in women who cannot tolerate or for whom estrogen is contraindicated; however, long-term safety profiles have not been well established
   a. Inhibits osteoclast activity, decreases bone turnover, and shifts the balance between bone formation and resorption toward formation; classified as a resorption-inhibiting drug
   b. Not recommended for patients with creatinine clearance less than 35 mL per minute
   c. Dosage: Alendronate 10 mg QD; initiate gradually
   d. Because of gastric and esophageal adverse reactions the following patient education is recommended (see following table)

EDUCATION FOR PATIENTS TAKING ALENDRONATE (FOSAMAX)

1. Take drug first thing in morning, at least 30 minutes prior to eating or drinking anything other than water; must take on an empty stomach as the drug binds with food and beverages
2. Take drug with at least 6-8 ounces of water to wash drug completely through esophagus and into stomach
3. Do not lie down for a least 30 minutes after taking drug; lying down would allow drug to pool in esophagus whereas staying erect allows gravity to help drug reach stomach
4. Stop taking drug and call health care provider if any of the following symptoms develop: difficulty or pain on swallowing, chest pain, or new and/or severe heartburn
5. Important to take calcium supplementation along with drug

---

3. Salmon calcitonin (Calcimar, Miacalcin) is another therapy; effectiveness is less than estrogen and alendronate but it has a good safety profile
   a. Inhibits activity of osteoclasts, inhibits bone resorption, and slows remodeling; classified as a resorption-inhibiting drug
   b. Because of the analgesic properties, it is the drug of choice for patients with recent fractures and pain
   c. Prescribe either intranasal or parenteral (SQ or IM) calcitonin; both routes are equally effective but intranasal route has less side effects and is less expensive
      (1) Intranasal calcitonin: 200 IU QD (one spray in one nostril, alternating nostrils daily)
      (2) Parenteral calcitonin: 100 IU/day SQ, daily or 3 times/week (available 200 Units/mL); bedtime injections are recommended because of possible adverse reactions of nausea and face flushing
4. Although they do not carry a specific indication for osteoporosis, the following FDA-approved therapies are also available
   a. Slow release fluoride preparation has the greatest effect on bone density but its safety profile has not been established
      (1) Unique action of stimulating osteoblast proliferation which increases bone formation
      (2) Disadvantage is that high doses may increase incidence of hip fractures
      (3) When FDA approves, dosage will be Fluoride, slow release (Slow Fluoride) 25 mg BID, along with 400 mg calcium BID in 14 month cycles (12 months on drug regime and 2 months on no drugs)
      (4) Important to stress that calcium supplementation must be taken along with fluoride; bone can be resorbed if calcium intake is insufficient
   b. Vitamin D metabolites calcifediol (Calderol) and calcitriol (Rocaltrol) may be beneficial for persons who have calcium malabsorption problems
   c. The bisphosphonate, etidronate disodium (Didronel), may be helpful in treatment of corticosteroid-induced osteoporosis but it can cause impaired mineralization; typically prescribed in cycles of 400 mg/day for 2 weeks followed by calcium only for 12 weeks; then repeat cycle for a total of 150 weeks
   d. Tamoxifen citrate (Nolvadex) is a selective estrogen reuptake inhibitor which is rarely used because of adverse effects (increases the risk of endometrial proliferation, endometrial polyp, and adenocarcinoma)

C. Treat back pain from vertebral fracture with analgesics, heat/cold and massage
   1. To decrease spinal stress when resting on back, place thin pillows under head and legs; when resting on side, place a thin pillow between legs and keep both hips slightly flexed
   2. Early extension exercises rather than flexion exercises may be beneficial in preventing future fractures
   3. Calcitonin may provide symptomatic relief in acute stages

D. Men with osteoporosis
   1. Preventive strategies should include calcium 1.0-1.5 grams per day or higher, regular exercise, possibly Vitamin D supplementation, and avoidance of excessive alcohol and cigarette smoking
   2. Treatment includes alendronate (although not FDA approved for men) and calcitonin for men with painful vertebral osteoporosis
   3. For hypogonadal men, testosterone is the drug of choice

E. Treatment of steroid-induced osteoporosis
   1. Order DEXA at baseline, before patients begin corticosteroid therapy
   2. Recommend preventive therapies
      a. Calcium and Vitamin D supplementation; American College of Rheumatology recommended 1500 mg of elemental calcium per day along with 800 IU of vitamin D; daily dosage should be divided into at least three equal doses
      b. Weight-bearing exercise program
      c. Sex hormone replacement
         (1) Consider oral contraceptives in premenstrual women (no conclusive evidence to support this practice)
         (2) Hormone replacement therapy for postmenopausal women
         (3) Testosterone for men with low serum levels
   3. Thiazide diuretics and sodium restriction are helpful in reducing the hypercalciuria that accompanies corticosteroid use; reducing hypercalciuria improves calcium balance; consider prescribing hydrochlorothiazide (Thiazide) 25 mg/day
   4. For patients who have low bone density or who cannot tolerate preventive therapies, consider prescribing alendronate and calcitonin

F. Follow Up
   1. Patients who are prescribed HRT, alendronate, salmon calcitonin, and fluoride should return in 1-2 months and have regular follow up visits every 3-6 months.
   2. Annual visits are needed for patients on prophylactic therapy

RHEUMATOID ARTHRITIS

I. Definition: A chronic inflammatory disease which primarily affects joints but may have generalized manifestations

II. Pathogenesis

A. Autoimmune disorder of unknown etiology; immunologic changes due to multiple factors

B. Inflammation of synovial membranes results in panus or thickened synovium which adheres to articular cartilage and later erodes cartilage and underlying bone

C. Adhesions between opposing joint surfaces and/or cysts develop

III.   Clinical Presentation

A.   Criteria for diagnosis (see following table)

REVISED CRITERIA FOR CLASSIFICATION OF RHEUMATOID ARTHRITIS* (AMERICAN RHEUMATOLOGY ASSOCIATION, 1987)
• Morning stiffness -- at least one hour before maximal improvement (6 weeks)†.
• Arthritis of 3 or more joint areas (6 weeks)†.
• Arthritis of hand joints (wrist, metacarpophalangeal joints or proximal interphalangeal joints) (6 weeks)†.
• Symmetric arthritis -- simultaneous involvement of same joint areas on both sides of body (6 weeks)†.
• Rheumatoid nodules.
• Rheumatoid factor in serum.
• Radiologic changes (hand x-ray changes typical of RA must include erosions or unequivocal bony decalcification).

*Diagnosis of rheumatoid arthritis if satisfies 4 criteria
†This symptom must be present for at least 6 months to be considered a positive criterion.

Adapted from Arnet, F.C. (1989). Revised criteria for classification of rheumatoid arthritis. Bulletin on Rheumatic Diseases, 38(5), 1-6.

B.   Three times more common in women than men; peak age of onset is 20-30 years

C.   Onset usually is insidious but may be acute following stress, surgery, infection, trauma or pregnancy

D.   Course of rheumatoid arthritis (RA) is highly variable
   1.   Approximately 50% of patients have a progressive disease, but only about 3% have erosive, destructive arthritis
   2.   The following predict a poor prognosis: earlier age at onset, high titer of rheumatoid factor, elevated sedimentation rate, swelling of >20 joints and extraarticular manifestations

E.   Joint involvement
   1.   Swelling is soft and spongy, not bony as in osteoarthritis.
   2.   May have carpal tunnel syndrome, shoulder bursitis, Baker's cyst behind knee, hallux valgus, temporomandibular joint problems, and atlantoaxial (C1-C2) subluxation.

F.   Extra-articular involvement
   1.   Rheumatoid nodules over extensor surfaces of elbows, forearms and hands
   2.   Vasculitis, pleurisy, keratoconjunctivitis, pericarditis, peripheral neuropathy
   3.   Felty's syndrome may occur in older population with rheumatoid arthritis, splenomegaly and leukopenia
   4.   Systemic symptoms may include fever, fatigue, weight loss, anorexia, sweats and Raynaud's phenomenon
   5.   Osteoporosis may develop due to the sedentary lifestyle of many RA patients and the drugs used to treat the disease, particularly corticosteroids

IV.   Diagnosis/Evaluation

A.   History
   1.   Exactly determine duration, location and characteristics of pain, tenderness, inflammation and morning stiffness
   2.   Question about systemic symptoms such as weight loss, fever, and fatigue
   3.   Inquire about associated symptoms such as nodules, eye pain, or conjunctivitis
   4.   Ask about past medical history and medication use
   5.   Inquire about family medical history
   6.   Specifically determine degree of limitation in patient's activities of daily living

B. Physical Examination
1. Measure vital signs
2. Count number of swollen joints, noting bilateral symmetry of joint involvement
3. Check for various deformities of the hand such as swan-neck deformity, mallet finger, Boutonnière deformity
4. Carefully palpate joints noting tenderness, temperature, and swelling
5. Apply traction maneuvers to determine joint stability
6. Assess muscular strength, particularly grip strength
7. A complete physical examination is often needed because of systemic problems such as pleurisy, pericarditis, splenomegaly

C. Differential Diagnosis (see section on JOINT PAIN)
1. Polymyalgia rheumatica
2. Reiter's syndrome
3. Systemic lupus erythematosus
4. Gouty arthritis, gonococcal arthritis, psoriatic arthritis
5. Lyme disease
6. Acute rheumatic fever
7. Ulcerative colitis and Crohn's disease

D. Diagnostic Tests
1. Baseline laboratory information in patient suspected of RA includes CBC with differential, erythrocyte sedimentation rate, urinalysis, rheumatoid factor titer
2. Before initiating any drugs it is important to get the following: electrolytes, serum creatinine, liver function tests, hepatic panel, urinalysis, stool guiac
3. In selected patients, consider ordering the following:
   a. Synovial fluid analysis to rule out other diseases; may need repeated during disease flares to rule-out septic arthritis
   b. X-rays of selected joints; limited diagnostic value early in disease, but helpful in establishing a baseline to periodically monitor progression and response to therapy
   c. Additional serological studies such as antinuclear antibodies (ANAs) and serum hemolytic complement (CH50) may be needed to rule-out other diseases

V. Plan/Management: Goals are to relieve pain, preserve joint function, and prevent further disease progression

A. Initially, patients are treated by specialists; consultation is also needed when patients have exacerbations or flares of their symptoms

B. Patient education includes discussion of chronicity of disease and ways to decrease exacerbations and prevent deformities
1. Maintain ideal body weight
2. Exercise with emphasis on joint extension (physical therapy is always helpful)
3. Receive adequate rest with naps
4. Perform correct body mechanics
5. Always use of large joints, such as shoulders or hands, rather than fingers to carry pail of water, etc.

C. Early referral to physical therapists and occupational therapists is beneficial; splints and protheses are often prescribed to protect joints, to keep in functional position, and to reduce pain

D. Hot and cold therapy, ultrasound, electrical stimulation with transcutaneous nerve stimulator are often beneficial

E. Visual imagery, massage, acupuncture and hypnosis may be helpful

F. Drug therapy
1. General principles
   a. In past, a pyramid approach was used in which NSAIDS were used for at least 3-6 months and then other drugs were added

b.   A more aggressive pharmacological plan is recommended today because of the following reasons
   (1)   NSAIDS are more toxic than previously believed
   (2)   NSAIDS may provide relief from pain but do prevent further joint damage or delay progression of disease
   (3)   Disease-modifying antirheumatic drugs (DMARDs) are less toxic than once thought and may forestall progression of disease
2.   To reduce joint pain and swelling, initially select a NSAID or a Cox-2 inhibitor, celecoxib (Celebrex), which may have fewer GI side effects
   a.   Select drug based on dosing regimen, efficacy, toxicity, tolerance, costs, patient's age, comorbidities, concurrent medications and patient preference
   b.   Avoid combination of two or more NSAIDS
   c.   Possible NSAIDS: Ibuprofen (Motrin, Advil) 800 mg TID or Sulindac (Clinoril) 200 mg BID
3.   Prescribe a DMARD if RA remains active despite treatment with NSAIDS. **DO NOT delay treatment beyond 3 months** of established diagnosis if patient has pain, morning stiffness, fatigue or persistent elevation of ESR or C-reactive protein; goal of therapy is to intervene in RA before joints are damaged
   a.   Common characteristic of all DMARDs is that they are slow acting; clinical response may not be evident for 1-6 months
   b.   DMARDs have potential to delay or prevent joint damage
   c.   DMARDs have adverse effects and many need frequent monitoring (see table below on RECOMMENDED MONITORING STRATEGIES)

RECOMMENDED MONITORING STRATEGIES FOR DMARDS

Drugs	Toxicities requiring monitoring	Baseline evaluation	Monitoring
Nonsteroidal antiin-flammatory drugs	Gastrointestinal ulceration and bleeding	CBC, creatinine, AST, ALT	CBC yearly, LFTs, creatinine testing may be required
Hydroxychloroquine	Macular damage	None unless patient is >40 years or has previous eye disease	Funduscopic and visual fields every 6-12 months
Sulfasalazine	Myelosuppression	CBC, and AST or ALT in patients at risk, G6PD	CBC every 2-4 weeks for first 3 months, then every 3 months
Methotrexate	Myelosuppression, hepatic fibrosis, cirrhosis, pulmonary infiltrates or fibrosis	CBC, chest radiography, hepatitis B and C serology in high-risk patients, AST or ALT, albumin, alkaline phosphatase, and creatinine	CBC, platelet count, AST, albumin, creatinine every 4-8 weeks
Gold, intramuscular	Myelosuppression, proteinuria	CBC, platelet count, creatinine, urine dipstick for protein	CBC, platelet count, urine dipstick every 1-2 weeks for first 20 weeks, then at the time of each injection
Gold, oral	Myelosuppression, proteinuria	CBC, platelet count, urine dipstick for protein	CBC, platelet count, urine dipstick for protein every 4-12 weeks
D-penicillamine	Myelosuppression, proteinuria	CBC, platelet count, creatinine, urine dipstick for protein	CBC, urine dipstick for protein every 2 weeks until dosage stable, then every 1-3 months
Azathioprine	Myelosuppression, hepatotoxicity, lympho-proliferative disorders	CBC, platelet count, creatinine, AST or ALT	CBC and platelet count every 1-2 weeks with changes in dosage, and every 1-3 months thereafter
Cyclophosphamide	Myelosuppression, myeloproliferative disorders, malignancy, hemorrhagic cystitis	CBC, platelet count, urinalysis, creatinine, AST or ALT	CBC and platelet count every 1-2 weeks with changes in dosage, then every 1-3 months, urinalysis and urine cytology every 6-12 months
Corticosteroids (oral ≤10 mg of prednisone or equivalent)	Hypertension, hyperglycemia	BP, chemistry panel, bone densitometry in high-risk patients	Urinalysis for glucose yearly, BP at each visit

Adapted from American College of Rheumatology Ad Hoc Committee on Clinical Guidelines. (1996). Guidelines for monitoring drug therapy in rheumatoid arthritis. Arthritis and Rheumatism, 39, 723-731.

d. For milder disease prescribe one of following
    (1) Hydroxychloroquine (Plaquenil) 200 mg QD or BID; free of side effects but only modestly effective
    (2) Sulfasalazine (Azulfidine): Begin 500 mg BID to maximum of 1.5 gram BID; safest drug but can cause annoying adverse effects
e. For more severe disease, methotrexate (Rheumatrex) is often prescribed, particularly if there is presence of RF positivity, erosions, or extraarticular problems
    (1) Start orally at dosage of 7.5 mg/week. The 2.5 mg tablets should be taken in 3 separate doses, 12 hours apart once a week or take all 3 tablets in a single dose
    (2) Methotrexate is the DMARD with the most predictable benefit
    (3) Disadvantages: expensive, needs frequent laboratory monitoring
f. Gold IM is effective but is expensive, inconvenient, and needs frequent monitoring; Gold sodium thiomalate (Myochrysine) and aurothioglucose (Solganal) 25-50 mg IM are given weekly up to a total dose of 1000 mg, then 50 mg monthly
g. Oral gold, auranofin (Ridaura) 3 mg BID is often less toxic and less effective than Intramuscular gold
h. Leflunomide (Arava) is a new drug approved by the FDA; it is as effective as methotrexate with few serious side effects; contraindicated in pregnant women and premenopausal women should use birth control
i. Others DMARDs that can be prescribed: d-penicillamine, cyclophosphamide, and azathioprine
j. If the patient's disease remains active or is progressing, the following options should be considered:
    (1) Increase DMARD dosage
    (2) Change DMARD
    (3) Combine two or three DMARDs; following are possible combinations:
        (a) Hydroxychloroquine and sulfasalazine
        (b) Methotrexate plus sulfasalazine plus hydroxychloroquine
        (c) Methotrexate plus cyclosporine
        (d) Gold plus hydroxychloroquine
    (4) Initiate or increase dose of oral glucocorticoid (see V.F.4)
4. Low-dose oral glucocorticoids and local intra-articular injections of glucocorticoids are highly effective in relieving symptoms and can be used with DMARDs
    a. For uncomplicated RA, prescribe low-dose oral prednisone (do not give dosage higher than 10 mg daily)
        (1) Beneficial during the period before DMARD has gained full effect or when symptoms are severe (some patients may need maintenance therapy to control symptoms)
        (2) Limit prednisone to short course, or, if maintenance dose is needed, use at the lowest possible dosage
        (3) Consider osteoporosis prophylaxis for all corticosteroid-treated patients (see V.E. in section on OSTEOPOROSIS)
    b. Intra-articular injections can treat most symptomatic joints early in the disease and can be used to treat flares in one or more joints
        (1) Rule-out infection in joint before injecting
        (2) Do not inject joint more than once within 3 months

G. Surgery is needed if there is marked structural damage on x-ray, lack of response to medical therapy, or significant pain and loss of function

H. Future antirheumatoid therapies:
1. Minocycline and doxycycline have been found to decrease cartilage damage by inhibiting metalloproteinases in animal models
2. Other future therapies include cytokine antagonist, an oral type II collagen derived from sternal cartilage of chicks, recombinant human interleukin 1ra, antibodies to TNF-α, and autologous stem cell transplantation

I.   Follow Up
      1.   When initiating new drug therapies, patient should be seen every 1-2 weeks
      2.   Interval between follow up visits depends upon patient's condition and monitoring
            recommendations of medications (see preceding table on RECOMMENDED
            MONITORING STRATEGIES)

SHOULDER PAIN

I.   Definition: Pain in the shoulder that is either acute or chronic

II.   Pathogenesis

      A.   Acute shoulder pain
            1.   Fractures, dislocations, sprains and strains are the most common causes
            2.   Trauma is usually responsible

      B.   Chronic shoulder pain
            1.   The rotator cuff, the dynamic stabilizer of the glenohumeral joint, is composed of four
                  muscles--the subscapularis, the supraspinatus, the infraspinatus, and the teres minor,
                  along with their musculotendinous attachments
            2.   Rotator cuff injury or dysfunction occurs in many circumstances in which the space
                  between the undersurface of the acromion and the superior aspect of the humeral head
                  becomes so narrowed that there is impingement of the acromion onto the rotator cuff
                  tendons (this impingement occurs during forward shoulder elevation that takes place in
                  many overhead activities relating to occupational and recreational pursuits)

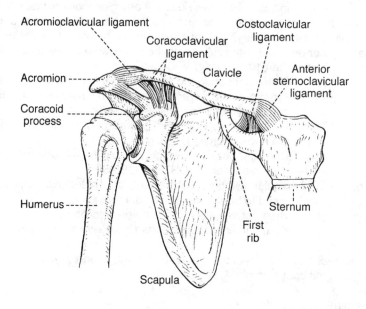

Figure 17.15. Shoulder Bones and Joints

III.   Clinical Presentation

      A.   Shoulder problems are one of the most common orthopedic complaints in primary care

      B.   Most common fractures of the shoulder involve the proximal humerus and the clavicle (fractures
            of the scapula are infrequent and are usually associated with multiple fractures relating to severe
            trauma)

C. Fractures of the proximal humerus most often occur in older patients who fall on an outstretched hand
    1. Incidence increases with age and women are twice as likely as men to sustain this type of fracture
    2. Patient typically presents with complaints of pain, tenderness, and swelling in the shoulder region in the area of the greater tuberosity
    3. Crepitus may or may not be present

D. Fractures of the clavicle are by far the most common fracture that occurs in childhood; in recent decades, this type fracture has become much more common in adults secondary to motor vehicle accidents and participation in contact sports
    1. Mechanisms of injury are usually either a fall on outstretched hand or a direct blow to the shoulder
    2. Considerable force is needed to crack the clavicle in an adult; therefore, if trauma is minor, look for an underlying cause (neoplastic disease, infection)
    3. Patient usually presents with pain at the fracture site; a displaced fracture may be obvious
    4. Patient may avoid moving the arm or may angle head toward the injured side to relax the pull of the trapezius to limit pain

E. Dislocations make up about 25% of all shoulder injuries, with about 95% being anterior glenohumeral dislocations
    1. Anterior dislocations occur when the arm is forcefully elevated and pulled backwards
    2. First-time dislocations are always the result of significant trauma; once glenohumeral instability is present, however, dislocations tend to recur
    3. Patient usually presents with the affected arm in external rotation and abduction
    4. Shoulder is painful, especially with passive range of motion; active range of motion may be very difficult due to muscle spasm

F. Sprains of the shoulder are most often due to a fall on the point of the shoulder
    1. Direct force of the fall is usually transmitted through the acromioclavicular (AC) joint into the clavicle; if a fracture of the clavicle does not occur from the force of the fall, the result is a sprain or a tear of the supporting AC joint ligaments and capsule
        a. Patients with sprains most often experience point tenderness directly over the joint; there is very little if any deformity
        b. Patients with tears usually have a noticeable bump at the AC joint

G. The diagnosis of shoulder strain is a diagnosis of exclusion and is reserved for a muscle injury, usually involving the large deltoid muscle

H. The most frequent cause of chronic shoulder pain is injury to the rotator cuff with pain, weakness, and loss of motion usually reported
    1. Most common among patients 40 years of age and older
    2. Many activities of daily living including combing hair, putting on a coat, reaching high shelves, and driving a car can place demands on the rotator cuff
    3. Occupations that require repetitive overhead work such as painting and carpentry place extra demands on the shoulder
    4. Many sports such as tennis, swimming, football, and basketball require constant overhead positioning of the arms and shoulders; sports such as golf require external rotation of the shoulders

I. Rotator cuff impingement syndrome (and associated tears of the rotator cuff) is usually classified into three stages (see following table)

STAGES OF ROTATOR CUFF IMPINGEMENT SYNDROME	
Stage I	❖ Usually involves patients <25 years of age ❖ Most often occurs in athletes, with pain developing after exercise ❖ Pain is dull, aching, and diffuse ❖ Rotator cuff edema and hemorrhage may by present ❖ Process is reversible at this point
Stage II	❖ Typically occurs in laborers aged 25-40 ❖ Work requires repeated and constant overhead reach for many hours during the day ❖ Pain occurs both during and after activity ❖ Pain frequently occurs at night, interfering with sleep ❖ Pathologic changes become evident and include fibrosis and irreversible tendon changes
Stage III	❖ Final stage usually occurs in patients >50 years of age ❖ Usually, person has been a laborer for many years ❖ In addition to the pain described under stage II, above, additional complaints of stiffness and weakness may be present ❖ Patients present with a long history of shoulder problems ❖ May also present with sudden, severe episode of pain with resultant shoulder disability from an apparently minor recent trauma ❖ Rotator cuff is either partially or completely torn ❖ Damage is irreversible at this stage

IV.   Diagnosis/Evaluation

   A.   History
      1.   Acute shoulder pain
         a.   Ask about the onset (sudden or gradual), duration, location, and intensity of pain (have patient rate on a scale of 1 to 10 with 1 being no pain at all and 10 being the worst pain the patient has ever experienced)
         b.   Ask if the onset of pain is related to a single event (macrotrauma) or reinjury of a chronically symptomatic joint
         c.   If macrotrauma involved, ask about the activity or sport being performed at the time of the injury and the exact mechanism of injury. Ask if there was a direct blow to the shoulder or an indirect injury such as falling on the elbow or arm
         d.   If macrotrauma involved, determine if there was immediate pain, swelling, or deformity
         e.   If reinjury of a chronically symptomatic joint is suspected, ask what activities were being engaged in when pain started (was the patient lifting overhead, pulling, throwing, or was there no apparent cause for the reinjury?) [**Note**: If no apparent cause, consider systemic arthritis, neoplasm, infection, or cardiac disease]
         f.   Ask what reduces the pain and what makes it worse
         g.   Ask if the shoulder feels loose or unstable
         h.   Inquire about treatments that have been initiated by patient or another provider
         i.   Obtain past medical history (including past surgeries for orthopedic problems) and medication history; ask about allergies
         j.   Complete a ROS focusing on pathology in other body systems that could cause referred pain to the shoulder
      2.   Chronic shoulder pain
         a.   Ask about the onset (sudden or gradual) duration, location, and usual intensity of pain (have patient rate on a scale of 1 to 10 with 1 being no pain at all and 10 being the worst pain the patient has ever experienced) [**Note**: Gradual onset of pain is the hallmark of impingement syndrome]
         b.   Determine if pain awakens patient from sleep and if lying on the affected shoulder is avoided because of discomfort
         c.   Ask appropriate questions to grade the patient's overuse pain in terms of impact on function (from less to most impact)
            (1)   Grade 1: Pain occurs only after activity (implies early inflammatory activity)
            (2)   Grade 2: Pain during activity but not restricting performance
            (3)   Grade 3: Pain during activity and restricting performance
            (4)   Grade 4: Pain chronic and unremitting, even at rest

d. Ask if the shoulder feels loose or unstable; if there is shoulder weakness or stiffness; if there is swelling or deformity

e. Determine source of microtrauma or repetitive overload of shoulder joint: Is it related to patient's occupation or to leisure activities?

f. Ask about exacerbating and ameliorating factors

g. Ask about previous treatments (including diagnostic testing, hospitalizations, surgeries, and pain management)

h. Ask about problems with other joints, especially the neck and elbow

i. Obtain complete neurologic history for the upper extremity to include paresthesia, weakness, or radiating pain

j. Obtain a complete ROS to detect remote, nonshoulder sources of symptoms (with a focus on respiratory, cardiovascular, gastrointestinal systems); ask about systemic symptoms including fevers, night sweats, and weight loss

k. Obtain past medical history, social history, medication history, and allergies

B. Physical Examination

1. Acute shoulder pain

a. Inspect the affected shoulder from both front and back for swelling, discoloration, deformity, abrasions, and lacerations

b. Palpate the entire shoulder for point tenderness, subtle deformities, or bony crepitus; palpate the area distal and proximal to the pain location

c. Assess for nerve injury
   (1) Sensation in the arm and hand on the affected side should be evaluated
   (2) Muscles that are innervated by the major nerves of the extremity should be examined for motor function

d. Assess for arterial blood flow
   (1) Assess for circulatory compromise on the affected side
   (2) Color, warmth, and nail bed capillary refill time should be assessed in each finger
   (3) Radial, ulnar, and brachial pulses should be evaluated

e. **Note**: Examination of the unaffected shoulder should be performed at each step of the exam for comparison with the involved shoulder

f. In the absence of trauma (i.e., patient denies a precipitating event for the acute onset of shoulder pain), it is important to carefully check the neck, chest, heart, and abdomen for sources of referred pain

2. Chronic shoulder pain

a. Observe the height of the shoulders and scapulae, the symmetry of the contours, and muscle bulk (common for the dominant shoulder to be slightly lower). This is best done with patient standing, facing both toward and away from the examiner

b. Perform muscle strength testing as weakness is often both the underlying cause and the result of injury (on a standard scale of 0 to 5, results of muscle testing should be in 4 to 5 range)

c. Palpation should be done with patient at rest and with shoulder movement
   (1) Bony structures and joints should be palpated with the patient at rest
   (2) Palpation during active ROM may reveal grinding, popping, and snapping in the AC or glenohumeral joints

d. **Note**: Examination of the unaffected shoulder should be performed at each step of the exam in order to compare it with the involved shoulder

e. Perform maneuvers to screen for cervical spine pathology and to reproduce shoulder pain as described in the following table

MANEUVERS TO ASSESS SUBACUTE SHOULDER PAIN

Test	Description	Interpretation
Maneuver to Screen for Cervical Spine Pathology		
Head compression test	◆ With patient sitting on low stool, stand behind patient, lock hands together, and then apply gentle but firm downward pressure on head, using both hands locked together (see A below)	◆ Pain localized to neck suggests disk degeneration or facet joint arthritis ◆ Burning pain or pain radiating to involved shoulder suggests nerve root involvement ◆ If test is negative (shoulder pain is not reproduced), continue with exam
Maneuvers to Test Range of Motion		
Scratch test	◆ Evaluate adduction and internal rotation by having patient place arm and hand behind back and reach toward the opposite scapula with the thumb pointed up (see B below) ◆ Evaluate abduction and external rotation by having patient place the hand behind the neck and touch the border of the scapula on the opposite side (see C below)	◆ Repeat with the unaffected side and compare differences ◆ Adhesive capsulitis reduces range of motion on the affected side
Painful arc test	◆ Patient begins test with arm held at side, and then lifts arm to position over head. At 45 degrees of abduction, pain is felt when inflamed tissue is forced under the acromion; pain continues until the 120 degree point on the arc is reached; then, pain subsides as the inflamed tissue passes from beneath the acromion as the arm moves into full abduction (see D below)	◆ This pattern of pain strongly supports impingement

C. Differential Diagnosis
1. Acute shoulder pain: Necessary to differentiate among intrinsic causes (fracture, dislocation, strains and sprains) and to determine if pain is being referred from areas such as the chest, abdomen, or cervical spine
2. Chronic shoulder pain: Many conditions can mimic impingement (examples are adhesive capsulitis, biceps tendon rupture, glenohumeral arthritis, septic arthritis, gout, rheumatoid arthritis, cervical radiculopathy, avascular necrosis, tumor)

D. Diagnostic Tests
    1. All patients with acute shoulder pain should be evaluated via x-ray; for suspected proximal humeral and clavicle fractures, AP and lateral (Y view) x-rays made in the scapular plane are recommended; for suspected dislocations and shoulder sprains, an AP view is usually diagnostic, but in anterior dislocation, the axillary view is the test of choice (**Note**: If systemic disease is suspected, perform appropriate tests to detect abnormalities)
    2. For patients with chronic shoulder pain, the following diagnostic testing is recommended
        a. The routine radiograph or x-ray film should be used first before consideration of more sophisticated and expensive studies
        b. The standard views include the anteroposterior and lateral views (can disclose basic bony structures but not helpful in viewing the coracoacromial arch or the glenohumeral joint)
        c. Scapular Y (outlet) view discloses the coracoacromial arch as well as the supraspinatus outlet
        d. West Point axillary view can be used to rule out dislocation and assess for avulsion fractures of the glenoid caused by dislocation
    3. Further imaging studies such as MRI and arthrography should be done by the specialist to whom patients with Stages II and III impingement syndrome are referred

V. Plan/Management

    A. All patients with acute shoulder pain should be referred to an orthopedist for management

    B. Patients who are determined to have Stage I impingement (pain is Grade 1 or 2 which suggests mild to moderate inflammation) can be managed conservatively with the goal of decreasing the inflammation that is compressing the subacromial space before irreversible damage occurs

---

CONSERVATIVE TREATMENT FOR STAGE I SHOULDER IMPINGEMENT
ADVICE THAT SHOULD BE GIVEN TO PATIENT

✔ **Rest without** immobilization
✔ **Use** arm and shoulder in activities that do not require overhead motion
✔ **Refrain** from activities that precipitated the injury
✔ **Apply ice** as often as desired and as long as inflammation is present
  (**Note**: Ice is a potent anti-inflammatory agent that can both reduce pain and muscle spasm)
✔ **Use** nonsteroidal anti-inflammatory drugs (NSAIDs) for 2-4 weeks
✔ **Visit** physical therapist for therapeutic modalities such as high-voltage electrical stimulation and ultrasound, and training in stretching and strengthening exercises

---

    C. Patients with Stage I impingement that does not respond to conservative therapy in 4 weeks should be referred for further evaluation and possible corticosteroid injections

    D. Patients with Stages II and III impingement syndrome require referral to an orthopedist

    E. Follow Up
        1. For patients with acute shoulder pain, should be to specialist to whom patient was referred
        2. For patients with Stage I impingement syndrome (chronic pain) follow up should be in 4 weeks to assess the efficacy of conservative management
        3. For patients with Stages II and III impingement syndrome, follow up should be with specialist to whom patient was referred

WRIST PAIN

I.   Definition: Chronic or recurrent pain or discomfort of the hand or wrist caused by selected common problems

II.   Pathogenesis

   A.   Carpal tunnel syndrome
      1.   An entrapment neuropathy involving the median nerve of the wrist
      2.   Conditions that cause a decrease in the size of the carpal tunnel (such as Colles' fracture, rheumatoid arthritis), enlargement of the median nerve (such as endoneural edema in diabetes mellitus), or increase in the volume of other structures within the tunnel (such as tenosynovitis [most often due to forceful repetitive wrist and hand movements], urate deposits in gout, fluid retention in pregnancy) may compromise median nerve function

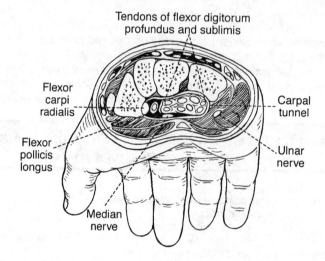

Figure 17.16. Cross Section of the Wrist Illustrating Location of the Median Nerve in the Carpal Tunnel.

   B.   De Quervain's tenosynovitis
      1.   Subacute or chronic inflammation of the extensor tendons within the first dorsal compartment of the wrist
      2.   Usually precipitated by excessive repetitive handwork involving hobby or occupation

   C.   Ganglion cysts
      1.   Believed to result from an out pouching of the wrist capsule; cysts contain fluid very similar to joint fluid
      2.   May be caused by damage to the scapholunate ligament, either from trauma or overuse

III. Clinical Presentation

   A.   Carpal tunnel syndrome is the most common entrapment neuropathy
      1.   Affects nearly 1% of the general population in the US
      2.   Most common among women, industrial workers, and persons whose hobby or occupation requires forceful repetitive wrist and hand movements or the use of vibratory tools

3. The typical presenting symptoms are pain and hand numbness or dysesthesia extending into the radial three digits of the hand
   a. Early in the course of the disorder, pain and numbness that awaken the patient from sleep are common (shaking the hands and stretching the wrists are reported to relieve the discomfort); these early symptoms are usually exertional in nature and are provoked by specific activities
   b. As the condition progresses, the patient often describes a fixed sensory loss and a feeling of loss of strength in the hand; symptoms remain relatively stable and unrelated to any specific activities at this point

B. De Quervain's tenosynovitis is one of the most commonly encountered wrist problems
   1. Involves the tendons within the first dorsal compartment of the wrist
   2. Excessive repetitive handwork such as involved in knitting, peeling vegetables aggravates the condition
   3. Pain is exacerbated by use of the thumb and is reproducible by having patient tuck his/her thumb into palm, making a fist, and then ulnarly deviating and palmar flexing the wrist

C. Ganglion cysts are extremely common, solitary, fluid-filled cysts found in a number of sites, most often the dorsum of the wrists between the midcarpal and radiocarpal joints
   1. In many cases, patients are unable to link the ganglia with a specific traumatic event
   2. Many ganglia are asymptomatic and resolve spontaneously; others produce mild to moderate pain
   3. The cysts are benign, feel soft to palpation, and fluctuate in size

IV. Diagnosis/Evaluation

A. History
   1. Determine onset, duration, and location of all symptoms related to the presenting problem
      a. If pain present, ask if it disturbs sleep and if it is relieved by shaking hands and wrists
      b. If numbness present, ask about location and whether it is constant or recurring
      c. If weakness or loss of strength in hand, ask patient to describe
      d. If mass on wrist is present, determine if it is painful and if it changes in size
   2. Ask about recent trauma to wrist, hand, or elbow
   3. Determine if patient engages in activities requiring repetitive movements or use of vibratory tools as part of work or hobby
   4. Obtain past medical history to determine if patient has any condition (including pregnancy) that might compromise median nerve function (see II.A above for conditions that might impact the carpal tunnel)
   5. Obtain medication history
   6. Inquire about what makes the condition better or worse (do symptoms increase with activity and improve with rest?)
   7. Ask about treatments tried and their results (both what patient has tried and what treatments have been received in the past from another provider)

B. Physical Examination
   1. Inspect hands and wrists in resting position with wrists in the neutral position; observe the bone and soft-tissue contours of the forearm, wrist, and hand, for any deviations, comparing both sides
   2. Note any muscle wasting on the thenar eminence (median nerve) or hypothenar eminence (ulnar nerve) that may indicate nerve injury
   3. Observe for any localized swellings or masses; palpate the mass to determine if it is soft and easy to manipulate (**Note**: A mass that is firm and fixed, and lies blow the level of the fascia is not likely to be a ganglia); transilluminate the mass if it is large enough (ganglia usually contain clear fluid and will often transilluminate)
   4. Palpate the proximal forearm for tenderness in the area where the median nerve passes beneath the pronator teres
   5. Palpate the forearm just proximal and radial to the anatomic "snuff box" for tenderness
   6. Perform Finkelstein test to reproduce pain characteristic of De Quervain's tenosynovitis

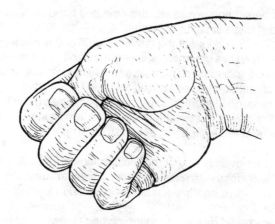

Figure 17.17. Finkelstein Test.

Have patient tuck thumb into palm and make a fist as illustrated. Then ulnarly deviate and palmar flex the wrist; pain with this maneuver is a positive test.

7.   To test for carpal tunnel syndrome, perform the following two tests
    a.   Gently tap the carpal tunnel at and just distal to the flexor crease near the palmaris longus tendon (Tinel's sign); positive sign is a tingling sensation in the sensory distribution of the median nerve (thumb, index finger, and the middle and lateral half of the ring finger)

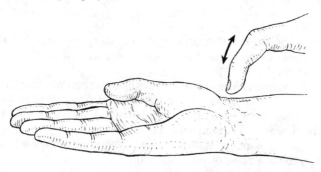

Figure 17.18. Tinel's Sign

    b.   Position the patient with elbows placed on a flat surface and the forearms held in a vertical position; the wrists are then acutely flexed. The test is positive if pain, numbness, or tingling is produced or made worse within 60 seconds (considered one of the most sensitive tests)

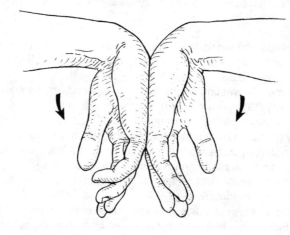

Figure 17.19. Test for Carpal Tunnel Syndrome

Test designed to reproduce numbness and tingling when carpal tunnel syndrome is present.

8.   Motor evaluation: Evaluate motor function of the hand by asking patient to abduct the thumb, index, and little fingers against resistance

9.   Sensory Evaluation: Evaluate sensation at the dorsal web space between thumb and index finger (radial nerve), the tip of the long finger (median nerve), and the tip of the little finger (ulnar nerve)

C.   Differential Diagnosis
1.   Fracture of the scaphoid or radial styloid
2.   Cervical disk herniation
3.   Mucous cysts
4.   Brachial plexopathy

D.   Diagnostic Tests: Variable depending upon diagnosis
1.   Consider wrist x-ray to rule out fracture of the scaphoid or radial styloid
2.   Needle aspiration of ganglia is the most definitive method of diagnosing a suspected ganglia (may also be therapeutic, but ganglia often return)
3.   Electrophysiologic testing to confirm focal median nerve conduction delay within the carpal canal (beneficial especially in patients considering surgical intervention)

V.   Plan/Management
A.   Carpal tunnel syndrome
1.   For patients with mild symptoms (intermittent numbness, tingling, and pain in wrist and hands) likely to respond to conservative therapy
a.   Wrist splinting with wrist in the neutral position; response to splinting is variable among patients
b.   Use of NSAIDs is also important; splinting combined with use of NSAIDs provides relief in most patients
c.   Patients should be assisted to use proper body mechanics at work if repetitive use is believed to be part of the etiology; if possible, encourage patient to rotate jobs to reduce the amount of time spent on activities that expose the hypothenar area to vibration or pressure
2.   If conservative therapy fails to provide relief, refer the patient for corticosteroid injection of the carpal canal which has the advantage of both confirming the diagnosis and reduces the symptoms
3.   Patients with more severe symptoms such as those described below should be referred for surgery without attempts at conservative management
a.   Patients with persistent symptoms that include hyperesthesia, clumsiness, and loss of dexterity and pinch strength
b.   Burning pain that increases at night and with hand use
c.   Patients with thenar muscle atrophy and motor weakness noted on physical examination

B.   De Quervain's tenosynovitis
1.   Conservative therapy involves rest, use of a thumb spica splint to immobilize the thumb, and oral NSAIDs
2.   If conservative therapy fails to provide relief, refer the patient to an orthopedist for corticosteroid injection under the pulleys of the abductor pollicis longus and the extensor pollicis brevis

C.   Ganglion cyst
1.   Needle aspiration is both diagnostic and therapeutic; although cysts frequently return after being evacuated
2.   Recurrent ganglions that are recurrent may best be managed surgically; refer patient to a hand surgeon who can now resect ganglions arthroscopically with good results and very few recurrences

D.   Follow Up: In one month to evaluate therapy and determine need for referral except for those patients who were immediately referred to a specialist who should receive follow up by specialist

REFERENCES

Alvarez, J.A., & Hardy, R.H. (1998). Lumbar spine stenosis: A common cause of back and leg pain. <u>American Family Physician, 57,</u> 1825-1834.

Andrews, W.C. (1998). What's new in preventing and treating osteoporosis? <u>Postgraduate Medicine, 104,</u> 89-97.

American College of Rheumatology Ad Hoc Committee on Clinical Guidelines. (1996). Guidelines for management of rheumatoid arthritis. <u>Arthritis and Rheumatism, 39,</u> 713-722.

American College of Rheumatology Ad Hoc Committee on Clinical Guidelines. (1996). Guidelines for monitoring drug therapy in rheumatoid arthritis. <u>Arthritis and Rheumatism, 39,</u> 723-731.

American College of Rheumatology Task Force on Osteoporosis Guidelines. (1996). Recommendations for the prevention and treatment of glucocorticoid-induced osteoporosis. <u>Arthritis & Rheumatism, 39,</u> 1791-1800.

Arnett, F.C. (1989). Revised criteria for the classification of rheumatoid arthritis. <u>Bulletin on the Rheumatic Diseases, 38</u>(5), 1-6.

Bach, B.R. (1997). Acute knee injuries: When to refer. <u>The Physician and Sportsmedicine, 25,</u> 39-50.

Baker, D.G. & Schumacher, H.R. Jr. (1993). Acute monarthritis. <u>The New England Journal of Medicine, 329</u>(14), 1013-1020.

Ballas, M.T., Tytko, J., & Cookson, D. (1997). Common overuse running injuries: Diagnosis and management. <u>American Family Physician, 55,</u> 2473-2480.

Ballas, M.T., Tytko, J., & Mannarino, F. (1998). Commonly missed orthopedic problems. <u>American Family Physicians, 57,</u> 267-274.

Ballinger, S.H., & Bowyer, S.L. (1997). Fibromyalgia: The latest "great imitator." <u>Contemporary Pediatrics, 14,</u> 140-154.

Berarducci, A., & Lengacher, C.A. (1998). Osteoporosis in perimenopausal women. <u>The American Journal for Nurse Practitioners, 2</u> (9), 9-14.

Bergfeld, J., Ireland, M.L., Wojtys, E.M., & Glaser, V. (November 15, 1997). Pinpointing the cause of acute knee pain. <u>Patient Care,</u> 100-117.

Bigos, S., Bowyer, O., Braen, G., et al. (1994). <u>Acute low back problems in adults. Clinical practice guideline No. 14.</u> AHCPR Publication No. 95-0642. Rockville, MD: Agency for Health Care Policy and Research, Public Health Service, U.S. Department of Health and Human Services.

Blackburn, W.D. (1996). Management of osteoarthritis and rheumatoid arthritis: Prospects and possibilities. <u>The American Journal of Medicine, 100</u>(suppl 2A), 2A-24S-2A-30S.

Branstetter, B. (1998). Practical solutions to the mystery of fibromyalgia. <u>Journal of American Association of Physicians Assitants, 11,</u> 27-37.

Brunet, M.E., Norwood, L.A., & Sykes, T.F. (1997, January). What to do for the painful shoulder. <u>Patient Care,</u> 56-83.

Brunet, M.E., Norwood, L.A., & Sykes, T.F. (1997, November). A systematic approach to acute shoulder pain. <u>Patient Care,</u> 34-51.

Carey, T.S., Garrett, J., Jackman, A., et al. (1995). The outcomes and costs of care for acute low back pain among patients seen by primary care practitioners, chiropractors, and orthopedic surgeons. <u>New England Journal of Medicine, 333,</u> 913-917.

Creamer, P. & Hochberg, M.C. (1997). Osteoarthritis. <u>Lancet, 350,</u> 503-508.

Daniels, J.M. (1997). Treatment of occupationally acquired low back pain. <u>American Family Physician, 55,</u> 587-596.

Davidson, K. (1993). Patellofemoral pain syndrome. <u>American Family Physician, 48</u>(7), 1254-1262.

Deal, C.L. (1997). Osteoporosis: Prevention, diagnosis, and management. American Journal of Medicine, 102(suppl 1A), 35S-39S.

Eastell, R. (1998). Treatment of postmenopausal osteoporosis. The New England Journal of Medicine, 338, 736-746.

Ethridge, C.P., Maddox, M., & Ruch, D. (1997, November). Handling common wrist complaints. Patient Care, 56-75.

Fongemie, A.F., Buss, D.D., & Rolnick, S.J. (1998). Management of shoulder impingement syndrome and rotator cuff tears. American Family Physician, 57, 667-674.

Gillette, R.D. (1996). A practical approach to the patient with back pain. American Family Physician, 53, 670-676.

Goroll, A.H., May, L.A., & Mulley, Jr., A.G. (1995). Evaluation of acute monoarticular arthritis. In A.H.Goroll, L.A. May, A.G.Mulley, Jr., Primary care medicine, (3rd ed.). Lippincott: Philadelphia.

Goroll, A.H., May, L.A., & Mulley, Jr., A.G. (1995). Evaluation of polyarticular complaints. In A.H.Goroll, L.A. May, A.G.Mulley, Jr., Primary care medicine, (3rd ed.). Lippincott: Philadelphia.

Gotzsche, P.C., & Johansen, H.K. (1998). Meta-analysis of short term low dose prednisolone versus placebo and non-steroidal anti-inflammatory drugs in rheumatoid arthritis. British Medical Journal, 316, 811-818.

Gremillion, R.B., & van Vollenhoven, R.F. (1998). Rheumatoid arthritis: Designing and implementing a treatment plan. Postgraduate Medicine, 103, 103-123.

Haefner, J.K., & Fitzsimmons, M.S. (1997). Carpal tunnel syndrome. The Female Patient, 22, 21-31.

Hochberg, M.C., Altman, R.D., Brandt, K.D., Clark, B.M., Dieppe, P.A., Griffin, M.R., Moskowitz, R.W. & Schnitzer, T.J. (1995). Guidelines for the medical management of osteoporosis, Part I: Osteoarthritis of the hip, Part II: Osteoarthritis of the knee. Arthritis and Rheumatism, 38, 1535-1541.

Howard, T.M., & O'Connor, F.G. (1997). The injured shoulder: Primary care assessment. Archives of Family Medicine, 6, 376-384.

Isenbarger, D.W., & Chapin, B.L. (1997). Osteoporosis: Current pharmacologic options for prevention and treatment. Postgraduate Medicine, 101, 129-142.

Jones, A.K. (1997). Primary care management of acute low back pain. Nurse Practitioner, 22(7), 50-73.

Jupiter, J.B. (1995). Approach to minor orthopedic problems of the foot and ankle. In A.H. Goroll, L.A. May, & A.G. Mulley, Jr. (Eds). Primary care medicine, Philadelphia: Lippincott.

Karol, L.A. (1997). Rotational deformities in the lower extremities. Current Opinion in Pediatrics, 9, 77-80.

Kleerekoper, M. (1998). Detecting osteoporosis: Beyond the history and physical examination. Postgraduate Medicine, 103, 45-68.

Klipper, A.R. (1998). Gout. Lippincott's primary care practice, 2, 93-96.

Lane, N.E., & Thompson, J.M. (1997). Management of osteoarthritis in the primary-care setting: An evidence-based approach to treatment. American Journal of Medicine, 103(6A), 25S-30S.

Loder, R. (1998). Slipped capital femoral epiphysis. American Family Physician, 57, 2135-2142.

Lucas, K.H., & Davis, S.M. (1998). Calcium in corticosteroid-induced osteoporosis. The Annals of Pharmacotherapy, 32, 970-972.

Lufkin, E.G., & Zilkoski, M. (1996). Diagnosis and management of osteoporosis. American Family Physician, monograph, No. 1, 1-20.

Maffie-Lee, J. (1997). Osteoporosis: Assessment, prevention, and intervention. Clinical Excellence for Nurse Practitioners, 1, 221-230.

Magee, D.J. (1992). Orthopedic physical assessment. Philadelphia: Saunders.

Malmivaara, A., et al. (1995). A treatment of acute low back pain--bed rest, exercises, or ordinary activity. New England Journal of Medicine, 332, 351-355.

Mankin, K.P., & Zimbler, S. (1997). Gait and leg alignment: What's normal and what's not. Contemporary Pediatrics, 14(11), 41,45-46, 51-58, 62-70.

Marlow, S.M. (1998). Evaluating rheumatic complaints. Lippincott's primary care practice, 2, 3-19.

Maurizio, S.J., & Rogers, J.L. (1997). Recognizing and treating fibromyalgia. Nurse Practitioner, 22(12), 18-31.

Millard, P.S., Rosen, C.J., & Johnson, K.H. (1997). Osteoporotic vertebral fractures in postmenopausal women. American Family Physician, 55, 1315-1322.

Mikuls, T., & O'Dell, J.R. (1998). Today's approach to managing rheumatoid arthritis: The goal of medical therapy is disease remission. Women's Health in Primary Care, 1 614-626.

Morgan, R.L., & Linder, M.M. (1997). Common wrist injuries. American Family Physician, 56, 857-865.

Nattiv, A. (1998). Osteoporosis: Its prevention, recognition, and management. Family Practice Recertification, 20(2), 17-28, 33-36, 41.

Oddis, C.V. (1996). New perspectives in osteoarthritis. American Journal of Medicine, 100(suppl 2A), 2A-10S-2A-15S.

Reilly, B.M. (1991). Low back pain. In B.M. Reilly (Ed.), Practical strategies in outpatient medicine. Philadelphia: Saunders. Saunders.

Roberts, W.N. (1998). Hyperuricemia and gout. 1998 Conn's current therapy. Philadelphia: Saunders.

Ross, C. (1997). A comparison of osteoarthritis and rheumatoid arthritis: Diagnosis and treatment. Nurse Practitioner, 22(9), 20-39.

Rothenberg, M.I., & Graf, B.K. (1993). Evaluation of acute knee injuries. Postgraduate Medicine, 93 75-86.

Schiff, M. (1997). Emerging treatments for rheumatoid arthritis. American Journal of Medicine, 102 (suppl 1A), 11S-15S.

Seiler, J.G. (1997, May). Carpal tunnel syndrome: Update on diagnostic testing and treatment options. Consultant, 1233-1242.

Slemenda, C., Brandt, K.D., Heilman, D.K. et al. (1997). Quadriceps weakness and osteoarthritis of the knee. Annals of Internal Medicine, 127, 97-104.

Stiell, I.G., Wells, G.A., Hoag, R.H., et al. (1993). Decision rules for the use of radiography in acute ankle injuries: Refinement and prospective validation. Journal of American Medical Association, 269, 1127-1132.

Tan, E.M., Cohen, A.S., Fries, J.F., et al. (1982). The 1982 revised criteria for the classification of systemic lupus erythematosus. Arthritis Rheumatology, 25, 1275-1277.

Trovato, D., Mroczek, K.J., & Splain, S. (1998, March). The painful shoulder. Emergency Medicine, 78-100.

Waddell, G., Feder, G., & Lewis, M. (1997). Systematic reviews of bed rest and advice to stay active for acute low back pain. British Journal of General Practice, 47, 647-652.

Wexler, R.K. (1998). The injured ankle. American Family Physician, 57, 474-480.

Wheeler, A.H. (1995). Diagnosis and management of low back pain and sciatica. American Family Physician, 52, 1333-1341.

Wolfe, F., et al. (1990). The American College of Rheumatology 1990 criteria for the classification of fibromyalgia. Arthritis and Rheumatism, 33(2), 160-172.

Neurologic Problems

ALZHEIMER'S DISEASE

I. Definition: The most common type of dementia; there is progressive and irreversible deterioration in intellectual abilities so severe that it interferes with the person's usual social and occupational functioning

II. Pathogenesis

    A. Alzheimer's disease (AD) selectively damages critical clusters of neurons in the cortex and limbic structures of the central nervous system, particularly the basal forebrain, amygdala, hippocampus, and cerebral cortex
        1. These areas are associated with functions of higher learning, memory, reasoning, behavior, and emotional control
        2. There are four major alterations in these brain structures: cortical atrophy, degeneration of cholinergic and other neurons, presence of neurofibrillary tangles (NFTs), and accumulation of neuritic plaques

    B. As AD progresses, the neurons in these areas, which integrate the complex functions of memory and learning, atrophy and eventually die

    C. Widespread cell destruction leads to a variety of neurotransmitter deficits, with the cholinergic pathways most profoundly damaged

    D. Neurofibrillary tangles (NFTs) and neuritic plaques are present in normal brains and increase in number with aging
        1. In AD, the numbers of these lesions increase dramatically, especially in areas associated with memory and cognition--the hippocampus, amygdala, and cerebral cortex
        2. NFTs are located intracellularly and disrupt cell structure causing improper cell function and cell death
        3. Neuritic plaques (also called amyloid plaques) are extracellular lesions that are comprised of a core of beta amyloid protein
        4. NFTs and neuritic plaques substantially interfere with neuronal transmission

    E. Recent research has identified at least three autosomal-dominant forms of Alzheimer's disease, all with early-onset symptoms, involving chromosomes 1, 14, and 21

    F. Alleles of the apolipoprotein E gene locus on chromosome 19 have been associated with late-onset Alzheimer's disease

III. Clinical Presentation

    A. The most common of the dementing disorders affecting an estimated 4 million persons in the US

    B. Onset most often occurs in late life, generally after the age of 60, but in rare cases the disorder can begin as early as age 30

    C. Progression is gradual but steadily downward, with an average duration from onset of symptoms to death of 8 to 10 years; plateaus may occur, but progression usually resumes after a period of months or a few years (range of 3 to 20 years duration from diagnosis to death)

    D. Manifestations of AD in the early stages of the disease
        1. Memory impairment is the most prominent early symptom
            a. Effect on recent memory is most pronounced
            b. Remote memory is less affected
        2. Cognitive impairments create problems with functioning in daily life; for many patients and families, the functional impairments are the first sign that there is a problem

3. Attention impairment occurs and is manifest by difficulty with competing stimuli and in changing mental set
4. Visual-spatial functioning is affected and patients experience difficulty with drawing and route finding (diminishes ability to safely drive a motor vehicle)
5. Both problem-solving and calculations are affected as abstract thinking and judgment become impaired
6. Deficits in executive function (e.g., performing tasks involving multiple steps, such as planning and preparing a meal, organizing a shopping trip) are typically seen
7. Personality changes or increased irritability may be exhibited
8. Generally, there is relative preservation of motor and sensory functions until the later stages
9. Language and social skills may be fairly well preserved so that casual observer would be unaware that the person is experiencing cognitive impairment

E. By the middle and late stages of the disease, a number of mental and physical disabilities occur
1. Agitation (a range of behavioral disturbances including aggression, combativeness, shouting, hyperactivity, and disinhibition) is the most commonly occurring behavioral change, with as many as 50% of patients, particularly in middle and later stages of the illness, exhibiting this behavior
2. Psychotic symptoms (paranoia, delusions, and hallucinations) are far less frequent than agitation, but are much more dangerous to the patient and alarming to the family
3. Patients may also develop wandering behaviors which place them in great jeopardy of injury
4. Gait, motor disturbance, and incontinence may also occur in later stages

F. A variety of diagnostic classification schemes for AD exist; these diagnostic criteria include different combinations of impairment in cognitive, emotional, and social abilities, often reflecting a focus on different clinical features
1. Correctly diagnosing dementia in its early stages is often difficult; in many cases, dementing disorders are misdiagnosed or unrecognized
2. The tendency among many clinicians is to regard mild deficits that occur in the early stages of dementia as inevitable consequences of aging

G. Diagnostic criteria for dementia of the Alzheimer's type as set forth in the <u>Diagnostic and Statistic Manual of Mental Disorders, 4th ed.</u> (1994) are often used by clinicians and are contained in the following table

---

DIAGNOSTIC CRITERIA FOR DEMENTIA OF THE ALZHEIMER'S TYPE

The development of multiple cognitive deficits that is manifested by both of the following
- ◆ Memory impairment (both in learning new information and recalling previously learned information)
- ◆ One of more of the following cognitive disturbances
  - ❖ Aphasia (disturbance in language)
  - ❖ Apraxia (inability to carry out motor activities despite intact motor function)
  - ❖ Agnosia (inability to recognize objects despite intact sensory function)
  - ❖ Disturbances in executive functioning (planning, organizing, sequencing)

The cognitive deficits described above cause significant impairment in social or occupational functioning and represent a significant decline from previous functioning

The course is characterized by both gradual onset and continuing decline

The cognitive deficits described above are not due to any of the following
- ◆ Other central nervous system conditions that cause progressive decline in memory and cognition such as cerebrovascular disease, Huntington's disease, and Parkinson's disease
- ◆ Systemic conditions known to cause dementia such as hypothyroidism, vitamin B_{12} or folic acid deficiency, neurosyphilis, and HIV infection
- ◆ Substance-induced conditions

The deficits do not occur exclusively during the course of a delirium

The disturbance is not better accounted for by another disorder such as major depressive disorder or schizophrenia

Adapted from American Psychiatric Association. (1994). <u>Diagnostic and statistical manual of mental disorders</u>, (4th ed.). Washington, DC: Author.

H. The Agency for Health Care Policy and Research (AHCPR) has developed a clinical practice guideline to assist with the initial assessment of Alzheimer's disease
    1. The guideline contains a clinical tool to aid in the recognition of dementia in its early stages
    2. While this list of symptoms that might indicate dementia are not considered diagnostic criteria in the formal sense, the clinical tool is nonetheless very helpful for the primary care clinician
    3. The following table contains the symptoms that might indicate dementia as formulated by the clinical practice guideline panel of the Agency for Health Care Policy and Research (AHCPR) [1996]. The guideline recommends that six signs and symptoms be the focus of history taking and thereby provide the diagnostic criteria when evaluating patients in whom AD is suspected

---

CLINICAL GUIDE FOR RECOGNITION AND INITIAL ASSESSMENT OF DEMENTIA

Does the person have increased difficulty with any of the activities listed below?

Learning and retaining new information	Is repetitive; has trouble remembering recent conversations, events, appointments; frequently misplaces objects
Handling complex tasks	Has trouble following a complex train of thought or performing tasks that require many steps such as balancing a checkbook or cooking a meal
Reasoning ability	Is unable to respond with a reasonable plan to problems at work or home, such as knowing what to do if the bathroom is flooded; shows uncharacteristic disregard for rules of social conduct
Spacial ability and orientation	Has trouble driving, organizing objects around the house, finding way around familiar places
Language	Has increasing difficulty with finding the words to express what he or she wants to say and with following conversations
Behavior	Appears more passive and less responsive; is more irritable than usual; is more suspicious than usual; misinterprets visual or auditory stimuli

Interpretation: Positive findings in any of these areas generally indicate the need for further assessment for the presence of dementia

Source: US Department of Health and Human Services, Public Health Service, Agency for Health Care Policy and Research. (1996). Recognition and initial assessment of Alzheimer's disease and related dementias. Clinical Practice Guideline No. 19. Rockville, MD: Author.

I. The diagnosis of AD is one of inclusion, not exclusion, and in approximately 90% of cases, the diagnosis can be made on the basis of history, physical examination, and neuropsychological testing

IV. Diagnosis/Evaluation

    A. History
        1. The history should be obtained from the patient and a **reliable informant**
            a. Validity of patient reports are often limited by memory loss and lack of insight
            b. To increase accuracy of reporting, information from more than one family member may be helpful
            c. Patient should be informed that others may be interviewed to help with understanding of symptoms
            d. Dignity of the patient should be preserved!
            e. In evaluating informant reports, keep in mind that family members may have questionable motives which may lead to exaggerating or minimizing patient symptoms
        2. Using the clinical tool from AHCPR contained in the table above, document the presence and chronology of each of the six areas (DSM-IV criteria may also be used, but AHCPR was selected for use here)

3. Systematically, ask about the presence of each of the six symptom areas, beginning with establishing that the symptom is present (see table on page 678)
   a. For **Area 1, Learning and retaining new information**, Ask, "Do you (or interviewing the informant, "Does [patient's name]) have trouble remembering recent conversations, events, or appointments?"
   b. Ask about onset: "Was it abrupt or gradual?"
   c. Ask about progression "Is it getting worse?" "Is it improving?"
   d. Ask about duration: "How long has this been going on?"
4. Repeat this process for each of the **six areas** with both patient and the informant
5. Obtain medical history including any systemic diseases, psychiatric disorders, any known neurological disorders, history of head trauma
6. Obtain social history including alcohol, tobacco, drug use
7. Ask about occupational or recreational exposures to toxic substances
8. Determine what medications the patient is taking, including prescription products, over-the-counter drugs, and vitamin and herbal remedies
9. Obtain an in-depth family history with a focus on presence in the family of early-onset Alzheimer's disease or rare genetic conditions such as Huntington's disease
10. A functional status assessment should be part of the initial assessment
    a. The Functional Activities Questionnaire, which evaluates performance on 10 complex, higher-order activities, is recommended as the best approach to measurement of functional abilities
    b. This is an **informant-based** measure (must be completed by informant, not patient)

SUMMARY OF THE FUNCTIONAL ACTIVITIES QUESTIONNAIRE (FAQ)

- Bill paying
- Assembling records relating to business affairs
- Shopping alone
- Playing a game of skill
- Performing a task involving multiple steps (writing letter, stamping envelope, place in mailbox)
- Preparing a balanced meal
- Being aware of current events
- Understanding and discussing TV program, book, newspaper article
- Remembering and keeping appointments
- Driving, arranging to take bus, or walking to familiar places

In normal persons, all 10 activities are performed; the fewer activities that the person can perform independently, the more dependent he/she is

The Functional Activities Questionnaire was developed by R.I. Pfeiffer, T.T. Kurosake, & C.H. Harrah and is available in the Journal of Gerontology, Volume 37, pages 323-329, 1982. Administration and scoring of the instrument is explained in the article

---

11. Screen for abuse/neglect by asking the SAFE questions (see section on DOMESTIC VIOLENCE: ELDER AND DISABLED ADULT ABUSE AND NEGLECT)

B. Physical Examination
   1. Vital signs should be measured first, with blood pressure measured with patient supine and standing
   2. Assessment of vision and hearing should be completed
   3. A complete physical examination should be done with focus on cardiovascular, respiratory, and neurological systems
      a. Assess the cranial nerves, the motor system, the sensory system, and reflexes (during early stage, motor, sensory, and cerebellar portions of the exam are usually normal)
      b. Assess mental status using the Mini-Mental State Examination (MMSE) [see table on page 680]
      c. Normal MMSE scores vary according to age and education
      d. Cognitive measures such as the MMSE are probably **most** useful in terms of measuring change over time
   4. Pay particular attention for signs of abuse and neglect

OVERVIEW OF THE MINI-MENTAL STATE EXAMINATION		
Function	**Test**	**Maximum Score**
Orientation	• Ask date including year, season, date, day, month	5
	• Ask where presently located, including state, county, city	5
Registration	• Ask patient to repeat the name of three objects you have just named (Example--bird, ring, boat)	3
Attention and Calculation	• Ask the patient to begin with 100 and count backwards by 7 (stop after five subtractions); alternately ask to spell "world" backwards	5
Recall	• Ask patient to repeat the three objects named in Registration above	3
Language	• Point to familiar objects like clock and pencil; ask patient to name	2
	• Ask patient to repeat this sentence after you "No ifs, ands, or buts"	1
	• Direct patient to follow a 3-stage command "Take a paper in your right hand, fold it in half, and put it on the floor"	3
	• Ask patient to read and obey the following statement: "Close your eyes"	1
	• Ask patient to write a sentence; do not dictate sentence	1
	• Ask patient to copy a drawing of intersecting pentagons	1

Generally, a score of <26 indicates cognitive impairment, but this is only a crude indicator of functioning

Assess level of consciousness along a continuum from alert, to drowsy, to stupor, to coma

The Mini-Mental State Examination was developed by M.F. Folstein, S.E. Folstein, & P.R. McHugh. A copy of the instrument including instructions for administration and scoring is available in _Journal of Psychiatric Research_, Volume 12, pages 196-198, 1975.

C. Differential Diagnosis

1. **Depression.** Often mistaken for dementia; when depression is suspected based on history, symptoms consistent with depression should be sought (see section on DEPRESSION for diagnostic criteria)

2. **Delirium.** Often difficult to differentiate from dementia because both are marked by global disturbances in cognition and the conditions may occur together
   a. Clinical course of delirium is one in which features develop over a short period of time (usually hours to days) and there are significant fluctuations in degree of cognitive impairment over the course of the day
   b. Person who develops sudden onset of cognitive impairment, disorientation, and perceptual disturbances (such as hallucinations) is likely to have delirium
   c. Delirium is a medical emergency requiring immediate evaluation and treatment of the underlying cause, some of which can be fatal (e.g., bacterial meningitis or hypoglycemia)

3. **Vascular (multi-infarct) dementia.** Due to the effects of strokes on cognitive function; typically an abrupt onset and course within the context of cerebrovascular disease documented by history, focal neurological signs and symptoms and imaging studies

4. **Dementia due to Parkinson' s disease.** Dementia associated with Parkinson's disease (a slowly progressive condition characterized by tremor, rigidity, bradykinesia, and postural instability) has an insidious onset and slow progression; other signs and symptoms of Parkinson's are present

5. **Dementia due to Pick's disease and other frontal lobe dementias.** Characterized in early stages by changes in personality, executive dysfunction, deterioration of social skills (frontal lobe changes); difficult to distinguish clinically from atypical AD; brain imaging reveals prominent frontal and/or temporal atrophy with relative sparing of parietal and occipital lobes

6. **Dementia associated with Lewy bodies (DLB).** A recently recognized disorder that is clinically similar to AD, but tends to have earlier and more prominent visual hallucinations and Parkinsonian features, and a more rapid evolution; positive diagnosis requires both a finding of dementia and at least one of three core symptoms: detailed visual hallucinations, Parkinsonian signs, and alterations of alertness or attention

7. **Dementia due to other causes.** A number of general medical conditions can cause dementia including structural lesions, head trauma, endocrine conditions, nutritional conditions, infectious conditions, and toxic effects of long-standing substance abuse, especially alcohol

D. Diagnostic Tests
1. Laboratory assessment is performed to identify reversible or coexisting illnesses
2. Should be individualized based on history and physical examination, but **basic testing** usually includes those listed in the following table
3. Other studies may be indicated such as magnetic resonance imaging (MRI) if vascular dementia is suspected
4. Neuropsychological testing and evaluation should be performed on all patients in whom the diagnosis remains unclear after an initial assessment

BASIC LABORATORY ASSESSMENT FOR PATIENTS BEING EVALUATED FOR AD	
Blood studies	CBC Sedimentation rate Chemistry profile Liver function tests Thyroid function test (TSH) Syphilis serology Vitamin B_{12} and folate levels HIV testing
Radiologic studies	Chest x-ray Computed tomography (CT) of the brain
Other studies	Electrocardiogram Urinalysis

V. Plan/Management

A. The overall goal of care for patients with this progressive and irreversible disease is to improve quality of life for both the patient and family by maximizing the patient's cognition, mood, and behavior, and thereby his/her functional ability
1. Pharmacologic therapies for cognitive impairment and nonpharmacologic and pharmacologic treatments for the behavioral problems associated with dementia can have a significant impact on quality of life
2. Interventions of various types for family members who are caregivers are extremely important as nearly half of all caregivers become depressed

B. Improvement of central cholinergic neurotransmission with the use of cholinesterase inhibitors is the only treatment currently available for cognitive impairment
1. Substantial improvement is not a characteristic outcome with these agents, but they are believed to slow the rate of deterioration
2. The cholinesterase inhibitors--tacrine and donepezil--are described in a table that follows
3. Other agents that are currently being evaluated for their effectiveness in the treatment of cognition in AD are also briefly described on page 682

PHARMACOLOGIC THERAPY: COGNITIVE AND FUNCTIONAL ENHANCERS

Cholinesterase Inhibitors	<ul><li>Only treatment currently available for the cognitive impairment of AD</li><li>Improves central cholinergic neurotransmission</li><li>Two agents with labeling for treatment of AD, tacrine and donepezil, have been approved by the FDA</li><li>May improve cognitive functioning or delay decline; may also have beneficial effects on behavioral symptoms in some patients</li><li>Effects on patients with more severe disease have not been assessed</li><li>Monitoring effectiveness of these drugs: Serial evaluations of cognitive functioning (using an instrument such as the MMSE) and functional status (using the FAQ) can be helpful in determining effectiveness</li></ul>
Tacrine (Cognex)	<ul><li>Starting dose is 10 mg QID, which can be increased up to maximum dose of 40 mg QID</li><li>Nausea and vomiting are very common</li></ul> **Note**: Patients receiving this drug must have baseline and frequent follow-up alanine aminotransferase determinations! Recommended schedule is baseline and every other week for at least the first 15 weeks after the initiation of tacrine treatment, after which point monitoring may be less frequent
Donepezil (Aricept)	<ul><li>Second generation cholinesterase inhibitor</li><li>Has a longer duration of inhibitory action than tacrine and has greater specificity for brain tissue</li><li>Starting dose is 5 mg/day which may be increased to 10 mg/day after one month</li><li>Higher dose is more efficacious, but adverse effects such as nausea, diarrhea, and insomnia are very difficult for the patient to tolerate and occur especially often when dose is increased too rapidly</li><li>Many experts believe donepezil should be used as **first-line therapy** because of once a day dosing and regular monitoring of liver function is not required</li></ul>

PHARMACOLOGIC THERAPY: OTHER AGENTS UNDER INVESTIGATION

NSAIDs have been studied to determine if they can lower the risk of AD onset
- ❖ Rationale for use of NSAIDs is based on possibility that the amyloid peptide deposition and acute phase reactants in the neuritic plaques are indicative of an inflammatory process

Estrogen replacement has been associated with a delay in onset or reduced risk of AD
- ❖ The mechanism of the apparent protective effect of estrogen has been speculated to be based on the role of estrogens as trophic hormones to cholinergic neurons

Selegiline and vitamin E have been studied to determine if they benefit patients with AD
- ❖ These substances were selected for study because of the possibility that oxidative stress and accumulation of free radicals contribute to the neural degeneration in AD
- ❖ Vitamin E exerts antioxidant activity, and it is believed that selegiline has a similar antioxidant activity; in addition, selegiline may exert benefit by elevating catecholamine levels in the brain
- ❖ Many experts recommend vitamin E 400 IU tabs 2-3 x/day even though the benefits remain questionable

Gingko biloba has been used extensively in Europe to enhance memory and improve cognitive function with benefits attributed to antioxidant activity

C. Nonpharmacologic management of behavioral problems are summarized here
1. Encourage caregivers to modulate the environment, guided by the principle that patients with dementia are sensitive to their environments and often do best with moderate stimulation; too much stimulation may increase agitation and confusion while too little may lead to withdrawal
2. Familiar routines are comforting to the patient through promotion of a sense of security and predictability
3. Stimulation-oriented treatment such as use of art and other expressive recreational activities can improve mood
4. An exercise program should be instituted that includes outdoor daily walking if possible (**Note**: The role of daily exercise in the improvement of mood and behavior is critically important and cannot be overemphasized)
5. Caregivers can help with memory and orientation through encouraging patient to read newspapers and watch television programs which are educational and help link the patient with the outside world
6. Important family events can provide positive experiences for both the patient and family
7. The use of frequent reminders about the content of a conversation, if done in a kind way, can be very helpful to the patient in social situations

8. Psychotherapeutic techniques employed by expert therapists include reality orientation and memory retraining and may be of some limited benefit to some patients (many specialists believe the potential risks--frustration and depression in the patient and caregiver--may outweigh the benefits)

D. Pharmacologic management of behavioral problems
    1. Patients with depressive symptoms such as depressed mood, anorexia, insomnia, fatigue, irritability, and agitation should be considered for treatment with antidepressants even if they fail to meet criteria for depressive syndromes
        a. Selective serotonin reuptake inhibitors (SSRIs) are first-line treatment
        b. Tricyclic antidepressants, because of their significant anticholinergic activity are not recommended
        c. See the section on DEPRESSION for details on prescribing SSRIs in the elderly
    2. Patients should be evaluated for sleep disturbances and insomnia
        a. See section on INSOMNIA for recommendations regarding sleep hygiene
        b. Medications should be used only as a last resort

E. From a management standpoint, early diagnosis of AD is extremely important
    1. Patient and family are better able to cope with the disease once they are provided with information, can anticipate and plan for future medical, legal, and financial challenges, and have access to formal support services
    2. Cognition enhancing drugs are more likely to be effective early rather than late in the course of the illness when neurons become severely damaged

F. A team approach involving the primary care provider, social worker, nurse, and community agencies can best address problems of patients with AD and their families; unfortunately, the team is used only in times of crisis by many families rather than used for continuity of care

G. After the diagnosis of possible or probable AD has been made, a meeting with the patient and family should be held in which the following topics are addressed
    1. A discussion of the diagnosis and education about the illness and its treatment
    2. The probable course of the illness should be explained
    3. The availability of support groups and educational resources (see table at end of section, RESOURCES FOR PATIENTS WITH AD AND THEIR FAMILIES)
    4. The overall plan in terms of follow-up appointments over the next year; emphasize that you are available to supervise care and to provide support to patient and family
    5. Need for consultation with attorney or financial advisor for advice on legal and financial issues
    6. **Note**: It is very difficult to deal with all of these issues in a single visit; thus, judgment should be used regarding which topics to address first and which ones to address after the family has had time to reflect on the situation

H. **Management of mildly impaired patients and their families**
    1. A major focus at this time is dealing with loss and the perceived stigma of the illness
    2. It is important to highlight remaining abilities while assisting with specific impairments
    3. Risk of driving should always be discussed; there is no consensus on this issue, but concern for the safety of the patient and others should be discussed with recommendations on how to handle this situation
    4. Nonpharmacologic strategies may decrease behavioral problems and improve mood in the patient (see above recommendations under V.C.)
    5. Pharmacologic therapy with cognitive and functional enhancers may be instituted at this time
    6. Patients with depressive symptoms may benefit from treatment with a selective serotonin reuptake inhibitor (SSRI) as described above

I. **Management of moderately impaired patients and their families**
   1. A major focus at this time is on keeping the patient safe and requires working closely with the family; patients in this stage are likely to require more supervision
      a. Accidents relating to forgetfulness are likely to occur
      b. There is the possibility of wandering
      c. Patients in this stage should strongly be urged not to drive
   2. Another focus at this time is respite care for the caregiver; home health care, or day care should be considered for part of the day so that the caregiver is not overburdened
   3. Families should begin to consider options for care including placement in a long-term care facility
   4. Suggest the nonpharmacologic strategies listed above, if not done previously
   5. Pharmacologic therapy with cognitive and functional enhancers may be instituted at this time, if not done previously
   6. Patients with depressive symptoms may benefit from treatment with a selective serotonin reuptake inhibitor (SSRI) as described above
   7. Patients with psychosis and agitation are best managed by a specialist

J. **Management of profoundly impaired patients and their families**
   1. At this stage, patients are almost completely dependent on others for help with the activities of daily living
   2. Families typically struggle greatly when a family member is in this stage of the disease
      a. Most caregivers benefit from a frank discussion of their feelings of grief, guilt, and resentment
      b. Families should be assisted in locating additional resources during this stage; hopefully, most families will already have been involved with support services prior to this stage
      c. The decision to continue cognitive and functional enhancing medications at this time should be made on an individual basis
      d. Patients in this category may require referral to a specialist for management

K. Follow Up
   1. Regular patient monitoring is important and should be at least every 3 to 6 months for all patients
   2. Patients with complex or potentially dangerous symptoms, who are on medications that require frequent monitoring of effectiveness and of side effects such as hepatotoxicity must be followed up every one to two weeks (see recommendations regarding monitoring of transaminase levels in patients receiving tacrine in the table above, PHARMACOLOGIC THERAPY: COGNITIVE AND FUNCTIONAL ENHANCERS)

RESOURCES FOR PATIENTS WITH AD AND THEIR FAMILIES

Organizations providing consumer education, research, and support programs and activities for patients and families include the following
   + Alzheimer's Association   1-800-272-3900
   + Geriatric Psychiatry Alliance   1-888-463-6472
   + American Geriatrics Society   (212) 308-1414
   + Alzheimer's Disease Education & Referral Center   1-800-438-4380

The readings listed below may be helpful to families of persons with AD
   + *Failure-Free Activities for the Alzheimer's Patient.* San Francisco, CA: Cottage Books, 1987
   + *Reminiscence: Uncovering a Lifetime of Memories.* San Francisco, Ca: Elder Press, 1991
   + *Living in the Labyrinth: A Personal Journey Through the Maze of Alzheimer's.* San Francisco, CA: Elder Press, 1993
   + *The 36 Hour Day.* Baltimore, MD: Johns Hopkins University Press, 1981

BELL'S PALSY (PERIPHERAL FACIAL PALSY)

I. Definition: Acute, unilateral paralysis of facial muscles due to inflammation and swelling of the 7th (the facial) cranial nerve

II. Pathogenesis

    A. An Idiopathic lower motor neuron disease

    B. Condition is believed to be viral in origin and may be related to reactivation of herpes simplex virus (HSV)

    C. Damage to the intraneural capillaries is believed to be caused by viral infection of the nerve
        1. Fluid effusion is generated
        2. Subsequently, edema induces paralysis

III. Clinical Presentation

    A. Affects all age groups but most commonly affects young and middle-aged adults

    B. In the majority of patients, stress, fever, or an upper respiratory infection precedes the onset of the disorder

    C. Typical presentation is loss of facial expression, loss of voluntary movement of facial and scalp muscles on affected side, inability to close one eye, and numbness of the face

    D. May have loss of taste, be hypersensitive to sound, and have excessive tearing

    E. May have pain behind ear or over the cheek near the ear

    F. May have facial sagging from loss of muscle tone in severe cases, but this is rare

    G. Most patients recover completely within weeks to a few months, but some have residual effects

    H. Recurrent facial nerve palsy is unusual and if patient has more than two episodes of the condition, the possibility of sarcoidosis, leukemia, or tumor should be suspected

IV. Diagnosis/Evaluation

    A. History
        1. Question about onset of symptoms as paralysis in Bell's palsy is abrupt and does not occur gradually over days or weeks
        2. Include careful questioning about neurological symptoms in other areas of face and body
        3. Inquire about cerebrovascular and cardiac risk factors
        4. Ask about predisposing factors such as infection or trauma

    B. Physical Examination
        1. Measure vital signs, noting elevations in blood pressure and temperature
        2. Observe general appearance including gait, evidence of trauma or distress
        3. Inspect skin for herpetic lesions or characteristic lesions of Lyme disease
        4. Carefully examine the head, ears, eyes, nose, and throat
        5. Special attention should be given to assessment of the cranial nerves and the neurological examination
        6. Use a grading system such as the one in the following table to classify paralysis of the face

GRADING SYSTEM TO CLASSIFY FACIAL PARALYSIS	
Grade 1	• Normal
Grade 2	• No synkinesis (movement in a paralyzed muscle accompanying motion in another part) • Good facial and scalp movement with preserved eyelid closure
Garde 3	• Dyskinesis, or difficulty in performing voluntary movements may or may not be present • Differences between sides of face are apparent
Grade 4	• Incomplete eye closure is present (eyes normal at rest)
Grade 5	• Incomplete eye closure is present (eyes are asymmetric at rest)
Grade 6	• Complete paralysis

    C.   Differential Diagnosis: Simultaneous bilateral facial palsies, unilateral facial weakness that slowly progresses over 3 weeks with or without facial hyperkinesis, and failure of facial function to return within 6 months after acute onset suggests a diagnosis other than Bell's palsy; possible alternative diagnoses are the following
        1.   Stroke
        2.   Tumor
        3.   Infectious processes, viral, bacterial, or spirochete
        4.   Trauma
        5.   Guillain-Barré syndrome (typically has symmetric bilateral weakness)
        6.   Neurofibromatosis (typically has café au lait spots and cutaneous neurofibromas)

    D.   Diagnostic Tests
        1.   Diagnostic tests are not needed unless there is uncertainty about the diagnosis
        2.   Obtain Lyme titer if there is a history of exposure to ticks
        3.   Consider computerized tomography (CT) scan or magnetic resonance imaging (MRI) to rule out tumor and stroke
        4.   Electromyographic (EMG) testing occasionally is done to predict prognosis and progression of disease
        5.   An audiogram can detect hearing loss which is inconsistent with the diagnosis of Bell's palsy

V.   Plan/Management

    A.   Explain to the patient that symptoms usually resolve in 3-4 weeks without any treatment and with no sequelae

    B.   Maintain normal conjunctival moisture when there is loss of lid function with eye drops such as Tears Naturale II ophthalmic solution, 1-2 drops as needed

    C.   Affected eye may need to be taped, especially at night, to reduce eye damage

    D.   A physical therapy referral may be beneficial; usually involves heat therapy, electrical stimulation, or massage

    E.   Use of corticosteroids is controversial, but is commonly used nonetheless, particularly in patients who present with moderate to severe paralysis
        1.   If there are no contraindications, initiate short-term treatment with prednisone (60 mg/day in divided doses for 4 days), and then tapered and discontinued over the next 6 days)
        2.   Corticosteroids should be started as soon as possible after the onset of facial paralysis
        3.   Initiation of therapy within 3 days is considered optimal

    F.   Follow Up
        1.   For patients with moderate or severe symptoms, reevaluate in at 3-4 days, and then in 2-4 weeks
        2.   Patients taking steroids should be seen after completion of course of therapy

3. Patients with mild symptoms should be told to return immediately if symptoms worsen or do not resolve completely in 3-4 weeks
4. Patients who have delayed or incomplete recovery should be referred to a specialist for treatment; Botulinum toxin type A injection has produced good results

HEADACHES

I. Definition: Diffuse pain in the head

II. Pathogenesis

    A. Primary headaches are caused by traction on pain sensitive structures, inflammation of vessels and meninges, vascular dilation, excessive muscle contraction, and dysregulation of the ascending brain stem serotonergic system

    B. Secondary headaches are due to an underlying organic cause; less than 2-10% of headaches are secondary

    C. International Headache Society Classification (1988)
        1. Migraine with aura and unaccompanied by aura
        2. Tension-type headache
        3. Cluster and chronic paroxysmal hemicrania
        4. Head trauma and post-traumatic headache
        5. Vascular disorders such as severe hypertension, temporal arteritis
        6. Nonvascular intracranial disorders such as brain tumor
        7. Substances or their withdrawal such as pain from caffeine withdrawal or use of nitrates
        8. Noncephalic infections such as otitis media, sinusitis, influenza
        9. Metabolic disorders such as pheochromocytoma
        10. Disorders of face, neck or cranial structures such as cervical radiculopathy, temporomandibular joint (TMJ) dysfunction, eyestrain, acute narrow angle glaucoma, dental problems
        11. Cranial neuralgias such as trigeminal neuralgia
        12. Other types such as psychogenic headaches

    D. In the elderly, headaches are more likely secondary due to disease such as giant cell arteritis, intracranial masses, ischemic cerebrovascular disease, chronic obstructive lung disease with hypercapnia or prescription/other-the-counter medications

III. Clinical Presentation of Primary Headaches

    A. Migraines
        1. More common in females than males
        2. Episodes often begin in adolescence or early adulthood; often remit by age 50 or 60
        3. Frequently there is a positive family history
        4. Females often report a relationship between the migraine and their menses; headaches often remit after menopause
        5. Often unilateral, throbbing and accompanied with nausea, vomiting, phonophobia, photophobia, and perspiration
        6. Subdivided into two categories:
            a. Migraine accompanied with an aura such as visual prodromes (flashing lights, zigzags, illusions of distorted shapes, strange odors, or paresthesias); previously referred to as a classic migraine
            b. Migraine without an aura; previously referred to as common or nonclassic migraine
        7. Complicated migraines are characterized by persistent neurologic symptoms
        8. Research indicates that migraines may increase stroke risk

B. Tension-type
1. Most common headache type, with a lifetime prevalence of 69% in men and 88% in women
2. Often slowly progressing, bilateral, non-throbbing, or patient complains of dull pressure or band-like sensation about head
3. Pain is usually mild to moderate
4. Patients usually do not get nausea, vomiting, photophobia, or phonophobia and headache is not aggravated by physical activity
5. The International Headache Society distinguishes between patients with episodic tension-type headaches and chronic tension-type headaches (head pain must be present for 15 days a month for at least 6 month to be considered chronic)
6. Depression, anxiety, and chronic headaches may coexist together
7. May have combination migraine and tension-type headache

C. Cluster
1. Severe, unilateral burning or stabbing pain behind eye
2. Accompanied with at least one of the following on the headache side: ptosis, miosis, redness/edema of eyelid, conjunctival injection, lacrimation, nasal congestion, rhinorrhea, forehead and facial sweating
3. Cluster headaches often begin in the 4th decade of life (30s)
4. Attacks occur in a series which may last months to weeks
5. Attacks may be as short as 15 minutes or last more than 2-3 hours; attacks may occur once a day or as frequently as 8 times a day

IV. Diagnosis/Evaluation

A. History
1. Ask about onset of headache; ask about the patient's age at the time of their first headache
2. Ask patients to rate their headaches on a scale from 1 to 10
3. Question about symptoms which are related to ominous causes (see section V.A.)
4. Focus on temporal pattern of headaches, associated symptoms, and characteristics of pain such as location and whether headache is throbbing, dull, or burning
5. Inquire about an aura and prodromal symptoms
6. Determine whether there is a seasonal relationship to the headaches
7. Ask about precipitating factors such as stress, diet, physical exertion, sleep problems, or menses
8. Inquire about medication use, particularly birth control pills, which often cause headaches
9. Ask about previous trauma to the head
10. Determine how much caffeine is consumed each day
11. Question about past medical history including mental health problems
12. Carefully document family medical history, especially history of migraine headaches
13. Explore present and previous treatments and responses to treatments including over-the-counter medications and home remedies
14. Determine impact of headaches on patient's quality of life and daily functioning
15. Patients with chronic headaches should keep a diary documenting their symptoms and the circumstances surrounding the symptoms

B. Physical Examination
1. Observe general appearance, noting signs of acute distress, anxiety, or depression
2. Measure blood pressure, pulse, pulse pressure
3. Inspect head for signs of trauma and deformities
4. Palpate temporal arteries for tenderness (patients with temporal arteritis have firm, tender, enlarged arteries)
5. Palpate sinuses and temporomandibular joint (TMJ)
6. Perform complete eye exam with funduscopy; check pupils for size, shape, accommodation, and response to light

7. Examine mouth and teeth
8. Check for nuchal rigidity, cervical bruits, cervical vertebrae radiculopathy
9. Auscultate and palpate peripheral pulses
10. Perform complete neurological exam including careful assessment of cranial nerves

C. Differential Diagnosis:
 1. Determine whether headache is a secondary headache due to an organic cause or a primary headache; consider the following questions:
   a. Does the patient have risk for secondary causes such as diabetes and hyperlipidemia which may be associated with headaches due to stroke?
   b. Do the associated symptoms suggest a secondary cause?
     (1) Meningitis/encephalitis (fever, nuchal rigidity)
     (2) Sinusitis (frontal tenderness, fever, nasal discharge)
     (3) Narrow angle glaucoma (cloudy vision)
     (4) TMJ syndrome (pain with chewing)
     (5) Cervical radiculopathy (pain with neck movement)
   c. Are the headaches related to precipitating factors such as cold or hot foods and drinks which may be associated with trigeminal neuralgia?
 2. Brain tumors are always a consideration; patients with traction headaches due to intracranial lesions have the following signs and symptoms:
   a. Gradual onset of deep, aching pain which is often worse in morning and aggravated by coughing or straining for stool
   b. May have signs of increased intracranial pressure such as papilledema, and widening pulse pressure
 3. Headaches that are sudden in onset and described as the "worst headache" may be due to a subarchnoid hemorrhage
 4. If the secondary cause of headache is excluded, determine which type of primary headache is causing the pain

D. Diagnostic Tests
 1. Order computerized tomography (CT) scan or magnetic resonance imaging (MRI):
   a. When there is suspicion of the following: intracranial tumor, cerebellar hemorrhage or infarction, stroke, intracerebral hemorrhage
   b. When there has been head trauma with findings of increased intracranial pressure, depressed or open skull fracture, and penetrating head injury
 2. Other diagnostic tests should be ordered on the basis of the history and physical examination; the following are examples, but not an exhaustive list of possible tests:
   a. CBC with differential and immediate lumbar puncture if infection is suspected
   b. Erythrocyte sedimentation rate, temporal artery biopsy, and antinuclear antibody to detect temporal arteritis
   c. Magnetic resonance angiography if aneurysm is suspected
   d. Cervical spine x-rays to detect cervical radiculopathy
   e. X-rays of the temporomandibular joints if TMJ syndrome is suspected
 3. CT, MRI, spectroscopy and PET are sometimes ordered for headaches without clinical findings when the diagnosis is uncertain
 4. Consider screening EKG if triptan or ergotamine will be prescribed

V. Plan/Management

A. Consider referral to a specialist if the patient has a complicated migraine or any of the following ominous signs (see table)

OMINOUS SIGNS OF HEADACHE
❖ Abnormal physical signs
❖ New-onset, unilateral headache, particularly in patients over age 35
❖ Severe headache or headache different from previous ones
❖ Headaches becoming more continuous and intense
❖ Headaches accompanied by vomiting but not nausea

B. Acute therapy for migraines in adults
1. Limit all medications to those absolutely necessary to prevent transforming migraines to chronic, daily, intractable head pain or to avoid rebound headaches
2. Antiemetics administered orally, intramuscularly or by rectal suppository may offset nausea and enhance the effectiveness of analgesic drugs; prescribe one of the following:
   a. Metoclopramide (Reglan) 10 mg PO every 6 hours increases gut motility which may counteract the gastric stasis that often accompanies migraine attacks; use sparingly because of possible dystonia effects
   b. Alternatively, prescribe prochlorperazine (Compazine) 5-10 mg TID/QID PO, 5-10 mg IM every 3-4 hours, or 25 mg BID rectally
3. For mild attacks prescribe one of the following:
   a. Aspirin 325-400 mg tablets, 2 tablets PO every 4 hours
   b. Excedrin Migraine which contains 250 mg acetaminophen, 250 mg aspirin, 65 mg caffeine is the first over-the-counter analgesic to be cleared by the FDA for treatment of mild-to-moderate migraine pain; recommend 2 tabs every 6 hours as needed with maximum of 8 tabs per day
   c. Nonsteroidal anti-inflammatory drugs (NSAIDs) such as naproxen sodium (Anaprox), 275 mg tablets, 2 tabs initially followed by 1 tab every 6-8 hours
4. For moderate and severe attacks prescribe one of the following drugs:
   a. Sumatriptan (Imitrex), a selective serotonin 5-HT 1D receptor agonist, is the agent of choice for adults
      (1) Prescribe one of the following administration routes:
          (a) 6 mg subcutaneous injection (available 6mg/0.5 mL); onset of action is rapid; may repeat injection in 1 hour, with a maximum of 2 doses in 24 hours
          (b) 25-100 mg PO (available 25 & 50 mg tabs) -- 50 mg dose recently found to be most effective; may give second dose 2 hours after first with additional doses at two hour intervals if needed; maximum is 300 mg/day or 200 mg/day if injection was also used; take with fluids
          (c) 5 mg, 10 mg, or 20 mg intranasally (available 5 mg & 20 mg per spray); dose is administered into single nostril, unless patient is using 10 mg dose, which requires 5 mg sprayed in each nostril; may repeat dose once after 2 hours; maximum of 40 mg/day and treatment of 4 headaches within 30 days
      (2) First dose of injectable sumatriptan should be given under medical supervision and possibly monitored with an electrocardiogram; cautiously prescribe to patients who are likely to have unrecognized coronary artery disease, such as postmenopausal women, men over 40 years, and patients with risk factors for coronary vascular disease
      (3) Contraindicated in patients with history of myocardial infarction, symptomatic ischemic heart disease, Prinzmetal's angina or uncontrolled hypertension
      (4) Do not use sumatriptan with vasoconstrictor drugs or within 2 weeks of therapy with monoamine oxidase inhibitors, and use of ergotamine derivatives within the previous 24 hours
      (5) Advantages: medication is effective in relieving pain when given at any time during the attack and it is helpful in relieving nausea
      (6) Disadvantages are that it is expensive, headaches tend to recur, and side effects such as flushing, throat discomfort, neck and chest tightness or pain, tingling can occur
   b. Other selective serotonin 5-HT 1D receptor agonists are available for patients categorized as poor responders to other treatments including sumatriptan (see following table)

COMPARISON OF NEW TRIPTANS			
Drug	**Dosing**	**Administration**	**Comment**
Naratriptan tablets (Amerge)	1 or 2.5 mg with fluid. Repeat once after 4 h when necessary. Maximum dosage: 5 mg/24 h	Maximum dosage in patients with mild to moderate renal or hepatic impairment is 2.5 mg/24 h. Consider a lower starting dose. Contraindicated in patients with severe kidney or liver disease.	Long onset of action; long elimination half life; helpful for patients with long migrainous episodes; may have slightly lower rate of recurrence of migraine than other triptans; favorable side effect profile.
Rizatriptan (MAXALT, MAXALT-MLT)	5 or 10 mg by mouth. Repeat once after at least 2 h when necessary. Maximum dosage: 30 mg/24 h; for patients using propranolol, 15 mg/24 h.	Patients should be advised to consult the health care provider before administering a second dose if the first has had no effect. Make sure patients know that the conventional tablet must be swallowed with liquid. The fast-melting form, packaged in blisters, will dissolve with saliva.	More rapid onset of action than oral sumatriptan.
Zolmitriptan tablets (Zomig)	2.5 mg or less to start-- tablets can be broken in half, but response is better with 2.5- or 5-mg strengths. Dose can be repeated after 2 h. Maximum dosage: 10 mg/24 h.	Liver disease hinders clearance of zolmitriptan, a situation that can push up BP. Caution is warranted in patients with hepatic dysfunction--individual doses should be <2.5 mg.	More rapid onset of action than oral sumatriptan; favorable side effect profile.

Adapted from Starr, C. (1998). Emerging migraine treatments. Patient Care Nurse Practitioner, 10-26.

    c.   Ergotamine tartrate, a serotonin agonist, is a second-line abortive agent
        (1)   Prescribed one of the following administration routes (rectal route may be best if patient is nauseous):
            (a)   Ergotamine tartrate with caffeine (Cafergot) 1 suppository per rectum; may insert 2nd suppository after 60 minutes up to 2 per day or 5 per week; best absorbed of all nonparenteral preparations
            (b)   Ergotamine tartrate 1 mg, caffeine 100 mg (Wigraine): take 2 tabs; may repeat 1 tab every 30 minutes up to 6 mg per attack or 10 mg per week
            (c)   Ergotamine tartrate (Ergostat): 2 mg under tongue; may repeat every 30 minutes up to 6 mg per day or 10 mg per week
        (2)   Must take these agents early in the attack to be effective
        (3)   With all routes of administration, there should be a 5-day hiatus between treatment days
        (4)   Not adhering to dosage guidelines should be avoided to prevent rebound headaches which are common with these agents
        (5)   Contraindications include coronary or peripheral vascular disease, uncontrolled hypertension, impaired hepatic or renal disorders; some experts avoid giving this drug to elderly patients
        (6)   Side effects include nausea, vomiting, diarrhea, cramping dizziness, transient paresthesias, vasoconstrictive complications, tachycardia, bradycardia, localized edema or itching
    d.   Dihydroergotamine mesylate (D.H.E. 45, Migranal) is a derivative of ergotamine and is used for rapid control of migraines
        (1)   Dosage is dependent on route of administration
            (a)   D.H.E. 45: Give 1 mL IM or IV at onset of attack then 1 mL after one hour as needed; maximum is 2 mL IV or 3 mL IM per attack
            (b)   Migranal: One spray in each nostril; repeat 15 minutes later with maximum of 6 sprays in 24 hours and 8 sprays per week
        (2)   Contraindications and side effects are similar to ergotamine

     e.   Isometheptene mucate 65 mg, dichloralphenazone 100 mg, acetaminophen 325 mg tablets (Midrin) is a cerebral vasoconstrictor and a third-line agent
- (1) Usually recommended for patients who can't take sumatriptan or ergotamine
- (2) Less beneficial in patients with severe headaches
- (3) Prescribe 2 tabs initially followed by 1 every hour, maximum 5 per 12 hours
- (4) Contraindications: Glaucoma, severe renal, cardiac, hypertensive, or hepatic disease, concurrent MAOIs
- (5) Has fewer side effects than sumatriptan and ergotamine

     f.   Analgesics and sedatives are sometimes helpful but it is best to avoid regular use of them
- (1) Butorphanol tartrate nasal spray (Stadol NS) 1 mg: Spray in one nostril; if relief is not provided within 60-90 minutes an additional 1 mg may be given; repeat every 3-4 hours as needed
- (2) Fiorinal (combination of aspirin 325 mg, caffeine 40 mg, barbiturate 50 mg): Prescribe one to two tabs every four hours
- (3) Parenteral narcotics can be used for pain relief and to enable patient to sleep through the attack; minimize use to prevent abuse

C.   Treatment of severe, intractable migraine attacks
1. Ketorolac (Toradol) 30-60 mg IM is often used in emergency departments
2. Three dopamine-antagonist drugs given intravenously may be beneficial: metoclopramide (Reglan), chlorpromazine (Thorazine), prochlorperazine (Compazine)
3. IV dihydroergotamine and/or corticosteroid therapy (IM or IV) along with metoclopramide or another antiemetic may break the headache cycle

D.   Migraine preventive therapy in adults
1. Consider preventive therapy when the patient has >2 attacks per month, when attacks are severe or predictable, or when other therapies have failed or had serious side effects
2. General principles to follow when ordering preventive therapy:
   - a. Women of childbearing age should use barrier methods of contraception rather than oral birth control pills which often trigger headaches
   - b. Patients should discontinue all prior headache medications before prophylaxis therapy because previous medications may compete for monoamine-receptor sites with preventive drugs
   - c. Each preventive medication should be given for an adequate time to judge its effectiveness (i.e., 2-3 months)
   - d. Preventive medication is usually given for 6 months and then gradually withdrawn after the frequency of headaches diminishes
3. Common preventive medications are the following:
   - a. Aspirin 325-400 mg tabs, 1-2 tabs PO HS
   - b. Adrenergic blocking agents are especially beneficial for patients with concomitant hypertension, angina pectoris or thyrotoxicosis (avoid agents with intrinsic sympathomimetic activity)
     - (1) Contraindicated in patients with bronchospasm, congestive heart failure, cardiac arrhythmias, or a history of depression
     - (2) Propranolol (Inderal) is considered drug of choice: Start with 20 mg PO BID and increase gradually to maximum 160 mg/day
     - (3) Alternative drug is timolol (Blocadren): 10-20 mg/day
     - (4) Alternative drug (especially for asthmatics): Metoprolol (Lopressor) 100-200 mg/day in two divided doses
   - c. Divalproex sodium (Depakote), an anticonvulsant, is the first-line therapy for patients with concomitant seizures, mania, or anxiety; may also be given to patients without history of seizures
     - (1) Begin with 125-250 mg TID and increase gradually; average dose is 250-500 mg TID; prescribe twice daily for patients without seizures
     - (2) Order baseline CBC and liver function tests at frequent intervals, particularly in first 6 months
     - (3) Dose-related side effects are nausea, tremor, weight gain, hair loss

d. Tricyclic antidepressants such as amitriptyline (Elavil) 50-100 mg po HS are not first-line agents, but may be beneficial, particularly for patients with coexisting migraine and tension-type headaches

e. Calcium channel blockers are usually used after trials of the more effective beta blockers or amitriptyline; alternative to beta blockers in patients with asthma or chronic obstructive pulmonary disease; effective in patients with neurologic symptoms

    (1) Verapamil (Calan) is the best studied agent in this class; prescribe 120-480 mg/day

    (2) Use these agents with caution in patients with congestive heart failure

    (3) Avoid abrupt withdrawal of these agents because of the potential to induce chest pain, rebound angina, or exacerbation of symptoms

f. For headaches unresponsive to above therapies, consider use of methysergide (Sansert), 2 mg PO TID/QID

    (1) One of most effective agents but can cause retroperitoneal, pleural, and pulmonary valve fibrosis with extended use; monitor patient by assessing peripheral pulses and auscultating the chest monthly

    (2) Contraindicated in patients with vascular disease because of its vasoconstrictor action

    (3) Continue for 4 months then reduce slowly with gradual substitution of another prophylactic agent, so that one month elapses before resumption.

g. Other classes of drugs that may be used are nonsteroidal anti-inflammatory drugs (NSAIDs), clonidine (Catapres), and selective serotonin reuptake inhibitors (SSRIs) such as fluoxetine (Prozac)

E. Patients with menstrual migraines

1. Acute therapy is similar to treatment of migraines not associated with menses (see V.B.)

2. Prophylaxis with one of following drugs may be helpful when administered for one week during the luteal phase of the menses;

    a. Percutaneous estrogen in gel form or transdermal patches containing 0.05 mg of ethinyl estradiol (Climara, Estroderm) because migraines may be triggered by falling estrogen levels (start 2-3 days before expected headaches)

    b. NSAIDs such as mefenamic acid (Ponstel) 250 mg BID/TID

    c. Propranolol (Inderal) 20-120mg PO BID

    d. Amitriptyline 50-100 mg po HS

    e. Antiestrogen tamoxifen citrate (Nolvadex) 5-15 mg/day

    f. Bromocryptine mesylate (Parlodel) 2.5-5 mg/day

    g. Androgen derivative danazol (Danocrine) 200-600 mg/day

F. Migraine: Patient Education

1. Reduce precipitating factors such as stress, foods with nitrites (hot dogs), foods with monosodium glutamate (Chinese food), and tyramine containing foods (cheese, chocolate, red wine)

2. Limit caffeine to 2 beverages/day

3. Avoid alcoholic beverages, undersleeping, oversleeping, missing meals, smoking

4. Avoid craning neck forward

5. Avoid possible triggers such as glare or exposure to flickering lights, noise, or strong odors

6. Avoid analgesic, ergotamine, and decongestant overuse

7. Oral contraceptives should be discontinued; but hormone replacement therapy is usually helpful

8. Get regular aerobic exercise

9. Biofeedback, relaxation therapy

10. Rest in quiet dark room with topical ice to head or neck

11. For more information on migraines, consult the following organizations (see following table)

RESOURCES FOR INFORMATION ON MIGRAINES		
Organization	**Telephone Number**	**Website**
American Academy of Neurology	800/879-1960	http://www.aan.com
American Association for the Study of Headache	609/423-0043	http://www.aash.org
American Council for Headache Education	609/423-0258	http://www.achenet.org
American Medical Association	312/464-5000	http://www.ama-assn.org/migraine
American Neurological Association	612/545-6284	http://www.aneuroa.org
Migraine Awareness Group; a National Understanding for Migraineurs (MAGNUM)	703/739-9384	http://www.migraines.org
National Headache Foundation	800/843-2256	http://www.headaches.org

Adapted from Starr, C. (1998). Emerging migraine treatments. Patient Care Nurse Practitioner, 10-26.

G. Tension-type Headache Treatment
   1. Because of chronic nature of these headaches, try nonpharmacological approaches such as biofeedback, stress management, relaxation and exercise first
   2. Initiate drug therapy with least potent and least addictive medications such as acetaminophen, aspirin, and NSAIDS
   3. Use drugs for brief time period and limit to <15 pills per week; overuse of analgesics can lead to rebound headaches
   4. Chronic tension headache sufferers need evaluation for underlying anxiety and depression; antidepressant therapy with amitriptyline (Elavil) 50-100 mg PO HS or specific serotonin reuptake inhibitors such as Prozac may be a beneficial

H. Cluster Headache Treatment
   1. Inhalation of 100% oxygen administered no longer than 15 minutes at 6-8 liters/minute flow rate
   2. For acute therapy, sumatriptan and ergotamine are often used as well as the other medications recommended for treatment of migraine headaches (see V.B.)
   3. For preventive therapy the following are recommended:
      a. Verapamil (Calan) 80-120 mg TID
      b. Lithium initiated at 300-600 mg/day and increased to 600-1200 mg/day as needed in 2-4 divided dosed is effective
      c. Methysergide 2 mg QID is effective in shortening the course of headaches; doses should be tapered after 2-3 weeks of freedom from headaches
      d. Injectable or oral corticosteroids may be given for patients who do not respond to above preventive therapies; initiate prednisone at dose range of 40-60 mg per day in divided doses and taper over 1 month
      e. Other medications listed under preventive therapy for migraine headaches may also be effective for cluster headaches

I. Other therapies such as intranasal lidocaine and capsaicin nasal application have been effective in a few studies, but more research is needed before they can be recommended

J. Follow up for all types of headaches is to return if headache is unrelieved or if it increases in severity, duration or frequency from usual pattern

PARKINSON'S DISEASE

I.   Definition: Chronic, degenerative, and progressive central nervous system movement disorder

II.   Pathogenesis

    A.   Etiology of Parkinson's disease (PD) remains unclear, but numerous causes have been postulated including genetic factors, stress, depression, vascular accidents, brain trauma, tumor, metabolic, infectious disease, toxins, drugs, and aging

    B.   Degeneration of dopamine-producing cells in the substantia nigra is believed to be responsible for the clinical findings that characterize the disease

III. Clinical Presentation

    A.   PD is the most common movement disorder that is managed in the primary care setting

    B.   Approximately 50,000 new cases are diagnosed each year with men and women equally affected; the disease is less common among African Americans and Japanese

    C.   Age of onset is most often between ages 50 and 65; about 80% of affected persons are between the ages of 60 and 79

    D.   Cardinal manifestations or the classic tetrad of PD
        1.   Unilateral resting tremor
        2.   Rigidity or "cogwheel" resistance to passive movement in the limbs
        3.   Dyskinesias including bradykinesia, (slowness of voluntary movement), hypokinesia (decreased movement or function), and akinesia (inability to move)
        4.   Postural instability
            a.   Slow, shuffling gait with a tendency toward propulsion or retropulsion
            b.   Loss of postural "righting" reflexes which leads to development of a stooped or "simian" posture, with flexion of the knees, trunk, elbows, wrists, and metacarpophalangeal joints
            c.   Lacking the autonomic righting reflex, the patient may unconsciously drift sideways or backward when sitting or standing

    E.   Other clinical features of PD include the following
        1.   Motor symptoms such as intermittent immobility or "freezing," difficulty at halting steps while walking, termed "festination," and hypomimia or a masked quality to facial expression
        2.   Autonomic dysfunction which results in seborrhea and excessive perspiration, orthostatic blood pressure changes, sexual disturbances, bladder and anal sphincter dysfunction, and constipation
        3.   Mental status changes including confusion, dementia, and depression; dementia is estimated to be present in 15-30% of patients with PD

IV.   Diagnosis/Evaluation

    A.   History: Keep in mind that diagnosis is based on clinical criteria
        1.   Explore onset and progression of signs and symptoms, with focus on tremor, rigidity, dyskinesia, postural instability, manifestations related to autonomic dysfunction, and mental status changes
        2.   Determine patient's ability to perform physical activities of daily living (ADLs)--bathing, dressing, toileting, and eating
        3.   Determine patient's ability to perform instrumental ADLs through using the FUNCTIONAL ACTIVITIES QUESTIONNAIRE in section on ALZHEIMER'S DISEASE
        4.   Assess for depression (see section on DEPRESSION)

5. Ask the patient which symptoms of PD are the most bothersome (for example, is his or her job in jeopardy)
6. Carefully question about medication history, focusing on neuroleptic, gastrointestinal, and antihypertensive medications
7. Inquire about occupational, recreational, and environmental history to uncover exposure to toxins such as carbon monoxide, manganese or cyanide, licit and illicit drugs
8. Obtain complete past medical history, social history, and family history with a focus on any dementing illnesses or hereditary disorders

B. Physical Examination: Keep in mind that diagnosis is based on clinical criteria
   1. (**Note**: Obtaining a history and physical examination on a PD patient requires TIME and PATIENCE; bradykinesia causes patient to respond slowly to commands, and bradyphrenia causes the patient to require more time to process questions and respond)
   2. Observe for characteristic posture (simian) and gait (difficulty turning, absent arm swing, slow, shuffling gait, tendency toward propulsion or retropulsion)
   3. Observe for tremor, "pill rolling" motion (may also affect jaw, tongue, and lips, or may be absent)
   4. Perform orthostatic blood pressure and pulse readings to assess for autonomic dysfunction
   5. Perform mental status exam (see section on ALZHEIMER'S DISEASE for details on assessment of cognitive functioning)
   6. Assess cranial nerves
      a. Sense of smell is often lost
      b. Blink reflex often is reduced
      c. Extraocular movements are normal except for impairment in upward gaze (disturbance in ocular motility suggests progressive supranuclear palsy)
   7. Test motor and extrapyramidal systems
      a. Passively move limbs noting characteristic rigidity
      b. Observe for hand and foot posturing which is common
   8. Check reflexes which are usually normal but may be slightly hyperactive or difficult to elicit due to tremors and rigidity
   9. Examine sensory system for common peripheral neuropathies
   10. Examine skin for scaly, greasy lesions characteristic of seborrhea; check for excessive perspiration

C. Differential Diagnosis
   1. Essential tremor (patients usually have positive family history and an action tremor)
   2. Neuroleptic-induced Parkinsonism due to medication intake
   3. Progressive supranuclear palsy which usually has impaired vertical neck extension and early dysarthria and dysphagia
   4. Wilson's disease which occurs in younger persons and is characterized by copper accumulation throughout the body

D. Diagnostic Tests
   1. There are no specific diagnostic tests indicated as the diagnosis of Parkinson's disease is made on the basis of clinical criteria
   2. The history and physical examinations should guide decisions to order testing to rule out other conditions; in general, a CBC, chemistry profile, and urinalysis are ordered on all patients
   3. An imaging study, preferably magnetic resonance imaging (MRI) of the brain can evaluate for possible mass lesions or infarction

V. Plan/Management

A. Consultation with a neurologist should be considered when the diagnosis of PD is made so that the neurologist can confirm the diagnosis and develop a treatment plan; the primary care provider can then follow the patient and refer to the neurologist when difficulties in management occur (**Note:** The classic presentation of PD usually poses few problems in diagnosis, but some presentations are more difficult to recognize)

B. The management recommendations that are outlined here are general recommendations only; definitive treatment guidelines should be developed in consultation with a neurologist as there are controversies regarding how best to treat patients with pharmacotherapy

C. Once the diagnosis has been confirmed, it is important to discuss both the diagnosis and its implications with the patient and his/her family
   1. Important to emphasize that the goals of treatment are to enhance the quality of life
   2. A return to the patient's former level of functioning is not realistic
   3. Symptomatic therapy alone has been shown to improve the quality of life for some patients; patients should understand, however, that the ideal pharmacotherapy does not exist

D. Treatment is individualized and is based on a number of important factors that have implications for management
   1. Age of the patient, the severity of the disease/degree of functional impairment, and the expected benefits and risks of available pharmacologic agents must be considered in each case
   2. Guiding principle of care is to keep the patient functioning independently as long as possible
   3. Key to long-term success in treatment is to continue to maintain symptom-control but to limit complications of therapy

E. Age of the patient: Implications for management
   1. In patients ≤ 60 years of age without substantial impairment, a dopa-sparing strategy is often recommended as the likelihood of developing complications relating to levodopa (L-dopa) therapy is very high after a few years of use
   2. In patients ≥ 70 years of age, there is less need for a dopa-sparing strategy because of the shorter time horizon for this age group
   3. Further, in patients ≥70 years of age, there is greater susceptibility to the adverse effects of other antiparkinsonian drugs, although the second generation dopamine agonists have fewer serious side effects than the older drugs in this class

F. Severity of Parkinson's disease (and its impact on functional impairment) is generally divided into five stages according to a staging scheme devised by Hoehn and Yahr (1967): Implications for management
   1. Stage 1. Unilateral involvement
   2. Stage 2. Bilateral involvement but no postural abnormalities
   3. Stage 3. Bilateral involvement with mild postural imbalance; patient leads independent life
   4. Stage 4. Bilateral involvement with postural instability; patient requires substantial help
   5. Stage 5. Severe, fully developed disease; patient restricted to bed or wheelchair
   6. **Note**: For many patients, their symptoms may overlap into two stages, but these stages provide some framework for the clinician in managing patients as they progress from early to severe, late stage PD

G. Benefits and risks of available pharmacologic agents: Implications for management
   1. **Levodopa**. Patients respond to this drug almost immediately; however, almost all patients develop dyskinesia or motor fluctuations within 5 years of starting levodopa therapy
   2. **Selegiline**. An MAO-B inhibitor that may have neuroprotective or symptomatic effects in treatment of PD; may reduce free radical production by decreasing the oxidative metabolism of dopamine; usefulness of this therapy cannot be determined but its adverse-effect profile is generally benign and it is frequently employed both as monotherapy and as combination therapy to extend the duration of action of L-dopa
   3. **Dopamine agonists**. These drugs have a potentially protective effects on dopamine neurons; often used as monotherapy early in the disease, particularly in younger patients; also used as adjunct therapy to levodopa in patients with motor fluctuations; many adverse events associated with use of this class of drugs including hypotension, nausea, vomiting, constipation, dry mouth, hallucinations; psychiatric adverse events are especially common in the elderly and in those with a history of mental illness

4. **Anticholinergic drugs**. Help restore motor function by blocking muscarinic cholinergic receptors within the striatum; useful in patients with PD who have predominant tremor; adverse effects severely limit usefulness

5. **Amantadine**. An antiviral agent that is believed to work via blockage of the re-uptake of dopamine into presynaptic neurons and by directly stimulating postsynaptic receptors; useful in patients with early PD, especially for bradykinesia or tremor and in more advanced disease as adjunct therapy to L-dopa; adverse effects include restlessness, confusion, depression, nausea, and hypotension

6. **Catechol-*O*-methyl transferase (COMT) inhibitors**. Selective inhibition of COMT may increase levels of levodopa in the brain; the drug is administered with L-dopa to prolong the effects of L-dopa

H. **Treatment of early or newly diagnosed (Stage 1) Parkinson's disease**
1. Earliest stage of PD is when symptoms are present but not yet particularly troublesome
2. Experts agree that symptomatic treatment is not necessary at this point; a reasonable approach to management is the use of the following drug which may have a neuroprotective effect
   a. Selegiline (Eldepryl), a relatively selective inhibitor of the enzyme MAOB
      (1) Dose of selegiline should not exceed 10 mg/day, given in two doses, with the first dose in AM and the second dose at noon
      (2) A single 5 mg dose in AM may be sufficient for many people; the drug has a long half life, and the stimulatory effect of the drug may produce insomnia in some persons
   b. Patients taking selegiline do not have to be on an MAO inhibitor diet so long as the dose does not exceed 10 mg day (tyramine-containing foods can cause hypertensive crisis in patients taking MAO inhibitors); patients cannot take meperidine while taking this drug because of risk of severe adverse events
   c. Whether selegiline slows the progression of the disease is controversial

I. **Treatment of mild (Stage 2) Parkinson's disease**
1. At this stage, symptoms begin to interfere with daily activities and the risks and benefits of symptomatic management should be discussed with the patient; controversy remains regarding optimal treatment at this stage
2. If the symptoms are not severe enough to require levodopa, a dopa-sparing approach should be considered in younger patients (≤60 years)[L-dopa monotherapy may be indicated in patients >70 because of the shorter time horizon for treatment]
   a. Dopamine agonist monotherapy may be used; select **one** of the available drugs in this category
      (1) Pergolide (Permax); initiate with 0.05 mg at bedtime x 3 days, then switch from bedtime to daytime dosing for the remainder of the first week; the daily dose can be increased gradually on a weekly basis to the usual therapeutic dose of 1.0 - 4 mg day divided TID (**Note**: Dosage must be individualized; consult PDR for more information)
      (2) Bromocriptine (Parlodel); initiate with 1.25 mg at bedtime x 3 days, then switch from bedtime to daytime dosing for the remainder of the first week; the daily dose can be increased gradually on a weekly basis to a usual therapeutic dose of 10-40 mg, divided TID
      (3) Ropinirole (Requip) [a second-generation dopamine agonist that is a complete, rather than partial, agonist]; initiate with 0.25 mg TID for the first week, gradually increasing dose at weekly intervals to a usual therapeutic dose of 3 - 12 mg per day, divided TID
      (4) Pramipexole (Mirapex) [a second-generation dopamine agonist similar to pergolide and bromocriptine but with fewer side effects]; pramipexole must be dosed based on creatinine clearance results with the starting dose gradually increased to therapeutic levels at intervals of 5-7 days
      (5) For all drugs in this class, use the lowest dose that provides adequate benefit

          (6)   Dopamine agonists are less likely than levodopa to cause adverse motor effects, but more like to cause neuropsychiatric effects

          (7)   Use with caution in older patients and in all patients with a history of psychiatric disorders

    b.   Another choice for patients with mild (Stage 2) PD is amantadine (Symmetrel), a mild indirect dopaminergic which also has some anticholinergic properties

          (1)   Usual dosage is 100 mg BID; a higher dose (up to 300mg/day) may be necessary in some patients

          (2)   This drug is especially useful in patients with bradykinesia and tremor

          (3)   This drug is useful not only in mild disease, but also in the **advanced stage of the disease as an adjunctive drug to levodopa** and the dopamine agonists

          (4)   Use with **caution** in patients with renal impairment!

    c.   Anticholinergic drugs are not as effective as the dopamine agonists, improving Parkinsonism in only about 20% of patients

          (1)   Some clinicians use this class of drugs to control tremor not relieved by an agonist or levodopa (a drug from this class is added to the treatment regime); an anticholinergic can also be used as monotherapy for tremor

          (2)   Commonly used agents are trihexyphenidyl (Artane) and benztropine mesylate (Cogentin)

               (a)   Usual starting dose of Artane is 1 mg QD, increasing gradually over several weeks to 2 mg TID

               (b)   Usual starting dose of Cogentin is 0.5 mg at bedtime, increasing gradually to 1 mg BID

J.   **Treatment of moderate (Stages 2-3) Parkinson's disease**

    1.   Treatment with levodopa is necessary to control symptoms in this stage of the disease; levodopa remains the most effective agent for treatment of PD even though most levodopa-treated patients eventually develop fluctuations and dyskinesias

    2.   The rule of thumb is to use the lowest dose that controls symptoms rather than the highest dosage that the patient can tolerate

    3.   Levodopa is combined with carbidopa which blocks the peripheral conversion of L-dopa to dopamine, thus increasing the amount of L-dopa transported to the brain

    4.   Carbidopa/levodopa is available in both standard release (Sinemet) and controlled-release form (Sinemet CR)

        a.   Usual starting dose of Sinemet (standard form) is one-half to one tablet of 25/100 mg increasing by 25/100 mg per day each week until TID dosing is achieved (slowly titrate up to 300-400 mg of L-dopa per day)

        b.   Not every symptom responds equally as well, with bradykinesia and rigidity responding best, and tremor responding the least

        c.   After 3 or more years of treatment, approximately one-third of patients receiving this drug begin to develop involuntary movements and to have very short-duration responses to the medication

    5.   There is controversy regarding timing of adjunctive dopamine agonist therapy

        a.   Traditionally, the approach has been to introduce a dopamine agonist when fluctuations emerge

        b.   Recently, however, the trend has been to add a dopamine agonist to the L-dopa therapy earlier in the disease course (in moderate rather than in advanced disease)

        c.   One approach that is frequently used is to add a dopamine agonist when a patient is taking L-dopa in the range of 400 to 600 mg/day and needs incremental therapy

        d.   The goal of early combination therapy is to use more conservative doses of L-dopa while maintaining adequate symptom control

K.   **Treatment of advanced (Stages IV-V) Parkinson's disease**

    1.   In this stage of the disease, there is significant disability and loss of independence in spite of levodopa therapy; there is loss of postural reflexes, the freezing phenomenon has developed, there is pronounced flexed posture, or complications from levodopa (fluctuations, dyskinesia, psychosis) have developed so that the complications of treatment become the focus

2. A pattern of progressively worsening motor complications usually occurs in patients who are on chronic levodopa therapy
3. Patients who begin treatment with levodopa typically experience a long duration of response to the drug in the first few years
   a. Over time, response fluctuations begin to occur so that there is a wearing off or end-of-dose failure in response to a previously adequate dosage of levodopa
   b. The "offs" tend to be mild at first, but progress to become deeper with more severe Parkinsonism and the duration of the "on" response becomes shorter
   c. Many patients who develop response fluctuations also develop abnormal involuntary movements
4. When the wearing off phenomenon is mild, a decrease in the dosing interval, or addition of selegiline (initiated at 2.5 mg daily, and gradually increasing to 5 mg BID) may be helpful
   a. A lower dose of levodopa may be necessary
   b. Sinemet CR (controlled-release) may also be helpful in this situation, especially in patients with mild wearing-off; gradually switch from standard carbidopa-levodopa to Sinemet CR
5. Dopamine agonists can also be used in combination with standard Sinemet or Sinemet CR to reduce the severity of the "off" states; levodopa dosage may need to be reduced
6. Tolcapone (Tasmar) is the first COMT(catechol-O-methyl transferase) inhibitor to be approved for use with levodopa in both non-fluctuating patients (those whose response to levodopa is relatively stable) and in fluctuating patients with the "wearing-off" and "on-off" phenomena and dyskinesia; usual dose is 100-200 mg TID with a maximum daily dose of 600 mg
7. Because of the complexity in management of patients with advanced Parkinson's disease who frequently have comorbidities which increase the risk of adverse events and drug interactions, referral to a specialist is necessary

L. Surgical therapy for PD includes thalamotomy and deep brain stimulation, pallidotomy, and neural tissue transplantation

M. Treatment of depression, a common nonmotor symptom in PD is important; all patients should be evaluated for depression and appropriate treatment should be initiated before pharmacotherapy for PD is initiated
1. Use of the tricyclic antidepressant amitriptyline, with its anticholinergic and soporific effects can be useful
2. The use of selective serotonin reuptake inhibitors such as fluoxetine and sertraline are also effective but may aggravate Parkinsonism if antiparkinsonian drugs are not being used concurrently

N. Referrals to physical, speech, or occupational therapists are often needed

O. Follow up is variable depending on involvement of the neurologist, patient's degree of disability and the need to monitor adverse events and renal functioning in patients on certain medications

SEIZURES AND EPILEPSY

I. Definitions

A. Seizures: Paroxysmal alteration in consciousness or other cerebral cortical function

B. Epilepsy: More than one unprovoked seizure in lifetime

II. Pathogenesis

A. Initiated by electrochemical abnormalities in brain such as alterations in concentration of excitatory or inhibitory neurotransmitter

B. Abnormal electrical discharge from one site is rapidly transmitted to other parts of the brain, producing disturbances in perception, motor control, attention, and consciousness

C. Major causes of seizure by age group are as follows
    1. Young adults
        a. Idiopathic
        b. Alcohol or drug related
        c. Trauma
        d. Infection
    2. Older adults and elderly
        a. Alcohol or drug related
        b. Brain tumor
        c. Circulatory causes
        d. Metabolic causes
        e. Infection

III. Clinical Presentation

A. Seizures affect about 1% of the population in the US

B. Adults are most likely to have seizures secondary to a traumatic or infectious cause, a preexisting known illness, a mass lesion, or drug or alcohol use
    1. Traumatic causes, most often from accidental injuries
        a. Birth and perinatal injuries can cause seizures but these are usually diagnosed early in life
        b. Head trauma from MVAs, falls, and sports injuries are common causes, with the more severe the head injury, the greater the likelihood of developing posttraumatic seizures
    2. Infectious causes, including infection of the brain, encephalitis; septic emboli and abscesses associated with endocarditis
        a. Presence of an epidemic of encephalitis, recent history of febrile illness, and changes in mental status suggest an infectious cause
        b. History of parenteral drug use, AIDS, recent dental work, and murmur or valvular heart disease also point to an infectious cause
    3. Circulatory and metabolic disorders can cause seizures
        a. In older adults, circulatory abnormalities account for many seizures
        b. Hypoxemia in pulmonary disease and metabolic disorders such as occur in uremia, in hypoglycemia, and liver failure can cause seizures
    4. Mass lesions (both benign and malignant), are responsible for a significant number of seizures in older adults
        a. Patients often have a history of malignancy
        b. Focal findings on neurologic examination and documentation of mass or masses via neuroimaging help make the diagnosis
    5. Alcohol and drug related seizures occur via a number of mechanisms
        a. Alcohol can cause seizures due to malnutrition, because the alcoholic is at increased risk of head trauma, and during withdrawal
        b. Cocaine and other stimulants are associated with increased risk of seizure; withdrawal from barbiturates can also cause seizures

C. International classification of seizures is based on mode of seizure onset and spread; an abbreviated version of the classification appears in the following table

D. Partial seizures begin in one hemisphere of the brain and result in an asymmetric seizure (unless there is secondary generalization); this type seizure usually begins with an aura (commonly reflecting the focal nature of the epileptic discharge at its onset)
   1. Present as alterations in motor functions, sensory or somatosensory symptoms, or autonomic symptoms
   2. Are classified as simple, partial, complex partial depending on whether there is an impairment of consciousness, and partial seizures with secondary generalization
   3. Partial seizures are the most common type of seizure

E. Generalized seizures involve both hemispheres with motor involvement that is bilateral and there is an impairment in consciousness; types of generalized seizures are listed below
   1. Absence seizures are manifest by sudden onset, an interruption of activity in which the person is engaged, and a blank stare (also called behavior arrest)
   2. Tonic-clonic seizures are manifest by loss of consciousness; most often without warning, but with an aura in some patients; tonic refers to stiffening and clonic to contraction with tonic stiffening usually occurring first followed by clonic contractions; patient may fall, lose sphincter control, bite tongue, or develop cyanosis; a patient frequently falls into deep sleep after the seizure
   3. Tonic and clonic seizures may occur separately and thus are classified as separate types
   4. Myoclonic seizures are brief shock-like muscular contractions of the face, trunk, and extremities; may be isolated events or occur repetitively
   5. Atonic seizures are characterized by sudden loss of muscle tone; may be a head drop, a limb drop, or total body drop to the floor or ground

F. Unclassified seizures include all seizures that cannot be classified because of inadequate or incomplete data

IV. Diagnosis/Evaluation

   A. History
      1. History should include information to help determine if a seizure has occurred and the probable type of seizure
         a. Important to question family members and witnesses as well as patient (for much of the history, witnesses are better sources than patients, but patients are the best source for presence and type of aura)
         b. Explore precipitating factors
         c. Describe the focal onset, duration, and seizure characteristics
         d. Inquire about the setting in which episode occurred

e. Determine whether the patient completely lost consciousness and/or was incontinent

f. Determine if there was an aura, antigrade amnesia, or postictal period

2. Ask if there was a history of trauma; ask about alcohol or drug use and withdrawal from alcohol or drugs; enquire about exposures to toxins, including occupational, recreation, or accidental exposures

3. Obtain complete medical history, including history of any pulmonary, hepatic, cardiac, renal, or endocrine disease; ask about history of cancer

4. Obtain complete medication history and ask about allergies

5. Question about family history of seizures

6. For patients with known epilepsy who present with seizures, determine the following:
   a. Precipitating factors
   b. Similarity and differences between these seizures and ones in the past
   c. Medications currently taking and adherence with regime
   d. If the seizures are occurring more frequently

B. Physical Examination
1. Assess vital signs and evaluate for orthostatic hypotension
2. Perform a complete physical examination with a focus on cardiovascular and neurological systems
   a. Examine the heart for signs of valvular disease and arrhythmia
   b. Perform a neurologic exam including assessment of the head, eye grounds, cranial nerves, neck, speech, gait, mental status, motor (including cerebellar), sensory, and deep tendon reflexes (**Note**: A normal neurologic exam is often found in persons with idiopathic seizures)

C. Differential Diagnosis
1. Most common causes of seizures are listed under II.C. above and must be considered
2. Syncope does not cause seizures but is often confused with this disorder
   a. Whereas patients with syncope may exhibit repetitive clonic, myoclonic, or dystonic movements, these movements rarely last beyond 5-10 seconds and do not exhibit the organized progression from tonic to clonic phase seen in convulsive seizures
   b. Incontinence does not occur with syncope but may occur with seizures
   c. Tongue biting does not occur with syncope but may occur with seizures
   d. A few minutes of confusion immediately following the event is not likely with syncope but is likely with seizures

D. Diagnostic Tests
1. Basic laboratory evaluation should focus on detecting systemic disorders sometimes associated with seizures
   a. CBC
   b. Chemistry profile
   c. Liver function tests
   d. Toxicology screen
   e. Electroencephalography (EEG) [Multiple EEGs increase their diagnostic utility]
2. Most authorities recommend that all patients who experience an unprovoked seizure undergo a brain imaging study to detect any cerebral lesions (tumor, abscess, vascular malformation, stroke, traumatic injury)
   a. In nonurgent presentations, the imaging study of choice is magnetic resonance imaging (MRI) because it is more sensitive than computed tomography (CT)
   b. In emergent cases, in which the history or physical examination suggest new focal deficits, altered mental status, fever, persistent headache, recent trauma, history of cancer, immunosuppression, emergency imaging is required, most often with a CT scan (better at detection of acute hemorrhage than MRI)
   c. If an infection in the nervous system is suspected, lumbar puncture should be performed

V.   Plan/Management

A.   Some seizures are from correctable etiologies and the underlying problem must be identified and corrected in those cases

B.   Goal of treatment of patients with epilepsy is to provide optimal control of seizures without producing unacceptable side effects

C.   Decision to treat **initial or first-time** seizures with medications is controversial and patients with first seizure should be referred to a neurologist in the following instances
   1.   There is uncertainty regarding whether event was actually a seizure
   2.   For evaluation of focal seizures
   3.   If the neurologic examinations is abnormal
   4.   When the EEG shows focality
   5.   When special diagnostic procedures are indicated (MRI, CT scan, sleep-deprived EEG)

D.   Selection of an antiepileptic drug (AED) that is appropriate for the patient's type of epilepsy is the cornerstone of treatment
   1.   From the appropriate drugs, select one that best fits the patient based on both patient and medication characteristics including side-effect profile
   2.   Initiate and titrate the medication at the correct dosage, and make incremental changes that will enhance effectiveness and tolerability
   3.   A general rule of thumb is to initiate therapy with one-fourth to one-third of the anticipated maintenance dose and increase the dose to maintenance over a 3-4 week period
   4.   Increase the medication dosing until complete seizure control occurs or until side effects that are persistent and nontolerable occur
   5.   If adequate seizure control--defined as complete seizure control for most persons--is not attained at the maximum tolerated dosage of the first medication that is prescribed two approaches can be considered
      a.   First, consideration should be given to referring the patient for neurologic consultation if such consultation has not already been sought
      b.   A second option is to start a second drug and taper the first. As the dosage of the new medication is titrated up, the original medication is gradually tapered until monotherapy with the new agent is achieved. If control is not obtained with monotherapy with a second drug, then refer to a neurologist (**Note:** Dual therapy should never be used until adequate trials of at least two or three drugs as monotherapy have been attempted)
      c.   Never abruptly withdraw any drug; gradually taper

E.   Treatment should begin with one AED, preferably the drug of choice
   1.   Common epilepsy types with the first- and second-choice AED treatments are listed in the following table
   2.   The advantage of using one drug is that patient adherence is increased, the management of toxicity is easier, side effects are easier to monitor and control, drug interactions are avoided, and it is less expensive

Seizure Type	Drugs of Choice	Alternative Drugs
Generalized Seizures		
Primary generalized, tonic-clonic	Valproic acid (Depakene)	Carbamazepine (Tegretol), Phenytoin (Dilantin), Primidone (Mysoline), Phenobarbital
Primary generalized, absence	Ethosuximide (Zarontin), valproic acid	Clonazepam (Klonopin)
Primary myoclonic	Valproic acid, clonazepam	Phenytoin, phenobarbital
Partial Seizures		
Partial simple and complex, and secondarily generalized epilepsy	Carbamazepine, phenytoin	Valproic acid, phenobarbital, primidone
Mixed Forms	Valproic acid, clonazepam	Carbamazepine, phenytoin, phenobarbital

F.   Patient's age, seizure type, daily activities, and economic considerations should influence selection of AED
    1.   Primidone and phenobarbital may cause excess sedation, behavioral problems such as irritability, and cognitive impairment
    2.   Phenytoin is a poor first choice for young adults because of the consequences of long-term use which may include coarsening of the facial features, gingival hyperplasia, hirsutism, and enlargement of the lips
    3.   For some adults, phenytoin is an attractive choice because of its once-daily dosing and low cost
    4.   Carbamazepine, particularly the new extended-release preparation, may be a good choice for adults with focal seizures

G.   The newer AEDs include tiagabine, gabapentin, lamotigine, felbamate, and topiramate; these drugs are used primarily as adjunctive therapy in refractory patients
    1.   **Tiagabine** (Gabitril) is used as adjunctive therapy in patients ≥12 years of age with localization-related epilepsy; drug selectively inhibits uptake of gamma aminobutyric acid (GABA) and prolongs the duration of inhibitory activity at postsynaptic receptors
    2.   **Gabapentin** (Neurontin) is used as adjunctive therapy in patients ≥12 years of age with localization-related epilepsy; works well in patients in whom drug-drug interactions must be avoided such as persons with comorbidities and the elderly on multiple medications
    3.   **Lamotrigine** (Lamictal) is used as adjunctive therapy in adults with localization-related epilepsy and also as an alternative in patients with localization-related or generalized epilepsies; has been associated with severe, potentially life-threatening rashes, including Stevens-Johnson syndrome and toxic epidermal necrolysis; not licensed for use in children
    4.   **Felbamate** (Felbatol) is used as adjunctive therapy or monotherapy in adults with localization-related epilepsy and as adjunctive therapy in children with Lennox-Gastaut syndrome (symptomatic generalized epilepsy consisting of multiple types of generalized seizures); felbamate has been associated with aplastic anemia and fulminant hepatic failure and this drug should only be used by an epileptologist in patients in whom the benefits outweigh the risks
    5.   **Topiramine** (Topamax) is used as adjunctive therapy in adults with localization-related epilepsy and may also be useful in some patients with certain types of generalized epilepsies; cognitive effects constitute the main dose-limiting toxicity that is known at this time

H.   Dosages for the most commonly used AEDs
    1.   Carbamazepine : Tegretol, 100, 200 mg tabs, and 100 mg chewable tabs; Tegretol suspension, 100 mg/5 mL
        a.   Dosage: Begin with 200 mg BID and increase dose weekly if needed by increments of 200 mg/day in 3-4 divided doses (Maximum daily dose is 1.6 g)
        b.   Tegretol-XR, 100, 200, 400 mg tabs: Same beginning dose and weekly rate of increase as described above **except** dosing should be BID

2.	Phenytoin: Dilantin, 30, 100 mg caps, and 50 mg chewable tabs; Dilantin suspension, 125 mg/5 mL
   a.	Dosing: Begin with 100 mg TID and can increase weekly to a maximum of 200 mg TID
   b.	Once daily dosing ONLY for sustained release caps for patients controlled on 300 mg a day
3.	Ethosuximide: Zarontin, 250 mg caps; Zarontin suspension, 250 mg/5mL
   a.	Dosing: Begin with 250 mg BID, increasing by 250 mg/day every 4-7 days if needed (Maximum daily dose is 1.5 g, in divided doses)
   b.	Used only for absence seizures, thus rarely used in adults as few adults have this seizure type
4.	Valproic acid: Depakene 250 mg caps; Depakene syrup, 250 mg/5 mL
   a.	Dosing: Initially, 15 mg/kg/day in 3 divided doses; increase weekly if needed by 5-10 mg/kg/day
   b.	Maximum daily dose is 60 mg/kg/day in divided doses
5.	Clonazepam: Klonopin, 0.5, 1, 2 mg tabs
   a.	Dosing: Initially, not greater than 0.5 mg TID; increase if needed every 3 days by 0.5-1 mg daily
   b.	Maximum daily dose is 20 mg/day in divided doses
6.	Phenobarbital: Begin with 30 mg BID; maintenance dose is usually 60-300 mg QD
7.	Titrate dosages to achieve adequate blood concentrations
   a.	Because all drugs have central nervous system effects, begin therapy with low doses
   b.	Use therapeutic range in combination with clinical response to determine appropriate dosage
8.	Patients at high risk for recurrent seizures should be treated for two year period
9.	Prior to initiation of any antiepileptic medication, the following laboratory studies should be done: CBC with differential and platelet count, electrolytes, and liver enzymes
10.	Repeat studies during the early weeks of treatment (for example, at one and three months) are also recommended

I.	Patient Education is summarized below
   1.	Understanding the disorder and the prescribed medications by both the patient and family is of the utmost importance; non-adherence to the medication regime has been identified as the single most common reason for treatment failure
      a.	Teach patient regarding dosing, actions, side effects, and drug interactions of the particular AED that is being prescribed
      b.	For women of childbearing age or who are taking oral contraceptives, emphasize that AEDs are teratogenic and that they also reduce the effectiveness of oral contraceptives
      c.	Patient education must be continuous and must be addressed on every visit
   2.	Instruct families regarding the fundamentals of emergency management of seizures
   3.	Review the law in your state concerning operating a motor vehicle by persons with seizure disorders
   4.	If patient has good control of seizures, minimum restrictions are needed such as swimming with a buddy or wearing a helmet with some sports
   5.	Review factors that are sometimes associated with seizures such as stimulants, alcohol, caffeine, inadequate sleep or fever
   6.	Discuss the emotional stress that often occurs in family related to social stigma and unpredictability of seizure activity in some patients
   7.	Patients may ask about the ketogenic diet, a diet that mimics the mebatolic effects of fasting that is sometimes used in the treatment of children (and more recently adults) to treat refractory epilepsy; this diet must be supervised by experts and used only in patients with refractory epilepsy
   8.	Refer the patient and family to the Epilepsy Foundation of American (EFA), an organization dedicated to countering societal misconceptions and prejudices about epilepsy as well as improving the quality of life for persons affected by seizures
      a.	The national office can be contacted by writing EFA, 4351 Garden City Drive, Landover, MD 20785-2267 or by calling 301/459-3700 or 1-800-EFA-1000

    b.   The Internet Web sites is http://www.efa.org

    c.   Most states have local affiliates which provide community outreach programs, support groups, information and referral, employment services, respite care for families, and help with living arrangements

J.   Follow Up

    1.   Follow-up visits should be weekly during period of adjusting medication dose, then every 3 months for the next 6 months, and then every six months thereafter

    2.   AEDs may not need to be given for a lifetime

        a.   Factors promoting complete withdrawal from medication include a seizure-free period of 2-4 years, complete seizure control within 1 year of onset, an onset of seizures after age 2 but before age 35, and a normal EEG

        b.   The withdrawal of therapy should be gradual and at a mutually agreed upon time with the patient

        c.   Review state laws regarding operation of a motor vehicle as related to tapering of seizure medication

    3.   Patients on carbamazepine

        a.   May need to monitor more frequently than recommended under V.H. (above); consult PDR for recommendations

        b.   Leukopenia is the most common hematologic side effect of carbamazepine

    4.   Patients on phenytoin

        a.   Monitor serum drug concentrations 2-4 weeks after any dose increase

        b.   Obtain periodic serum drug concentrations

        c.   Annual CBC, LFTs and platelet

    5.   Patients on long-term phenobarbital: Annual CBC and LFTs

    6.   Patients on long-term ethosuximide: Periodic CBC

    7.   Patients on long-term Valproic acid: Baseline LFTs; repeat every 2-3 months x 2

STROKE AND TRANSIENT ISCHEMIC ATTACK

I.   Definitions

    A.   Stroke: An episode of focal cerebral ischemia that has not resolved completely after three weeks

    B.   Transient ischemic attack (TIA): Transient episode of focal cerebral dysfunction that lasts from 2-15 minutes, resolves completely within a few hours and is presumed to be due to embolic or thromboembolic vascular disease

    C.   Reversible ischemic neurologic deficits (RINDs): An episode of focal cerebral dysfunction that lasts > 24 hours but resolves completely within three weeks

    D.   These disorders are further classified as either ischemic or hemorrhagic disorders

        1.   Ischemic disorders are caused by diseases of large vessels, small deep vessels, (lacunar infarcts) or cardiogenic emboli

        2.   Hemorrhagic disorders are either intraparenchymal hemorrhage or subarachnoid hemorrhage

II.   Pathogenesis

    A.   Ischemia is the most frequent cause of cerebrovascular dysfunction; approximately 85% of all strokes are ischemic strokes

        1.   Atherosclerosis is the underlying process resulting in ischemic cerebrovascular disease in most patients

            a.   Larger vessels at base of brain and in neck at bifurcations are most commonly affected

      b.   Narrowed sites in the affected vessels collect atherosclerotic plaque, cholesterol debris, platelet-fibrin material, a process that over time leads to significant stenosis and cerebral ischemia

      c.   Lacunar events are small infarcts caused by thrombotic occlusion of the small, deep penetrating vessels in the deeper, subcortical parts of the cerebrum and brain stem

2.   Embolic strokes occur when a thrombus is released from a proximal site and lodges in a distal vessel, compromising blood flow; the most common sources of emboli are the heart and major vessels (carotid and vertebral arteries) with stenotic lesions

      a.   Cardiac sources of emboli include myocardial infarction, valvular heart disease, ventricular septal defects with thrombus formation, and arrhythmias, especially atrial fibrillation which accounts for 65% of all embolic strokes

      b.   Rare causes of emboli include endocarditis and fat emboli secondary to long bone fractures

B.   Both TIA and stroke result from focal ischemia, which manifests itself neurologically

C.   Hemorrhage is the other main type of cerebrovascular dysfunction and results from leakage of blood outside normal vessels

1.   In a subarachnoid hemorrhage, bleeding occurs within the surrounding membranes and cerebrospinal fluid

2.   An intracerebral hemorrhage occurs when bleeding is directly into the cerebral parenchyma; the majority of cases of intracerebral hemorrhage are associated with chronic hypertension

III.   Clinical Presentation

A.   Stroke is the most common cause of major neurologic disability and third most common cause of death in the US among persons ≥65 years of age

B.   Cerebrovascular disorders including TIAs and stroke occur most often in those >65 years of age with risk factors of hypertension (the major risk factor), atherosclerosis, smoking, and hyperlipidemia; male gender and diabetes mellitus are also important risk factors

C.   Nearly all thrombotic strokes are preceded by a TIA affecting the same region as the ensuing stroke; the exact incidence of TIAs progressing to full strokes is unknown

D.   Symptoms, signs, course, and prognosis are dependent on the type and location of the cerebrovascular event, whether TIA or stroke

E.   With large vessel ischemia, symptoms develop gradually or in a step-wise fashion and correspond to which vessels in the vascular distribution of the brain are affected

1.   Occlusion in the anterior circulation or carotid artery syndrome is most common

      a.   Sudden dimness or loss of vision, especially in one eye

      b.   Speech disorders, primarily expressive aphasia

      c.   Sudden severe headache with no known cause

      d.   Sudden weakness or numbness of the face, arm, or leg

      e.   Unexplained dizziness, unsteadiness, or sudden falls

2.   Occlusion in the posterior circulation or the vertebral-basilar syndrome is less common

      a.   Bilateral disturbance of vision; diplopia

      b.   Speech disorder is likely to be dysarthria, due to poor control of palatal muscles

      c.   Simultaneous motor and sensory deficits on both sides of body

      d.   Vertigo, ataxia, tinnitus, nystagmus, extra-ocular movement dysfunction, nausea, vomiting, dysphagia, and drop attacks

F.   Symptoms and signs of cardiogenic embolisms have abrupt onset and often occur with activity; symptoms and signs depend on location of clot and are similar to those of large arterial cerebral thrombosis

G. Hemorrhagic events usually have abrupt onset with deficits rapidly evolving
1. Subarachnoid hemorrhages often occurs in a younger population (50% of patients under age 55) and the first symptom may be a sudden, severe headache followed by fever, sweating, tachycardia and altered levels of consciousness
2. Symptoms and signs of intracerebral hemorrhage are variable resulting in minor, focal problems to coma

IV. Diagnosis/Evaluation: Patients who are experiencing an ischemic stroke or "brain attack," must be immediately transported for emergency care because the window of opportunity for treatment with a thrombolytic agent is **three hours** after onset

A. History
1. For patients presenting with possible TIAs in which the symptoms have resolved by time of presentation, carefully determine severity, duration, and frequency of symptoms (**Note:** Patient who has had several TIAs over the past few months, with progressively shorter intervals between the attacks are experiencing crescendo TIAs and is at very high risk for stroke)
2. Inquire about symptoms such as transient blindness, double vision, dizziness, headache, sensory deficiencies, dysphagia, speech problems, motor difficulties, and weakness/numbness
3. Question about risk factors such as hypertension, smoking, hyperlipidemia, cardiac disease, diabetes mellitus, and heredity
4. Involve family members in history taking because patient is often unaware of the total clinical presentation

B. Physical Examination
1. Blood pressure readings both in lying and sitting positions
2. Funduscopy exam to determine ocular plagues in retinal artery branches
3. Auscultate carotid arteries for bruits
4. Complete cardiovascular exam including palpation and auscultation of peripheral pulses
5. Perform complete neurological examination
6. Complete a mental status examination using the Mini-Mental State Exam (see section on ALZHEIMER'S DISEASE)

C. Differential Diagnosis
1. Tumor (usually has very slow developing signs and symptoms)
2. Dissecting aortic aneurysm (discrepancy in blood pressure readings in arms)
3. Subdural hematoma (history of trauma)
4. Multiple sclerosis (usually involves a young adult or middle-aged adult who has multiple signs and symptoms which do not follow a predictable location or pattern)
5. Bell's palsy (often follows an infection; only sign is peripheral facial nerve weakness)
6. Focal seizures
7. Meniere's Disease (vertigo and hearing loss often present)
8. Hyperventilation can produce tingling and numbness

D. Diagnostic Tests
1. Diagnostic evaluation of patients with suspected stroke is not considered here as those patients must be referred immediately for rapid evaluation and, if indicated, aggressive intervention with t-PA; all patients evaluated for an acute stroke should have an emergency computed tomography (CT) of the brain to rule out other potential mimics of an ischemic event such as an intracranial tumor, abscess, hemorrhage (**Note:** Intracranial hemorrhage must be excluded prior to administration of thrombolytic agents)
2. For patients who present with a history suggesting prior TIAs, order CBC, platelet count, blood glucose, sedimentation rate, serological test for syphilis, urinalysis, ECG, to rule out other causes
3. Lipid studies should be considered to document risk factors
4. A CT scan is usually ordered and is best in distinguishing between ischemia, hemorrhage, and tumor

5. Echocardiogram should be ordered if cardiogenic source of emboli is being considered
6. Holter monitor should be ordered if arrhythmia is being considered
7. If the symptoms are characteristic of carotid disease, or if the patient is asymptomatic and routine physical examination detects a bruit in the arteries in the neck, assessment of carotid disease should be evaluated, beginning with a carotid duplex ultrasonographic scan

V. Plan/Management

A. Patients who present with an acute TIA should be treated with the same urgency as a completed stroke and must be immediately transported for care

B. Patients who are experiencing a pattern of crescendo TIAs by history should be immediately referred for emergent care

C. All patients who present with a history of continuing TIAs despite ongoing therapy with aspirin or ticlopidine should be referred for emergent care

D. Patients who present with a **history** of TIAs that are not of a crescendo pattern and who are not presently receiving antiplatelet therapy should be managed as follows
1. If symptoms are consistent with carotid disease, the patient should be evaluated with carotid duplex ultrasonographic scan for presence and degree of stenosis
2. Patients in whom carotid disease is confirmed should be considered for carotid endarterectomy (CEA)
   a. CEA is most cost-effective for treatment of patients with high-grade stenosis (greater than 70% blockage) and TIA or minor stroke
   b. CEA is not cost-effective for patients with low-grade stenosis (less than 30% blockage) or those without other signs or symptoms consistent with high risk for stroke
3. Patients who are nonsurgical candidates should be treated with aspirin or ticlopidine unless contraindicated
   a. Patients on aspirin should use an enteric coated variety that is less likely to be associated with gastrointestinal side effects
   b. Patients on ticlopidine should have a neutrophil count according to manufacturer directions
4. Patients with atrial fibrillation should be referred to a specialist for management with warfarin unless risk of stroke is low or use is contraindicated
5. Patients in whom the diagnosis remains uncertain after evaluation should be referred to a neurologist for evaluation

E. Patient education involves the following
1. All patients with risk of stroke should modify their risk factors through controlling hypertension, smoking cessation, weight reduction, reducing fats and lipids in the diet, and regular exercise
2. Stroke prophylaxis as described above under V.D. 3. should be followed

F. Follow Up
1. Dependent on severity, frequency and duration of TIAs
2. Patients with low and intermediate stenosis should be considered for follow-up serial duplex ultrasound in 3-4 months to evaluate for plaque instability
3. Annual duplex ultrasonographic evaluation should be adequate thereafter unless a change in symptoms or degree of arterial narrowing prompts more aggressive action

TREMOR

I.   Definition: Involuntary, rhythmic oscillatory movements of any body part

II. Pathogenesis

   A.   Tremors are produced by repetitive patterns of muscle contractions and relaxation

   B.   Pathophysiology of different tremors is poorly understood

   C.   Tremors are sometimes classified according to the conditions of rest, movement, and postural maintenance

   D.   Resting tremor may be due to one of the following:
      1.   Parkinson's disease
      2.   Related to ingestion of certain drugs such as phenothiazine, methyldopa, reserpine, or carbon monoxide
      3.   Tumor
      4.   Trauma
      5.   Wilson's disease

   E.   Intention tremor may be due to one of the following:
      1.   Cerebellar disease
      2.   Multiple sclerosis
      3.   Drugs and toxins such as alcohol, sedatives, phenytoin

   F.   Postural tremor
      1.   Physiologic tremor exaggerated under certain conditions
         a.   Stress
         b.   Caffeine ingestion
         c.   Fatigue
      2.   Endocrine disorders such as hyperthyroidism, hypoglycemia, pheochromocytoma
      3.   Essential tremor is a type of postural tremor
         a.   Familial or benign hereditary tremor
         b.   Senile

III. Clinical presentation of common tremors

   A.   Resting tremor of Parkinson's disease (see section on PARKINSON'S DISEASE)
      1.   Often begins with a "pill-rolling" tremor of one hand
      2.   Tremor often affects the legs, feet, toes and less frequently the lips, tongue or chin

   B.   Intention tremor results in oscillation of the limb as it approaches a target and is rarely the only presenting symptom of cerebellar dysfunction

   C.   Physiologic tremors are fine, barely visible, rapid tremors that sometimes occur when hands are outstretched

   D.   Essential tremors are the most common form of postural tremors
      1.   Increase with age, but can be seen in teenagers
      2.   Often characterized by bilateral and symmetrical involvement of hands but may be unilateral and involve the head, voice or lower extremities
      3.   Slow tremor which is absent or minimal at rest
      4.   Alcohol often suppresses the tremor
      5.   No neurologic abnormality is present

IV.   Diagnosis/Evaluation

    A.   History
        1.   Determine location, frequency, temporal onset and whether tremor occurs during rest, activity, or postural maintenance
        2.   Ask about associated neurological symptoms
        3.   Inquire about family history of tremors
        4.   Question about drug use
        5.   Ascertain whether alcohol suppresses tremor
        6.   Obtain complete medication history and history of allergies
        7.   Determine the impact of tremors on performing activities of daily living

    B.   Physical Examination
        1.   Ask patient to perform certain activities to determine whether tremor is better or worse with rest
            a.   Observe hands resting in patient's lap and with arms outstretched
            b.   Observe patient during performance of finger-to-nose and heel-to-shin maneuvers, rapid alternating movements, and handwriting
        2.   Assess functional competence by observing patient drink from cup or use a fork for eating
        3.   Watch patient discretely during history and physical, because calling attention to tremor may exaggerate it
        4.   Perform a complete neurological examination

    C.   Differential Diagnosis
        1.   Chorea is purposeless, involuntary movements of distal extremities and face and occurs in Huntington's disease
        2.   Asterixis is coarse, "flapping" movement seen in outstretched hands of patients with hepatic or metabolic encephalopathies
        3.   Motor tics often begin in childhood and are differentiated from tremors by their lack of rhythmicity, complexity of movement, and associations with vocalizations and behavioral disturbances
        4.   Myoclonus is a brief, rapid contraction of a muscle or group of muscles and is often related to metabolic disorders, degenerative diseases or trauma

    D.   Diagnostic Tests
        1.   Often no tests are needed because diagnosis is made on basis of history and physical examination
        2.   If diagnosis is uncertain, consider ordering thyroid stimulating hormone (TSH), liver function tests, and serum toxicology levels
        3.   EMG may be ordered to confirm the presence of a fine tremor at rest

V.   Plan/Management

    A.   Resting tremor (see section on PARKINSON'S DISEASE)

    B.   Tremor with cerebellar dysfunction needs referral to a neurologist

    C.   Physiologic tremor
        1.   Reduce precipitating factors such as caffeine, fatigue, or stress
        2.   For patients who have situational anxiety and concomitant exaggerated physiologic tremors, consider prophylactic treatment with propranolol (Inderal) 20-40 mg 1 hour before anxiety-producing event, if there are no contraindications

    D.   Essential tremor
        1.   When tremor begins to interfere with patient's ADLs or causes embarrassment consider medication therapy (**Note:** Treatment with a medication is rarely justified)
            a.   Younger adults, with no contraindications, use propranolol (Inderal) 10 mg TID per day for one week and advance slowly to a maximum of 200 mg per day

       (1)   Pulse rate should remain above 50 per minute and systolic blood pressure >110 mmHg

       (2)   If drug is discontinued, it must be slowly tapered; abrupt withdrawal can lead to MI

   b.   Older adults, with no contraindications, use primidone (Mysoline), 25 mg at HS and then titrate to tremor improvement versus side effect up to 150 mg/day in divided doses

   c.   Caution patient about risk of depression, confusion, urinary retention, and memory difficulties with use of primidone

2.   Patient education should include a discussion that usually tremor can only be reduced in severity, not totally abolished

E.   Follow Up
1.   Patients diagnosed with physiologic and essential tremors should be told to return to clinic if tremor worsens, changes in pattern and location, or neurological symptoms develop
2.   Scheduling of return visits will depend on the type of tremor the patient manifests and the type of medication or therapy that is prescribed

VERTIGO

I.   Definition: Sensation of abnormal movements of the body or surroundings

II.   Pathogenesis

A.   Usually a disturbance of the peripheral or central vestibular system which assists in the maintenance of spatial orientation and posture

B.   **Peripheral origin**: Dysfunction of structures peripheral to the brain stem
1.   Vestibular neuritis: May be of viral origin; affects the vestibular nerve
2.   Labyrinthitis: Presumed to be of viral origin with bacterial labyrinthitis extremely rare; may also occur secondary to trauma
3.   Meniere's disease: Unknown cause, but dilation of the endolymphatic systems of middle ear occurs
4.   Benign paroxysmal positional vertigo: Believed to result from calcium carbonate crystal deposition in inner ear
5.   Drug induced vertigo: Related to vestibulotoxic drugs such as furosemide, NSAIDs (especially indomethacin), cytotoxic agents, anticonvulsant (phenytoin, carbamazepine, and ethosuximide), and aminoglycosides

C.   **Central origin**: Involves disease processes affecting brain stem or cerebellum
1.   Acoustic schwannomas or meningiomas: Tumor affecting cranial nerve VIII
2.   Cerebellar pontine angle tumors: Tumors affecting cranial nerves V, VII, IX, and XII
3.   Cerebellar infarction
4.   Cerebellar hemorrhage
5.   Vertebrobasilar insufficiency

III.   Clinical Presentation of disorders based on origin--peripheral or central--is contained in the table below

CLINICAL PRESENTATION OF VERTIGO DISORDERS	
Type of Vertigo	**Typical Presentation**
Peripheral Vertigo	
Vestibular neuritis	Acute onset of vertigo with associated nausea and vomiting Head positioning worsens the symptoms; may be preceded by URI No hearing loss Vertigo may last for days or weeks
Labyrinthitis	Vertigo with associated hearing loss May occur (rarely) secondary to bacterial infection such as otitis media, mastoiditis May also occur secondary to trauma
Meniere's disease	Triad of hearing loss, tinnitus, and vertigo Most patients are >50 years Attacks range from several per week to every few years
Benign paroxysmal positional vertigo	Most common cause of vertigo in elderly Occurs when patient moves head No associated hearing loss or tinnitus
Drug induced vertigo	Acute onset related to medication use Nausea and vomiting are common Hearing loss can occur
Central Vertigo Acoustic schwannomas	Tumors have highest incidence in 5th decade of life Gradual onset of vertigo preceded by hearing loss
Cerebellar pontine angle tumors	Vertigo, hearing loss, and nystagmus Onset of symptoms is gradual
Cerebellar infarction	Sudden onset of vertigo Cranial nerve deficits are present as well as cerebellar signs
Cerebellar hemorrhage	Vertigo and an occipital headache Gaze is affected; patient cannot look toward side of lesion Other cranial nerves (in addition to the sixth) are often affected
Vertebrobasilar insufficiency	Disruption of both cranial nerve and cerebellar function Vertigo may occur

IV.   Diagnosis/Evaluation

    A.   History
        1.   Ask patient to describe in a few words the sensation he/she experiences
            a.   Vertigo always has a sensation of motion that things are spinning around the patient or that the patient is spinning around the environment
            b.   Lightheadedness or feeling that one is about to faint is referred to as syncope or near syncope (see section on SYNCOPE/NEAR SYNCOPE)
            c.   Disequilibrium or a sensation of feeling drunk, unsteady on one's feet, or imbalance suggests a syndrome of multiple sensory deficits, vertebrobasilar insufficiency, anxiety, or motor gait disorder such as Parkinson's disease or cerebellar degeneration
        2.   Ask about symptom patterns
        3.   If possible obtain a description of the episode and events preceding the vertigo from a witness
        4.   Inquire about past medical history including past episodes of vertigo, recent respiratory, gastrointestinal, or ear infections, trauma, risk factors for cardiovascular disease such as smoking, diabetes, hyperlipidemia
        5.   Obtain a complete medication history with a focus on medications known to produce vertigo

B.	Physical Examination
　　1.	Measure vital signs; assess for orthostatic hypotension (see section on SYNCOPE for measurement procedure)
　　2.	Complete ear examination
　　　　a.	Observe TM for loss of landmarks, erythema, or cholesteatoma
　　　　b.	Perform hearing, Rinne and Weber tests
　　3.	Nystagmus is objective marker for new onset vertigo
　　　　a.	Look for spontaneous nystagmus in 5 positions of gaze
　　　　b.	Reproduce nystagmus with Bárány maneuver. (Sitting, turn head to right and quickly lower to supine position with head over edge 30° below horizontal level and observe for nystagmus. Repeat on other side) [see Figure 18.1]

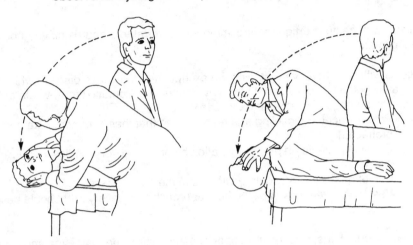

Figure 18.1. Nylen-Bárány Maneuver.

Source: Reilly, B.M. (1991). Practical strategies in outpatient medicine. Philadelphia: Saunders, p. 204. Reprinted by permission.

　　4.	Auscultate neck for carotid bruits
　　5.	Perform a complete cardiovascular exam
　　6.	Do a careful neurological examination to determine if the condition is central or peripheral in origin
　　　　a.	Test cranial nerves (**Note**: Any cranial nerve abnormality suggests a central process)
　　　　b.	Test cerebellar function and the Romberg test
　　7.	Symptom reproduction with hyperventilation may also be helpful

C.	Differential Diagnosis
　　1.	Includes all conditions listed under pathogenesis as well as syncope, multiple sensory defects, and various neurologic disorders
　　2.	The major challenge is differentiating peripheral and central vertigo; clinical features of both types are compared in the following table

DIFFERENTIATING PERIPHERAL AND CENTRAL VERTIGO		
Characteristics	**Peripheral Vertigo**	**Central Vertigo**
Onset	Abrupt	Insidious
Intensity	Moderate to severe	Mild to moderate
Nausea & Vomiting	Common	Not common
Positionally related	Usually	Not usually
Hearing loss	Common	Not common
Neurologic deficits	No	Yes
Nystagmus	Fatigable and inhibited by ocular fixation	Nonfatigable Not inhibited by ocular fixation

D. Diagnostic Tests
1. Cerebral imaging is required for patients with central vertigo to rule out tumor, hemorrhage, or infarction; MRI is usually the test of choice
2. For patients in whom a peripheral etiology is suspected, the following testing may be considered
    a. Audiometry may be ordered and is abnormal with Meniere's disease and acoustic neuroma
    b. Special vestibular function tests may be ordered
        (1) Caloric stimulation
        (2) Electronystagmography

V. Plan/Management

A. Patients with central vertigo require immediate referral to a neurologist/neurosurgeon for management

B. Patients with peripheral vertigo (with the exception of Meniere's disease which is discussed separately below) usually benefit from hydration, symptomatic therapy with antivertiginous and antiemetic drugs, and vestibular exercises
1. Patients need counseling and reassurance that their symptoms are benign but may be protracted
2. Counsel patients on proper hydration by providing very explicit instructions regarding fluid intake
3. Use of medications should be limited to the acute phase
4. Vestibular exercises offer the best approach to recovery and should be instituted as soon as possible

C. Antivertiginous drugs, through a number of mechanisms, decrease the imbalance resulting from a vestibular disorder; prescribe one of the following:
1. Meclizine (Antivert) 12.5-25 PO QD or QID with dosage tapered as symptoms improve
2. Dimenhydrinate (Dramamine) 50 mg PO, Q 4-6 hours
3. Scopolamine transdermal disc (Transderm-Scop) 1 disc applied behind ear, leave in place for 3 days

D. Antiemetic drugs suppress the brain emetic centers or input to these centers, including signals from the vestibular nuclei; prescribe one of the following if nausea and vomiting are a problem; can be combined with an antivertiginous medication
1. Prochlorperazine (Compazine) 5-10 mg PO Q 6 hours as needed; also available in suppository: 25 mg Q 12 hours as needed
2. Promethazine (Phenergan) 25 mg PO Q 6 hours; also available in suppository form: 50 mg Q 12 hours as needed

E. Vestibular exercises are designed to speed the compensation for interruptions in vestibular input
1. Should be begun as soon as possible after the acute stage of nausea and vomiting has resolved
2. Many of the exercises result in dizziness, a sensation that is a necessary stimulus for developing compensatory mechanisms
3. The exercises should be done under the supervision of a trained therapist
4. Compensation development often requires 2 to 6 months

F. Patients with Meniere's disease should receive therapy aimed at reducing the inner ear fluid pressure and controlling the vertigo
1. A sodium-restricted diet (1500 mg per day), use of caffeine and alcohol in moderation, and avoidance of nicotine
2. Management of body fluids via diuretic therapy (Dyazide, Maxzide) with frequent electrolyte monitoring
3. Use of antivertiginous, antiemetic drugs, and vestibular exercises described above are also an integral part of the management

G.   Follow Up: Symptoms that fail to improve with pharmacologic therapy and vestibular exercises should be reevaluated in 2-4 weeks; patients who develop worsening symptoms should return immediately for further evaluation

REFERENCES

Agency for Health Policy and Research. (1995). Stroke prevention: Recommendations. Silver Spring, MD: Author.

Allen, T. (1997, Oct). Seizure disorders: A primary care guide. Advance for Nurse Practitioners, 32-66.

American Psychiatric Association. (1994). Diagnostic and statistical manual of mental disorders, (4th ed.). Washington, DC: Author.

American Psychiatric Association. (1997). Practice guideline for the treatment of patients with Alzheimer's disease and other dementias of late life. Washington, DC: Author.

Aminoff, M.J., Burns, R.S, & Silverstein, P.M. (1997, May). Update of Parkinson's disease. Patient Care, 12-25.

Baloh, R.W. (1998, Jun). Dizzy patients: The varieties of vertigo. Hospital Practice, 55-77.

Barnett, H.J., Cooley, D.A. Perler, B.A., & Rubin, B.G. (1997, Nov). Who can benefit from carotid endarterectomy? Patient Care, 58-75.

Billue, J.S. (1997). Bell's palsy: An update on idiopathic facial paralysis. The Nurse Practitioner, 22(8), 88-107.

Bleicher, J.N., Hamiel, S., Gengler, J.S., & Antimarino, J. (1996). A survey of facial paralysis: Etiology and incidence. Ear, Nose, & Throat Journal, 75, 355-358.

Broderick, J.P. (1998). Practical considerations in the early treatment of ischemic stroke. American Family Physician, 57, 73-80.

Commission on Classification and Terminology of the International League Against Epilepsy. (1981). Proposal for revised clinical and electroencephalographic classification of epileptic seizures. Epilepsia, 22, 480-490.

Cummings, J.L. (1998, Feb). New developments in the treatment of Alzheimer's disease. Medicine and Behavior, 29-34.

Curry, W.J., & Kulling, D.I. (1998). Newer antiepileptic drugs: Gabapentin, lamotrigine, felbamate, topiramte and fosphenytoin. American Family Physician, 57, 513-520.

Davis, W.M. (1997, November). Advances in the pathophysiology and pharmacotherapy of epilepsy. Drug Topics, 110-117.

Delagarza, V.W. (1998). New drugs for Alzheimer's disease. American Family Physician, 58, 1175-1182.

Diamond, S., & Diamond, M.L. (1997). Emergency treatment of migraine: Insights into current options. Postgraduate Medicine, 101, 169-179.

Edmeads, J. (1997). Headaches in older people: How are they different in this age group? Postgraduate Medicine, 101 (5), 91-100.

Erkinjuntti, T., Ostbye, T., Steenhuis, R., & Hachinski, V. (1997). The effect of different diagnostic criteria on the prevalence of dementia. New England Journal of Medicine, 337, 1667-1674.

Fettes, I. (1997). Menstrual migraine: Methods of prevention and control. Postgraduate Medicine, 101, 67-75.

Finkel, A.G. (1997). Headache. In L. Dornbrand, A.J. Hoole, & R.H. Fletcher (Eds.). Manual of clinical problems in adult ambulatory care. (3rd ed.)

Froehling, D.A. Silverstein, M.D., Mohr, D.N., & Beatty, C.W. (1994). Does this dizzy patient have a serious form of vertigo? JAMA, 271, 385-389.

Gambert, S.R. (1997). Is it Alzheimer's disease?: Primary care physicians' growing responsibility for diagnosis. Postgraduate Medicine, 101(6), 42-56.

Hamalainen, M.L., et al. (1997). Ibuprofen or acetaminophen for the acute treatment of migraine in children. Neurology, 46, 103-107.

Hams, R.J. (1997). After the diagnosis: Supporting Alzheimer's patients and their families. Postgraduate Medicine, 101(6), 57-70.

Headache Classification Committee of the International Headache Society. (1988). Classification and diagnostic criteria for headache disorders, cranial neuralgias and facial pain. Cephalalgia, 8 (Suppl. 7), 1-96.

Hilton, G. (1997). Seizure disorders in adults: Evaluation and management of new onset seizures. The Nurse Practitioner, 22(9), 42-59.

Hoehn, M.M., & Yahr, M.D. (1967). Parkinsonism: Onset, progression, and mortality. Neurology, 17, 427-442.

Imke, S. (1998, January). Parkinson's disease. A medical management update. Advance for Nurse Practitioners, 24-28.

Kakaiya, R. (1997, Aug). Bell's palsy: Update on causes, recognition, and management. Consultant, 2217-2227.

Knox, G.W., & McPherson, A. (1997). Meniere's disease: Differential diagnosis and treatment. American Family Physician, 55, 1185-1190.

Koller, W.C., & Montgomery, E.B. (1997). Issues in the early diagnosis of Parkinson's disease. Neurology, 49(Suppl 1), S10-S25.

Leston, J.A. (1996). Migraine and tension-type headache are not separate disorders. Cephalagia, 16 (4), 220-222.

Levine, S.F. (1997, Nov). Thrombolytic therapy for stroke: The new paradigm. Hospital Practice, 57-73.

Lewis, E.D., Ford, B., Lee, H., Andrews, H., & Cameron, G. (1998). Diagnositic criteria for essential tremor. Archives of Neurology, 55, 823-828.

Marks, W.J., & Garcia. (1998). Management of seizures and epilepsy. American Family Physician, 57, 1589-1600.

Merikangas, K., et al. (1997). Association between migraine and stroke in a large-scale epidemiological study of the United States. Archives of Neurology, 54, 362-368.

Moore, K.L. (1997). Drug treatment of migraine: Part I. Acute therapy and drug-rebound headache. American Family Physician, 56, 2039-2048.

Moore-Sledge, C.M. (1997). Evaluation and management of first seizures in adults. American Family Physician, 56, 1113-1120.

Mosier, W., & Schymanski, T.J. (1997, Oct). Quieting neuronal storms: Understanding seizure disorders. Advance for Physician Assistants, 24-28.

National Institute of Neurological Disorders and Stroke (NINDS) rt-PA Stroke Study group. (1997). Systems approach to immediate evaluation and management of hyperacute stroke: Experience at eight centers and implications for community practice and patient care. Stroke, 28, 1530-1540.

Noble, S.L. & Moore, K.L. (1997) Drug treatment of migraine: Part II. Preventive therapy. American Family Physician, 56, 2279-2287.

Plantz, S.H., & Adler, J.N. (1998). Emergency medicine. Baltimore: Williams & Wilkins.

Reilly, B.M. (1991). Practical strategies in outpatient medicine. Philadelphia: Saunders.

Richman, E. (1996, Apr). Acute stroke interventions. Clinician Reviews, 79-94.

Schacter, S.C., & Yerby, M.S. (1997). Management of epilepsy: Pharmacologic therapy and quality of life issues. Postgraduate Medicine, 101(2), 133-153.

Schneck, M.J. (1998, Jan). Acute stroke: An aggressive approach to intervention and prevention. Hospital Medicine, 11-28.

Selman, W.R., Tarr, R., & Landis, DM. (1997). Brain attack: Emergency treatment of ischemic stroke. American Family Physician, 55, 2655-2662.

Selwyn, A. (1998, April). New concepts in parkinsonism. Cortlandt Forum, 168-179.

Sirven, J.I., & Liporace, J.D. (1997). New antiepileptic drugs: Overcoming the limitations of traditional therapy. Postgraduate Medicine, 102(1), 147-162.

Sloane, P.D. (1998). Advances in the treatment of Alzheimer's disease. American Family Physician, 58, 1577-1586.

Small, G.W., Rabins, P.V., Barry, P.P, Buckholz, N.S., DeKosky, S.T., Ferris, S.H., et al. (1997). Diagnosis and treatment of Alzheimer disease and related disorders: Consensus statement of the American Association for Geriatric Psychiatry, the Alzheimer's Association, and the American Geriatrics Society. JAMA, 278, 1363-1371.

Smith, A.L., & Whitehouse, P.J. (1998, Mar). Progress in the management of Alzheimer's disease. <u>Hospital Practice</u>, 151-166.

Sperling, M.R., Bucurescu, G., & Kim, B. (1997). Epilepsy management: Issues in medical and surgical treatment. <u>Postgraduate Medicine, 102</u>(1), 102-118.

Starr, C. (1998). Emerging migraine treatments. <u>Patient Care Nurse Practitioner</u>, 10-26.

Stern, M.B. (1997). The changing standard of care in Parkinson's disease: Current concepts and controversies. <u>Neurology, 49</u>(Suppl 1), S1-S7.

Tapper, V.J. (1997). Pathophysiology, assessment, and treatment of Parkinson's disease. <u>Nurse Practitioner, 22</u>(7), 76-95.

Tariot, P.N., Schneider, L., & Porteinsson, A.P. (1997). Treating Alheimer's disease:Pharmacologic options now and in the near future. <u>Postgraduate Medicine, 101</u>(6), 73-99.

Tariot, P.N., & Suderland, T. (1997). <u>Aggression in patients with dementia</u>. Champaign, IL: Abcomm., Inc.

Unger, J. (1998, March). Diagnosis and management of Parkinson's disease. <u>The Clinical Advisor</u>, 26-38.

US Department of Health and Human Services, Public Health Service, Agency for Health Care Policy and Research. (1996). Recognition and initial assessment of Alzheimer's disease and related dementias. <u>Clinical Practice Guideline No. 19.</u> Rockville, MD: Author.

Waters, C.H. (1997). Managing the late complications of Parkinson's disease. <u>Neurology, 49</u>(Suppl 1), S49-S57.

Watts, R.L. (1997). The role of dopamine agonists in early Parkinson's disease. <u>Neurology, 49</u>(Suppl 1), S34-S48.

Wells, B.G. (Ed.). (1998). Headache: Migraine and cluster. In B.G. Wells, J.T. DiPiro, T.L. Schwinghammer, & C.W. Hamilton (Eds.). <u>Pharmacotherapy Handbook</u>. Stamford, Connecticut: Appleton & Lange.

Wells, B.G. (1998). Epilepsy. In B.G. Wells, J.T. DiPiro, T.L. Schwinghammer, & C.W. Hamiliton (Eds.). <u>Pharmacotherapy handbook</u>. Stamford, CT: Appleton & Lange.

CHAPTER 19

Hematologic Problems

Anemia of Chronic Disease
Iron Deficiency Anemia
Megaloblastic Anemia

ANEMIA OF CHRONIC DISEASE

I. Definition: A hypoproliferative anemia associated with infectious, inflammatory, or neoplastic disorders that last >1-2 months

II. Pathogenesis

    A. The cause of anemia of chronic disease (ACD) is uncertain but the result is a decreased RBC life span as well as a reduction in the production or action of erythropoietin

    B. The basic defect is in the iron utilization for erythropoiesis
        1. For unknown reasons the delivery of iron from the reticuloendothelial iron stores to the developing red cell is blocked (defect in release mechanism)
        2. Consequently, the red cells are deficient in iron, whereas the body stores have abundant iron

    C. When the primary disease is controlled, the anemia is reversible

III. Clinical Presentation

    A. Clinical presentation is similar to that of iron deficiency anemia, but physical findings depend more on the nature of the underlying disease than on the anemia

    B. Anemia is usually mild and asymptomatic

    C. Laboratory findings are as follows:
        1. Usually, the peripheral blood smear shows a normochromic, normocytic picture, but in advanced states, the appearance may be hypochromic and microcytic (though not as severe as with iron deficiency anemia)
        2. Anemia is usually moderate, and if hematocrit is <25%, another explanation should be sought
        3. Serum iron and total iron-binding capacity (TIBC) are low; low TIBC helps differentiate this disorder from iron deficiency anemia
        4. Serum ferritin is increased, with values to 50-2000 µg/mL; this point can be used to discriminate between anemia of chronic disease and iron deficiency anemia since serum ferritin values are <10 µg/mL in iron deficiency states

IV. Diagnosis/Evaluation

    A. History
        1. Determine onset, duration of symptoms
        2. Obtain complete medical history to determine if chronic disorder present
        3. Obtain medication history

    B. Physical Examination: Guided by the history since numerous inflammatory processes, chronic infections, and malignant neoplasms can produce the anemia; **always** obtain stool for occult blood

    C. Diagnostic Tests
        1. CBC with peripheral smear to classify the category of anemia
        2. Iron studies in the anemia of chronic disease include serum iron (should be low), TIBC (should be low), serum ferritin (should be normal or increased), free erythrocyte protoporphyrin (should be high), Hemoglobin A2 (should be normal), Hemoglobin F (should be normal), red cell distribution width (RDW) [should be normal]
        3. Obtain stool for occult blood x 6
        4. A this point, should also order appropriate tests to determine underlying cause (based on findings from history and physical exam) or can wait for results of CBC and iron studies before proceeding

D. Differential Diagnosis
    1. Must be differentiated from other types of anemia with most common types in differential being iron deficiency, α-thalassemia, β-thalassemia, and sideorblastic anemia
    2. Numerous underlying causes including chronic infection, inflammatory processes, and malignant neoplasms

V. Plan/Treatment

A. No specific therapy for ACD

B. Successful treatment of the underlying disease leads to resolution of the anemia

C. Red cell transfusions are effective, but should be limited to situations in which oxygen transport is inadequate due to other medical problems

D. Consult specialist regarding use of erythropoietin (EPO) to stimulate erythropoiesis; patients with ACD have a relatively impaired response to erythropoietin and treating with EPO may not be successful

E. Follow Up: Variable depending on underlying disorder causing the anemia

IRON DEFICIENCY ANEMIA

I. Definition: Anemia characterized by small (microcytic), pale (hypochromic), RBCs, and depletion of iron (Fe) stores

II. Pathogenesis

A. Regulation of iron balance occurs mainly in the GI tract through absorption

B. When iron loss exceeds intake, storage iron (ferritin) is progressively depleted

C. As storage iron is depleted, a compensatory increase in absorption of dietary Fe and in the concentration of transferrin occurs

D. When iron stores are no longer able to meet the needs of the erythroid marrow; the plasma-transferrin level increases, the serum Fe concentration declines, resulting in a decrease in Fe available for RBC formation

III. Clinical Presentation

A. Anemia is frequently discovered during a routine evaluation

B. Iron deficiency anemia (IDA) is the most common known form of nutritional deficiency; prevalence is highest among young children and women of childbearing age, particularly pregnant women

C. In adulthood (excluding pregnancy), by far the most common cause of iron deficiency anemia is blood loss
    1. In adult men and in post-menopausal women, bleeding is usually from the GI tract
    2. In premenopausal women, menstrual loss may be the underlying mechanism, but other sites of bleeding must always be considered

D. Other causes of IDA in adults include increased demand (as often occurs with pregnancy), inadequate absorption from the gastrointestinal tract (as can occur with malabsorption syndromes, postgastrectomy states, or unrelenting diarrhea) and uncommonly from dietary deficiencies (for example, in vegetarians, food faddists, or anorectics)

E. Iron deficiency anemia is usually slow in onset, allowing for compensatory mechanisms to develop so that symptoms may be minimal until significant anemia develops

F. Clinical presentation depends on severity, age, and ability of the cardiovascular and pulmonary systems to compensate for decreasing oxygen carrying capacity of the blood

G. There are few symptoms when hematocrit (HCT) is 30 or above in otherwise healthy individuals and anemia is frequently discovered during routine health maintenance visits; as HCT falls, dyspnea and mild fatigue with exercise may occur

H. Nonspecific complaints of headache, poor concentration, palpitations, anorexia can also occur

I. Signs of anemia include pallor, best seen in the conjunctiva

J. In very severe anemia, atrophic glossitis, cheilitis, and koilonychia may appear

K. Laboratory indices that reflect an iron-deficient state are listed here
    1. Low mean red cell volume
    2. Reduced serum ferritin level
    3. Reduced serum iron level
    4. Increased serum iron-binding capacity
    5. Increase in hemoglobin concentration after the institution of iron therapy

L. The earliest laboratory change associated with iron-deficiency anemia is decreased serum ferritin; the absence of storage iron, as defined as a serum ferritin level below 20 μg per liter in an anemic patient is **conclusive evidence** of iron deficiency anemia

M. In mild forms of iron-deficiency anemia, the laboratory values of iron-deficiency and iron-sufficiency may overlap considerably, thus presenting a diagnostic challenge

IV. Diagnosis/Evaluation

A. History
    1. Inquire about onset and duration of symptoms
    2. Ask if there has recently been an unintended weight loss
    3. Obtain a careful history of gastrointestinal complaints that might suggest gastritis, peptic ulcer disease, or other conditions that might produce gastrointestinal bleeding
    4. Ask if there has been change in stool patterns or color and if there are hemorrhoids present (**Note**: Black tarry stools usually indicate an upper GI source of bleeding, while stool streaked with red blood is more often associated with colorectal bleeding [or bleeding from hemorrhoids])
    5. In menstruating women, ask about blood loss during menses
    6. Ask about dietary intake of iron rich foods and pica
    7. Obtain medication history, particularly use of aspirin and other NSAIDs; ask about past history of GI bleeding

B. Physical Examination
    1. Obtain weight and compare with previous weight
    2. Observe for pallor, particularly the conjunctiva
    3. Examine tongue, corners of mouth, and nails for characteristic changes
    4. Perform abdominal exam for tenderness on palpation and enlargement of the spleen
    5. Auscultate heart for systolic flow murmurs
    6. Obtain stool for occult blood

C. Differential Diagnosis
    1. Inadequate intake of iron
    2. Any condition that causes acute or chronic blood loss
    3. Hemolytic diseases such as sickle cell
    4. Megaloblastic anemias
    5. Anemia of chronic disease

D. Diagnostic Tests
1. CBC and peripheral smear
2. Serum ferritin level is considered the single most powerful test for the diagnosis of iron deficiency anemia (after bone marrow aspiration)
3. Menstruating women who are found to have microcytic anemia with reticulocytopenia and there is no reason to suspect GI blood loss usually do not require additional evaluation
4. Additional evaluation is needed for adult men and postmenopausal women
5. Consider iron studies which include measurement of serum iron, total iron-binding capacity, transferrin saturation and serum ferritin
6. In men and postmenopausal women who are asymptomatic (no weight loss, abdominal pain, or report of black, tarry stools or frank blood in stools) obtain stool for occult blood x 6; patient is directed to collect two samples of stools on each of 3 days during which specific dietary, medication, sample collection, and storage guidelines are followed
7. In men and postmenopausal women who are symptomatic or in whom occult blood is found in the stool, either colonoscopy or endoscopy of the upper GI tract is indicated (based on history) to look for the source of bleeding
8. Urinalysis for blood loss from the urinary tract (a much less common source of bleeding) should also be performed

V. Plan/Treatment

A. The World Health Organization hemoglobin (Hb) and hematocrit (HCT) cut-points for diagnosing anemia in adults have been widely adopted
1. In men, anemia is defined as a Hb level of less than 13 g/dL or Hct level of less than 41%
2. In menstruating women, anemia is defined as a Hb level of less than 12 g/dL or Hct of less than 36%
3. Cigarette smokers and persons living at high altitudes (>3000 feet) tend to have higher levels of Hb and HCT

B. A therapeutic trial of oral iron therapy (200 mg of elemental iron per day) is justified for menstruating women who are determined to be anemic based on the values listed above
1. Products available include Nu-Iron 150 capsules which contain 150 mg of elemental iron and may be dosed once daily OR
2. Feosol tablets which contain 65 mg of elemental iron and is given TID

C. In adult men, non-menstruating, and non-pregnant women, **source of bleeding must be identified**: See Diagnostic Tests in section IV.D. above

D. Follow up for menstruating women who have been placed on a therapeutic trial of iron therapy
1. In 4 weeks for repeat examination and hemoglobin
a. A hemoglobin response of less than 2 g/100 mL over a 4-week period is unacceptable and the patient should be reevaluated at that point
b. Restoration of iron stores is the goal of iron replacement therapy; the time required to accomplish this goal varies from patient to patient; in general, approximately 3 to 6 months of therapy is necessary
2. A reticulocytosis occurs within 7-10 days after initiation of iron therapy, but a reticulocyte count is not usually ordered unless there are concerns about the diagnosis; if the patient does not develop reticulocytosis, the diagnosis should be reevaluated
3. Common causes of treatment failure include noncompliance with therapy, misdiagnosis, and malabsorption
4. The therapeutic trial should not be continued beyond 1 month if the hemoglobin concentration has not increased appropriately and the patient has been compliant with the treatment regimen; referral to an expert for further evaluation is indicated

E. Follow up of iron deficiency anemia in adult men and postmenopausal women is variable depending on cause of anemia (source of blood loss, cause of malabsorption, or dietary deficiency)

MEGALOBLASTIC ANEMIAS

I. Definition: Anemia related to vitamin B_{12} (cobalamin) or folate deficiency or defects in their transport or metabolism

II. Pathogenesis

    A. Folic acid and vitamin B_{12} are cofactors for the pyrimidine synthesis of DNA

    B. The deficiency of these factors alters the synthesis of DNA, resulting in a decreased rate of cellular duplication

    C. Abnormal amounts of DNA and proteins are produced resulting in the morphologic changes of megaloblastosis

    D. Vitamin B_{12} deficiency can result from inadequate intake, decreased absorption, or inadequate utilization
        1. Pernicious anemia (PA) is the most common cause of vitamin B_{12} deficiency; PA is an autoimmune disease characterized by production of autoantibodies to gastric parietal cells and their secretory product, intrinsic factor, which is necessary for absorption of B_{12}
        2. Other conditions that interfere with absorption and utilization include Crohn's disease, Whipple's disease, sprue, and gastrectomy
        3. Poor intake is extremely rare, but can occur in strict vegetarians
        4. Many drugs interfere with the cobalamin-folate-dependent metabolic pathway, especially chemotherapeutic agents such as methotrexate and fluorouracil
        5. Animal products are the primary dietary source of vitamin B_{12}
            a. The recommended daily dietary allowance of the vitamin is 2.4 μg
            b. The average Western diet provides an excess of the vitamin (3 to 9 μg per day) which is stored mainly in the liver); body stores can hold up to a three year reserve (between 7-9 mg)

    E. Folic acid deficiency may result from inadequate intake, deceased absorption, hyperutilization, or inadequate utilization
        1. Inadequate intake, usually encountered in those with very poor diets such as elderly, chronically ill, food faddists, and alcoholics is a very common cause
        2. Malabsorption syndromes such as tropical and nontropical sprue are also causative factors
        3. Hyperutilization of folic acid may occur in physiologic states (such as pregnancy, and the growth spurts seen in infancy and adolescence) and in disease states such as malignancy, chronic inflammatory disorders such as Crohn's disease and rheumatoid arthritis
        4. Many drugs interfere with the cobalamin-folate-dependent metabolic pathway, especially chemotherapeutic agents such as methotrexate and fluorouracil
        5. Food sources for folate include green vegetables, yeast, and liver
            a. The recommended daily dietary allowance of folate is 400 μg with increased requirements in pregnancy and lactation
            b. The average Western diet supplies 400-600 μg of folate daily
            c. Body stores can reach 5 mg, a 3-4 month supply; thus folate deficiency can develop quickly with dietary deficiency

III. Clinical Presentation

    A. Vitamin B_{12} deficiency due to pernicious anemia
        1. Onset is insidious, usually occurring in fifth and sixth decades of life with the median age at diagnosis being 60 years
        2. Slightly more women than men are affected

3. Earlier studies suggested that the disorder was largely restricted to Northern Europeans; more recent studies have reported the disease in black and Latin-American persons with an earlier age of onset in black women
4. The usual presentation is with symptoms of anemia
5. Gastrointestinal manifestations include several abnormalities
   a. A smooth and beefy red tongue due to atrophic glossitis is a common finding
   b. Megaloblastosis of the epithelial cells of the small intestine may produce malabsorption and diarrhea
6. Peripheral neuropathy and lesions in the posterior and lateral columns of the spinal cord and in the cerebrum are neurologic complications that may occur
   a. The most frequent manifestations of peripheral neuropathy are paresthesia and numbness
   b. Manifestations of a lesion in the spinal cord can produce loss of vibration and position sense, sensory ataxia with positive Romberg's sign, and limb weakness, spasticity, and extensor plantar responses
   c. Cerebral manifestations can range from mild personality changes and memory loss to psychosis

B. Folic acid deficiency occurs most often from dietary deficits
   1. Elderly, alcoholics, and indigents may have inadequate intake due to poor diet
   2. Clinical features are similar to those with B_{12} deficiency with one important difference -- neurologic symptoms do not occur

C. The morphology of the peripheral blood and bone marrow is identical in both folic acid and vitamin B_{12} deficiencies

IV. Diagnosis/Evaluation

A. History
   1. Inquire about onset, duration of symptoms
   2. If gastrointestinal complaints, inquire about presence of red, burning tongue, abdominal complaints, presence of diarrhea or constipation
   3. If neurologic complaints, inquire about presence of pins-and-needles paresthesia and weakness, unsteadiness due to proprioceptive difficulties, and memory loss
   4. Inquire about dietary intake, using 24-hour recall
   5. Ask about alcohol consumption
   6. Obtain medication history with a focus on drugs commonly implicated in interference with absorption or utilization of cobalamin or folate
   7. Obtain past medical history, specifically if history of gastrectomy, resection of ileum

B. Physical Examination
   1. Examine oral cavity for characteristic red, shiny tongue
   2. Perform abdominal exam for tenderness, organomegaly
   3. Perform neurologic exam with a focus on uncovering abnormal findings described under III.A.6 above

C. Differential Diagnosis
   1. The many causes of anemia should be grouped according to the red cell indices and peripheral blood smear results into microcytic, normochromic-normocytic, and macrocytic as a beginning point (see following table)
   2. Based on the grouping, differential diagnosis of anemia by red cell morphology can be undertaken (see the table that follows)
   3. Once the patient is determined to have macrocytic anemia, the primary differential diagnostic approach is the identification of vitamin B_{12} or folate deficiency

> **Microcytic (MCV 50-82, MCHC 24-32)**
> * Iron deficiency
> * Thalassemia
> * Chronic disease
>
> **Normochromic-Normocytic (MCV 82-92, MCHC 32-36)**
> * Hemorrhage
> * Hemolysis
> * Chronic disease
> * Early iron deficiency
> * Aplastic anemia
>
> **Macrocytic (MCV>100, MCHC >36)**
> * B_{12} deficiencies
> * Folic acid deficiencies
> * Antimetabolites

D. Diagnostic Tests
1. CBC and peripheral smear should be done to determine classification of anemia to facilitate work-up
2. Red cell distribution width (RDW) can assist in detecting red cell heterogeneity, previously available only by exam of the peripheral smear (this helps overcome the problems of detecting a coexisting microcytic and macrocytic anemia)
3. The most common method of establishing B_{12} deficiency is by measurement of serum B_{12} level
   a. Vitamin B_{12} deficiency as the cause of megaloblastic anemia is established by a low serum B_{12} concentration and normal serum folate concentration
   b. A Shilling test will confirm that the vitamin B_{12} deficiency is a result of intestinal malabsorption due to intrinsic factor deficiency
   c. Confirmation of the diagnosis of intrinsic factor deficiency can also be accomplished by detection of serum intrinsic-factor autoantibodies
4. The most common method of establishing folate deficiency is by measurement of serum folate levels

V. Plan/Management

A. Treatment of vitamin B_{12} deficiency
1. A commonly used regimen is initiation of therapy with daily injections of 800-1000 μg of vitamin B_{12} for 1-2 weeks which should saturate B_{12} stores and resolve clinical manifestations of the deficit
2. After that initial 1-2 week period, the dose should be reduced to 100-1000 μg once weekly until normalization of the hemoglobin and hematocrit occurs
3. Thereafter, monthly injections of 100-1000 μg should be administered to be continued for the rest of the patient's life

B. Treatment of folic acid deficiency
1. To replenish stores, therapy should be initiated with 0.5 mg folic acid orally for 2 days, followed by 2 mg orally twice a week or 0.5-1 mg daily
2. Therapy should be continued for approximately 4 months
3. Taking a multivitamin containing 0.4 mg daily may need to be continued if the patient is not eating an adequate diet, or if underlying cause cannot be corrected
4. Dietary counseling regarding foods high in folic acid should be provided (important sources are liver, wheat bran, leafy green vegetables, beans, grains)

C. With both types of anemia, treatment brings about the following results
1. A rapid reticulocytosis following treatment (peaks in 5-8 days)
2. A rise in hematocrit and hemoglobin values in 1 week
3. In uncomplicated cases, hematocrit should reach normal levels within two months

D. Follow Up
   1. Patients with vitamin B_{12} deficiency must be seen in 2 weeks to determine response to treatment
      a. Patient should experience an increased sense of well being and appetite in 2-3 days and a diminution in neurologic signs/symptoms
      b. Increased reticulocyte count and increased hematocrit as described above should also occur
      c. The patient should be followed monthly for B_{12} injections
   2. Patients with folic acid deficiency must be seen in 2 weeks to determine response to treatment, and then monthly until condition stabilizes; symptomatic improvement as evidenced by increased alertness, appetite and cooperation are often noted early during the course of treatment

REFERENCES

Barkin, J.S., Green, R., Johnson, B., & Krantz, S. (1998, March). A practical workup for the patient with anemia. Patient Care, 70-90.

Borman, R.J., & McGuire, S.M. (1997). In R.B. Taylor (Ed.), Manual of family practice. Boston: Little, Brown.

Carmel, R. (1996). Prevalence of undiagnosed pernicious anemia in the elderly. Archives of Internal Medicine, 156, 1097-2000.

Hamilton, C.W. (1998). Hematologic disorders. In B.G. Wells, J.T. DiPiro, T.L. Schwinghammer, & C.W. Hamilton (Eds.), Pharmacotherapy handbook. Stamford, CT: Appleton & Lange.

Paulman, P.M. (1997). Pernicious anemia and other macrocytic anemias. In R.B. Taylor (Ed.), Manual of family practice. Boston: Little, Brown.

Shine, J.W. (1997). Microcytic anemia. American Family Physician, 55, 2455-2462.

Spruill, W.J., & Wade, W.E. (1997). Anemia. In J.T. DiPiro, R.L. Talbert, G.C. Yee, G.R. Matzke, B.G. Wells, & L. M. Posey (Eds.), Pharmacotherapy: A pathophysiologic approach. Stamford, CT: Appleton & Lange.

Toh, B., Van Driel, I.R., & Gleeson, P.A. (1997). Pernicious anemia. New England Journal of Medicine, 337, 1441-1448.

US Department of Health and Human Services. (1994). Clinician's handbook of preventive services: Put prevention into practice. Washington, DC: Author.

US Preventive Services Task Force. (1996). Guide to clinical preventive services. Baltimore: Williams & Wilkins.

Volterra, F. (1997). Hematology. In L.M. Rucker (Ed.), Essentials of adult ambulatory care. Baltimore: Williams & Wilkins.

Emergencies

AVULSED TOOTH

I. Definition: A total displacement of a tooth out of its socket

II. Pathogenesis

   A. Trauma to mouth resulting in displacement of tooth

   B. Teeth not fully erupted have loosely structured periodontal ligaments; thus these are the teeth most likely to be displaced when trauma to mouth occurs

III. Clinical Presentation

   A. An upper central incisor is the most frequently avulsed tooth

   B. Children are more likely to have avulsed teeth, but avulsion can also occur in adults

IV. Diagnosis/Evaluation

   A. Determine if the avulsed tooth is a primary or a secondary tooth; primary teeth should not be reimplanted because they often ankylose or fuse to the bone

   B. Defer history and physical since immediate reimplantation of the tooth is necessary to maintain vitality of the tooth (each minute the tooth remains out if its socket greatly reduces the likelihood that implantation will be successful)

   C. Go immediately to treatment

V. Plan/Treatment

   A. The avulsed tooth should be replanted immediately if possible
      1. If the tooth was displaced from the mouth and has collected debris from the ground or floor, rinse gently with sterile water holding the tooth by the crown. (DO NOT TOUCH ROOT SURFACE)
      2. Holding the tooth by the crown, gently tease it back onto the socket and cover with gauze; instruct patient to gently bite down on gauze during transport to dentist office
      3. If the avulsed tooth cannot be placed into socket for transport, store tooth in physiologic medium to preserve vitality of tooth
      4. Milk is an ideal storage medium; physiologic saline is also a satisfactory storage medium
      5. Saliva is a less desirable storage medium, but if milk and saline are not available, and placement back into socket cannot be done, placement of the tooth under the patient's tongue is better than allowing to air dry which is destructive to the tooth (irreversible damage to the periodontal cells occurs in 30 minutes of air drying)
      6. Transport to the dentist must be immediate

   B. Follow Up: By dentist to whom the patient was referred for reimplantation

BITE WOUNDS

I. Definition: Mechanical trauma to skin and/or underlying tissue from bite of an animal or human

II. Pathogenesis

    A. Transmission of bacteria from animal's or human's mouth into wound may produce infection
        1. *Pasteurella multocida* is the causative agent in 20-50% of infections from dog bites and 80% of infections from cat bites
        2. Dog and cat bites also become infected with *Staphylococcus aureus*, *Streptococcus epidermidis*, and *Enterobacter* species
        3. Enteric gram-negative bacteria and anaerobes are likely to cause infection from reptile bites
        4. Rats and mice bites may become infected from *Streptobacillus moniliformis*
        5. Streptococci, *Staphylococcus aureus*, *Eikenella corrodens,* or anaerobes are likely to cause infection from human bites
            a. Hepatitis B can be transmitted by human bites; especially consider this if the biter is within a high-risk group
            b. Transmission of human immunodeficiency virus (HIV) is low but is a risk if the biter is HIV infected; especially consider this if biter is from a high-risk group

    B. Rabies, an acute viral illness, may be transmitted to human beings by infected saliva or other secretions after an animal bite or by licking mucosa of an open wound; airborne transmission has been reported in bat-infested caves

III. Clinical Presentation

    A. Dog bites account for over 90% of mammal bites

    B. Most bites are minor and may include scratches, abrasions, lacerations, and puncture wounds

    C. Human bites; "Clenched-fist" injuries that occur during fistfights can cause potential tendon or joint capsule injuries and often require hospitalization

    D. Potential complications of bites include to the following:
        1. Infection is the most common problem
            a. Cat bites become infected more frequently than dog bites because they are often deep puncture wounds
            b. Bites on the hand have the highest infection rate; bites on the face have the lowest infection rate
            c. Cellulitis and abscesses are common; infections of tendons, periosteum, and joint spaces can be devastating infections
        2. Rabies may occur after a bite
            a. Rabies in small rodents is rare
            b. Rabies in domestic animals has been decreasing, but rabies in wild animals is on the increase
            c. Skunks, bats, raccoons, bobcats, coyotes, and foxes may harbor the virus and may also bite and infect domestic dogs, cats, horses, and cows
            d. Infection with rabies produces an acute febrile illness with central nervous system problems and death if untreated
        3. Bites of large dogs and other animals may produce crush injuries, avulsions, and fractures

IV.   Diagnosis/Evaluation

   A.   History
      1.   Inquire about type of mammal which bit patient
      2.   Ask if attack was provoked or unprovoked
      3.   If animal is known to the patient, obtain name and telephone number(s) of owner
      4.   Ask about condition of animal such as was animal acting strangely or did animal appear ill
      5.   Determine the amount of time which has elapsed since the bite
      6.   If patient receives a human bite, determine whether the biter is HIV infected or has hepatitis B or if biter is from a high risk group
      7.   Inquire about all self-treatments of injury
      8.   Determine immune status of the animal or human biter
      9.   Inquire about tetanus immunization status and prior rabies immunizations
      10.   Inquire about patient's past medical history, especially diseases such as diabetes mellitus and immunodeficiencies which would place patient at risk for infection

   B.   Physical Examination
      1.   Check distal to the injured site for neurovascular status and motor function
      2.   Determine extent and depth of wound; check for foreign body
      3.   In patients with old wounds, check for signs of infection

   C.   Differential Diagnosis: See Pathogenesis

   D.   Diagnostic Tests
      1.   Order x-rays if bony injury or presence of a foreign body such as tooth is suspected
      2.   Obtain wound cultures in following cases:
         a.   If wound is ≥8 hours and <24 hours from time of injury
         b.   All cases in which there are signs of infections regardless of time from injury
      3.   To determine if an animal is rabid, brain tissue can be examined by fluorescent microscopy

V.   Plan/Management

   A.   Wound care
      1.   Sponge away visible dirt
      2.   Irrigate wound with copious amounts of saline; do not irrigate puncture wounds
         a.   Irrigate under pressure with either a 18 gauge needle and a 35 mL syringe or a Water-Pik
         b.   Use at least 500-1000 mL of solution for irrigation and direct stream at all surfaces of wound
      3.   Scrub the surrounding area
      4.   Debride all wounds to reduce risk of infection unless they are small and superficial
      5.   Trim jagged edge of wound

   B.   Open-wound management versus sutures
      1.   Do not suture wounds that are likely to become infected such as the following:
         a.   Hand bites
         b.   Bites that are older than 8 hours
         c.   Deep or puncture bites
         d.   Bites with extensive injury
      2.   See section on WOUNDS for suturing procedure

   C.   Antibiotic prophylaxis of bite wounds to prevent infection
      1.   Following type of wounds need prophylaxis:
         a.   All wounds with signs of infections
         b.   Moderate or severe wounds, especially if edema or crush injury is present
         c.   Puncture wounds, especially if bone, tendon sheath, or joint penetration may have occurred
         d.   Facial bites

e.　Hand and foot bites
　　　f.　Genital area bites
　　　g.　Wounds in immunocompromised and asplenic persons
　2.　Selection of antimicrobial agent is based on organism likely to cause infection and should be modified after culture results (see following table for antibiotics)

ANTIBIOTICS FOR ANIMAL OR HUMAN BITE WOUNDS			
	Dog/Cat	Reptile	Human
Oral Route	Amoxicillin-clavulanate**	Amoxicillin-clavulanate**	Amoxicillin-clavulanate**
Oral Alternatives for Penicillin-Allergic Patients*	Extended spectrum cephalosporin or trimethoprim-sulfamethoxazole **PLUS** clindamycin	Extended spectrum cephalosporin or trimethoprim-sulfamethoxazole **PLUS** clindamycin	Trimethoprim-sulfamethoxazole **PLUS** clindamycin
Intravenous Route	Ampicillin-sulbactam	Ampicillin-sulbactam **PLUS** gentamicin **OR** ticarcillin-clavulanate	Ampicillin-sulbactam
Intravenous Alternative for Penicillin-Allergic Patients*	Extended spectrum cephalosporin or trimethoprim-sulfamethoxazole **PLUS** clindamycin	Clindamycin **PLUS** gentamicin	Extended spectrum cephalosporin or trimethoprim-sulfamethoxazole **PLUS** clindamycin

*In patients with history of allergy to penicillin, a cephalosporin or other β-lactam class drug may be acceptable. However, these drugs should not be used in patients with an immediate hypersensitivity (anaphylaxis) to penicillin because approximately 5% to 15% of penicillin-allergic patients also will be allergic to the cephalosporins.

**Prescribe amoxicillin/clavulanate (Augmentin) 250-500 mg every 8 hours for 3-7 days

Adapted from American Academy of Pediatrics. (1997). Bite wounds. In G. Peter (Ed.). Red book: Report of the committee on infectious diseases (24th ed., pp. 125). Elk Grove Village, IL: American Academy of Pediatrics.

　D.　Prescribe appropriate tetanus prophylaxis; see WOUND section for guidelines

　E.　If there is a high risk or known exposure to hepatitis B after a human bite, provide passive prophylaxis with hepatitis B immune globulin (HBIG) 0.06 mL/kg intramuscularly and begin hepatitis B vaccination three-shot series

　F.　Consult infectious disease specialist if there is a high risk or known exposure to HIV after a human bite

　G.　Control measures related to rabies
　　1.　Contact personnel in local health department who can provide information on the risk of rabies in a particular area for each species of animals (unprovoked attack is more suggestive of rabid animal than provoked attack; properly immunized domestic animals have only a minimal chance of developing rabies)
　　2.　A suspected domestic animal should be caught, confined, and observed by a veterinarian for 10 days; if animal develops signs of rabies it should be killed and its head removed and shipped to laboratory for examination. No treatment is necessary if examination of brain is negative
　　3.　A suspected wild animal should be killed and its brain examined for evidence of rabies. No treatment is necessary if examination of brain is negative
　　4.　Patients with bites from bats and wild carnivores need rabies prophylaxis if the offending animal cannot be caught

　H.　Care of patients exposed to rabies; after local wound care, use both passive and active immunoprophylaxis as soon as possible after exposure, ideally within 24 hours, but even patients who have been exposed >24 hours should still be given therapy
　　1.　Active immunization: Human diploid cell vaccine (HDCV) or rhesus diploid cell vaccine, rabies vaccine absorbed (RVA) 1.0 mL is given intramuscularly in the deltoid on first day of treatment, and repeat doses are administered on days 3, 7, 14, and 28

2. Passive immunization: Rabies immune globulin (Human) (RIG) should be used simultaneously with first dose of HDCV or RVA; recommended dose 20 IU of RIG per kilogram of weight; approximately one half of RIG is infiltrated into wound and the remainder is given intramuscularly

I. Patient Education
1. Teach patient to watch for signs of infection
2. Educate about bite prevention
   a. Caution against approaching unknown dogs, cats, and wild animals and avoid contact when animals are eating
   b. Secure garbage containers so that raccoons and other animals will not be attracted to home
   c. Chimneys and other potential portals of entry for wild animals should be identified and covered

J. Referral/consultation is needed in the following cases:
1. Bites of ears, face, genitalia, hands and feet
2. Large, contaminated wounds

K. Follow Up: Inspect wound for signs of infection within 48 hours

BURNS, MINOR

I. Definition: Lesions caused by heat or other cauterizing agents; the following are considered minor burns:

A. First- or second-degree burns covering <15% in adults

B. In addition, third-degree burns of less <2% TBSA when they do not involve the eyes, ears, face or genitalia

II. Pathogenesis

A. As a result of excessive heat energy which is transferred into the skin, cellular protein coagulation and destruction of enzyme systems occur

B. Common agents causing burns include the following:
1. Scalds or burns from wet heat
2. Direct burns from flames; matches and cigarettes are common sources; irons and ovens are other sources
3. Chemicals
4. Electricity
5. Radiation; burns caused by exposure to sunlight

III. Clinical Presentation

A. Depth of burn will depend on the intensity of the burning agent and the amount of time the burning agent is in contact with skin
1. First degree burns cause no skin loss and have erythema only; heal without scarring
2. Second degree burns (partial thickness) involve the upper layers of the epidermis and present with tender, erythematous, weeping skin and blisters
3. Third degree burns (full thickness) involve the entire thickness of the skin down to the subcutaneous tissues; sensation is absent and skin is charred or whitish in appearance

B.   Scalds are the most common type of burn injury and generally result in superficial skin loss

C.   Burns from flames are the second most common cause of burns; burns in which clothing is caught on fire is almost always third degree and serious

D.   The severity of chemical burns depends on the type of chemical, its concentration and the contact time; cement and phenol are common sources

E.   Electricity burns often cause small, punctate, deep burns at the entry point; electrical burns across the chest can cause cardiac problems

F.   Radiation burns due to sun exposure are always superficial but can be extensive, painful, and result in hospitalization

G.   Minor burns do not result in systemic problems (shock, acute renal failure, hypothermia, and severe depression of the immune systems) which may occur with severe burns

H.   Other injuries may accompany minor burns and include trauma and smoke inhalation; carbon monoxide and cyanide poisoning may occur with more extensive burns

I.   Bacterial infection is a complication of minor burns

IV.   Diagnosis/Evaluation

A.   History
   1.   Ask what caused the burn or how the burn was acquired
   2.   Query about length of the time the skin was in contact with the burning agent
   3.   Determine how much time has elapsed from burn occurrence to seeking of treatment
   4.   Question about occurrence of smoke inhalation
   5.   Ask about associated injuries
   6.   When chemicals are involved ask the name and concentration of the chemical
   7.   Ask patients with electrical injury about the amount of voltage involved and whether there was loss of consciousness at time of injury
   8.   Ask about tetanus status
   9.   Ask about past medical history, particularly cardiac valvular disease
   10.   Inquire about history of alcohol and narcotic abuse; this information is important in managing the patient's pain
   11.   Ask about recent streptococcal infection
   12.   Because of possibilities of abuse and neglect, ask about prior injuries and burns; documentation of quotes should be recorded

B.   Physical Examination; important to remove all clothing, dressings, jewelry, dentures and prostheses to thoroughly assess burns and any associated injuries
   1.   Observe general appearance for distress
   2.   Observe for any signs that suggest abuse such as scald burns consistent with "dipping" injuries of the buttocks or arms and legs, cigarette burns, and iron burns
   3.   Measure vital signs
   4.   Estimate the area of burn from Lund-Browder burn charts
   5.   Determine depth of burn
   6.   Assess sensation in the burn area by using a blunt sterile needle or pin
   7.   Check distal to the burn site for neurovascular status and motor function
   8.   Perform a complete exam of the lung and heart
   9.   Other body systems should be examined depending on location and extent of burn and to determine any associated injuries such as fractures and dislocations from jumping from windows in house fires
   10.   In old burns, assess for signs of infection

C.   Differential Diagnosis: Always consider possibility of abuse or neglect, particularly if location of burn is inconsistent with the history

D.   Diagnostic Tests: None usually needed

V. Plan/Management

A. Refer following patients to a burn center
   1. Patients 11-49 years with partial-thickness burns ≥20% TBSA
   2. Patients <10 years and/or >50 years with partial-thickness burns ≥10% TBSA
   3. Patients of any age with full-thickness burns ≥5% TBSA
   4. Patients with partial- or full-thickness burns to hands, feet, face, eyes, ears, perineum and/or major joints
   5. Patients with electrical injuries, including lightning injuries
   6. Patients with significant burns from caustic chemicals
   7. Patients with burns complicated by multiple trauma in which the burn poses the greatest risk of morbidity
   8. Patients with significant inhalation injury
   9. Patients with co-morbid conditions that could complicate the management
   10. Patients who need social or emotional support and/or long-term rehabilitative support including suspected family violence

B. Emergency treatment of severe burns while waiting transport of the patient to a burn center or an emergency department includes prompt IV fluid resuscitation with lactated Ringer's solution, elevating the burned areas, and administering 100% oxygen if inhalation injury is present

C. First aid consists of removing the burning agent and lavaging burned area with cool water or normal saline; chemical burns require extensive lavaging (at least 15 minutes)

D. Treatment of first degree burns from all causes except radiation
   1. Cleanse with mild detergent such as phisohex and water or saline
   2. May use topical anesthetic such as dibucaine (Nupercainal) cream or benzocaine (Americaine) spray 3-4 times a day as needed for pain
   3. No dressings needed

E. Treatment of second degree burns from all causes except radiation
   1. Cleanse burned areas with mild detergent such as phisoHex and sterile saline (may need to sedate patient with codeine or chloral hydrate 30 minutes before cleansing and debridement)
   2. Leave blisters intact unless they are large and thin-walled (may aspirate blister with 19-gauge hypodermic needle)
   3. Remove blistered skin that is almost detached and other devitalized skin
   4. For small burns on face cover with bacitracin ointment and leave open; for other small burns cover with bacitracin and apply nonadherent dressing and a bulky dressing to absorb drainage from burn
   5. For larger burns:
      a. Cover burned area with a thin layer of silver sulfadiazine 1% cream (Silvadene)
      b. For sulfa-allergic patients, use nitrofurazone (Furacin) cream
      c. Apply nonadherent gauze and bulky dressing to absorb drainage from burn
      d. Other appropriate dressings include transparent adhesive dressings (OpSite, Tegaderm) or a biosynthetic compound (Biobrane) that is applied directly to burn and wrapped in gauze

F. For mild sunburns use cool compresses and topical, dexamethasone aerosol spray every 3 hours; most effective if treatment is started within 12 hours of injury

G. Pain management of all types of burns is important; recommend regular use of aspirin, acetaminophen or a nonsteroidal anti-inflammatory drug

H. Tetanus prophylaxis is needed if the patient has not received either a course of immunizations or a booster within 10 years; see guidelines for tetanus prophylaxis in the WOUND section

I. Systemic antibiotics are given only if patient has a valvular disease or a concomitant streptococcal infection

J. Patient Education
   1. Teach patient to clean burned area completely twice a day with gentle soap and water, dry burn well, and reapply ointment or cream and dressing
   2. Keep dressing and/or burn clean and dry
   3. Increase fluid intake
   4. Elevate affected parts
   5. Maintain active range of motion of all joints with overlying burns
   6. Teach signs and symptoms of infection and need to return to provider if they occur

K. Follow Up
   1. Patients should be reevaluated in 24-48 hours for evidence of infection and change of dressing
   2. At least once a week, burn should be assessed for signs of complications at the health care site

CORNEAL ABRASION

I. Definition: Partial or complete removal of a focal area of epithelium on the cornea

II. Pathogenesis

   A. The cornea is composed of three principal layers: epithelium (the outer layer), stroma, and endothelium

   B. Disruption of the epithelium on the cornea by mechanical or chemical factors results in corneal abrasion

   C. Because the epithelium is richly innervated with sensory nerve endings, even the tiniest injuries are painful

III. Clinical Presentation

   A. Corneal injuries are very painful, with the degree of pain generally related to the amount of epithelial disruption

   B. Patients usually complain of a scratchy, gritty sensation (foreign body sensation) that develops suddenly and worsens with blinking

   C. Redness of the eye follows corneal insult due to the reactive conjunctival vasodilation (injection)

   D. Photophobia is often present and occurs because the disruption in the optical surface causes light to be scattered within the eye rather than focused so that bright light sources have a glaring appearance

IV. Diagnosis/Evaluation

   A. History
   1. Ask which eye is injured
   2. Determine how, when, and where the eye was injured
   3. Ascertain if eye pain or vision loss is present
   4. Ask if any eye protection was being used at time of injury and if anyone witnessed the injury
   5. Ask if contact lenses are being worn (or were being worn at time of injury)
   6. Ask about tetanus immunization status

B. Physical Examination
1. Measure visual acuity (**Note**: Even in the case of trauma, it is critically important to know visual ability is present; if patient is unable to read chart, acuity may be grossly evaluated by finger counting)
2. Evert the eyelids and examine the conjunctival fornices for foreign body (The presence of a foreign body under the upper lid should <u>always</u> be looked for in the presence of a suspected corneal abrasion)
3. Examine cornea for abrasions using the technique described in the following table:

FLUORESCEIN STAINING TO ASSESS CORNEAL EPITHELIAL INTEGRITY

Technique

▲ Instill 1 or 2 drops of a rapid onset and short duration topical anesthetic (e.g., proparacaine HCl 0.5% [Ophthetic])

▲ Moisten the fluorescein strip with sterile normal saline (can also touch strip to the tear film in the lower cul de sac of affected eye)

▲ Touch moistened fluorescein strip to lower conjunctiva of the eye being inspected (If used tear film to moisten, this step is unnecessary as dye has already been placed in eye)

▲ Ask patient to blink eye

▲ Illuminate the eye with cobalt blue light and inspect for patterns of fluorescence

▲ Remove excess dye with sterile saline and remind patient not to rub eye

Interpretation

▲ If the corneal epithelium has been disturbed, fluorescein will pool within these areas and stain the hydrophilic stroma; the resultant brighter fluorescence of these pools will delineate the corneal abrasion from surrounding intact epithelium

▲ The size and pattern of the defect depends on nature and extent of injury

▲ A characteristic pattern that suggests the presence of a foreign body trapped underneath the upper lid is a faint vertically- oriented pattern on the cornea

---

C. Differential Diagnosis
1. Corneal foreign body
2. Viral keratitis
3. Corneal laceration

D. Diagnostic Tests: None indicated beyond fluorescein staining described above

V. Plan/Management

A. Instil an antibiotic ointment such as erythromycin ophthalmic ointment (Ilotycin) OR gentamicin ophthalmic ointment (Garamycin) into the affected eye

B. Instruct patient to close injured eye and then apply a two-pad pressure dressing over the closed lids of the affected eye
1. The patch must be firm and tight such that the eye cannot be opened beneath it
2. Leave pad in place for 24 hours
3. Instruct patient to return to clinic after 24 hours for removal of dressing
4. Prescribe topical antibiotic ointment such as either of the ointments listed above, or drops such as sulfacetamide sodium solution (Sulamyd). Small amount of ointment or 2-3 drops should be used 4x/day x 5 days
5. Administer tetanus immunization if indicated

C. If the type of injury sustained is chemical, thermal, or a mechanical injury that has qualities of both blunt and sharp trauma, immediate transport to an ophthalmologist is required because of threat to vision

D. Follow Up: In 24 hours to remove patch and evaluate healing

HEAD TRAUMA, MINIMAL AND MILD

I. Definition: Trauma to the head; simple linear skull fractures and concussions are the most common examples of minor head injuries

    A. Simple linear skull fractures: small break in skull that is not associated with depressed bone fragments and underlying brain injury

    B. Concussion: Trauma-induced alteration in mental status that may or may not involve loss of consciousness (previously, to be diagnosed with a concussion, the patient had to have a loss of consciousness)

    C. Classification of head injuries (see following table)

CLASSIFICATION OF HEAD INJURIES		
Minimal	**Mild**	**Moderately or Potentially Severe**
All of the following:	Any of the following:	Any of the following:
* No loss of consciousness or amnesia * Glasgow Coma Scale score of 15 * Normal alertness and memory * No focal neurologic deficit * No palpable depressed skull fracture	* Brief (<5 min.) loss of consciousness * Amnesia for the event * Glasgow Coma Scale score of 14 * Impaired alertness and memory	* Prolonged (>5 min.) loss of consciousness * Glasgow Coma Scale score of <14 * Focal neurologic deficit * Posttraumatic seizure * Intracranial lesion detected on CT scan

Adapted from Smith, E.E. (1993). Minor head injury: A proposed strategy for emergency management. Annals of Emergency Medicine, 22, 1193-1196.

II. Pathogenesis:

    A. The most common cause of traumatic head injuries in all ages is falls; other common causes in adults are auto accidents, assaults, and sports injuries

    B. Outcomes following head trauma:
        1. Seriousness of the head injury is related to the nature and extent of the cerebral injury rather than the damage to the overlying scalp or skull structures
        2. Clinical course is dependent on the degree of acute injury to brain at the time of the accident (primary brain injury) and to delayed neurochemical and metabolic changes that result during the initial hours and days after the injury (secondary brain injury)
        3. Even minimal head injuries can result in a secondary brain injury which involves tissue injury, swelling, and ischemia
            a. Delayed cerebral edema may occur within 8-12 hours
            b. Maximal cerebral edema occurs within 48-72 hours after the injury
        4. "Second impact syndrome" occurs when a person (particularly an athlete) has a second concussion without recovering from the first; may lead to massive acute-brain swelling and ultimately, death; multiple head injuries can result in chronic impairment of brain function

III. Clinical Presentation

    A. Epidemiology
        1. Head injury is the most common cause of traumatic mortality in the U.S.
        2. Most patients with head injuries are between 15-24 years of age
        3. Males are 2-3 times more likely to have a head injury than females
        4. In 50-60% of adult cases with head injuries, a positive blood alcohol is detected

B. Simple or linear skull fractures
   1. Patients with linear fractures are usually asymptomatic, but any fracture requires close observation because the force required to fracture a skull is significant
   2. Skull fractures with underlying lacerations may predispose the patient to meningitis

C. Concussion
   1. Hallmarks are confusion and amnesia which occur immediately after injury or several minutes later
   2. Early symptoms (first few minutes or hours) include headache, dizziness or vertigo, lack of awareness of surroundings, and nausea and vomiting
   3. Postconcussive syndrome may occur and includes low-grade headaches, light-headedness, poor attention and concentration, memory dysfunction, reduced energy levels, intolerance of bright lights and noise, sleep disturbances, and irritability and depression; symptoms may last as long as 3 months post injury
   4. A grading scale based on severity of the injury is in the following table:

SCALE FOR GRADING THE SEVERITY OF CONCUSSION		
Grade 1	Grade 2	Grade 3
1. Transient confusion 2. No loss of consciousness 3. Concussion symptoms or mental status abnormalities on examination **resolve in *less* than 15 minutes**. Grade 1 concussion is the most common yet the most difficult form to recognize.	1. Transient confusion 2. No loss of consciousness 3. Concussion symptoms or mental status abnormalities on examination last *more* than 15 minutes. Grade 2 symptoms (greater than 1 hour) warrant medical observation.	1. Any loss of consciousness either brief (seconds) or prolonged (minutes). Grade 3 concussion is usually easy to recognize--the patient is unconscious for any period of time.

Adapted from American Academy of Neurology, Quality Standards Subcommittee: Practice parameter. (1997). The management of concussion in sports (summary statement). Neurology, 48, 581-585.

IV. Diagnosis/Evaluation

   A. History: Important to obtain information from the patient as well as a person at the scene of the injury as the patient may be amnestic or confused
      1. Determine how the injury occurred and the incidents surrounding the injury
      2. Ask whether the patient had a loss of consciousness and amnesia
      3. Inquire about symptoms after the injury such as vomiting, headaches, confusion, drowsiness, or abnormal behaviors
      4. Determine if there is any neck pain or pain in other areas of the body
      5. Inquire about other injuries
      6. Ask about self treatments
      7. Always ask about previous head injuries, particularly in athletes, to determine "second impact syndrome"

   B. Physical Examination
      1. To quickly rule out a serious injury which needs immediate intervention, perform the following
         a. Assess airway patency, breathing, and circulation
         b. Assess level of consciousness
         c. Measure vital signs
         d. Stabilize neck and check for signs of neck injury which often accompany head trauma
         e. Assess the thorax for hemothorax and pneumothorax
         f. Examine abdomen for signs of bleeding such as fullness and rigidity
         g. Signs of increased intracranial pressure are listed in the following table

<table>
<tr><td colspan="2">SIGNS OF INCREASED INTRACRANIAL PRESSURE[†]</td></tr>
<tr><td>* Papilledema
* Elevated systolic pressure
* Wide pulse pressure</td><td>* Decreased pulse
* Slow respirations</td></tr>
</table>

2. A rapid system for evaluating athletes who suffer injuries during an event is presented in the following table

QUICK EVALUATION OF ATHLETES WITH HEAD INJURIES DURING THE SPORTS EVENT

Mental Status Testing

Orientation	Time, place, person, and situation (circumstances of injury)
Concentration	Digits backward (e.g., 3-1-7, 4-6-8-2, 5-3-0-7-4) Months of the year in reverse order
Memory	Names of teams in prior contest; recall of 3 words and 3 objects at 0 and 5 minutes Recent newsworthy events; details of the contest (plays, moves, strategies, etc)
External Provocative Testing	40-yard sprint; 5 push ups; 5 sit ups; 5 knee bends (any appearance of associated symptoms is abnormal, e.g., headaches, dizziness, nausea, unsteadiness, photophobia, blurred or double vision, emotional lability, or mental status changes)

Neurologic Tests

Pupils	Symmetry and reaction
Coordination	Finger-nose-finger, tandem gait
Sensation	Finger-nose (eyes closed) and Romberg

Source: McCrea, M., Kelly, J.P., Kluge, J., Ackley, B., & Randolph, C. (1997). Standardized assessment of concussion in football players. Neurology, 48, 586-588.

3. After determining that the patient is not in acute distress, perform the following at frequent intervals:
   a. Use the Glasgow coma scale to quantitate mental status which can be used later to evaluate the patient's progress (see following table)

GLASGOW COMA SCALE FOR EVALUATING ADULTS*

Eye-Opening Response

Score	Response
4	Spontaneous
3	To verbal command
2	To pain
1	None

Motor Response

Score	Response
6	Obeys commands
5	Localizes pain
4	Withdraws from pain
3	Displays abnormal flexion to pain (decorticate rigidity)
2	Displays abnormal extension to pain (decerebrate rigidity)
1	None

Verbal Response

Score	Response
5	Is oriented and converses
4	Conversation is confused
3	Words are inappropriate
2	Sounds are incomprehensible
1	None

*Score of less than 8 denotes severe head injury

Adapted from Simon, J. (1992). Accidental injury and emergency medical services for children. In R.E. Behrman (Ed.). Nelson textbook of pediatrics. Philadelphia: WB Saunders.

      b.   Observe gait
      c.   Examine the eyes
          (1)   Evaluate pupillary size, equality, and reaction to light
          (2)   Perform funduscopy to detect retinal hemorrhage and papilledema
      d.   Carefully inspect and palpate head, noting wounds, indentations
      e.   Examine nasopharynx and ears for evidence of fresh blood
      f.   Palpate abdomen for signs of bleeding
      g.   Perform a complete neurologic examination including assessment of cranial nerves, reflexes, motor functioning, sensory functioning, and coordination
      h.   Assess mental status
      i.   Assess memory

C.   Differential Diagnosis: Crucial to identify persons who are at risk for development of complications such as intracranial mass lesions, intracranial edema, and delayed neurological deterioration

    1.   Age, co-morbidity, and mechanism of the injury are potential risk factors for severe head injuries (see following table)

RISK FACTORS FOR SEVERE HEAD INJURIES		
Mechanism	**Age**	**Medical Condition**
* High speed motor vehicle accident * Fall of more than 8 feet * Injury with extensive damage to other areas of body	* Greater than 65 years	* Long-term anticoagulant therapy * Presence of cerebrovascular malformation

Adapted from Marion, D.W. (1998). Acute head injuries in adults. In R.E. Rakel (Ed.), 1998 Conn's current therapy. Philadelphia: WB Saunders.

    2.   Common causes of serious head trauma include the following:
      a.   Basilar skull fractures
          (1)   Bruising around the eye (raccoon sign), blood in external auditory canal (Battle's sign), cerebrospinal fluid leakage in the ear or nose, and cranial nerve palsies often occur
          (2)   Fractures may not be present on plain x-rays, but are apparent on computed tomography (CT)
      b.   Cerebral contusion or laceration results from edema, hemorrhage and possibly necrosis
          (1)   Associated with trauma directly beneath the site of blunt or penetrating injury (coup) or may result from indirect trauma contralateral to the injury (contré coup)
          (2)   Typically, the patient has loss of consciousness for >2 minutes
          (3)   May result in death or severe residual neurologic deficits such as post-traumatic epilepsy
      c.   Acute epidural hemorrhage results from a tear in the meningeal artery, vein, or dural sinus and is usually associated with a skull fracture
          (1)   Several hours after injury the patient may have a headache, confusion, somnolence, seizures, or focal deficits
          (2)   Without treatment, coma, respiratory arrest, and death follow
      d.   Acute subdural hematoma is due to a tear in veins from cortex to superior sagittal sinus or from cerebral laceration
          (1)   More common injury than acute epidural hemorrhage
          (2)   The symptoms and complications are similar to an epidural hemorrhage but the interval before onset of symptoms is longer
      e.   Cerebral hemorrhage develops immediately after the injury with symptoms of intracranial pressures and distress; a hematoma is usually visible on CT scan
    3.   Typical characteristics of severe head injuries include the following:
      a.   Loss of consciousness associated with one or more neurologic deficits
      b.   Glasgow Coma Scale score of less than 8
      c.   Alterations in mental status

        d.   Prolonged memory deficit

        e.   Persistent vomiting and severe headache

        f.   Seizures

        g.   Signs of primary brainstem injury include coma, irregular breathing, fixation of pupils to light, and diffuse motor flaccidity

    4.   Family violence should always be included in differential diagnosis

D.   Diagnostic Tests:

    1.   No tests are needed in patients with minimal head trauma (see classification system in I.C.) who have no abnormal neurological signs but monitoring for neurological abnormalities should extend for at least 48 hours after the injury

    2.   CT scan is the most efficacious test for detecting intracranial injury but a skull x-ray is helpful in the following cases: penetrating injuries, possible depressed fractures, or suspected nonaccidental injuries; consider ordering skull x-rays in patients who have point tenderness or scalp hematomas

    3.   Order CT scans in patients who are classified as having mild, moderate, or severe head injuries (see I.C.) and patients with minimal head trauma if they have evidence of a skull fracture on x-ray or if they later develop abnormal neurological symptoms and signs

    4.   Always consider ordering cervical spine films or other radiographs for any patient depending on the mechanism and circumstances surrounding the injury

    5.   Consider ordering a blood alcohol

V.   Plan/Management

A.   Hospitalization

    1.   For patients with simple fractures and concussions without abnormal neurologic signs and symptoms, hospitalization is not required

    2.   Hospitalization is recommended in the following situations:

        a.   Suspicion of family violence

        b.   All head injuries categorized as mild, moderate, or severe

        c.   Injuries accompanied with a neurologic deficit

        d.   Any mechanism severe enough to cause concern of secondary brain injury

B.   For patients who are not hospitalized, careful monitoring for delayed abnormal signs and symptoms is essential; patient education includes the following:

    1.   Teach family members that there is a need for thorough, frequent observation and precautions for at least 48 hours after the injury; recommend the following:

        a.   Check whether pupils are equal and react to light

        b.   Determine arousability and coherence by waking patient every 4 hours

        c.   Time respiratory rate and check whether respiratory pattern is regular

    2.   Call health care provider for any of the following:

        a.   Headaches which worsen

        b.   Vomiting becomes more frequent

        c.   Pupils are unequal or do not react to light

        d.   Symptoms such as seizures, neck pain, drowsiness, confusion, difficulty walking, talking, or visualizing occur

        e.   Respirations increase, decrease, or become irregular

    3.   Instruct family members that patient should be observed for the development of complications for at least 2 weeks after the injury; signs of complications include drowsiness, vomiting, gait disturbance, or severe headache

    4.   Emphasize to family members of athletes, that repeat head injuries can lead to permanent brain damage

C.   Guidelines for the management of sports-related concussions were developed by the American Academy of Neurology

    1.   Initial management following the head injury depends on the grade of the concussion (see III.C.4)

        a.   Athletes with Grade 1 injuries may return to play the same day if the following are met: Normal on-site evaluation (see IV.B.2) while at rest and with exertion, including a normal, detailed mental status examination

b. Athletes with Grade 2 and Grade 3 injuries must have a complete neurologic examination and may not return to play the same day

2. Decisions on when to return to play after removal from the athletic event are based on grade of the concussion and whether previous head injuries have occurred (see table that follows)

RECOMMENDATIONS ON ATHLETE'S RETURN TO PLAY	
Grade of Concussion	Time Until Return to Play*
Multiple Grade 1 concussions	1 week
Grade 2 concussions	1 week
Multiple Grade 2 concussions	2 weeks
Grade 3--brief loss of consciousness (seconds)	1 week
Grade 3--brief loss of consciousness (minutes)	2 weeks
Multiple Grade 3 concussions	1 month or longer, based on clinical decision of evaluating health care provider

*Only after being asymptomatic with normal neurologic assessment at rest and with exercise.

Adapted from American Academy of Neurology, Quality Standards Subcommittee: Practice parameter. (1997). The management of concussion in sports (summary statement). Neurology, 48, 581-585.

D. Prevention of head injuries
1. Remind patients to wear safety belts in motor vehicles and helmets when riding a bike or motorcycle
2. Proper safety equipment is needed for even recreational sports
3. Measures to prevent falls in the household such as removing loose carpets and maintaining uncluttered, well-lit walkways are important

E. Follow Up
1. Frequent monitoring of all head injuries is important
2. Communicate with family members within first 4-12 hours after the injury and then periodically depending on the clinical condition of the patient

INSECT STING AND BROWN RECLUSE SPIDER BITE

I. Definition: A sting or bite in which there is secretion of venom into skin by insect or spider

II. Pathogenesis

A. Insect Sting
1. Honeybees, bumblebees, wasps, hornets, and yellow-jackets (hymenoptera) embed a firm, sharp stinger in the skin; venom is secreted
2. Honeybees leave their stingers in the skin (with venom sac attached; other hymenoptera have a retractable stinger and thus may sting many times)
3. The injected venoms are proteins with enzyme activity that can cause local or general reactions, or both; reactions are classified as toxic or allergic

B. Brown Recluse Spider Bite
1. Of the 50 or so species known to bite humans, the brown recluse spider (*Loxosceles reclusa*) is one of two species in the US (black widow is the other) capable of producing severe reactions

2. Brown recluse spider is small (1.5 cm or less) light brown, and lives in dark areas such as closets, under porches, or in basements; usually found in river country of mid-America, most commonly in the south-central US
3. Spider venom is composed of enzyme-spreading factor hyaluronidase, and a toxin distributed by the enzyme
4. The venom of the spider is antigenic and once a person has been bitten, subsequent bites are not severe
5. Spider bite can cause local or general reactions, but does not cause allergic reactions

III. Clinical Presentation

A. Insect Sting
1. A sharp, pinprick sensation is felt at the instant of stinging followed by burning pain at site
2. A red papule or weal appears, enlarges, then subsides within hours
3. Multiple stings can cause a toxic reaction producing symptoms such as syncope, dizziness, vomiting, diarrhea, and headache because of the large toxin load
4. Allergic reactions begin as localized toxic reactions but quickly (within minutes or hours) produce an exaggerated urticarial response
5. Generalized reactions begin 2-60 minutes after sting and range from a few hives to anaphylaxis; forty percent of persons with generalized allergic reactions have a previous history of similar reaction
6. Anaphylaxis symptoms include generalized itching, hypotension, shortness of breath, and wheezing which may subside spontaneously or progress to edema of upper airway causing obstruction and death

B. Brown Recluse Spider Bite
1. Bite may feel sharp, or it might cause little or no pain; subsequent minor swelling and erythema at site often occur
2. Severity of local reaction appears to depend on site of bite with fatty areas of body developing more severe reactions
3. Tissue necrosis in bite area may develop as early as four hours after bite
4. Cutaneous changes at the site include a blue-gray, macular halo around puncture site; emergence of pustule, or vesicle/bulla at site; widening of macule and sinking of center of lesions producing a "sinking infarct;" sloughing of tissue leaving a deep ulcer which takes weeks or months to heal
5. In a few cases, within 12 hours after bite, systemic symptoms of fever, chills, nausea, vomiting, and generalized weakness may appear; rarely severe systemic reactions of generalized hemolysis, disseminated intravascular coagulation, and renal failure occur (usually only in children)

IV. Diagnosis/Evaluation

A. History
1. Quickly question regarding type of bite or sting, time of occurrence, and location of bite/sting
2. If sting, quickly determine if allergic reaction is present (generalized itching, shortness of breath, and wheezing)
3. If sting, question about history of previous allergic reactions

> ***** **ALERT** *****
> **If allergic reaction is present or anticipated based on history,**
> **go immediately to treatment.**

4. If bite, determine type of spider if patient can describe
5. If bite, ask about presence of systemic symptoms such as fever, chills, nausea, vomiting, and weakness

B. Physical Examination
   1. If history suggests a severe anaphylactic reaction is imminent, do not complete exam or wait for symptoms to develop, institute treatment immediately (See V.B., below)
   2. If sting with no allergic reaction evident or anticipated based on history, take pulse, respirations, and blood pressure
   3. Examine site of bite or sting for characteristic erythema and edema. If spider bite which occurred within hours, examine for characteristic progression of site described under Brown Recluse Spider bite, above

C. Differential Diagnosis
   1. Vasovagal attacks: May follow pain or upset and be accompanied by nausea, diaphoresis and hypotension; lasts only a few minutes and relieved by lying down
   2. Hyperventilation episodes: Accompanied by tachypnea, perioral tingling, but BP is maintained and other signs of anaphylaxis are absent

D. Diagnostic Tests: None indicated for bites or stings with no systemic symptoms

V. Plan/Treatment

A. Treatment of anaphylactic reactions is based on type of reaction which can range from mild to life-threatening; in all cases, epinephrine is the drug of choice

B. Treatment of mild anaphylaxis is outlined in the table that follows

TREATMENT OF MILD ANAPHYLAXIS
For mild symptoms of pruritus, erythema, urticaria, and wheezing, treat with epinephrine injected subcutaneously, followed by diphenhydramine, hydroxyzine, or other antihistamine given orally or parenterally
Epinephrine, 1:1000 (aqueous) 0.01 mL/kg per dose, administered subcutaneously. Usual dose for adults: 0.3-0.5 mL
Repeat in 10-20 minutes; monitor patient's condition constantly, and monitor BP every 10 minutes
Antihistamine: Give **one** of the following: Hydroxyzine, Oral or IM: Give 0.5-1 mg/kg/dose (100 mg maximum single dose) Diphenhydramine, Oral, or IM: Give 1-2 mg/kg/dose (100 mg maximum single dose)
If symptoms improve with this management, give a long-acting epinephrine injection (Sus-Phrine) as a single dose, 0.005 mL/gm. Usual dose for adults: 0.15-0.25 mL
Also, give oral antihistamines for next 24 hours; see dosing above
Observe patient in clinic for several hours before discharging to home. Instruct patient to apply ice to site and elevate the affected extremity to control local reaction
Follow Up: By telephone in 12-24 hours.

C. For severe and potentially life-threatening systemic anaphylaxis (bronchospasm, laryngeal edema, hypotension, shock, and cardiovascular collapse) institute the following and call 911 for immediate transport

TREATMENT OF SEVERE ANAPHYLAXIS
Promptly institute airway maintenance and oxygen therapy **Give Intravenous (IV) epinephrine**
A slow continuous infusion is preferable to repeated bolus administration. For a continuous infusion, add one milligram (1 mL) of 1:1000 dilution of epinephrine to 250 mL of 5% dextrose in water, resulting in a concentration of 4 μg/mL; initially infuse at a rate of 0.1 μg/kg/minute and increase gradually to 1.5 μg/kg/minute to maintain blood pressure
If bronchospasm is prominent, inhaled β_2 agonist: Albuterol (Ventolin) should be administered via nebulizer. Usual dose for adults: 2.5 mg (0.5 cc of 0.5% solution) in 2 cc saline
Transport to emergency department

D. Prevention of recurrence in patients with mild to severe anaphylactic reactions
1. Refer patient for allergy testing with insect venom to identify the venom responsible for sensitization
2. Five venoms are commercially available for this purpose: honeybee, yellow jacket, yellow hornet, white-faced hornet, and Polistes wasps
3. If skin tests produce ambiguous results, a RAST can be performed to detect IgE antibody to venoms
4. Immunization with insect venom can prevent future systemic reactions in patients with a previously documented reaction

E. Emergency treatment kits (available by prescription) for self-treatment before reaching medical help should be obtained by all persons at risk for anaphylaxis from insect stings
1. Patients should be prescribed 3 kits: one for home, one for car, and one to carry
2. Ana-Kit (Hollister-Stier, Spokane, WA) contains a preloaded syringe; refill syringes (Ana-Guard) are available
3. Epi-Pen or Epi-Pen Junior are spring-loaded automatic injectors for individuals reluctant to perform self-injection

F. Patients should also wear a medical alert tag

G. For insect stings which are localized with mild urticaria
1. Remove stinger if present using forceps, or by scraping out (do not attempt to squeeze out)
2. Wash the wound thoroughly and apply ice packs
3. Prescribe oral antihistamines (see above for dosing of hydroxyzine and diphenhydramine) to relieve local reaction and discomfort
4. Recommend continued use of ice packs and elevation for the next 8-12 hours

H. For moderate swelling, the interventions outlined above should be used. In addition, a short course (5 days) of oral steroids is also recommended

I. Treatment of the brown recluse bite is somewhat controversial; there are no accepted, conclusively established guidelines
1. All experts recommend the following conservative treatment
a. Gentle cleansing with soap and water
b. Apply ice and elevate
c. Avoid strenuous exercise
d. AVOID APPLICATION OF HEAT
e. Give tetanus toxoid if indicated
2. Controversy surrounds which drugs, if any, are indicated
a. No drug treatments are indicated, according to most experts (excellent outcomes usually occur without any pharmacologic interventions)
b. Some experts recommend systemic steroids for patients who are seen within 24 hours of the bite; methylprednisolone, 100 mg IV, followed by oral prednisone for 5 days
c. Some experts recommend Dapsone, 50-200 mg per day, even though it has many side effects and must be used with extreme caution
d. Antibiotic treatment may be helpful, but use is recommended only in treating secondary infection (prophylactic use has not been proven to be of any benefit)
(1) If secondary infection present, erythromycin is a good choice
(2) Dosing: Erythromycin (as base) [E-Mycin] 250 mg QID x 10 days
e. Use of oral and intralesional steroids have not been shown to decrease progressive reaction in patients with clinically significant bites (necrosis >1 cm)
3. In previous years, early debridement was the most commonly advocated brown recluse spider bite therapy; this is no longer done as no evidence supports the belief that this procedure promotes healing and reduces complications

Follow Up
  1. Stings: In 24-24 hours (may be by telephone) for patients with mild anaphylactic symptoms; none indicated for those with localized reactions only
  2. Brown recluse spider bite: No follow up is needed, but patients must be instructed to report any systemic problems such as headache, myalgia, fever, chills, gastrointestinal complaints, rash and darkening of urine (the presentation of hemolysis is within the first weeks); complications of wound healing may occur at any time until resolution and patients must be instructed in signs and symptoms of wound infection

OCULAR FOREIGN BODY

I. Definition: Presence of a foreign body in the cul-de-sacs and under the upper lid or on the cornea

II. Pathogenesis

  A. A foreign body of the conjunctiva occurs when particles become entrapped under the upper lid or in the cul-de-sacs

  B. Most often occurs with blowing dirt or sand; there is usually no trauma involved

  C. A foreign body of the cornea occurs when substances become embedded in the corneal epithelium most often due to some traumatic event

  D. A sudden event such as an explosion, or an accident involving metal grinding may scatter small fragments onto the cornea

III. Clinical Presentation

  A. The most common conjunctival foreign bodies are dust, sand, and contact lenses

  B. The most common foreign bodies found on the cornea are metallic, often rusty particles

  C. Foreign bodies may be single or multiple, easily seen without magnification or barely detectable with slit-lamp examination

  D. Symptoms are photophobia, lacrimation, and foreign body sensation

IV. Diagnosis/Evaluation

  A. History
    1. Ask which eye is injured
    2. Determine how, when, and where the eye was injured
    3. Ascertain if eye pain or vision loss is present
    4. Ask if any eye protection was being used at time of injury and if anyone witnessed the injury (important for medicolegal reasons)
    5. Ask if contact lenses are in place (or were in place at time of injury)
    6. Ask about tetanus immunization status
    7. Note: Based on history, if foreign body is result of explosion, blunt or sharp trauma, (i.e., if corneal foreign body is suspected) eye should be protected from further damage by placing eye shield over eye (or if shield not available, a paper cup to prevent rubbing eye) at this point and person transported for emergency care

B. Physical Examination
   1. Measure visual acuity (Note: Even in the case of trauma, it is critically important to know visual ability is present; if patient is unable to read chart, acuity may be grossly evaluated by finger counting)
   2. Evert the eyelids and examine for foreign body
   3. Technique for everting the eyelid is as follows:

EVERSION OF THE UPPER LID
▲ Instill 1 or 2 drops of a rapid onset, short duration topical ophthalmologic anesthetic such as proparacaine HCl (Ophthetic, 0.5%) into the affected eye
▲ Ask patient to look down
▲ Grasp the lashes with one hand and apply gentle pressure on the lid above the tarsal plate with a cotton-tip applicator with the other hand
▲ Foreign bodies such as soft contact lenses and grit are often found in superior temporal cul-de-sac of the orbit

   4. Examine the inferior cul-de-sac by having the person look up while the lower lid is pulled down

V. Plan/Management

   A. When foreign body is visualized, sweep sterile cotton-tipped swab moistened with topical anesthetic across conjunctival area to remove the object
      1. If there is difficulty with removal or if patient complains of severe pain, attempts should be discontinued
      2. Refer to ophthalmologist

   B. After removal of conjunctival foreign body (or if conjunctival foreign body cannot be located), determine if corneal abrasion present (See CORNEAL ABRASION)
      1. If no corneal abrasion present, prescribe topical antibiotic ointment or drops such as sulfacetamide sodium (Sulamyd); apply small amount of ointment or 2-3 drops to affected eye 4x/day x 5 days
      2. If corneal abrasion present, see CORNEAL ABRASION for treatment recommendations
      3. Provide tetanus immunization if indicated

   C. Follow Up: In 24 hours

SUBCONJUNCTIVAL HEMORRHAGE

I. Definition: A flat, bright-red hemorrhage under the conjunctiva

II. Pathogenesis

   A. May occur spontaneously, with raised venous pressure from a forced Valsalva maneuver (as in coughing, sneezing)

   B. May occur with minor or major trauma

III. Clinical Presentation

   A. Presents as a striking flat, deep-red hemorrhage under the conjunctiva and may become sufficiently severe to cause a "bag of blood" to protrude over lid margin

   B. Subconjunctival hemorrhage is usually asymptomatic

IV.   Diagnosis/Evaluation

    A.   History
       1.   Determine which eye affected how, when, and where the injury occurred
       2.   Ascertain if eye pain, discharge of secretions, or vision loss is present
       3.   Ask if patient has had previous symptoms or complaints similar to the current complaint

    B.   Physical Examination
       1.   Measure visual acuity
       2.   Examine lids and the adnexa for symmetry, swelling, abnormal discharge, and erythema
       3.   Palpate the soft tissue of the orbit, lids, and zygoma
       4.   Inspect the conjunctiva and sclera for localized swelling, signs of hemorrhage
       5.   Examine pupils for size, shape, reaction to light, and perform funduscopic exam

    C.   Differential Diagnosis
       1.   Conjunctivitis
       2.   Conjunctival laceration

    D.   Diagnostic Tests: None indicated

V.   Plan/Management

    A.   With no other signs and symptoms, no treatment is required; the patient should be reassured that the blood will clear over a 2-3 week period

    B.   If trauma with a sharp object is suspected, or if there is impaired vision, eye pain, foreign body sensation, discharge of secretions from the eye, change in the appearance of the globe, patient should be referred to an ophthalmologist for evaluation

    C.   Follow Up: None required; for patients with signs and symptoms described under V.B. above, follow-up should be by the ophthalmologist to whom the patient was referred

WOUNDS

I.   Definition: Breach in the external surface of the body

II.   Pathogenesis

    A.   Wounds such as lacerations and abrasions typically heal through a 3 stage process: clotting, inflammatory and proliferative stages

    B.   Devitalized tissue, oral secretions, toxic solutions, soil and dirt, and injurious forces can impede the healing process and possibly cause infection

    C.   *Staphylococcus aureus* and *β-hemolytic streptococcus* are the most common pathogens causing wound infection

    D.   Tetanus can also occur due to multiplication of *Clostridium tetani*, producing a toxin which can block motor neurons

III.   Clinical Presentation

    A.   Mechanism of injury is important in determining likelihood of infection and tissue damage
       1.   Sharp objects often make smooth cuts which can penetrate deep structures
       2.   Crushing injuries often damage underlying tissues and can result in fractures

3. Human bites have the greatest risk of bacterial infection and can also transmit hepatitis B and possibly human immunodeficiency virus (HIV)

B. Location or environment in which the wound occurred suggests potential problems; wounds which occur in dirty soil such as farmyards are at risk for contamination with spores of *Clostridium tetani*

C. The time interval between when the wound first occurred to when the patient received appropriate care affects the chances of infection; if 6 hours have elapsed, bacterial multiplication is likely

D. Site of the wound influences rate of healing and potential for complications:
   1. Due to rich vascular supply, wounds on face heal rapidly, but may create future cosmetic problems
   2. Hands are used extensively; wounds on hands have increased risk for reinjury and infection

E. Certain types of wounds may be problematic
   1. Dirty wounds are more at risk for infection
   2. Deep wounds can cause underlying tissue destruction and also have increased risk of contamination
   3. Wounds with untidy edges often heal slowly and may heal with disfigurement
   4. Wounds with tissue necrosis have potential for infection and delayed healing

F. Characteristics of the patient are also factors in wound healing; elderly patients, undernourished patients, patients on corticosteroids and chemotherapeutic agents, and patients with underlying illnesses have the greatest risk for adverse sequela from wounds

G. Tetanus is a rare but dangerous complication of a wound and is characterized by trismus and severe muscular spasms

IV. Diagnosis/Evaluation

A. History
   1. Ask patient to explicitly describe how the wound occurred
   2. Determine where the injury was sustained
   3. Question how much time has elapsed since the wound occurred
   4. Ascertain tetanus immunization status
   5. Ask about allergies to drugs, dressings, and local anesthetics
   6. Ask about current medication use, especially steroid and anticoagulant therapy
   7. Inquire about past medical history to determine if patient has underlying illness such as immunodeficiency which could affect healing process
   8. Ask whether the patient has a tendency to form keloids, because this could result in a poor scar

B. Physical Examination: Always use sterile technique when examining wounds; it may be necessary to apply local or regional anesthesia prior to the examination
   1. Measure wound
   2. Assess depth of wound
   3. Explore wound for foreign bodies
   4. Fully examine underlying structures
   5. Assess circulation, sensation and movement distal to wound
   6. Palpate underlying bone
   7. Assess range of motion and strength against resistance of all body parts surrounding wound site
   8. Examination of the patient with an old wound includes the following:
      a. Carefully inspect wound and surrounding area
      b. Palpate for local lymphadenopathy
      c. Measure patient's temperature

C. Differential Diagnosis: Always consider the possibility of non-accidental injury (see following table)

INDICATORS OF POSSIBLE NON-ACCIDENTAL INJURY
• Delay between injury and seeking treatment
• The history of the accident does not match the observed injury
• The history changes
• Other injuries, especially if at different stages of healing
• Signs of general neglect or failure to thrive
• Signs of family tension or indications of alcohol or drug abuse

Adapted from Wardrope, J., & Smith, J.R.R. (1992). The Management of wounds and burns. New York: Oxford.

D. Diagnostic Tests
1. Order x-rays for crushing, and deep penetrating wounds
2. Obtain wound swabs for culture on any wound which is slow to heal; fresh wounds do not require a culture

V. Plan/Management

A. The following wounds should be managed by an health care provider with extensive experience in wound management
1. Wounds involving nerve, tendon, or bone damage
2. Wounds with full thickness skin loss
3. Facial and hand wounds (small, superficial wounds, however, may be treated in outpatient setting)

B. Wound-cleansing is the first step of wound care
1. Irrigate wound with one of the following:
    a. Normal saline is an economical and effective irritant
    b. Povidone-iodine, hydrogen peroxide, and other detergents can cause tissue toxicity and should not be used
    c. Use high-pressure irrigation which can be achieved with a 35- or 65-ml syringe and a 16- or 19- gauge needle; higher pressure may result in tissue trauma and should be reserved for highly contaminated wounds
2. Apply mechanical force to clean wound: may use a fine-pore sponge such as an Optipore with a surfactant such as poloxamer 188 (Shur Clens)

C. Preparation of the wound site is next
1. Debridement of devitalized tissue is important
2. Clip, do not shave, surrounding hair as close to skin surface as possible

D. After appropriately preparing the wound, the next step is to decide whether to apply sutures; the following wounds require open-wound management:
1. Abrasions and superficial lacerations
2. Wounds with a great deal of tissue damage
3. Wound which have a low risk for infection of >12-24 hours of age
4. Wounds which have a high risk for infection of >6 hours of age
5. Wounds contaminated by feces, human or animal saliva, or large amounts of soil or dirt
6. Abrasions or wounds involving large superficial denudement of skin

E. Wound dressings: Best environment for wounds which are not sutured is a moist one; the following occlusive or semiocclusive dressings can promote a moist environment and all are effective
1. Occlusive dressings such as duoderm, telfa, and Opsite can be used
2. Hydrocolloid dressing is another possible choice (good for leg ulcers and pressure sores)
3. Hydrogel dressing such a Vigilon may be selected
4. Foam dressings are another choice

F.   Closure of the wound with tape (Steri-strip) is appropriate if the wound is superficial, has little tension, the edges are well approximated, and the injured area has full range of motion

G.   Other wounds require sutures
1.   Anesthesia
a.   Inject 1% buffered lidocaine hydrochloride (Xylocaine) or 0.25% or 0.50% bupivacaine (may cause less discomfort than lidocaine)
b.   Topical anesthetics such a mixture of tetracaine, adrenaline, and cocaine (TAC) are generally not recommended because they are expensive, not reliable when used below the head, may be toxic to the tissue, and cause other complications
c.   Do not use any anesthetic containing epinephrine in an area in which circulation is easily compromised such as fingers, toes, nose, penis or ears
2.   Wound edge approximation should be achieved with little or no tension to the surrounding area. Tension would be indicated by puckering of the skin
a.   In patients with a history of keloid formation, close skin with minimal tension and consider applying a pressure dressing for 3-6 months
b.   Many different suture techniques are available; suturing technique will depend on site and extent of injury
c.   Different suture materials are available
(1)   Skin is usually closed with nonabsorbable suture material such as nylon, prolene, or silk
(2)   Subcutaneous tissue and mucosal surfaces are usually closed with absorbable material, such as Dexon, Vicryl, or plain or chromic gut
(3)   Rapidly dissolving suture forms may be used to close the skin in some patients to avoid the discomfort associated with follow up suture removal
3.   Delayed primary closures with sutures
a.   This technique is used for wounds that cannot be closed initially because of gross contamination, potential injury to joints or other deep structures, retained foreign bodies, host immune status or an inability to adequately cleanse the wound
b.   Consider closing wound in 3-5 days when the risk of infection decreases
4.   Care of wound after suturing
a.   For simple lacerations, place gauze over suture line and cover with occlusive dressing for 24-48 hours. For more complex lacerations, immobilize injured body part for 5-7 days and apply bulky dressing; some advocate wound closure tape directly over the sutures
b.   Splint sutured wounds which are over or around a joint
c.   Instruct patient to keep wound clean and dry for at least 48 hours

H.   Tissue adhesives or glue such as cyanoacrylates have been used in Europe and Canada and are under review by the Food and Drug Administration (FDA)
1.   Apply adhesive by approximating wound margins with one hand and applying adhesive with the other; apply just enough adhesive to close the wound
2.   Application is rapid and painless
3.   Suture removal is not necessary as adhesives slough off in 7-10 days
4.   Adhesives act as their own dressings and have antimicrobial effects against gram-positive organisms
5.   Disadvantages are that adhesives have lower tensile strength than sutures and may break over high-tension areas such as joints

I.   Certain types of wounds require different therapy
1.   Puncture wounds should have very high-powered irrigation with saline; do not close puncture wounds with sutures
2.   Flap wounds which have edges which are not approximated should be cleaned, non-viable fat should be removed, and steristrips should be applied to appose but not close the wound

J.   Topical antibiotic ointments can be applied to open or sutured wounds
1.   Polysporin, bacitracin, and mupirocin are appropriate choices
2.   Avoid neosporin because it may cause allergies

K. Oral antibiotics are sometimes used for prophylactic purposes to prevent infection
    1. Prophylactic antibiotics should be given in the following cases:
        a. Most mammal bites (see section on BITE WOUNDS)
        b. Puncture wounds in which cleansing was difficult
        c. Patients with valvular disease or implants who are at risk for bacteremia
    2. Also, consider prophylactic antibiotics in the following cases:
        a. Heavily contaminated wounds
        b. Wounds with delayed treatment
        c. Wounds with tissue necrosis
    3. Choose one of the following antibiotics for prophylaxis
        a. Amoxicillin-clavulanate (Augmentin) can be used as prophylactic antibiotic; Prescribe 250-500 mg every 8 hours.
        b. For patients with penicillin allergies, prescribe erythromycin (E-Mycin) 250 mg QID for 7-10 days

L. Prevention of tetanus is important (following table provides guidelines on tetanus prophylaxis)

GUIDE TO TETANUS PROPHYLAXIS IN WOUND MANAGEMENT				
History of Tetanus Immunization (doses)	Clean, Minor Wounds		All Other Wounds**	
	Td*	TIG*	Td*	TIG*
Uncertain or <3	Yes	No	Yes	Yes
3 or More[†]	No[‡]	No	No[§]	No

*Td = adult-type tetanus and diphtheria toxoids. TIG = tetanus immune globulin.
**Such as, but not limited to, wounds contaminated with dirt, feces, soil, and saliva; puncture wounds; avulsions; and wounds resulting from missiles, crushing, burns, and frostbite
[†]If only 3 doses of fluid toxoid have been received, a fourth dose of toxoid, preferably an adsorbed toxoid, should be given.
[‡]Yes, if >10 years since the last dose.
[§]Yes, if >5 years since the last dose.

Adapted from American Academy of Pediatrics. (1997). Tetanus. In G. Peter (Ed.), 1997 red book: Report of the Committee on Infectious Disease. 24th ed. Elk Grove Village, IL: American Academy of Pediatrics.

M. Patient Education
    1. Teach patient to return if wound is increasingly painful, if there is significant discharge or if there is spreading of redness around wound or a red streak developing from the wound in the direction of the heart
    2. Inform patient that appearance of the wound and subsequent scar will change substantially during the year after the injury; thus, decisions for scar revision should be made after one year
    3. Advise patients to avoid sun exposure of their wounds to reduce the risk of developing hyperpigmentation

N. Follow Up
    1. On return visits evaluate and consider hospitalization or aggressive antimicrobial therapy if signs and symptoms of pyogenic abscess, cellulitis, and ascending lymphangitis (red line spreading proximally on a limb) are present
    2. Return for reevaluation, dressing change and/or suture removal in 2 days
    3. Time to remove sutures depends on wound location; apply surgical adhesives or tape after sutures are removed
        a. Facial wounds: 3-5 days
        b. Scalp wounds: 7-10 days
        c. Hand wounds: 10-14 days
        d. Lower legs: 14 days
        e. Other: 7-21 days

REFERENCES

Allwood, J.S. (1995). The primary care management of burns. <u>Nurse Practitioner, 20</u> (8), 74-87.

American Academy of Pediatrics. (1997). Bite wounds. In G. Peter (Ed.), <u>Red book: Report of the Committee on Infectious Diseases</u> (24th ed.). Elk Grove Village, IL: Author.

American Academy of Pediatrics. (1997). Rabies. In G. Peter (Ed.), <u>Red book: Report of the Committee on Infectious Diseases</u> (24th ed.). Elk Grove Village, IL: Author.

American Academy of Pediatrics. (1997). Tetanus. In G. Peter (Ed.), <u>Red book: Report of the Committee on Infectious Diseases</u> (24th ed.). Elk Grove Village, IL: Author.

American Academy of Pediatrics. (1997). Treatment of anaphylactic reactions. In G. Peter (Ed.), <u>Red book: Report of the committee on infectious diseases</u> (24th ed.). Elk Grove Village, IL: Author.

American Burn Association. (1996). <u>Guidelines for transfer of patients in burn centers.</u> New York: American Burn Association.

American Academy of Neurology, Quality Standards Subcommittee: Practice parameter. (1997). The management of concussion in sports (summary statement). <u>Neurology, 48,</u> 581-585.

Anderson, P.C. (1997). Spider bites in the United States. <u>Dermatologic Clinics, 15</u>(2), 307-311.

Arminoff, M.J. (1998). Nervous system. In L.M. Tierney, S.J. McPhee, & M.A. Papadakis (Eds.), <u>Current medical diagnosis and treatment 1998</u> (37th ed.). Stamford, CT: Appleton & Lange.

Cornell, S. (1997, August). When animals attack. <u>Advance for Physician Assistants</u>, 47-50.

Crown, L.A., Lofton, B., & Magill, E. (1998). A 20-year old woman with an insect bite. <u>Family Practice Recertification, 20</u>(4), 22-29.

Doody, D.P. (1999). Lacerations and abrasions. In R.A. Dershewitz (Ed.), <u>Ambulatory pediatric care</u>. Philadelphia: Lippincott.

Gruen, P., & Liu, C. (1998). Current trends in the management of head injury. <u>Contemporary Issues in Trauma, 16,</u> 63-83.

Hall, D.E. (1997). Head injuries. In R.A. Hoekelman (Ed.), <u>Primary pediatric care</u> (3rd ed.). St. Louis: Mosby.

Howell, J.M., & Chisholm, C.D. (1997). Wound care. <u>Emergency Medical Clinics of North America, 15,</u> 417-425.

Kelly, J.P., & Rosenberg, J.H. (1997). Diagnosis and management of concussion in sports. <u>Neurology, 48,</u> 575-580.

Lloyd, D.A., Carty, H., Patterson, M., Butcher, C.K., & Roe, D. (1997). Predictive value of skull radiography for intracranial injury in children with blunt head injury. <u>Lancet, 349,</u> 821-824.

Marion, D.W. (1998). Acute head injuries in adults. In R.E. Rakel (Ed.), <u>1998 Conn's current therapy</u>. Philadelphia: WB Saunders.

McCrea, M., Kelly, J.P., Kluge, J., Ackley, B., & Randolph, C. (1997). Standardized assessment of concussion in football players. <u>Neurology, 48,</u> 586-588.

Monafo, W.W. (1996). Initial management of burns. <u>New England Journal of Medicine, 335,</u> 1581-1586.

National Association of State Public Health Veterinarians, Inc. (1997). Compendium of animal rabies control 1997. <u>MMWR, 46</u> (RR-4), 1-15.

Pavan-Langston, D. (1996). <u>Manual of ocular diagnosis and therapy</u>. Boston: Little, Brown and Company.

Presutti, R.J. (1997). Bite wounds: Early treatment and prophylaxis against infectious complications. <u>Postgraduate Medicine, 101,</u> 243-253.

Singer, A.J., Hollander, J.E., & Quinn, J.V. (1997). Evaluation and management of traumatic lacerations. <u>New England Journal of Medicine, 337,</u> 1142-1148.

Smith, E.E. (1993). Minor head injury: A proposed strategy for emergency management. <u>Annals of Emergency Medicine, 22,</u> 1193-1196.

Trued, S.J. (1997). Minor soft tissue injuries and infections. In L. Dornbrand, A.J. Hoole, & R.H. Fletcher. (Eds.), <u>Manual of clinical problems in adult ambulatory care</u> (3rd ed.). Philadelphia: Lippincott-Raven.

Varma, R. (1997). <u>Essentials of eye care</u>. Philadelphia: Lippincott-Raven.

Wardrope, J., & Smith, J.A.R. (1992) <u>The management of wounds and burns</u>. New York: Oxford University Press.

Widell, T. (1998). Eye, ear, nose, throat, and dental emergencies. In S. H. Plantz, & J.N. Adler (Eds.), <u>Emergency medicine</u>. Baltimore: Williams & Wilkins.

Wipfler, E.J. (1998). Insect and arachnid bites and stings. In S. H. Plantz, & J.N. Adler (Eds.), <u>Emergency medicine</u>. Baltimore: Williams & Wilkins.

Zaveruha, A., Bishop, D., St. Clair, A., & Moreau, K. (1997). Rabies update for primary-care practitioners. <u>Clinical Excellence for Nurse Practitioners, 1,</u> 367-375.

INDEX

BARMARRAE BOOKS, INC.

ORDERING INFORMATION

1-888-276-7780

Credit card orders (VISA or MasterCard) or institutional purchase orders may be placed toll free 8 A.M. - 5 P.M. EST weekdays at the above telephone number.

Credit card orders (VISA or MasterCard) or institutional purchase orders may be faxed 24 hours to **1-352-378-1441**

OR

Please photocopy or clip the order form below and mail with your check, money order, or purchase order to:

BARMARRAE BOOKS, INC.
3017 NW 62ND TERRACE
GAINESVILLE, FL 32606

Note to Book Sellers:
All book returns require written permission and label from the publisher. Write to the address above or fax to the number above for permission.

Please photocopy this form or cut and mail to
Barmarrae Books, Inc., 3017 NW 62nd Terrace, Gainesville, FL 32606

ORDER FORM
BARMARRAE BOOKS, INC.
3017 NW 62ND TERRACE
GAINESVILLE, FL 32606

Order by mail, phone, or fax

Title	Unit Price	Qty	Total	
Clinical Guidelines in Family Practice ISBN 0-9646151-3-4	60.00			Name: _____
Clinical Guidelines in Adult Health ISBN 0-9646151-5-0	55.00			Address: _____
Clinical Guidelines in Child Health ISBN 0-9646151-4-2	55.00			City: _____ State/Zip _____
				Area Code/Phone No.: _____
Subtotal				Form of Payment: ❑ Check ❑ Money Order
Shipping and Handling (within the US)	5.00			❑ Purchase Order (Institutions Only) ❑ MasterCard ❑VISA
Shipping Outside US, add $15				Credit Card # _____
Florida residents, add 6% sales tax				Expiration Date _____
TOTAL DUE (US funds ONLY)				Signature _____

Mail Order to: BARMARRAE BOOKS, INC. 3017 NW 62nd Terrace Gainesville, FL 32606	Phone Order to: 1-888-276-7780 or 1- 352-378-5554 Fax Order to: 1-352-378-1441

BARMARRAE BOOKS, INC.

ORDERING INFORMATION

1-888-276-7780

Credit card orders (VISA or MasterCard) or institutional purchase orders may be placed toll free 8 A.M. - 5 P.M. EST weekdays at the above telephone number.

Credit card orders (VISA or MasterCard) or institutional purchase orders may be faxed 24 hours to **1-352-378-1441**

OR

Please photocopy or clip the order form below and mail with your check, money order, or purchase order to:

**BARMARRAE BOOKS, INC.
3017 NW 62ND TERRACE
GAINESVILLE, FL 32606**

Note to Book Sellers:
All book returns require written permission and label from the publisher. Write to the address above or fax to the number above for permission.

Please photocopy this form or cut and mail to
Barmarrae Books, Inc., 3017 NW 62nd Terrace, Gainesville, FL 32606

ORDER FORM
BARMARRAE BOOKS, INC.
3017 NW 62ND TERRACE
GAINESVILLE, FL 32606

Order by mail, phone, or fax

Title	Unit Price	Qty	Total
Clinical Guidelines in Family Practice ISBN 0-9646151-3-4	60.00		
Clinical Guidelines in Adult Health ISBN 0-9646151-5-0	55.00		
Clinical Guidelines in Child Health ISBN 0-9646151-4-2	55.00		

Name: _____

Address: _____

City: _____ State/Zip _____

Area Code/Phone No.: _____

Subtotal	
Shipping and Handling (within the US)	5.00
Shipping Outside US, add $15	
Florida residents, add 6% sales tax	
TOTAL DUE (US funds **ONLY**)	

Form of Payment: ❏ Check ❏ Money Order
❏ Purchase Order (Institutions Only) ❏ MasterCard ❏ VISA

Credit Card # _____

Expiration Date _____

Signature _____

Mail Order to: BARMARRAE BOOKS, INC.
3017 NW 62nd Terrace
Gainesville, FL 32606

Phone Order to: 1-888-276-7780 or
1- 352-378-5554
Fax Order to: 1-352-378-1441

BARMARRAE BOOKS, INC.

ORDERING INFORMATION

1-888-276-7780

Credit card orders (VISA or MasterCard) or institutional purchase orders may be placed toll free 8 A.M. - 5 P.M. EST weekdays at the above telephone number.

Credit card orders (VISA or MasterCard) or institutional purchase orders may be faxed 24 hours to **1-352-378-1441**

OR

Please photocopy or clip the order form below and mail with your check, money order, or purchase order to:

BARMARRAE BOOKS, INC.
3017 NW 62ND TERRACE
GAINESVILLE, FL 32606

Note to Book Sellers:
All book returns require written permission and label from the publisher. Write to the address above or fax to the number above for permission.

Please photocopy this form or cut and mail to
Barmarrae Books, Inc., 3017 NW 62nd Terrace, Gainesville, FL 32606

ORDER FORM
BARMARRAE BOOKS, INC.
3017 NW 62ND TERRACE
GAINESVILLE, FL 32606

Order by mail, phone, or fax

Title	Unit Price	Qty	Total	
Clinical Guidelines in Family Practice ISBN 0-9646151-3-4	60.00			Name: _____
Clinical Guidelines in Adult Health ISBN 0-9646151-5-0	55.00			Address: _____
Clinical Guidelines in Child Health ISBN 0-9646151-4-2	55.00			City: _____ State/Zip _____
				Area Code/Phone No.: _____

Subtotal		Form of Payment: ❑ Check ❑ Money Order
Shipping and Handling (within the US)	5.00	❑ Purchase Order (Institutions Only) ❑ MasterCard ❑VISA
Shipping Outside US, add $15		Credit Card # _____
Florida residents, add 6% sales tax		Expiration Date _____
TOTAL DUE (US funds ONLY)		Signature _____

Mail Order to:	BARMARRAE BOOKS, INC. 3017 NW 62nd Terrace Gainesville, FL 32606	Phone Order to:	1-888-276-7780 or 1- 352-378-5554
		Fax Order to:	1-352-378-1441

BARMARRAE BOOKS, INC.

ORDERING INFORMATION

1-888-276-7780

Credit card orders (VISA or MasterCard) or institutional purchase orders may be placed toll free 8 A.M. - 5 P.M. EST weekdays at the above telephone number.

Credit card orders (VISA or MasterCard) or institutional purchase orders may be faxed 24 hours to **1-352-378-1441**

OR

Please photocopy or clip the order form below and mail with your check, money order, or purchase order to:

BARMARRAE BOOKS, INC.
3017 NW 62ND TERRACE
GAINESVILLE, FL 32606

Note to Book Sellers:
All book returns require written permission and label from the publisher. Write to the address above or fax to the number above for permission.

Please photocopy this form or cut and mail to
Barmarrae Books, Inc., 3017 NW 62nd Terrace, Gainesville, FL 32606

ORDER FORM
BARMARRAE BOOKS, INC.
3017 NW 62ND TERRACE
GAINESVILLE, FL 32606

Order by mail, phone, or fax

Title	Unit Price	Qty	Total
Clinical Guidelines in Family Practice ISBN 0-9646151-3-4	60.00		
Clinical Guidelines in Adult Health ISBN 0-9646151-5-0	55.00		
Clinical Guidelines in Child Health ISBN 0-9646151-4-2	55.00		

Name: _____

Address: _____

City: _____ State/Zip _____

Area Code/Phone No.: _____

Subtotal	
Shipping and Handling (within the US)	5.00
Shipping Outside US, add $15	
Florida residents, add 6% sales tax	
TOTAL DUE (US funds **ONLY**)	

Form of Payment: ❑ Check ❑ Money Order

❑ Purchase Order (Institutions Only) ❑ MasterCard ❑ VISA

Credit Card # _____

Expiration Date _____

Signature _____

Mail Order to: BARMARRAE BOOKS, INC. 3017 NW 62nd Terrace Gainesville, FL 32606	**Phone Order to:** 1-888-276-7780 or 1- 352-378-5554 **Fax Order to:** 1-352-378-1441

BARMARRAE BOOKS, INC.

ORDERING INFORMATION

1-888-276-7780

Credit card orders (VISA or MasterCard) or institutional purchase orders may be placed toll free 8 A.M. - 5 P.M. EST weekdays at the above telephone number.

Credit card orders (VISA or MasterCard) or institutional purchase orders may be faxed 24 hours to **1-352-378-1441**

OR

Please photocopy or clip the order form below and mail with your check, money order, or purchase order to:

BARMARRAE BOOKS, INC.
3017 NW 62ND TERRACE
GAINESVILLE, FL 32606

Note to Book Sellers:
All book returns require written permission and label from the publisher. Write to the address above or fax to the number above for permission.

Please photocopy this form or cut and mail to
Barmarrae Books, Inc., 3017 NW 62nd Terrace, Gainesville, FL 32606

ORDER FORM
BARMARRAE BOOKS, INC.
3017 NW 62ND TERRACE
GAINESVILLE, FL 32606

Order by mail, phone, or fax

Title	Unit Price	Qty	Total	
Clinical Guidelines in Family Practice ISBN 0-9646151-3-4	60.00			Name: _____
Clinical Guidelines in Adult Health ISBN 0-9646151-5-0	55.00			Address: _____
Clinical Guidelines in Child Health ISBN 0-9646151-4-2	55.00			City: _____ State/Zip _____
				Area Code/Phone No.: _____
Subtotal				Form of Payment: ❑ Check ❑ Money Order
Shipping and Handling (within the US)	5.00			❑ Purchase Order (Institutions Only) ❑ MasterCard ❑ VISA
Shipping Outside US, add $15				Credit Card # _____
Florida residents, add 6% sales tax				Expiration Date _____
TOTAL DUE (US funds **ONLY**)				Signature _____

Mail Order to: **BARMARRAE BOOKS, INC.** 3017 NW 62nd Terrace Gainesville, FL 32606	**Phone Order to:** 1-888-276-7780 or 1- 352-378-5554 **Fax Order to:** 1-352-378-1441

BARMARRAE BOOKS, INC.

ORDERING INFORMATION

1-888-276-7780

Credit card orders (VISA or MasterCard) or institutional purchase orders may be placed toll free 8 A.M. - 5 P.M. EST weekdays at the above telephone number.

Credit card orders (VISA or MasterCard) or institutional purchase orders may be faxed 24 hours to
1-352-378-1441

OR

Please photocopy or clip the order form below and mail with your check, money order, or purchase order to:

BARMARRAE BOOKS, INC.
3017 NW 62ND TERRACE
GAINESVILLE, FL 32606

Note to Book Sellers:
All book returns require written permission and label from the publisher. Write to the address above or fax to the number above for permission.

Please photocopy this form or cut and mail to
Barmarrae Books, Inc., 3017 NW 62nd Terrace, Gainesville, FL 32606

ORDER FORM
BARMARRAE BOOKS, INC.
3017 NW 62ND TERRACE
GAINESVILLE, FL 32606

Order by mail, phone, or fax

Title	Unit Price	Qty	Total	
Clinical Guidelines in Family Practice ISBN 0-9646151-3-4	60.00			Name: _____
Clinical Guidelines in Adult Health ISBN 0-9646151-5-0	55.00			Address: _____
Clinical Guidelines in Child Health ISBN 0-9646151-4-2	55.00			City: _____ State/Zip _____
				Area Code/Phone No.: _____
Subtotal				Form of Payment: ❑ Check ❑ Money Order
Shipping and Handling (within the US)	5.00			❑ Purchase Order (Institutions Only) ❑ MasterCard ❑VISA
Shipping Outside US, add $15				Credit Card # _____
Florida residents, add 6% sales tax				Expiration Date _____
TOTAL DUE (US funds ONLY)				Signature _____

Mail Order to: BARMARRAE BOOKS, INC. 3017 NW 62nd Terrace Gainesville, FL 32606	**Phone Order to:** 1-888-276-7780 or 1- 352-378-5554 **Fax Order to:** 1-352-378-1441

BARMARRAE BOOKS, INC.

ORDERING INFORMATION

1-888-276-7780

Credit card orders (VISA or MasterCard) or institutional purchase orders may be placed toll free 8 A.M. - 5 P.M. EST weekdays at the above telephone number.

Credit card orders (VISA or MasterCard) or institutional purchase orders may be faxed 24 hours to 1-352-378-1441

OR

Please photocopy or clip the order form below and mail with your check, money order, or purchase order to:

**BARMARRAE BOOKS, INC.
3017 NW 62ND TERRACE
GAINESVILLE, FL 32606**

Note to Book Sellers:
All book returns require written permission and label from the publisher. Write to the address above or fax to the number above for permission.

Please photocopy this form or cut and mail to
Barmarrae Books, Inc., 3017 NW 62nd Terrace, Gainesville, FL 32606

ORDER FORM
BARMARRAE BOOKS, INC.
3017 NW 62ND TERRACE
GAINESVILLE, FL 32606

Order by mail, phone, or fax

Title	Unit Price	Qty	Total
Clinical Guidelines in Family Practice ISBN 0-9646151-3-4	60.00		
Clinical Guidelines in Adult Health ISBN 0-9646151-5-0	55.00		
Clinical Guidelines in Child Health ISBN 0-9646151-4-2	55.00		
Subtotal			
Shipping and Handling (within the US)			5.00
Shipping Outside US, add $15			
Florida residents, add 6% sales tax			
TOTAL DUE (US funds **ONLY**)			

Name: _____

Address: _____

City: _____ State/Zip _____

Area Code/Phone No.: _____

Form of Payment: ❑ Check   ❑ Money Order

❑ Purchase Order (Institutions Only) ❑ MasterCard ❑VISA

Credit Card # _____

Expiration Date _____

Signature _____

| **Mail Order to:** BARMARRAE BOOKS, INC. 3017 NW 62nd Terrace Gainesville, FL 32606 | **Phone Order to:** 1-888-276-7780 or 1- 352-378-5554 **Fax Order to:** 1-352-378-1441 |